Human Papillomavirus and Head and Neck Cancer

Human Papillomavirus and Head and Neck Cancer

Editor

Heather Walline

MDPI • Basel • Beijing • Wuhan • Barcelona • Belgrade • Manchester • Tokyo • Cluj • Tianjin

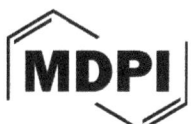

Editor
Heather Walline
Otolaryngology
University of Michigan
Ann Arbor
United States

Editorial Office
MDPI
St. Alban-Anlage 66
4052 Basel, Switzerland

This is a reprint of articles from the Special Issue published online in the open access journal *Cancers* (ISSN 2072-6694) (available at: www.mdpi.com/journal/cancers/special_issues/papillomavirus_cancer).

For citation purposes, cite each article independently as indicated on the article page online and as indicated below:

LastName, A.A.; LastName, B.B.; LastName, C.C. Article Title. *Journal Name* **Year**, *Volume Number*, Page Range.

ISBN 978-3-0365-6705-1 (Hbk)
ISBN 978-3-0365-6704-4 (PDF)

© 2023 by the authors. Articles in this book are Open Access and distributed under the Creative Commons Attribution (CC BY) license, which allows users to download, copy and build upon published articles, as long as the author and publisher are properly credited, which ensures maximum dissemination and a wider impact of our publications.

The book as a whole is distributed by MDPI under the terms and conditions of the Creative Commons license CC BY-NC-ND.

Contents

About the Editor vii

Christine Goudsmit, Felipe da Veiga Leprevost, Venkatesha Basrur, Lila Peters, Alexey Nesvizhskii and Heather Walline
Differences in Extracellular Vesicle Protein Cargo Are Dependent on Head and Neck Squamous Cell Carcinoma Cell of Origin and Human Papillomavirus Status
Reprinted from: *Cancers* **2021**, *13*, 3714, doi:10.3390/cancers13153714 1

Géraldine Descamps, Sonia Furgiuele, Nour Mhaidly, Fabrice Journe and Sven Saussez
Immune Cell Density Evaluation Improves the Prognostic Values of Staging and p16 in Oropharyngeal Cancer
Reprinted from: *Cancers* **2022**, *14*, 5560, doi:10.3390/cancers14225560 27

Marisa Mena, Xin Wang, Sara Tous, Beatriz Quiros, Omar Clavero and Maria Alejo et al.
Concordance of p16^{INK4a} and E6*I mRNA among HPV-DNA-Positive Oropharyngeal, Laryngeal, and Oral Cavity Carcinomas from the ICO International Study
Reprinted from: *Cancers* **2022**, *14*, 3787, doi:10.3390/cancers14153787 43

Harini Balaji, Imke Demers, Nora Wuerdemann, Julia Schrijnder, Bernd Kremer and Jens Peter Klussmann et al.
Causes and Consequences of HPV Integration in Head and Neck Squamous Cell Carcinomas: State of the Art
Reprinted from: *Cancers* **2021**, *13*, 4089, doi:10.3390/cancers13164089 55

Mehmet Gunduz, Esra Gunduz, Shunji Tamagawa, Keisuke Enomoto and Muneki Hotomi
Cancer Stem Cells in Oropharyngeal Cancer
Reprinted from: *Cancers* **2021**, *13*, 3878, doi:10.3390/cancers13153878 77

Tingting Qin, Shiting Li, Leanne E. Henry, Siyu Liu and Maureen A. Sartor
Molecular Tumor Subtypes of HPV-Positive Head and Neck Cancers: Biological Characteristics and Implications for Clinical Outcomes
Reprinted from: *Cancers* **2021**, *13*, 2721, doi:10.3390/cancers13112721 89

Malin Wendt, Lalle Hammarstedt-Nordenvall, Mark Zupancic, Signe Friesland, David Landin and Eva Munck-Wiklund et al.
Long-Term Survival and Recurrence in Oropharyngeal Squamous Cell Carcinoma in Relation to Subsites, HPV, and p16-Status
Reprinted from: *Cancers* **2021**, *13*, 2553, doi:10.3390/cancers13112553 111

Mark D. Wilkie, Emad A. Anaam, Andrew S. Lau, Carlos P. Rubbi, Nikolina Vlatkovic and Terence M. Jones et al.
Metabolic Plasticity and Combinatorial Radiosensitisation Strategies in Human Papillomavirus-Positive Squamous Cell Carcinoma of the Head and Neck Cell Lines
Reprinted from: *Cancers* **2021**, *13*, 4836, doi:10.3390/cancers13194836 123

Ramesh Paudyal, Milan Grkovski, Jung Hun Oh, Heiko Schöder, David Aramburu Nunez and Vaios Hatzoglou et al.
Application of Community Detection Algorithm to Investigate the Correlation between Imaging Biomarkers of Tumor Metabolism, Hypoxia, Cellularity, and Perfusion for Precision Radiotherapy in Head and Neck Squamous Cell Carcinomas
Reprinted from: *Cancers* **2021**, *13*, 3908, doi:10.3390/cancers13153908 139

Diego Camuzi, Luisa Aguirre Buexm, Simone de Queiroz Chaves Lourenço, Davide Degli Esposti, Cyrille Cuenin and Monique de Souza Almeida Lopes et al.
HPV Infection Leaves a DNA Methylation Signature in Oropharyngeal Cancer Affecting Both Coding Genes and Transposable Elements
Reprinted from: *Cancers* **2021**, *13*, 3621, doi:10.3390/cancers13143621 157

Adam Brewczyński, Beata Jabłońska, Agnieszka Maria Mazurek, Jolanta Mrochem-Kwarciak, Sławomir Mrowiec and Mirosław Śnietura et al.
Comparison of Selected Immune and Hematological Parameters and Their Impact on Survival in Patients with HPV-Related and HPV-Unrelated Oropharyngeal Cancer
Reprinted from: *Cancers* **2021**, *13*, 3256, doi:10.3390/cancers13133256 173

Anni Sjöblom, Ulf-Håkan Stenman, Jaana Hagström, Lauri Jouhi, Caj Haglund and Stina Syrjänen et al.
Tumor-Associated Trypsin Inhibitor (TATI) as a Biomarker of Poor Prognosis in Oropharyngeal Squamous Cell Carcinoma Irrespective of HPV Status
Reprinted from: *Cancers* **2021**, *13*, 2811, doi:10.3390/cancers13112811 193

Won Jin Cho, David Kessel, Joseph Rakowski, Brian Loughery, Abdo J. Najy and Tri Pham et al.
Photodynamic Therapy as a Potent Radiosensitizer in Head and Neck Squamous Cell Carcinoma
Reprinted from: *Cancers* **2021**, *13*, 1193, doi:10.3390/cancers13061193 207

Kim J. W. Chang Sing Pang, Taha Mur, Louise Collins, Sowmya R. Rao and Daniel L. Faden
Human Papillomavirus in Sinonasal Squamous Cell Carcinoma: A Systematic Review and Meta-Analysis
Reprinted from: *Cancers* **2020**, *13*, 45, doi:10.3390/cancers13010045 221

Marta Tagliabue, Marisa Mena, Fausto Maffini, Tarik Gheit, Beatriz Quirós Blasco and Dana Holzinger et al.
Role of Human Papillomavirus Infection in Head and Neck Cancer in Italy: The HPV-AHEAD Study
Reprinted from: *Cancers* **2020**, *12*, 3567, doi:10.3390/cancers12123567 239

About the Editor

Heather Walline

The main research areas in the Walline lab are, first, the contribution and mechanism of HPV in carcinogenesis, progression, and outcome in oropharyngeal and other virally induced cancers, and second, the clinical relevance of molecules from tumor extracellular vesicles (EV) in HNSCC, including early diagnosis, prognosis, and disease monitoring. Current projects include the molecular characterization of tumor EV oncogenic factors (protein, oncogenic transcripts, mutant DNA) from pretreatment patient saliva and plasma; the assembly of tumor EV profiles for diagnostic validation, patient-specific query in follow-up/post-treatment liquid biopsies, and treatment response/outcome; and mechanistic studies to improve our understanding of the tumor EV transfer of oncogenic factors to recipient cells.

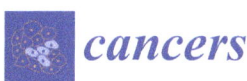

Article

Differences in Extracellular Vesicle Protein Cargo Are Dependent on Head and Neck Squamous Cell Carcinoma Cell of Origin and Human Papillomavirus Status

Christine Goudsmit [1], Felipe da Veiga Leprevost [2], Venkatesha Basrur [2,3], Lila Peters [1], Alexey Nesvizhskii [2,3] and Heather Walline [1,*]

[1] Department of Otolaryngology-Head and Neck Surgery, University of Michigan, Ann Arbor, MI 48109, USA; cgoud@umich.edu (C.G.); peters@umich.edu (L.P.)
[2] Department of Pathology, University of Michigan, Ann Arbor, MI 48109, USA; felipevl@umich.edu (F.d.V.L.); vbasrur@umich.edu (V.B.); nesvi@umich.edu (A.N.)
[3] Proteomics Shared Resource, Department of Pathology, University of Michigan, Ann Arbor, MI 48109, USA
* Correspondence: hwalline@umich.edu; Tel.: +1-734-647-7975

Simple Summary: Many individuals with head and neck cancer do not survive, even with intense treatment. Patients with HPV-positive tumors generally have better survival; however, for yet unknown reasons, a subset are unresponsive to therapy. One strategy to monitor cancers for progression and recurrence is evaluation of extracellular vesicles, released by tumor cells into the blood and other body fluids. We can also understand differences in tumors and their behavior by comparing the molecules packaged into vesicles that are released from tumor cells. Our study examined differences in the proteins contained within extracellular vesicles released from head and neck cancer cells. We found that key extracellular vesicle proteins differed based on HPV status of the originating cell line and tumor, as well as how responsive the originating tumor was to treatment. Our findings suggest that these extracellular vesicle proteins may be important markers for continued investigation.

Abstract: To identify potential extracellular vesicle (EV) biomarkers in head and neck squamous cell carcinoma (HNSCC), we evaluated EV protein cargo and whole cell lysates (WCL) from HPV-positive and -negative HNSCC cell lines, as well as normal oral keratinocytes and HPV16-transformed cells. EVs were isolated from serum-depleted, conditioned cell culture media by polyethylene glycol (PEG) precipitation/ultracentrifugation. EV and WCL preparations were analyzed by LC-MS/MS. Candidate proteins detected at significantly higher levels in EV compared with WCL, or compared with EV from normal oral keratinocytes, were identified and confirmed by Wes Simple Western protein analysis. Our findings suggest that these proteins may be potential HNSCC EV markers as proteins that may be (1) selectively included in EV cargo for export from the cell as a strategy for metastasis, tumor cell survival, or modification of tumor microenvironment, or (2) representative of originating cell composition, which may be developed for diagnostic or prognostic use in clinical liquid biopsy applications. This work demonstrates that our method can be used to reliably detect EV proteins from HNSCC, normal keratinocyte, and transformed cell lines. Furthermore, this work has identified HNSCC EV protein candidates for continued evaluation, specifically tenascin-C, HLA-A, E-cadherin, EGFR, EPHA2, and cytokeratin 19.

Keywords: HPV; head and neck squamous cell carcinoma; extracellular vesicle; proteomic

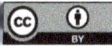

1. Introduction

Head and neck squamous cell carcinoma (HNSCC) is the sixth most common and eighth most fatal cancer worldwide and includes cancers of the oropharynx, larynx, hypopharynx, and oral cavity [1,2]. In 2018, there were 890,000 new cases and 450,000 deaths worldwide, and annual cases are expected to reach 1.08 million by 2030 [3]. Despite recent advances in treatment, including radiation, chemotherapy, surgery, concurrent chemoradiation, and immunotherapy, many tumors develop resistance and progress. Patients develop metastases or tumors recur locally or regionally; the 5-year overall survival rate for HNSCC is only 40–50% [4]. Furthermore, the majority of patients suffer at least one recurrence, typically within 2 years of treatment [5–7]. Factors that contribute to poor survival for patients with HNSCC include late stage diagnosis, lack of reliable markers for early stage detection, high level of biologic heterogeneity, and local recurrence and distant metastases after treatment [3].

There are subsets of HNSCC that respond better to therapy; 70–80% of HPV-positive oropharyngeal squamous cell carcinomas (OPSCCs) treated with concurrent chemotherapy and intensity-modulated radiation or surgery with lymph node dissection and postoperative radiation respond favorably. This improved outcome suggests that some patients could be treated with reduced-intensity treatments, sparing them the severe morbidities associated with current therapies [8,9]. However, de-escalation efforts risk increasing the current 20% of HPV-positive OPSCCs that are non-responsive to treatment. Unfortunately, regardless of treatment, many patients have tumors that progress or recur, and we are unable to distinguish those that are likely to respond to reduced treatment from tumors that will require additional or alternate therapies.

Extracellular vesicles (EVs) are membrane-enclosed particles released from a cell (constitutively, upon activation, or under hypoxic conditions), that contain various biological molecules, including signaling factors, proteins, nucleic acids, and lipids. The International Society of Extracellular Vesicles (ISEV) defines EVs as "particles released from a cell that are delimited by a lipid bilayer and cannot replicate (i.e., lack a functional nucleus)" [10]. These vesicles carry biologically active cytosolic and membrane components of the parent cell, allowing them to serve as originator surrogates [11]. They differ in size, density, function, and content, and include exosomes, microvesicles, and large oncosomes. Exosomes are small (40–150 nm) membrane-bound vesicles with a characteristic cup-shaped morphology that originate in the endosomes of cells, resulting in formation of multivesicular bodies, which are subsequently released into the extracellular space through fusion with the plasma membrane of the cell. Microvesicles and oncosomes are generated by outward budding from the plasma membrane of non-apoptotic cells, and are significantly larger than exosomes; microvesicles range in size from 0.1–10 µm, and oncosomes are 1–10 µm.

EVs are important because they are produced by both normal and tumor cells and have many functions, including roles in the immune response, inflammation, intercellular messaging, and transport [12,13]. Tumor extracellular vesicles (TEVs) are taken up by recipient cells locally in the primary tumor and tumor microenvironment (fibroblasts, endothelial cells, immune cells, or other tumor cells) as well as in distant cells and tissues, resulting in delivery of tumor molecules that can alter recipient cells [14–16]. Tumor cells are prolific vesicle producers, and TEVs have the capability to mediate pro-tumorigenic effects through immunomodulation, angiogenesis, promotion of tumor growth, modulation of the tumor microenvironment, and transport of oncogenic signals or active oncogenes from tumor cells to normal cells [11,13,17,18]. Extracellular vesicles affect recipient cells by docking to the surface to transmit signals or transferring their contents into the cell.

Proteins within EVs are protected from degradation in biological fluids, allowing for increased stability of these molecules for liquid biopsy evaluation compared with circulating tumor cells or cell-free circulating tumor molecules [19]. Some cancer-specific proteins released from HNSCC cells in culture have been previously identified, as well as proteins present in the saliva or circulation of HNSCC patients [20,21]. The goals of this study were to identify additional EV protein markers that may be (1) selectively included in EV cargo for export from the cell as a strategy for metastasis, tumor cell survival, or modification of tumor microenvironment, or (2) representative of originating cell composition, which may be developed for diagnostic or prognostic use in clinical liquid biopsy applications.

2. Materials and Methods

Cell culture: This study used 8 representative HNSCC cell lines (Table 1), one HPV-transformed cell line, HOK16b (Human Oral Keratinocytes-16A, RRID: CVCL_B404) [22], and two non-cancer oral keratinocytes, NOKsi (normal oral keratinocytes, spontaneously immortalized) [23] and HOKg (human oral keratinocytes from gingiva, Lifeline Cell Technologies Oceanside, CA), using methods established and optimized in our lab that adhere to the 2018 MISEV guidelines. The total number of cell lines used in the mass spec analysis [10] was chosen so that the samples could be assayed concurrently to reduce variation. These specific cell lines were chosen to include multiple HNSCC tumor sites (oral cavity, hypopharynx, larynx, and oropharynx) and HPV status. The non-responsive HNSCC cell lines (UM-SCC-38, UM-SCC-47, UM-SCC-118, UM-SCC-104, and UPCI:SCC152) were generated from more aggressive tumors that were resistant to treatment. These tumors were removed from patients with disease ultimately causal in their deaths. The responsive HNSCC cell lines (UM-SCC-17a, UM-SCC-105, and UM-SCC-92) were generated from tumors removed from patients with tumors responsive to treatment, and at last query the patients were alive with no evidence of disease.

Table 1. Head and Neck Squamous Cell Carcinoma Lines Used in the Study. Bold italics: HPV-positive.

Cell Line	Tumor Site	Tumor Stage	HPV Status	Patient Sex	Patient Age	Smoker?	Follow-Up
UM-SCC-38	Tonsil	T2N2aM0	Negative	Male	60	Yes	Patient died from disease one year after diagnosis
UM-SCC-47	Lateral Tongue	T3N1M0	HPV16	Male	53	Yes	Patient died from disease within a year of diagnosis
UM-SCC-118	Lateral Tongue	T4aN2M0	Negative	Female	23	No	Patient died from disease within a year of diagnosis
UM-SCC-104	Floor of Mouth	T4N2bM0	HPV16	Male	56	Yes	Patient died from disease within a year of diagnosis
UM-SCC-17a	Larynx	T1N0M0	Negative	Female	47	Yes	Patient alive with no evidence of disease 14+ years after diagnosis
UM-SCC-105	Larynx	T4N0M0	HPV18	Male	51	No	Patient alive with no evidence of disease 5+ years after diagnosis
UM-SCC-92	Tongue	T2N0M0	Negative	Female	38	No	Patient alive with no evidence of disease 4+ years after diagnosis
UPCI:SCC152	Recurrent Hypopharynx	T2N1M0	HPV16	Male	47	Yes	Patient died from disease 4 years after diagnosis

All cell lines were grown in T-150 flasks in 20 mL standard media containing serum. Upon reaching approximately 80% confluence, the media was removed, cells were rinsed twice with PBS, and exosome-depleted media (EDM) was added (Exosome-depleted Fetal Bovine Serum, Thermo Fisher #A2720801). Following 48 h of incubation, the conditioned cell culture media was collected for EV isolation. Three T-150 flasks were used for each HNSCC cell line, and 9 T-150 flasks were used for HOK16b and NOKsi cells.

Contamination testing and genetic assessment was performed on all cell lines prior to freezing, upon thawing, and monthly during the course of cell culture experiments. Cell lines were tested for mycoplasma contamination using the Lonza MycoAlert Mycoplasma Detection Kit and genotyped in the University of Michigan Genomics Core using Profiler-Plus, which interrogates 15 tetranucleotide short tandem repeats (STR), to confirm unique genotypes. The cell lines were also tested for known genetic characteristics including key mutations (using exon sequencing) and HPV status/type (using the HPV PCR-MassArray assay).

EV isolation by ultracentrifugation: Our EV ultracentrifugation method was modified from the isolation strategy described by Thery, et. al. [24]. Briefly, conditioned cell culture media was combined from replicate flasks, with each set including a 5 mL PBS wash (Corning #21-040-CV, without Calcium or Magnesium). Samples were precleared by centrifugation at $300 \times g$ for 10 min in 50 mL conical tubes, using an Eppendorf centrifuge (Model #5810R) at 4 °C. The supernatants were transferred to new tubes and centrifuged at $2800 \times g$ for 10 min with the same parameters as above. Supernatants were then transferred to ultracentrifuge tubes (OptiSeal Polypropylene Bell Top Tubes, Beckman Coulter #361625), and were centrifuged at $12,000 \times g$ for 30 min at 4 °C (SW 28 Swinging-Bucket Aluminum Rotor, Beckman Coulter #342204/Beckman Optima XL-100K Ultracentrifuge). Supernatants were transferred to new tubes (Quick-Seal Polypropylene Tubes, Beckman Coulter #342413) and centrifuged at $110,000 \times g$ for 90 min at 4 °C (Type 70 Ti Fixed-Angle Titanium Rotor, Beckman Coulter #337922/Beckman Optima XL-100K Ultracentrifuge). The supernatants were removed, and the pellets were resuspended in 1 mL PBS and transferred to fresh tubes. The original pellet tubes were washed twice with 1 mL PBS each time, and this was added to the resuspended pellets in the new tubes, for a combined total of 3 mL. The volume was brought to 13 mL with additional PBS before final centrifugation at $110,000 \times g$ for 90 min at 4 °C (Type 70 Ti rotor). Supernatants were removed and pellets were stored at -80 °C.

EV isolation by PEG precipitation/ultracentrifugation: This protocol was based on the PEG method from Rider et al. [25]. EVs were isolated by polyethylene glycol (PEG) precipitation followed by ultracentrifugation. Briefly, conditioned cell culture media was removed from the flasks, with each washed with 5 mL PBS and transferred to a 50 mL conical tube. Samples were precleared by centrifugation at $300 \times g$ for 10 min in 50 mL conical tubes using an Eppendorf centrifuge (Model #5810R) at 4 °C. Supernatants were transferred to new tubes and centrifuged at $2800 \times g$ for 10 min with the same parameters as above. Supernatants were then transferred to new 50 mL conical tubes and centrifuged at $10,000 \times g$ for 30 min at 4 °C (Sorvall ST 8R centrifuge with HIGHConic Fixed-Angle rotor).

Supernatants were combined with an equal volume of 16% PEG and 1 M NaCl, for a final concentration of 8% PEG, 0.5 M NaCl, and incubated overnight at 4 °C. The PEG precipitations were then pelleted at $3220 \times g$ for 60 min, using an Eppendorf centrifuge at 4 °C. The supernatants were removed and discarded, leaving approximately 2 mL on each of the pellets. The pellets were resuspended and transferred to ultracentrifuge tubes (Quick-Seal Polypropylene Tubes, Beckman Coulter #342413); the precipitation tubes were each washed twice with PBS and the washes were added to the pellet suspensions. The samples were each brought up to 13 mL total with PBS and centrifuged at $150,000 \times g$ for 120 min at 4 °C (Type 70 Ti rotor). Supernatants were removed and pellets were stored at -80 °C.

Electron microscopy: EVs were pelleted as described above and resuspended in 80 µL PBS. An amount of 10 µL of the resuspended pellet was fixed with an equal volume of 5% glutaraldehyde in 0.2 M cacodylate buffer, pH 7.2. After (10 µL/15 min) application to formvar/carbon coated EM grids (200 mesh copper), they were washed with dH$_2$O (3×1 min). Grids were then incubated for 5 min in 1% uranyl acetate for negative contrasting. Images were taken using a Jeol JEM-1400 Plus 120 keV transmission electron microscope equipped with C-MOS camera and AMT (Advanced Microscopy Technology) software (ver. 6.02).

Nanoparticle Tracking Analysis (NTA): EV size and concentration for each sample isolation was determined using a NanoSight NS300 instrument (NanoSight, Malvern, UK) using a Blue405 laser and sCMOS camera. Samples were diluted in PBS, and 100 µL aliquots were measured with three 60 s videos using a syringe pump speed of 100 at a controlled temperature of 25 °C. Videos were analyzed with NTA 3.2 Build 3.2.16 software to calculate particle size and concentration for each sample.

Protein extraction: EVs isolated by ultracentrifugation and associated whole cell lysates were prepared using 1% NP40 in PBS for mass spectrometry. EVs isolated by PEG precipitation/ultracentrifugation and associated whole cell lysates were prepared with Roche Complete Mini Protease Inhibitor Cocktail Tablets (catalog # 11836153001) for Western analysis, and quantified with the Bradford protein assay.

Mass spectrometry: Proteomic analysis was performed on EVs and whole cell lysates from the eight HNSCC cell lines, normal NOKsi cell line, and the transformed cell line, HOK16b. Relative quantitation of proteins using Tandem Mass Tag (TMT 10plex) and LC-Tandem MS was performed by the Proteomics Resource Facility at the Department of Pathology, University of Michigan, using an optimized protocol described by Tank et al. [26]. Briefly, equal amounts of each protein sample were digested, labeled with TMT 10plex reagents, and subjected to Multinotch MS3 method as previously described [27]. MS data analysis was performed using Proteome discoverer 2.1 (ThermoFisher (Waltham, MA, USA). Protein identification and relative quantification was achieved by searching the data against a Homo sapiens UniProtKB database (UP000005640) that was downloaded on 21 September 2018. Protein sequences from HPV16 and HPV18 were also added to the FASTA file bringing the total number of proteins to 73136. EV and whole cell lysate protein results were compared to identify differences between normal and carcinoma EVs and whole cell lysates, as well as between EVs from HPV-positive and –negative HNSCC cell lines.

Wes ProteinSimple Western: Protein was measured using a capillary-based electrophoresis instrument (Wes, ProteinSimple, San Jose, CA, USA). Protein amounts (0.25–1 µg) pre-optimized for specific antibodies were denatured using manufacturer-supplied reagents and loaded into multi-well plates. Protein separation and detection were performed via capillary electrophoresis, antibody binding, and HRP-conjugated visualization following the manufacturer's instructions. Thorough antibody optimization was completed for all proteins for which Wes analysis was performed to determine ideal input protein concentration/denaturation, specific antibody (supplier/clone), and dilution conditions. Antibodies used are listed in Table 2. Analysis was performed using the Compass software for Simple Western (ProteinSimple, San Jose, CA, USA).

Table 2. Wes Antibody Information.

Antibody	Clone	Supplier	Catalog #	Lot	Secondary
Annexin V	N/A	Novus	NB100-1930	4E15L33570	Rabbit
βCatenin	D10AB	Cell Signaling	8480	5	Rabbit
Calnexin	N/A	Novus	NB100-1965ss	D-2	Rabbit
CD59	N/A	R & D Systems	AF1987	KIF011911A	Goat
CD9	C-4	Santa Cruz	SC-13118	E1719	Mouse
Cyclin D1	H-295	Santa Cruz	sc-753	G2315	Rabbit
Cytokeratin 19	A53-B/A2	Santa Cruz	SC6278	D1618	Mouse
E-Cadherin	180215	R & D Systems	MAB1838	JAT0219051	Mouse

Table 2. Cont.

Antibody	Clone	Supplier	Catalog #	Lot	Secondary
EGFR	N/A	Origene	TA312545	20100915076	Rabbit
EPHA2	C-3	Santa Cruz	SC-398832	D2519	Mouse
HLA-A	EP1395Y	Abcam	ab52922	GR25873	Rabbit
HPV16 E7	N/A	Santa Cruz	SC-65711	I1216	Mouse
p16	N/A	Ventana	725-4793	E04025	Mouse
p53	DO-1	Neomarkers	MS-187-p	187p1201E	Mouse
Rb	1F8	Neomarkers	MS-107-p1	107p1607F	Mouse
STAT3	124H6	Cell Signaling	9139	7	Mouse
Tenascin-C	EPR4219	Abcam	ab108930	GR3209212-7	Rabbit

3. Results

3.1. Extracellular Vesicle Characterization

EV characterization was based on minimal information for studies of extracellular vesicles 2018 [1]. Representative TEM images are shown in Figure 1, revealing EVs that demonstrate classic EV cup-shape morphology and diameter range between 75 and 200 nm. NTA measurements at 10-fold and 100-fold dilutions indicated that EVs isolated from cell culture supernatants yielded an average particle size of 177 nm across the HNSCC lines measured (Figure 2), while the average concentration was 9.22×10^9 particles/mL.

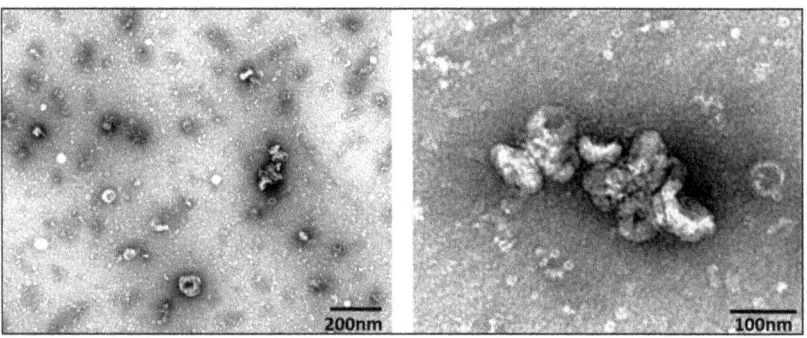

Figure 1. Representative TEM, UM-SCC-104, showing EVs 75–100 nm in diameter, with characteristic cup-shaped morphology.

3.2. Western Confirmation of EV Markers

(Figure 3) Positive EV marker CD9 was detected at 30 kDa in all of the EV lysates tested (HOK16b and HOKg bands are faint but present, see peak chemiluminescence, Figure S1, panel A). Similarly, AnnexinV, another positive EV marker, was detected at 38 kDa in all of the EVs tested (peak chemiluminescence shown in Figure S1, panel B). Calnexin, considered a negative marker for small EVs [10,28,29], was detected at 115 kDa in all of the whole cell lysates tested and none of the EV samples tested.

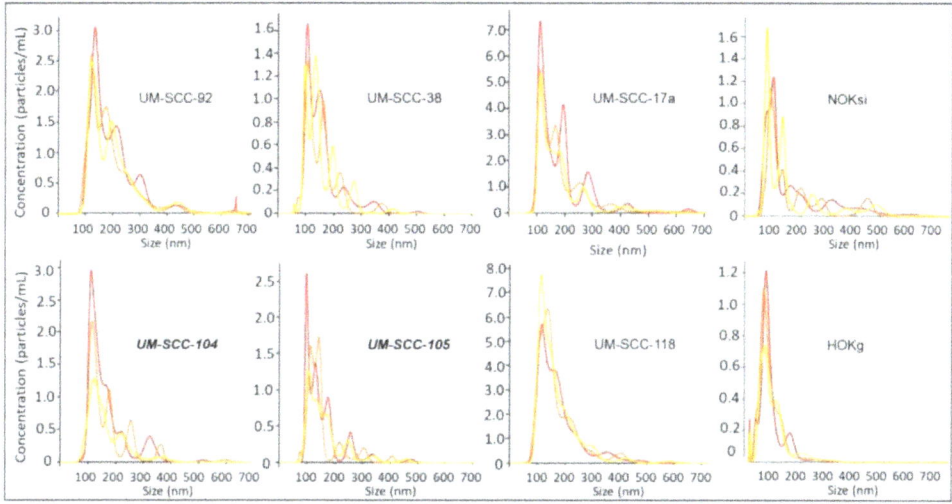

Figure 2. Nanoparticle tracking analysis, showing size and concentration for EVs from six representative HNSCC cell lines and two non-cancer cell lines measured. Bold italics: HPV-positive.

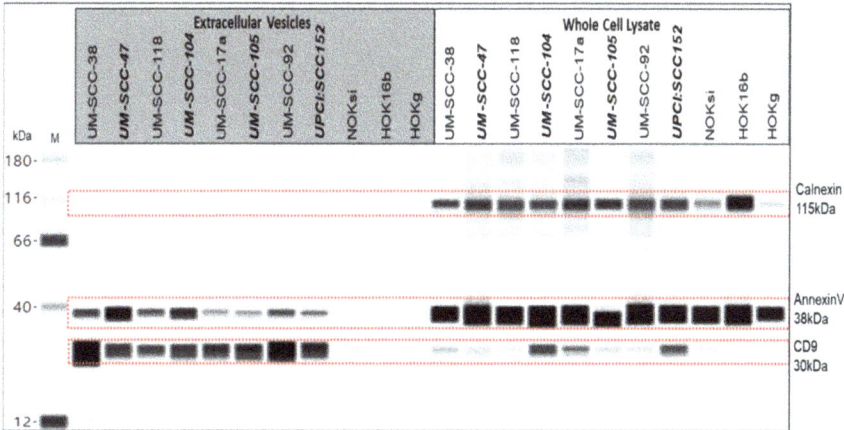

Figure 3. Wes protein analysis. Calnexin 1:50, 1 µg/µL protein; annexinV 1:200, 0.25 µg/µL protein; CD9 1:25, 1 µg/µL protein. Bold italics: HPV-positive.

3.3. Proteomic Analysis by Mass Spectrometry

The coverage—calculated by dividing the number of amino acids in all found peptides by the total number of amino acids in the entire protein sequence—of proteins were also taken into consideration for selection of potential protein markers, with higher coverage values considered to be more likely to yield promising candidates. A total of 4945 proteins were identified from the analysis of extracellular vesicles, and 5738 proteins were identified from the analysis of whole cell lysates. HNSCC EV fold-change peptide spectrum matches (PSM) for the EVs from the HNSCC lines compared with the EVs from the normal keratinocyte line (NOKsi) were averaged together. There were 149 proteins identified that were >2; these are represented in the cluster analysis (Figure 4) and listed in Table S1. Proteins in EVs released from HPV-positive and -negative HNSCC cell lines were further compared to determine proteins common to both groups or exclusive to EVs from either

HPV-positive or -negative lines (Figure 5). EVs from HPV-negative HNSCC cell lines exclusively contained 644 proteins; 133 proteins were detected exclusively in those from HPV-positive lines, and 562 were common in EVs from both HPV-positive and -negative HNSCC cell lines.

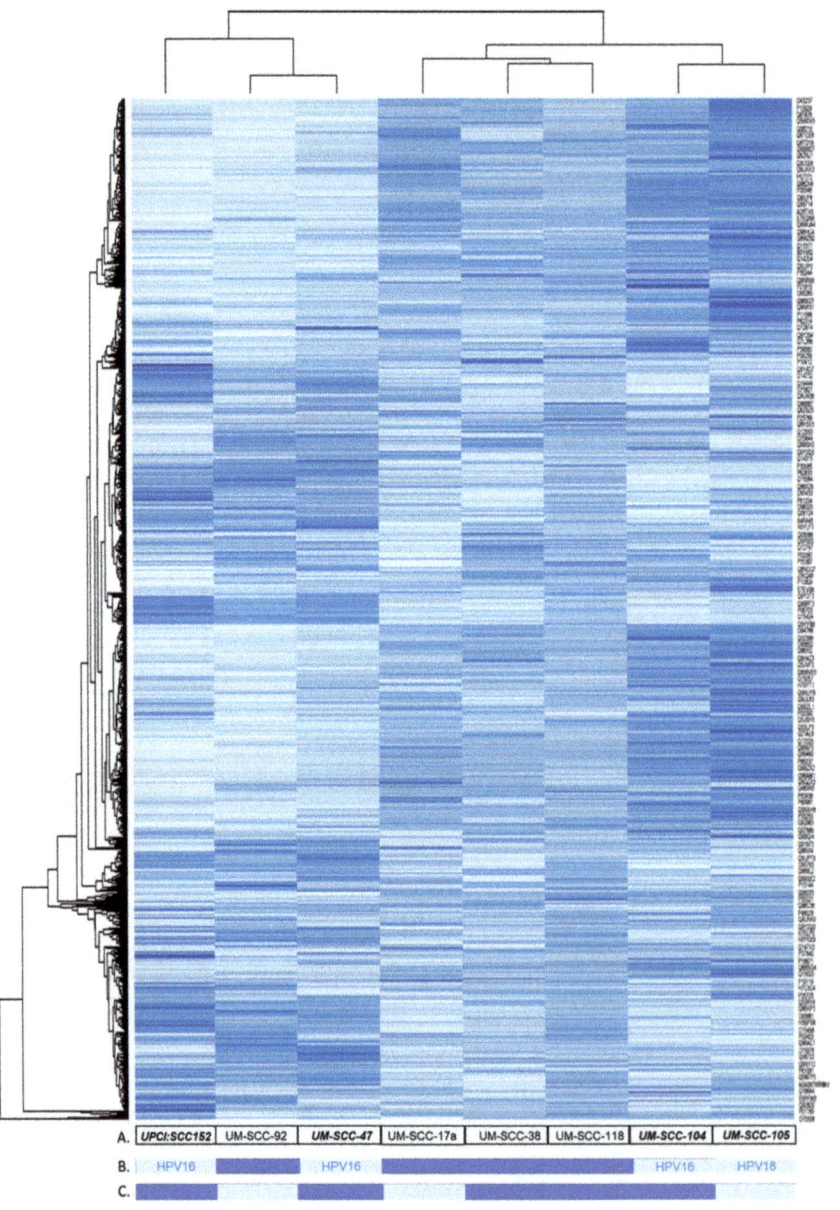

Figure 4. Cluster analysis of fold-change HNSCC EV protein abundance compared with NOKsi EV. protein. (**A**) UMSCC cell line EV identifier. (**B**) HPV status; light = HPV-positive, dark = HPV-negative. (**C**) Responsive/non-responsive origin tumor; light = responsive, dark = non-responsive. Bold italics: HPV-positive.

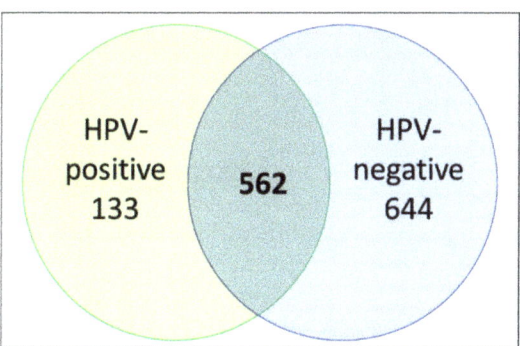

Figure 5. Venn diagram illustrating the distribution of proteins in EVs released from HPV-positive and HPV-negative HNSCC cell lines by averaged PSM values.

3.4. Western Analysis of Candidate Proteins

Candidate EV proteins were initially considered based on the proteomic analysis by mass spectrometry (using the coverage and comparative PSM values), and final candidates were selected by either previously reported involvement in tumors at multiple HNSCC sites, relationship with HPV tumorigenic pathways, or likelihood of EV association, including membrane proteins.

Protein results by ProteinSimple Wes analysis were not normalized to an internal control protein. Limitations inherent to working with EVs, recognized by the ISEV, prevent absolute normalization of expression data, due to variations in composition of EVs from different cell lines [30]. The ISEV recommends combining high-resolution imaging of isolated EVs with concentration measurements, as was performed in our study.

STAT3 (Figure 6A) was detected at 86 kDa in all of the whole cell lysates, with a much fainter band in the whole cell lysate from the normal NOKsi cell line. Overall, the STAT3 levels were generally detected at higher levels in EVs from the HPV-positive HNSCC lines compared with those from the HPV-negative lines. This was not the case for the whole cell lysates, where HPV-negative lines UM-SCC17A, UM-SCC-92, and UM-SCC-118 all had relatively high levels of STAT3 detected.

βCatenin (βCat) (Figure 6B) was detected at 92 kDa in all of the whole cell lysate samples tested. In the EVs, the only appreciable βCatenin signals were seen in the EVs from HPV-positive HNSCC lines UM-SCC-47, UM-SCC-105, and UPCI:SCC152, and those from the HPV-negative HNSCC line UM-SCC-17A.

EPHA2 (Figure 6C) was detected with a strong signal at 100 kDa in all of the whole cell lysates tested. The protein was detected at varying levels in EVs from all the cell lines tested with the exception of those from NOKsi, where no EPHA2 protein was detected.

CD59 (Figure 6D) was detected at 29 kDa in the whole cell lysates of all the lines tested, with the highest levels detected in the transformed cell line, HOK16a. This protein was detected in the EVs from all HNSCC lines, with the highest level seen in HPV-negative UM-SCC-38.

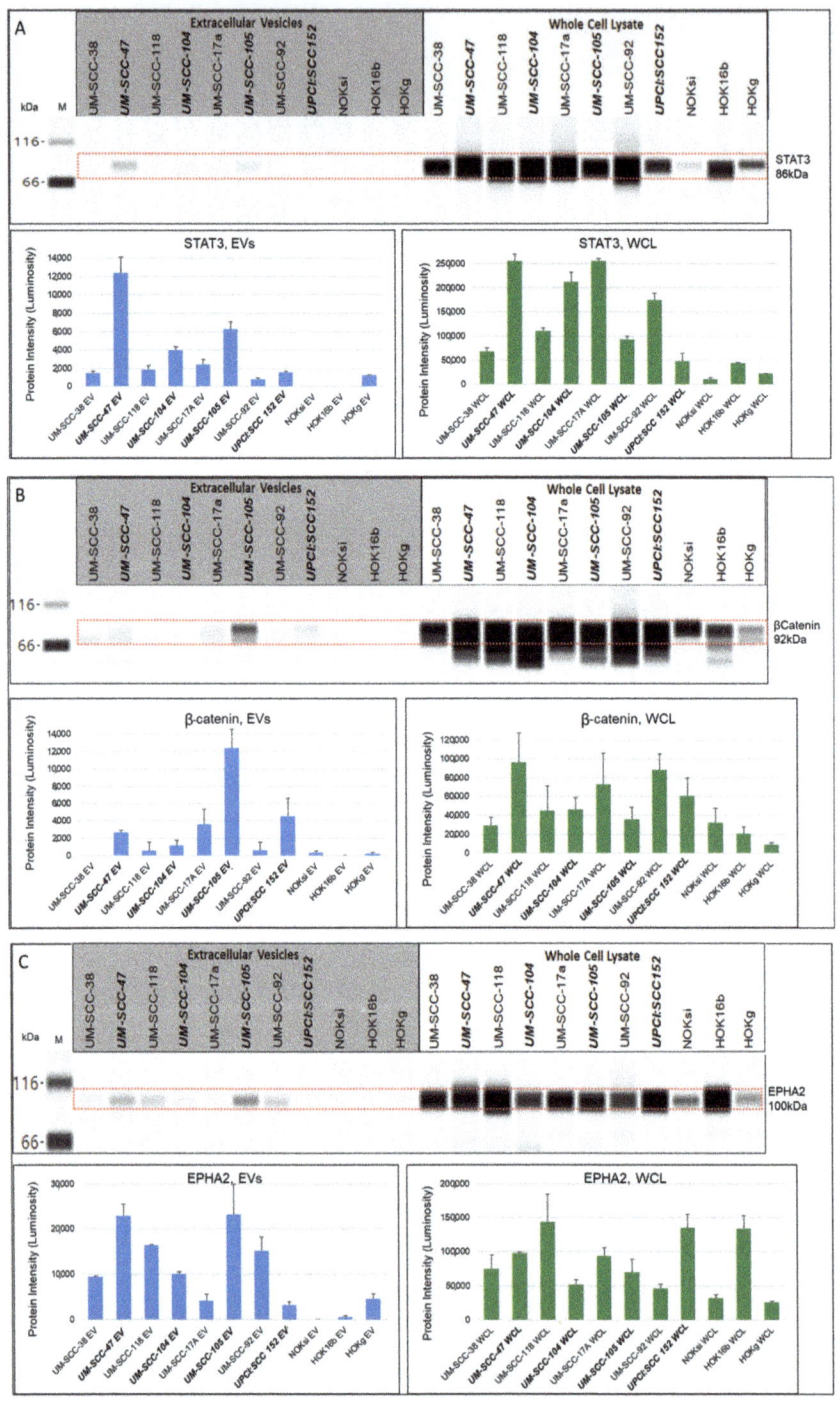

Figure 6. *Cont.*

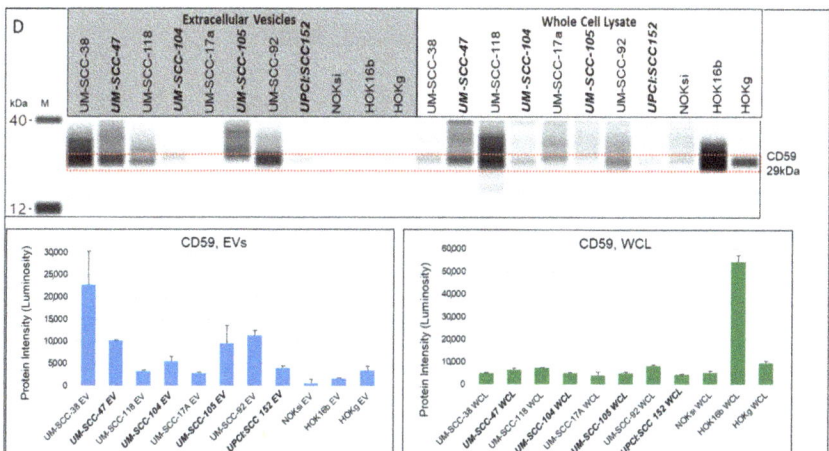

Figure 6. Wes protein gel and quantitative luminosity for extracellular vesicles and whole cell lysates from HNSCC, normal keratinocyte, and transformed cell lines. (**A**) STAT3 detected at 86 kDa, 1:25 antibody dilution, 0.5 µg/µL protein; (**B**) βCatenin detected at 92 kDa, 1:200 antibody dilution, 0.25 µg/µL protein; (**C**) EPHA2 detected at 100 kDa, 1:100 antibody dilution, 0.5 mg/mL protein; and (**D**) CD59 detected at 29 kDa, 1:100 antibody dilution, 1:7, 1 mg/mL protein. Bold italics: HPV-positive.

Despite tenascin-C (TNC) (Figure 7A) being detected in the whole cell lysate of only one (UM-SCC-118A) of the eleven cell lines tested, it was seen in several lines across the EV panel. Tenascin-C was detected at 266 kDa in EVs from the HPV-positive HNSCC lines, UM-SCC-47, UM-SCC-104, UM-SCC-105, and UPCI:SCC152, and at incredibly high levels in EVs from the HPV-negative cell line UM-SCC-118a. Fainter bands were detected in EVs from HPV-negative UM-SCC-38 and UM-SCC-92, and those from normal cell line HOKg.

HLA-A (Figure 7B) was detected at 54 kDa in all of the whole cell lysates with the highest intensity band in the whole cell lysate from the HPV-positive HNSCC cell line, UM-SCC-47. In the EVs, HLA-A was detected at the highest levels in EVs from the HPV-positive HNSCC lines, UM-SCC-47, UM-SCC-104, and UM-SCC-105. HLA-A was not detected in EVs from NOKsi or HOKg lines.

E-cadherin (E-Cad) (Figure 7C) was detected at 120 kDa in all of the whole cell lysates tested with the exception of the HPV transformed line, HOK16B. E-cadherin was also detected in all of the HNSCC EVs tested. Interestingly, the EVs from HPV-positive cell lines UM-SCC-47, UM-SCC-104, and UPCI:SCC152 (those generated from non-responsive tumors) had lower levels of E-cadherin detected than EVs from HPV-negative UM-SCC-17, or UM-SCC-92, or EVs from HPV18-positive UM-SCC-105 (generated from a responsive tumor).

EGFR (Figure 7D) was detected in all of the whole cell lysates tested. EGFR was detected in all of the HNSCC EVs. Two of the EV samples with the highest levels of EGFR were those from HPV18-positive UM-SCC-105 and HPV-negative UM-SCC-92; these cell lines were derived from tumors that were responsive to treatment and the patients are still alive.

Cytokeratin 19 (CK19) (Figure 7E) was detected at the highest levels in EV from HPV-negative cell lines UM-SCC-38 and UM-SCC-92, while the protein is also seen in the whole cell lysates of the HPV-negative cell lines as well as HPV-positive UM-SCC-47 and UM-SCC-105.

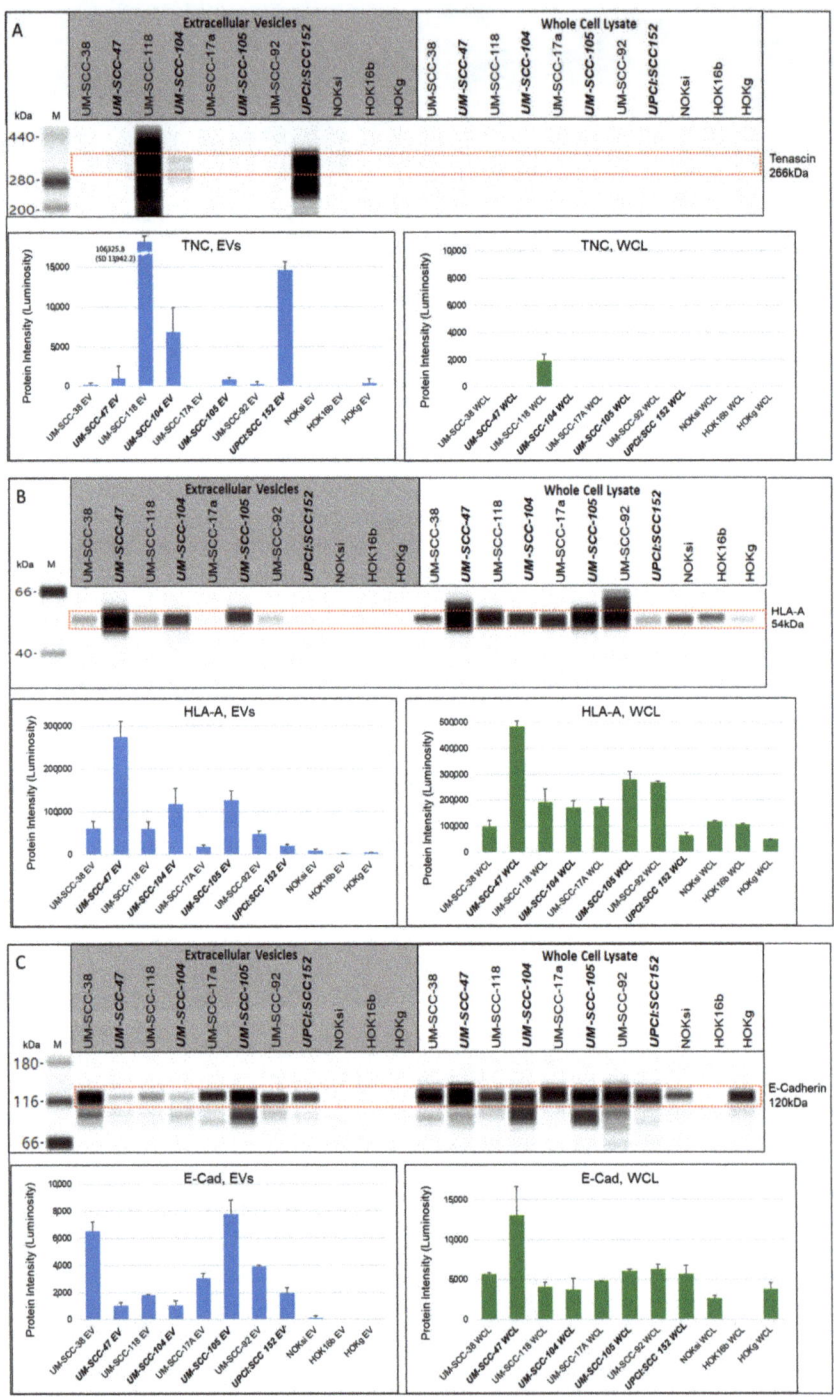

Figure 7. *Cont.*

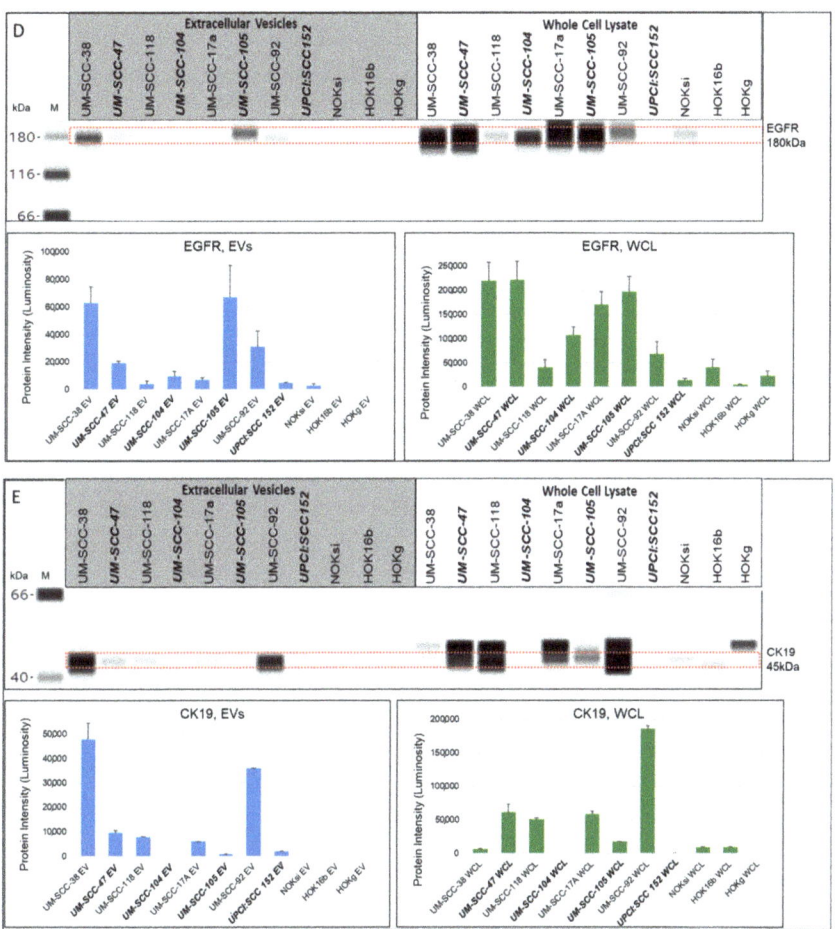

Figure 7. Wes protein gel and quantitative luminosity for extracellular vesicles and whole cell lysates from HNSCC, normal keratinocyte, and transformed cell lines. (**A**) Tenascin detected at 266 kDa, 1:200 antibody dilution, 0.5 µg/µL protein; (**B**) HLA-A detected at 54 kDa, 1:400 antibody dilution, 0.25µg/µL protein; (**C**) E-cadherin detected at 120 kDa, 1:250 antibody dilution, 0.5µg/µL protein; (**D**) EGFR detected at 180 kDa, 1:100 antibody dilution, 0.25 µg/µL protein; and (**E**) CK19 detected at 45 kDa, 1:100 antibody dilution, 0.25 mg/mL protein. Bold italics: HPV-positive.

HPV16 and associated proteins, RB, p53, CyclinD1, and p16 are shown in Figure 8. HPV16E7 was detected at 18 kDa in only the whole cell lysates of the HPV16-positive cell lines tested, UM-SCC-47, UM-SCC-104, UPCI:SCC152, and the HPV16-transformed cell line, HOK16b. HPV16E7 was not detected in any of the EVs tested.

The 112 kDa form of RB protein was detected in all of the whole cell lysates, and none of the EVs, from all of the eleven cell lines tested. The protein was detected at varying levels in the different whole cell lysates.

p53 was detected in only whole cell lysates from HPV-negative cell lines UM-SCC-38 (at 52 kDa and 60 kDa) and UM-SCC-17a (at 60 kDa), as well as whole cell lysates from the normal cell line NOKsi (at 48 kDa and 60 kDa). There was also a faint signal in the normal HOKg whole cell lysate sample at 60 kDa. p53 was not detected in any of the EVs tested.

CyclinD1 was detected at 40 kDa in all of the whole cell lysates tested with the exceptions of HPV-positive HNSCC cell lines UM-SCC-47 and UPCI:SCC152, where no

CyclinD1 protein was found. There was no CyclinD1 protein detected in any of the EVs tested.

None of the EVs tested contained detectable levels of p16 protein. We did identify p16 at 24 kDa in whole cell lysates of HPV-positive HNSCC cell lines UM-SCC-47, UM-SCC-104, UM-SCC-105, and UPCI:SCC152, as well as HPV-negative HNSCC line UM-SCC-92. The whole cell lysates of the transformed cell line HOK16b and normal HOKg cell line also contained p16 protein, although the lysate of the normal NOKsi line did not.

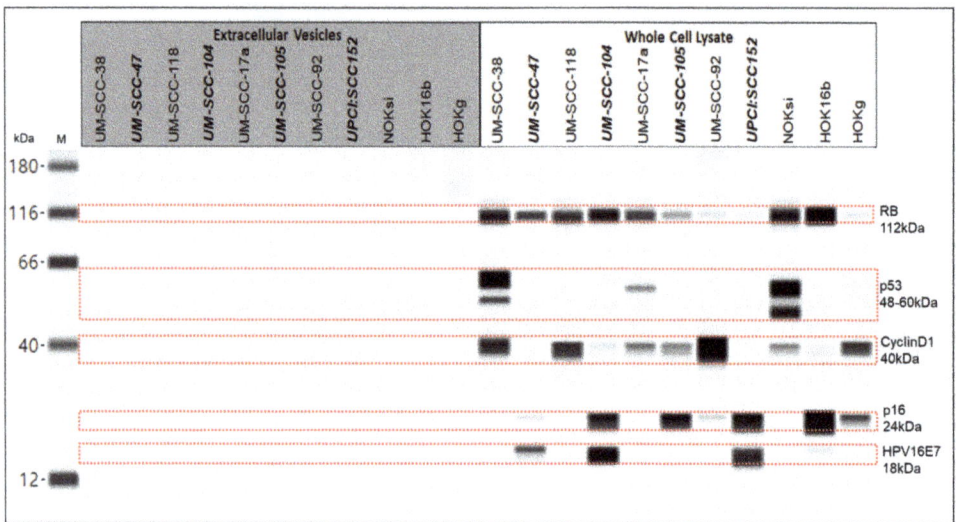

Figure 8. Wes protein gel for extracellular vesicles and whole cell lysates from HNSCC, normal keratinocyte, and transformed cell lines. RB detected at 112 kDa, 1:100 antibody dilution, 0.5 mg/mL protein; p53 detected at 60 kDa, 52 kda, and 48 kDa, 1:50 antibody dilution, 0.25 µg/µL protein; CyclinD1 detected at 40 kDa, 1:200 antibody dilution, 0.25 µg/µL protein; p16 detected at 24 kDa, no antibody dilution, 0.25 µg/µL protein; and HPV16E7 detected at 18 kDa, 1:100 antibody dilution, 1 µg/µL protein. Bold italics: HPV-positive.

4. Discussion

The proteins detected in the EVs from the HNSCC cell lines were expected to recapitulate the characteristics of the originating cells. This study suggests that this is frequently not the case, as seen in Figure 9, which illustrates the comparative protein levels detected in WCL and EV from HNSCC cell lines queried in this study. While the EV protein cargo does not consistently represent that of the parent cell, there are striking differences between EV proteins that could be important indicators of tumor cell behavior and these warrant further investigation. Furthermore, the proteins detected in EVs from tumor cells are likely purposely intended for transport from the cell as a mechanism for tumor cell survival, growth, or other advantage.

Tenascin-C is an extracellular matrix glycoprotein, expressed during embryogenesis, organogenesis, wound healing and inflammation [31–34]. TNC has been well studied, and has many known binding sites for cell surface receptors (including integrins) and extracellular matrix proteins (including fibronectin); multiple integrins and fibronectin were candidates in our proteomics analysis [31–35].

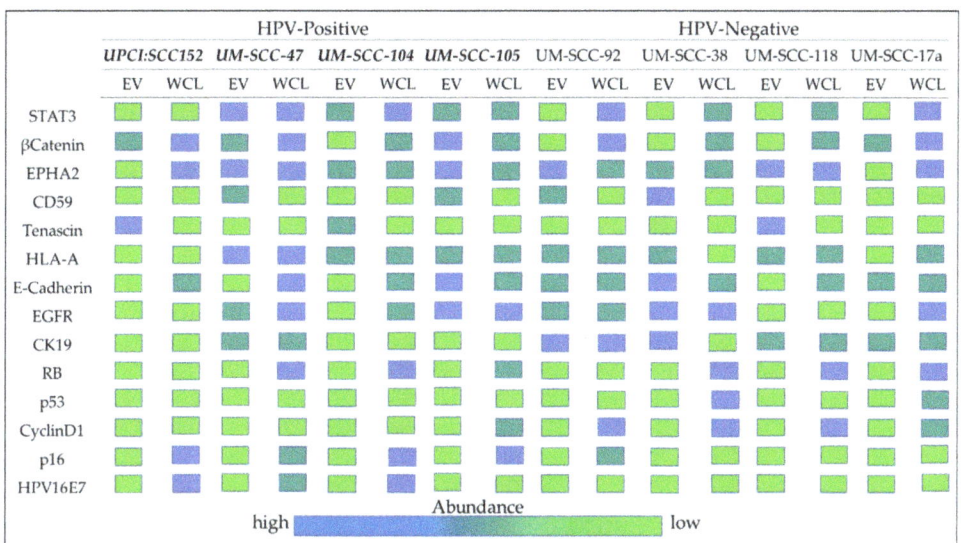

Figure 9. Relative abundance of the selected proteins detected by Wes protein analysis in EVs and WCL from HNSCC cell lines, by HPV status. Bold italics: HPV-positive.

Tenascin-C has been implicated in many cancer types: esophageal, breast, colorectal, bladder, Merkel cell carcinomas, glioma, malignant pleural mesothelioma, glioblastoma multiforme, malignant melanoma, and astrocytoma, and has been implicated in a variety of roles: tumorigenesis, angiogenesis, migration, proliferation, maintaining the stemness of cancer stem cells, and metastasis [31,32,36–41]. TCGA data have shown increased mRNA expression in HNSCC [37]. TNC has also been shown to suppress T cell activation [37,42]. TNC is implicated in HPV-positive cervical cancer, although its mechanism is still unknown [33,43]. TNC-containing exosomes were found in association with glioblastoma patients having a T cell-suppressive role [37]. Our Wes protein results showed TNC in two subsets: EVs from HNSCC cell line UM-SCC-118, generated from an HPV-negative tongue cancer, and EVs from all four HPV-positive HNSCC cell lines (UM-SCC-47, UM-SCC-104, UM-SCC-105, and UPCI:SCC152). TNC is seen more often in stroma cells than tumor cells, so it is not surprising that TNC was not detected in the majority of WCL, whether HPV-positive or -negative [44]. It is interesting that TNC expression was seen in UM-SCC-118 WCL, an HPV-negative cell line, and that the protein was detected in the EVs as well. The detection of TNC in HPV-positive EVs establishes the possibility of TNC as a marker for HPV-positive HNSCC. It has been studied previously as a biomarker for HNSCC (unrelated to HPV), with mixed results [35,40,45,46], while others have investigated TNC (associated with HPV) and found TNC to be involved but do not know the exact mechanism of action [33]. It is of particular interest that TNC was seen in such distinct EV groups, and makes this protein a candidate for further investigation.

The signal transducer and activator of transcription 3 (STAT3) is part of the signal transducer and activator of the transcription protein family. STAT3 plays a pivotal role in tumorigenesis through transcription regulation of genes having essential roles in cell proliferation, inflammation, differentiation, apoptosis, angiogenesis, immune response, and metastasis [47]. STAT3 has many known receptors including the Janus kinases, EGFR, and IL-6 [47–49]. In this study, STAT3 was detected in the EVs from all the HPV-positive HNSCC cell lines. The highest expression was in the EVs from UM-SCC-47, followed by those from UM-SCC-105, the only HPV18 positive line. Recent studies have shown that HPV18 causes activation of STAT3 through the HPV18 E6 protein [50,51]. There are also general implications that STAT3 is activated by viruses, which would account for the high levels of STAT3 in all of the HPV-positive whole cell lysates [52]. Based on these results, STAT3 would be a reasonable EV protein candidate for HPV-positive HNSCC, if it had not also been detected in the EVs from the non-cancer HOKg cell line, making this protein a less desirable candidate for progression in our studies.

HLA (human leukocyte antigen) is part of the MHC class I immune system. There are classical forms, HLA-A, HLA-B, and HLA-C, and non-classical forms, HLA-G, HLA-E, HLA-F, and HLA-H, of this protein; both have been identified in cancer with diverse roles [53–57]. In our study, we identified HLA-A in WCL from all of the lines tested and in EVs from all of the HNSCC lines. HLA-A was detected in the EVs from three of the HPV-positive HNSCC lines at higher levels than in EVs from the other HNSCC lines; this might support the use of HLA-A and allelotyping for prognosis in HPV-positive HNSCC, which is currently used in cervical carcinomas and to a lesser extent in HNSCC [53,58–66]. It would be worthwhile to look at these methods from the EV perspective to provide a less invasive predictive or prognostic biomarker. HLA-E has previously been suggested to offer a predictive prognosis in laryngeal lesions [53]. Although not tested by Wes protein analysis, many of the non-classical HLA forms were present in our EV MS proteomics data, with the exception of HLA-G. These non-classical HLA proteins participate in immune system evasion [54,56,57]. A recent study showed that the use of monalizumab blocked the binding of NKG2A in the presence of HLA-E, causing an increase in both natural killer and T cells. When used in combination with cetuximab, the authors showed a 31% objective response rate [67]. This study, taken together with our results, demonstrates that HLA proteins are robust EV protein candidates for continued investigation.

β-Catenin, together with the cadherin family of adhesion proteins, is part of the Wnt signaling pathway, and is thought to have roles in both HPV-positive and -negative HNSCC and be associated to de-differentiation and poor prognosis [68–71]. HPV-16 oncoprotein regulates the translocation of β-catenin via the activation of epidermal growth factor receptor. β-catenin is normally seen on cell membrane, but when it is cleaved from E-cadherin and not phosphorylated for degradation, it accumulates in the cytoplasm and is translocated to the nucleus by the T cell factor (TCF)/lymphoid enhancer-binding factor (LEF) transcriptional factors, ultimately leading to epithelial–mesenchymal transition (EMT) [71–74]. β-catenin has downstream targets associated with the tumor microenvironment including extracellular matrix components, laminin, and fibronectin; this relationship with the microenvironment may be supported through molecular transport by EVs [71]. The highest EV signal for β-catenin was seen in the EVs from HPV18-positive HNSCC UM-SCC-105, and was also detected in EVs from two other HPV-positive HNSCC lines.

E-cadherin is part of the cadherin family of proteins, and functions as a main adhesion protein of the epithelia with key roles in attachment with the formation of E-cadherin/β-catenin complex, polarity, and structure. Repression, downregulation, or loss of E-cadherin is correlated with metastasis and invasion and has been implicated in EMT [73,75–82]. E-cadherin is associated with a number of pathways, including Wnt/β-catenin, ERK, MAP kinase, and PI3K-Akt [77,83]. In HNSCC, reduced E-cadherin expression has been shown to be associated with poor prognosis, tumor aggressiveness, EMT completion, metastasis, and lower overall survival [80–82,84,85]. Historically, EPHA2 has been evaluated together with E-cadherin, as it is dependent on E-cadherin for localization to cell–cell sites. In the absence of E-cadherin, EPHA2 does not transfer to the cell–cell site and cells exhibit pro-metastatic behavior [86]. In HNSCC, loss of E-cadherin is characteristic of advanced tumor stage and metastatic potential [80–82,84,85]. In our study, E-cadherin was detected in the EVs from all of the HNSCC lines, but not the EVs from the normal keratinocyte lines. Furthermore, the E-cadherin levels detected in EVs from HPV-16 positive HNSCC lines UM-SCC-47, UM-SCC-104, and UPCI:SCC152 were overall lower than those in EVs from HPV-negative or HPV18-positive UM-SCC-17A, UM-SCC-105, and UM-SCC-92. This finding makes E-cadherin an especially attractive EV protein candidate for further investigation.

EphA2 is a receptor tyrosine kinase that binds to adjacent cells through binding to surface-associated Ephrin (Eph receptor interacting protein) ligands [87]. Dysfunction/dysregulation within the Eph family of proteins has been seen in several types of disease, ranging from cancer to inflammation and a variety of cell types with sometimes contradictory implications owning to its bidirectional and promiscuous signaling [87,88]. Eph proteins have been implicated in cellular adhesion, angiogenesis, cell migration and proliferation, survival, differentiation, and secretion [87–89]. Based on its involvement in carcinogenesis and other pathologies, EphA2 has been evaluated as a target for drug therapy [90–93]. In HNSCC, EphA2 has been further investigated for its role in inflammation, epithelial–mesenchymal transition, migration, proliferation, and point of viral entry [94–97]. The HNSCC TCGA subset showed EphA2 to be among the significantly mutated genes [98]. More recently, it has been suggested as a potential compensatory mechanism in MET inhibition [99]. In our study, EphA2 was detected in all of the whole cell lysates tested and all of the EVs tested with the exception of the EVs from one of the normal keratinocyte lines (NOKsi). Overexpressed EPHA2 is shown to increase resistance to common EGFR drug therapy, cetuximab, via EPHA2 mediated activation of the PI3K/AKT pathway [86]. Overexpression of EPHA2 is also seen in cells resistant to erlotinib, gefitinib, and afatinib. [100,101]. EPHA2 together with EGFR may be a feasible marker combination to predict anti-EGFR resistance, making both of these proteins attractive candidates for further investigation.

EGFR is a type I receptor tyrosine kinase with a structure that spans the cell membrane and includes an extracellular ligand-binding domain and an intracellular kinase domain. EGFR is expressed in most epithelial tissues, and is involved in multiple pathways, including PI3K/Akt/mTOR, JAK/STAT, and RAS/RAF/MEK/ERK [81,102,103]. Many of these pathways involve mutations that become carcinogenic drivers [104]. EGFR has been implicated in many other cancer types, including breast, cervical, astrocytoma, bladder, esophageal, gastric, lung adenocarcinoma, colorectal, ovarian, and others [105–113]. EGFR is frequently overexpressed in HNSCC and a variety of other cancers [114]. In HNSCC, EGFR plays roles in invasion, migration, survival, proliferation, and metastasis [81,102,115]. While EGFR is expressed in HPV-positive and -negative cell lines (as seen in whole cell lysates in our study as well), there has been an association shown between EGFR and high-risk HPV E5 proteins in HPV-positive tumors, with HPV E5 having a role in activating EGFR [116–119]. EGFR has been studied as a candidate for targeted drug therapy in HNSCC; however, while overexpression is seen in 80–90% of HNSCC, only 10–20% are responsive to anti-EGFR drug therapy [102,115,120,121]. In our data, we see the same overexpression of EGFR in the Wes results with WCL and EVs, but with an overall lower level of overexpression in the EVs when compared with WCL levels. In other studies, EGFR is linked to EPHA2, and EPHA2 signaling is suggested to contribute to anti-EGFR therapy resistance [86].

Cytokeratin 19 is part of the cellular cytoskeletal network of intermediate filaments (IF), in the sub-classification of type I epithelial keratins [122,123]. Keratins have a widely accepted role in protection and structure of the cell, but recently they have been investigated for involvement in different cancers [122–129]. CK19 plays a major role in wound healing and tissue remodeling and has a variety of responses to the stresses (both mechanical and non-mechanical) endured by cells, ranging from cell signaling, migration, cell growth, differentiation, post translational modification, protein regulation, transcriptional regulation, and even metastasis, but the mechanism of action is largely yet unknown [122–124,126,130–134]. Keratins are considered a marker for epithelial stem cells, and increased cytokeratin 19 expression has been shown to be a biomarker of highly invasive oral squamous cell carcinoma with metastatic potential, as well as higher tumor recurrence and lower survival [129,130,135–138]. The role of CK19 in HNSCC in liquid biopsies (and thus our interest in evaluating this protein in EVs) was prompted through the use of keratin proteins for immunohistochemical tumor diagnosis in carcinomas. In particular, CK5, CK7, CK8, CK18, CK19, and CK20 [122]. The majority of these were included in our proteomic analysis, and of these CK19 had the most robust PSM and coverage. In addition to CK19, several other keratin proteins were identified in our proteomic study, including CK17, CK14, CK8, CK18, and CK6A. The raw proteomic data suggest a possible pattern of keratins present in the EVs from a subset of cell lines. Furthermore, a group in Japan is using CK19 as a marker for HNSCC in liquid biopsies [139]. This is supported by our results, showing no cytokeratin 19 detected in any of the non-cancer EVs. Another interesting finding from our Wes results is the relatively low abundance of CK19 in the UM-SCC-38 whole cell lysate, while the protein is detected at the highest levels in EVs from that same cell line. This protein and other cytokeratin family members will be further investigated as possible EV proteins released from tumor cells to participate in modification of the tumor microenvironment or similar mechanisms for survival and metastasis.

CD59 is a cell surface inhibitor of the membrane attack complex present in most tissues and on all circulating cells [140,141]. It is overexpressed on tumor cells, enabling tumor cells to escape from complement-mediated killing, listed in the top 50 proteins in the human proteomic atlas as an unfavorable prognostic protein [140–143]. CD59 has been evaluated as a salivary biomarker for oral squamous cell carcinomas together with M2BP, S100A9/MRP14, and catalase, achieving diagnostic sensitivity of 90%, specificity of 83%, and AUROCC of 0.93 for OSCC detection [144,145]. CD59 has also been shown to be present in exosomes [146], consistent with our findings. Unfortunately, our study also detected CD59 by Wes in the EVs from the non-cancer HOKg cell line, making this protein a less desirable candidate for progression in our studies.

HPV and associated proteins, RB, p53, Cyclin D1, and p16, are common biomarkers for HPV-positive and -negative HNSCC. HPV16E7 is a viral oncoprotein expressed in the HPV16-positive HNSCC tumors and cell lines. We thought that it might be detected in the EVs from the HPV16-positive cell lines; however, it was identified only in the whole cell lysates, including the whole cell lysate of the HPV16-transformed cell line, HOK16b. Similarly, we did not detect HPV-associated proteins RB, p53, Cyclin D1, or p16 in any of the EVs tested. We will evaluate other HPV proteins (including HPV18E6 and E7, as appropriate, and HPV16E6) as potential EV markers, or perhaps investigate alternate antibodies, as HPV proteins and several of the other HPV-associated markers have previously been identified in EVs from HPV-positive cell lines [147]. It was somewhat surprising that HPV proteins (E6 and E7) were not detected by MS in EVs from the tested HPV-positive cell lines. Another group detected HPV proteins in exosomes from one of the same HPV-positive cell lines we tested, UM-SCC-47 [147]. This is not entirely unfounded, as the isolation methods used to obtain EVs, the type of vesicles extracted/evaluated, and the method of sample preparation used for MS were different between the studies.

5. Conclusions

We have demonstrated that proteins can be reliably detected in EVs and whole cell lysates from HNSCC, normal keratinocytes, and transformed cell lines, and that EVs released by HNSCC cells contain different proteins based on characteristics of the originating cell, including HPV status. Our work has importantly demonstrated that EVs released by tumor cells do not necessarily recapitulate the complete protein profile of the originating cell, and hypothesize that EV protein cargo is determined by other factors that are advantageous for the tumor cell, such as growth, immune evasion, modification of the tumor microenvironment, cell-to-cell communication, drug resistance, etc. Finally, this work has identified several protein candidates for continued evaluation for HNSCC EV markers, including tenascin-C, HLA-A, E-cadherin, EGFR, EPHA2, and cytokeratin 19.

Supplementary Materials: The following are available online at https://www.mdpi.com/article/10.3390/cancers13153714/s1, Table S1. Proteins from HNSCC cell line EVs with averaged fold-change peptide spectrum matches (PSM) >2 compared with the EVs from the normal keratinocyte line (NOKsi) (n = 149); Table S2.Wes protein intensity values for Figure 3; Table S3. Wes protein intensity values for Figure 8; Figure S1. CD9 and AnnexinV Wes protein quantitative luminosity for extracellular vesicles from HNSCC, normal keratinocyte, and transformed cell line; and Figure S2. All uncropped Wes gels showing protein bands and molecular weight markers.

Author Contributions: Conceptualization, C.G. and H.W.; data curation, C.G., L.P. and H.W.; formal analysis, F.d.V.L., V.B. and A.N.; funding acquisition, H.W.; investigation, C.G., L.P. and H.W.; methodology, C.G., F.d.V.L., V.B. and H.W.; project administration, H.W.; resources, H.W.; software, C.G., F.d.V.L., V.B., A.N. and H.W.; supervision, A.N. and H.W.; validation, C.G. and H.W.; visualization, C.G., F.d.V.L., V.B. and H.W.; writing—original draft, C.G. and H.W.; writing—review & editing, C.G., F.d.V.L., V.B. and H.W. All authors have read and agreed to the published version of the manuscript.

Funding: This research received no external funding and was performed with start-up funds provided by the University of Michigan Department of Otolaryngology.

Institutional Review Board Statement: Not applicable.

Informed Consent Statement: Not applicable.

Data Availability Statement: The data supporting the figures presented in this study are openly available in FigShare at [https://figshare.com/s/3d3cd935872558e323f2, accessed on 25 June 2021]. Public DOI 10.6084/m9.figshare.14378672.

Acknowledgments: The authors would like to acknowledge Arul M. Chinnaiyan for the use of the Wes instrument and thank Ingrid J. Apel for her generous assistance and expertise with the Wes system. Cell line UPCI:SCC152 was generously provided by S. Gollin from the University of Pittsburgh Cancer Institute.

Conflicts of Interest: The authors declare no conflict of interest.

References

1. Ferlay, J.; Soerjomataram, I.; Dikshit, R.; Eser, S.; Mathers, C.; Rebelo, M.; Parkin, D.M.; Forman, D.; Bray, F. Cancer incidence and mortality worldwide: Sources, methods and major patterns in GLOBOCAN 2012. *Int. J. Cancer* **2015**, *136*, E359–E386. [CrossRef] [PubMed]
2. Wong, N.; Khwaja, S.S.; Baker, C.M.; Gay, H.A.; Thorstad, W.L.; Daly, M.D.; Lewis, J.S.; Wang, X. Prognostic micro RNA signatures derived from The Cancer Genome Atlas for head and neck squamous cell carcinomas. *Cancer Med.* **2016**, *5*, 1619–1628. [CrossRef] [PubMed]
3. Johnson, D.E.; Burtness, B.; Leemans, C.R.; Lui, V.W.Y.; Bauman, J.E.; Grandis, J.R. Head and neck squamous cell carcinoma. *Nat. Rev. Dis. Prim.* **2020**, *6*, 1–22. [CrossRef]
4. Leemans, C.R.; Braakhuis, B.J.M.; Brakenhoff, R.H. The molecular biology of head and neck cancer. *Nat. Rev. Cancer* **2010**, *11*, 9–22. [CrossRef] [PubMed]
5. Applebaum, K.M.; Furniss, C.S.; Zeka, A.; Posner, M.R.; Smith, J.F.; Bryan, J.; Eisen, E.A.; Peters, E.S.; McClean, M.D.; Kelsey, K.T. Lack of Association of Alcohol and Tobacco with HPV16-Associated Head and Neck Cancer. *J. Natl. Cancer Inst.* **2007**, *99*, 1801–1810. [CrossRef]
6. Gillison, M.L.; D'Souza, G.; Westra, W.; Sugar, E.; Xiao, W.; Begum, S.; Viscidi, R. Distinct Risk Factor Profiles for Human Papillomavirus Type 16–Positive and Human Papillomavirus Type 16–Negative Head and Neck Cancers. *J. Natl. Cancer Inst.* **2008**, *100*, 407–420. [CrossRef]
7. Morris, L.G.; Sikora, A.G.; Patel, S.G.; Hayes, R.B.; Ganly, I. Second Primary Cancers after an Index Head and Neck Cancer: Subsite-Specific Trends in the Era of Human Papillomavirus–Associated Oropharyngeal Cancer. *J. Clin. Oncol.* **2011**, *29*, 739–746. [CrossRef] [PubMed]
8. Quon, H.; Cohen, M.A.; Montone, K.T.; Ziober, A.F.; Wang, L.P.; Weinstein, G.S.; O'Malley, B.W. Transoral robotic surgery and adjuvant therapy for oropharyngeal carcinomas and the influence of p16INK4a on treatment outcomes. *Laryngoscope* **2013**, *123*, 635–640. [CrossRef]
9. Haughey, B.H.; Hinni, M.L.; Salassa, J.R.; Hayden, R.E.; Grant, D.G.; Rich, J.T.; Milov, S.; Lewis, J.S.; Krishna, M. Transoral laser microsurgery as primary treatment for advanced-stage oropharyngeal cancer: A united states multicenter study. *Head Neck* **2011**, *33*, 1683–1694. [CrossRef]
10. Théry, C.; Witwer, K.W.; Aikawa, E.; Alcaraz, M.J.; Anderson, J.D.; Andriantsitohaina, R.; Antoniou, A.; Arab, T.; Archer, F.; Atkin-Smith, G.K.; et al. Minimal information for studies of extracellular vesicles 2018 (MISEV2018): A position statement of the International Society for Extracellular Vesicles and update of the MISEV2014 guidelines. *J. Extracell. Vesicles* **2018**, *7*, 1535750. [CrossRef] [PubMed]
11. Whiteside, T.L. The potential of tumor-derived exosomes for noninvasive cancer monitoring. *Expert Rev. Mol. Diagn.* **2015**, *15*, 1293–1310. [CrossRef]
12. Li, M.; Rai, A.J.; DeCastro, G.J.; Zeringer, E.; Barta, T.; Magdaleno, S.; Setterquist, R.; Vlassov, A.V. An optimized procedure for exosome isolation and analysis using serum samples: Application to cancer biomarker discovery. *Methods* **2015**, *87*, 26–30. [CrossRef] [PubMed]

13. Whiteside, T.L. Tumor-Derived Exosomes and Their Role in Cancer Progression. *Adv. Clin. Chem.* **2016**, *74*, 103–141. [CrossRef] [PubMed]
14. Rana, S.; Malinowska, K.; Zöller, M. Exosomal Tumor MicroRNA Modulates Premetastatic Organ Cells. *Neoplasia* **2013**, *15*, 281-IN31. [CrossRef]
15. Hannafon, B.N.; Ding, W.-Q. Intercellular Communication by Exosome-Derived microRNAs in Cancer. *Int. J. Mol. Sci.* **2013**, *14*, 14240–14269. [CrossRef] [PubMed]
16. Dhondt, B.; Rousseau, Q.; De Wever, O.; Hendrix, A. Function of extracellular vesicle-associated miRNAs in metastasis. *Cell Tissue Res.* **2016**, *365*, 621–641. [CrossRef]
17. Kalluri, R. The biology and function of exosomes in cancer. *J. Clin. Investig.* **2016**, *126*, 1208–1215. [CrossRef]
18. Koga, K.; Matsumoto, K.; Akiyoshi, T.; Kubo, M.; Yamanaka, N.; Tasaki, A.; Nakashima, H.; Nakamura, M.; Kuroki, S.; Tanaka, M.; et al. Purification, characterization and biological significance of tumor-derived exosomes. *Anticancer. Res.* **2005**, *25*, 3703–3707.
19. Jin, Y.; Chen, K.; Wang, Z.; Wang, Y.; Liu, J.; Lin, L.; Shao, Y.; Gao, L.; Yin, H.; Cui, C.; et al. DNA in serum extracellular vesicles is stable under different storage conditions. *BMC Cancer* **2016**, *16*, 753. [CrossRef]
20. Ralhan, R.; Masui, O.; DeSouza, L.V.; Matta, A.; Macha, M.; Siu, K.W.M. Identification of proteins secreted by head and neck cancer cell lines using LC-MS/MS: Strategy for discovery of candidate serological biomarkers. *J. Proteom.* **2011**, *11*, 2363–2376. [CrossRef]
21. Dowling, P.; Wormald, R.; Meleady, P.; Henry, M.; Curran, A.; Clynes, M. Analysis of the saliva proteome from patients with head and neck squamous cell carcinoma reveals differences in abundance levels of proteins associated with tumour progression and metastasis. *J. Proteom.* **2008**, *71*, 168–175. [CrossRef]
22. Park, N.-H.; Min, B.-M.; Li, S.-L.; Huang, M.Z.; Doniger, J. Immortalization of normal human oral keratinocytes with type 16 human papillomavirus. *Carcinogenesis* **1991**, *12*, 1627–1631. [CrossRef] [PubMed]
23. Castilho, R.M.; Squarize, C.; Leelahavanichkul, K.; Zheng, Y.; Bugge, T.; Gutkind, J.S. Rac1 Is Required for Epithelial Stem Cell Function during Dermal and Oral Mucosal Wound Healing but Not for Tissue Homeostasis in Mice. *PLoS ONE* **2010**, *5*, e10503. [CrossRef] [PubMed]
24. Théry, C.; Amigorena, S.; Raposo, G.; Clayton, A. Isolation and Characterization of Exosomes from Cell Culture Supernatants and Biological Fluids. *Curr. Protoc. Cell Biol.* **2006**, *30*, 1–29. [CrossRef] [PubMed]
25. Rider, M.A.; Hurwitz, S.N.; Meckes, D.G., Jr. ExtraPEG: A Polyethylene Glycol-Based Method for Enrichment of Extracellular Vesicles. *Sci. Rep.* **2016**, *6*, 23978. [CrossRef]
26. Tank, E.M.; Figueroa-Romero, C.; Hinder, L.M.; Bedi, K.; Archbold, H.C.; Li, X.; Weskamp, K.; Safren, N.; Paez-Colasante, X.; Pacut, C.; et al. Abnormal RNA stability in amyotrophic lateral sclerosis. *Nat. Commun.* **2018**, *9*, 1–16. [CrossRef]
27. McAlister, G.C.; Nusinow, D.; Jedrychowski, M.P.; Wühr, M.; Huttlin, E.; Erickson, B.; Rad, R.; Haas, W.; Gygi, S.P. MultiNotch MS3 Enables Accurate, Sensitive, and Multiplexed Detection of Differential Expression across Cancer Cell Line Proteomes. *Anal. Chem.* **2014**, *86*, 7150–7158. [CrossRef] [PubMed]
28. Martins, T.; Catita, J.; Rosa, I.M.; Silva, O.A.; Henriques, A.G. Exosome isolation from distinct biofluids using precipitation and column-based approaches. *PLoS ONE* **2018**, *13*, e0198820. [CrossRef]
29. Lässer, C.; Eldh, M.; Lötvall, J. Isolation and Characterization of RNA-Containing Exosomes. *J. Vis. Exp.* **2012**, *2012*, e3037. [CrossRef]
30. Hartjes, T.A.; Mytnyk, S.; Jenster, G.W.; Van Steijn, V.; Van Royen, M.E. Extracellular Vesicle Quantification and Characterization: Common Methods and Emerging Approaches. *Bioengineering* **2019**, *6*, 7. [CrossRef] [PubMed]
31. Midwood, K.S.; Hussenet, T.; Langlois, B.; Orend, G. Advances in tenascin-C biology. *Cell Mol. Life Sci.* **2011**, *68*, 3175–3199. [CrossRef] [PubMed]
32. Midwood, K.S.; Orend, G. The role of tenascin-C in tissue injury and tumorigenesis. *J. Cell Commun. Signal.* **2009**, *3*, 287–310. [CrossRef] [PubMed]
33. Maeda, N.; Maenaka, K. The Roles of Matricellular Proteins in Oncogenic Virus-Induced Cancers and Their Potential Utilities as Therapeutic Targets. *Int. J. Mol. Sci.* **2017**, *18*, 2198. [CrossRef] [PubMed]
34. Udalova, I.; Ruhmann, M.; Thomson, S.J.; Midwood, K.S. Expression and Immune Function of Tenascin-C. *Crit. Rev. Immunol.* **2011**, *31*, 115–145. [CrossRef] [PubMed]
35. Lyons, A.; Jones, J. Cell adhesion molecules, the extracellular matrix and oral squamous carcinoma. *Int. J. Oral Maxillofac. Surg.* **2007**, *36*, 671–679. [CrossRef]
36. Oskarsson, T.; Acharyya, S.; Zhang, X.; Vanharanta, S.; Tavazoie, S.F.; Morris, P.G.; Downey, R.J.; Manova-Todorova, K.; Brogi, E.; Massague, J. Breast cancer cells produce tenascin C as a metastatic niche component to colonize the lungs. *Nat. Med.* **2011**, *17*, 867–874. [CrossRef]
37. Mirzaei, R.; Sarkar, S.; Dzikowski, L.; Rawji, K.S.; Khan, L.; Faissner, A.; Bose, P.; Yong, V.W. Brain tumor-initiating cells export tenascin-C associated with exosomes to suppress T cell activity. *OncoImmunology* **2018**, *7*, e1478647. [CrossRef]
38. Nissen, N.I.; Karsdal, M.; Willumsen, N. Collagens and Cancer associated fibroblasts in the reactive stroma and its relation to Cancer biology. *J. Exp. Clin. Cancer Res.* **2019**, *38*, 1–12. [CrossRef]
39. Brown, Y.; Hua, S.; Tanwar, P.S. Extracellular matrix-mediated regulation of cancer stem cells and chemoresistance. *Int. J. Biochem. Cell Biol.* **2019**, *109*, 90–104. [CrossRef]

40. Sundquist, E.; Kauppila, J.H.; Veijola, J.; Mroueh, R.; Lehenkari, P.; Laitinen, S.; Risteli, J.; Soini, Y.; Kosma, V.-M.; Sawazaki-Calone, I.; et al. Tenascin-C and fibronectin expression divide early stage tongue cancer into low- and high-risk groups. *Br. J. Cancer* **2017**, *116*, 640–648. [CrossRef]
41. Lowy, C.M.; Oskarsson, T. Tenascin C in metastasis: A view from the invasive front. *Cell Adhes. Migr.* **2015**, *9*, 112–124. [CrossRef] [PubMed]
42. Hauzenberger, D.; Olivier, P.; Gundersen, D.; Ruegg, C. Tenascin-C inhibits beta1 integrin-dependent T lymphocyte adhesion to fibronectin through the binding of its fnIII 1-5 repeats to fibronectin. *Eur. J. Immunol.* **1999**, *29*, 1435–1447. [CrossRef]
43. Joo, J.; Omae, Y.; Hitomi, Y.; Park, B.; Shin, H.-J.; Yoon, K.-A.; Sawai, H.; Tsuiji, M.; Hayashi, T.; Kong, S.-Y.; et al. The association of integration patterns of human papilloma virus and single nucleotide polymorphisms on immune- or DNA repair-related genes in cervical cancer patients. *Sci. Rep.* **2019**, *9*, 1–9. [CrossRef] [PubMed]
44. Lacina, L.; Plzák, J.; Kodet, O.; Szabo, P.; Chovanec, M.; Dvořánková, B.; Smetana, K., Jr. Cancer Microenvironment: What Can We Learn from the Stem Cell Niche. *Int. J. Mol. Sci.* **2015**, *16*, 24094–24110. [CrossRef]
45. Tiitta, O.; Happonen, R.-P.; Virtanen, I.; Luomanen, M. Distribution of tenascin in oral premalignant lesions and squamous cell carcinoma. *J. Oral. Pathol. Med.* **1994**, *23*, 446–450. [CrossRef] [PubMed]
46. Atula, T.; Hedström, J.; Finne, P.; Leivo, I.; Markkanen-Leppänen, M.; Haglund, C. Tenascin-C expression and its prognostic significance in oral and pharyngeal squamous cell carcinoma. *Anticancer. Res.* **2003**, *23*, 3051–3056. [PubMed]
47. Xiong, A.; Yang, Z.; Shen, Y.; Zhou, J.; Shen, Q. Transcription Factor STAT3 as a Novel Molecular Target for Cancer Prevention. *Cancers* **2014**, *6*, 926–957. [CrossRef]
48. Grandis, J.R.; Drenning, S.D.; Chakraborty, A.; Zhou, M.Y.; Zeng, Q.; Pitt, A.S.; Tweardy, D.J. Requirement of Stat3 but not Stat1 activation for epidermal growth factor receptor- mediated cell growth In vitro. *J. Clin. Investig.* **1998**, *102*, 1385–1392. [CrossRef]
49. Geiger, J.L.; Grandis, J.R.; Bauman, J.E. The STAT3 pathway as a therapeutic target in head and neck cancer: Barriers and innovations. *Oral. Oncol.* **2016**, *56*, 84–92. [CrossRef]
50. Morgan, E.; Wasson, C.W.; Hanson, L.; Kealy, D.; Pentland, I.; McGuire, V.; Scarpini, C.; Coleman, N.; Arthur, J.S.C.; Parish, J.L.; et al. STAT3 activation by E6 is essential for the differentiation-dependent HPV18 life cycle. *PLOS Pathog.* **2018**, *14*, e1006975. [CrossRef] [PubMed]
51. Morgan, E.L.; Macdonald, A. Autocrine STAT3 activation in HPV positive cervical cancer through a virus-driven Rac1—NFκB—IL-6 signalling axis. *PLOS Pathog.* **2019**, *15*, e1007835. [CrossRef] [PubMed]
52. Suarez, A.A.R.; Van Renne, N.; Baumert, T.F.; Lupberger, J. Viral manipulation of STAT3: Evade, exploit, and injure. *PLOS Pathog.* **2018**, *14*, e1006839. [CrossRef]
53. Silva, T.G.; Crispim, J.C.O.; Miranda, F.A.; Hassumi, M.K.; De Mello, J.M.Y.; Simões, R.T.; Souto, F.; Soares, E.G.; Donadi, E.A.; Soares, C.P. Expression of the nonclassical HLA-G and HLA-E molecules in laryngeal lesions as biomarkers of tumor invasiveness. *Histol. Histopathol.* **2011**, *26*, 1487–1497. [PubMed]
54. Kochan, G.; Escors-Murugarren, D.; Breckpot, K.; Guerrero-Setas, D. Role of non-classical MHC class I molecules in cancer immunosuppression. *OncoImmunology* **2013**, *2*, e26491. [CrossRef]
55. Foroni, I.; Bettencourt, B.F.; Santos, M.; Lima, M.; Bruges-Armas, J. HLA-E, HLA-F and HLA-G—The Non-Classical Side of the MHC Cluster. In *HLA and Associated Important Diseases*; Xi, Y., Ed.; IntechOpen: London, UK, 2014.
56. Wischhusen, J.; Waschbisch, A.; Wiendl, H. Immune-refractory cancers and their little helpers—An extended role for immune-tolerogenic MHC molecules HLA-G and HLA-E? *Semin. Cancer Biol.* **2007**, *17*, 459–468. [CrossRef]
57. D'Souza, M.P.; Adams, E.; Altman, J.D.; Birnbaum, M.; Boggiano, C.; Casorati, G.; Chien, Y.-H.; Conley, A.; Eckle, S.B.G.; Früh, K.; et al. Casting a wider net: Immunosurveillance by nonclassical MHC molecules. *PLOS Pathog.* **2019**, *15*, e1007567. [CrossRef] [PubMed]
58. Hosono, S.; Kawase, T.; Matsuo, K.; Watanabe, M.; Kajiyama, H.; Hirose, K.; Suzuki, T.; Kidokoro, K.; Ito, H.; Nakanishi, T.; et al. HLA-A Alleles and the Risk of Cervical Squamous Cell Carcinoma in Japanese Women. *J. Epidemiol.* **2010**, *20*, 295–301. [CrossRef]
59. Ferns, D.M.; Heeren, A.M.; Samuels, S.; Bleeker, M.C.G.; De Gruijl, T.D.; Kenter, G.G.; Jordanova, E.S. Classical and non-classical HLA class I aberrations in primary cervical squamous- and adenocarcinomas and paired lymph node metastases. *J. Immunother. Cancer* **2016**, *4*, 78. [CrossRef]
60. Gensterblum-Miller, E.; Brenner, J.C. Protecting Tumors by Preventing Human Papilloma Virus Antigen Presentation: Insights from Emerging Bioinformatics Algorithms. *Cancers* **2019**, *11*, 1543. [CrossRef]
61. Liu, D.-W.; Yang, Y.-C.; Lin, H.-F.; Lin, M.-F.; Cheng, Y.-W.; Chu, C.-C.; Tsao, Y.-P.; Chen, S.-L. Cytotoxic T-Lymphocyte Responses to Human Papillomavirus Type 16 E5 and E7 Proteins and HLA-A*0201-Restricted T-Cell Peptides in Cervical Cancer Patients. *J. Virol.* **2007**, *81*, 2869–2879. [CrossRef]
62. Paaso, A.; Jaakola, A.; Syrjänen, S.; Louvanto, K. From HPV Infection to Lesion Progression: The Role of HLA Alleles and Host Immunity. *Acta Cytol.* **2019**, *63*, 148–158. [CrossRef] [PubMed]
63. Rooney, M.S.; Shukla, S.A.; Wu, C.J.; Getz, G.; Hacohen, N. Molecular and Genetic Properties of Tumors Associated with Local Immune Cytolytic Activity. *Cell* **2015**, *160*, 48–61. [CrossRef]
64. Eura, M.; Katsura, F.; Oiso, M.; Obata, A.; Nakano, K.; Masuyama, K.; Ishikawa, T. Frequency of HLA-A alleles in Japanese patients with head and neck cancer. *Jpn. J. Clin. Oncol.* **1999**, *29*, 535–540. [CrossRef] [PubMed]

65. Näsman, A.; Andersson, E.; Marklund, L.; Tertipis, N.; Hammarstedt-Nordenvall, L.; Attner, P.; Nyberg, T.; Masucci, G.V.; Munck-Wikland, E.; Ramqvist, T.; et al. HLA Class I and II Expression in Oropharyngeal Squamous Cell Carcinoma in Relation to Tumor HPV Status and Clinical Outcome. *PLoS ONE* **2013**, *8*, e77025. [CrossRef]
66. Tisch, M.; Kyrberg, H.; Weidauer, H.; Mytilineos, J.; Conradt, C.; Opelz, G.; Maier, H. Human Leukocyte Antigens and Prognosis in Patients With Head and Neck Cancer: Results of a Prospective Follow-up Study. *Laryngoscope* **2002**, *112*, 651–657. [CrossRef]
67. André, P.; Denis, C.; Soulas, C.; Bourbon-Caillet, C.; Lopez, J.; Arnoux, T.; Bléry, M.; Bonnafous, C.; Gauthier, L.; Morel, A.; et al. Anti-NKG2A mAb Is a Checkpoint Inhibitor that Promotes Anti-tumor Immunity by Unleashing Both T and NK Cells. *Cell* **2018**, *175*, 1731–1743.e13. [CrossRef]
68. Network, T.C.G.A. Comprehensive genomic characterization of head and neck squamous cell carcinomas. *Nat. Cell Biol.* **2015**, *517*, 576–582. [CrossRef]
69. Hu, Z.; Müller, S.; Qian, G.; Xu, J.; Kim, S.; Chen, Z.; Jiang, N.; Wang, D.; Zhang, H.; Saba, N.F.; et al. Human papillomavirus 16 oncoprotein regulates the translocation of β-catenin via the activation of epidermal growth factor receptor. *Cancer* **2015**, *121*, 214–225. [CrossRef]
70. Padhi, S.; Saha, A.; Kar, M.; Ghosh, C.; Adhya, A.; Baisakh, M.; Mohapatra, N.; Venkatesan, S.; Hande, M.P.; Banerjee, B. Clinico-Pathological Correlation of β-Catenin and Telomere Dysfunction in Head and Neck Squamous Cell Carcinoma Patients. *J. Cancer* **2015**, *6*, 192–202. [CrossRef]
71. Alamoud, K.; Kukuruzinska, M. Emerging Insights into Wnt/β-catenin Signaling in Head and Neck Cancer. *J. Dent. Res.* **2018**, *97*, 665–673. [CrossRef]
72. Zeisberg, M.; Neilson, E.G. Biomarkers for epithelial-mesenchymal transitions. *J. Clin. Investig.* **2009**, *119*, 1429–1437. [CrossRef]
73. Chen, C.; Zimmermann, M.; Tinhofer, I.; Kaufmann, A.M.; Albers, A.E. Epithelial-to-mesenchymal transition and cancer stem(-like) cells in head and neck squamous cell carcinoma. *Cancer Lett.* **2013**, *338*, 47–56. [CrossRef]
74. Medici, D.; Hay, E.D.; Goodenough, D.A. Cooperation between Snail and LEF-1 Transcription Factors Is Essential for TGF-β1-induced Epithelial-Mesenchymal Transition. *Mol. Biol. Cell* **2006**, *17*, 1871–1879. [CrossRef]
75. Chien, M.-H.; Chou, L.S.-S.; Chung, T.-T.; Lin, C.-H.; Chou, M.-Y.; Weng, M.-S.; Yang, S.-F.; Chen, M.-K. Effects of E-cadherin (CDH1) gene promoter polymorphisms on the risk and clinicopathologic development of oral cancer. *Head Neck* **2011**, *34*, 405–411. [CrossRef]
76. Takeichi, M. Cadherin cell adhesion receptors as a morphogenetic regulator. *Science* **1991**, *251*, 1451–1455. [CrossRef]
77. Loh, C.-Y.; Chai, J.; Tang, T.; Wong, W.; Sethi, G.; Shanmugam, M.; Chong, P.; Looi, C. The E-Cadherin and N-Cadherin Switch in Epithelial-to-Mesenchymal Transition: Signaling, Therapeutic Implications, and Challenges. *Cells* **2019**, *8*, 1118. [CrossRef]
78. Yao, D.; Dai, C.; Peng, S. Mechanism of the Mesenchymal–Epithelial Transition and Its Relationship with Metastatic Tumor Formation. *Mol. Cancer Res.* **2011**, *9*, 1608–1620. [CrossRef]
79. Mitra, A.; Mishra, L.; Li, S. EMT, CTCs and CSCs in tumor relapse and drug-resistance. *Oncotarget* **2015**, *6*, 10697–10711. [CrossRef]
80. Zhang, Z.; Filho, M.S.; Nör, J.E. The biology of head and neck cancer stem cells. *Oral Oncol.* **2012**, *48*, 1–9. [CrossRef]
81. Jimenez, L.; Jayakar, S.K.; Ow, T.J.; Segall, J.E. Mechanisms of Invasion in Head and Neck Cancer. *Arch. Pathol. Lab. Med.* **2015**, *139*, 1334–1348. [CrossRef]
82. Ihler, F.; Gratz, R.; Wolff, H.A.; Weiss, B.G.; Bertlich, M.; Kitz, J.; Salinas, G.; Rave-Fränk, M.; Canis, M. Epithelial-Mesenchymal Transition during Metastasis of HPV-Negative Pharyngeal Squamous Cell Carcinoma. *BioMed Res. Int.* **2018**, *2018*, 1–12. [CrossRef]
83. Wells, A.; Yates, C.; Shepard, C.R. E-cadherin as an indicator of mesenchymal to epithelial reverting transitions during the metastatic seeding of disseminated carcinomas. *Clin. Exp. Metastasis* **2008**, *25*, 621–628. [CrossRef]
84. Yazdani, J.; Ghavimi, M.A.; Hagh, E.J.; Ahmadpour, F. The Role of E-Cadherin as a Prognostic Biomarker in Head and Neck Squamous Carcinoma: A Systematic Review and Meta-Analysis. *Mol. Diagn. Ther.* **2018**, *22*, 523–535. [CrossRef]
85. Diniz-Freitas, M.; García-Caballero, T.; Antúnez-López, J.; Gándara-Rey, J.M.; Garcia-Garcia, A. Reduced E-cadherin expression is an indicator of unfavourable prognosis in oral squamous cell carcinoma. *Oral Oncol.* **2006**, *42*, 190–200. [CrossRef]
86. Cioce, M.; Fazio, V. EphA2 and EGFR: Friends in Life, Partners in Crime. Can EphA2 Be a Predictive Biomarker of Response to Anti-EGFR Agents? *Cancers* **2021**, *13*, 700. [CrossRef]
87. Pasquale, E.B. Eph-Ephrin Bidirectional Signaling in Physiology and Disease. *Cell* **2008**, *133*, 38–52. [CrossRef] [PubMed]
88. Soler, M.M.G.; Gehring, M.P.; Lechtenberg, B.C.; Zapata-Mercado, E.; Hristova, K.; Pasquale, E.B. Engineering nanomolar peptide ligands that differentially modulate EphA2 receptor signaling. *J. Biol. Chem.* **2019**, *294*, 8791–8805. [CrossRef] [PubMed]
89. Mateo-Lozano, S.; Bazzocco, S.; Rodrigues, P.; Mazzolini, R.; Andretta, E.; Dopeso, H.; Fernàndez, Y.; Del Llano, E.; Bilic, J.; Lopez, L.S.; et al. Loss of the EPH receptor B6 contributes to colorectal cancer metastasis. *Sci. Rep.* **2017**, *7*, 43702. [CrossRef] [PubMed]
90. Barquilla, A.; Pasquale, E.B. Eph Receptors and Ephrins: Therapeutic Opportunities. *Annu. Rev. Pharmacol. Toxicol.* **2015**, *55*, 465–487. [CrossRef]
91. Barile, E.; Wang, S.; Das, S.K.; Noberini, R.; Dahl, R.; Stebbins, J.L.; Pasquale, E.B.; Fisher, P.B.; Pellecchia, M. Design, Synthesis and Bioevaluation of an EphA2 Receptor-Based Targeted Delivery System. *ChemMedChem* **2014**, *9*, 1403–1412. [CrossRef]
92. Riedl, S.J.; Pasquale, S.J.R.A.E.B. Targeting the Eph System with Peptides and Peptide Conjugates. *Curr. Drug Targets* **2015**, *16*, 1031–1047. [CrossRef]
93. Boyd, A.W.; Bartlett, P.F.; Lackmann, M. Therapeutic targeting of EPH receptors and their ligands. *Nat. Rev. Drug Discov.* **2014**, *13*, 39–62. [CrossRef] [PubMed]

94. Zhang, H.; Li, Y.; Wang, H.-B.; Zhang, A.; Chen, M.-L.; Fang, Z.-X.; Dong, X.-D.; Li, S.-B.; Du, Y.; Xiong, D.; et al. Ephrin receptor A2 is an epithelial cell receptor for Epstein–Barr virus entry. *Nat. Microbiol.* **2018**, *3*, 164–171. [CrossRef]
95. Saloura, V.; Izumchenko, E.; Zuo, Z.; Bao, R.; Korzinkin, M.; Ozerov, I.; Zhavoronkov, A.; Sidransky, D.; Bedi, A.; Hoque, M.O.; et al. Immune profiles in primary squamous cell carcinoma of the head and neck. *Oral Oncol.* **2019**, *96*, 77–88. [CrossRef] [PubMed]
96. Wang, W.; Lin, P.; Sun, B.; Zhang, S.; Cai, W.; Han, C.; Li, L.; Lu, H.; Zhao, X. Epithelial-Mesenchymal Transition Regulated by EphA2 Contributes to Vasculogenic Mimicry Formation of Head and Neck Squamous Cell Carcinoma. *BioMed Res. Int.* **2014**, *2014*, 1–10. [CrossRef] [PubMed]
97. Brodie, T.M.; Tosevski, V.; Medova, M. OMIP-045: Characterizing human head and neck tumors and cancer cell lines with mass cytometry. *Cytom. Part A* **2018**, *93*, 406–410. [CrossRef]
98. Cheng, H.; Yang, X.; Si, H.; Saleh, A.D.; Xiao, W.; Coupar, J.; Gollin, S.M.; Ferris, R.L.; Issaeva, N.; Yarbrough, W.G.; et al. Genomic and Transcriptomic Characterization Links Cell Lines with Aggressive Head and Neck Cancers. *Cell Rep.* **2018**, *25*, 1332–1345.e5. [CrossRef] [PubMed]
99. Nisa, L.; Francica, P.; Giger, R.; Medo, M.; Elicin, O.; Friese-Hamim, M.; Wilm, C.; Stroh, C.; Bojaxhiu, B.; Quintin, A.; et al. Targeting the MET Receptor Tyrosine Kinase as a Strategy for Radiosensitization in Locoregionally Advanced Head and Neck Squamous Cell Carcinoma. *Mol. Cancer Ther.* **2019**, *19*, 614–626. [CrossRef]
100. Shang, X.; Lin, X.; Howell, S.B. Claudin-4 controls the receptor tyrosine kinase EphA2 pro-oncogenic switch through beta-catenin. *Cell Commun. Signal.* **2014**, *12*, 59. [CrossRef]
101. Zantek, N.; Azimi, M.; Fedor-Chaiken, M.; Wang, B.; Brackenbury, R.; Kinch, M.S. E-cadherin regulates the function of the EphA2 receptor tyrosine kinase. *Cell Growth Differ. Mol. Boil. J. Am. Assoc. Cancer Res.* **1999**, *10*, 629–638.
102. Li, Z.; Liao, J.; Yang, Z.; Choi, E.Y.; Lapidus, R.G.; Liu, X.; Cullen, K.J.; Dan, H. Co-targeting EGFR and IKKβ/NF-κB signalling pathways in head and neck squamous cell carcinoma: A potential novel therapy for head and neck squamous cell cancer. *Br. J. Cancer* **2019**, *120*, 306–316. [CrossRef]
103. Broek, R.V.; Mohan, S.; Eytan, D.; Chen, Z.; Van Waes, C. The PI3K/Akt/mTOR axis in head and neck cancer: Functions, aberrations, cross-talk, and therapies. *Oral Dis.* **2013**, *21*, 815–825. [CrossRef] [PubMed]
104. Sanchez-Vega, F.; Mina, M.; Armenia, J.; Chatila, W.K.; Luna, A.; La, K.C.; Dimitriadoy, S.; Liu, D.L.; Kantheti, H.S.; Saghafinia, S.; et al. Oncogenic Signaling Pathways in The Cancer Genome Atlas. *Cell* **2018**, *173*, 321–337.e10. [CrossRef] [PubMed]
105. Wang, X.; Zhang, S.; MacLennan, G.T.; Eble, J.N.; López-Beltrán, A.; Yang, X.J.; Pan, C.-X.; Zhou, H.; Montironi, R.; Cheng, L. Epidermal Growth Factor Receptor Protein Expression and Gene Amplification in Small Cell Carcinoma of the Urinary Bladder. *Clin. Cancer Res.* **2007**, *13*, 953–957. [CrossRef] [PubMed]
106. Milanezi, F.; Carvalho, S.; Schmitt, F.C. EGFR/HER2 in breast cancer: A biological approach for molecular diagnosis and therapy. *Expert Rev. Mol. Diagn.* **2008**, *8*, 417–434. [CrossRef] [PubMed]
107. Fuchs, I.; Vorsteher, N.; Bühler, H.; Evers, K.; Sehouli, J.; Schaller, G.; Kümmel, S. The prognostic significance of human epidermal growth factor receptor correlations in squamous cell cervical carcinoma. *Anticancer. Res.* **2007**, *27*, 959–963. [PubMed]
108. Voelzke, W.R.; Petty, W.J.; Lesser, G.J. Targeting the Epidermal Growth Factor Receptor in High-Grade Astrocytomas. *Curr. Treat. Options Oncol.* **2008**, *9*, 23–31. [CrossRef]
109. Tu, J.; Yu, Y.; Liu, W.; Chen, S. Significance of human epidermal growth factor receptor 2 expression in colorectal cancer. *Exp. Ther. Med.* **2015**, *9*, 17–24. [CrossRef]
110. Wei, Q.; Chen, L.; Sheng, L.; Nordgren, H.; Wester, K.; Carlsson, J. EGFR, HER2 and HER3 expression in esophageal primary tumours and corresponding metastases. *Int. J. Oncol.* **2007**, *31*, 493–499. [CrossRef]
111. Kim, M.A.; Lee, H.S.; Lee, H.E.; Jeon, Y.K.; Yang, H.K.; Kim, W.H. EGFR in gastric carcinomas: Prognostic significance of protein overexpression and high gene copy number. *Histopathology* **2008**, *52*, 738–746. [CrossRef]
112. Tang, X.; Varella-Garcia, M.; Xavier, A.C.; Massarelli, E.; Ozburn, N.C.; Moran, C.A.; Wistuba, I.I. Epidermal Growth Factor Receptor Abnormalities in the Pathogenesis and Progression of Lung Adenocarcinomas. *Cancer Prev. Res.* **2008**, *1*, 192–200. [CrossRef]
113. Lafky, J.M.; Wilken, J.A.; Baron, A.; Maihle, N.J. Clinical implications of the ErbB/epidermal growth factor (EGF) receptor family and its ligands in ovarian cancer. *Biochim. et Biophys. Acta (BBA) Bioenerg.* **2008**, *1785*, 232–265. [CrossRef]
114. Nicholson, R.; Gee, J.; Harper, M. EGFR and cancer prognosis. *Eur. J. Cancer* **2001**, *37*, 9–15. [CrossRef]
115. Bs, M.E.S.; Ferris, R.L.; Ferrone, S.; Grandis, J.R. Epidermal growth factor receptor targeted therapy of squamous cell carcinoma of the head and neck. *Head Neck* **2010**, *32*, 1412–1421. [CrossRef]
116. Rodriguez, I.; Finbow, M.E.; Alonso, A. Binding of human papillomavirus 16 E5 to the 16 kDa subunit c (proteolipid) of the vacuolar H+-ATPase can be dissociated from the E5-mediated epidermal growth factor receptor overactivation. *Oncogene* **2000**, *19*, 3727–3732. [CrossRef] [PubMed]
117. Williams, S.M.G. Requirement of Epidermal Growth Factor Receptor for Hyperplasia Induced by E5, a High-Risk Human Papillomavirus Oncogene. *Cancer Res.* **2005**, *65*, 6534–6542. [CrossRef]
118. Wetherill, L.; Holmes, K.K.; Verow, M.; Müller, M.; Howell, G.; Harris, M.; Fishwick, C.; Stonehouse, N.; Foster, R.; Blair, G.; et al. High-Risk Human Papillomavirus E5 Oncoprotein Displays Channel-Forming Activity Sensitive to Small-Molecule Inhibitors. *J. Virol.* **2012**, *86*, 5341–5351. [CrossRef]

119. Wasson, C.W.; Morgan, E.L.; Müller, M.; Ross, R.L.; Hartley, M.; Roberts, S.; Macdonald, A. Human papillomavirus type 18 E5 oncogene supports cell cycle progression and impairs epithelial differentiation by modulating growth factor receptor signalling during the virus life cycle. *Oncotarget* **2017**, *8*, 103581–103600. [CrossRef]
120. Cassell, A.; Grandis, J.R. Investigational EGFR-targeted therapy in head and neck squamous cell carcinoma. *Expert Opin. Investig. Drugs* **2010**, *19*, 709–722. [CrossRef] [PubMed]
121. Harari, P.M.; Wheeler, D.L.; Grandis, J.R. Molecular Target Approaches in Head and Neck Cancer: Epidermal Growth Factor Receptor and Beyond. *Semin. Radiat. Oncol.* **2009**, *19*, 63–68. [CrossRef]
122. Werner, S.; Keller, L.; Pantel, K. Epithelial keratins: Biology and implications as diagnostic markers for liquid biopsies. *Mol. Asp. Med.* **2020**, *72*, 100817. [CrossRef]
123. Karantza, V. Keratins in health and cancer: More than mere epithelial cell markers. *Oncogene* **2010**, *30*, 127–138. [CrossRef] [PubMed]
124. Yanagi, T.; Watanabe, M.; Hata, H.; Kitamura, S.; Imafuku, K.; Yanagi, H.; Homma, A.; Wang, L.; Takahashi, H.; Shimizu, H.; et al. Loss of TRIM29 Alters Keratin Distribution to Promote Cell Invasion in Squamous Cell Carcinoma. *Cancer Res.* **2018**, *78*, 6795–6806. [CrossRef] [PubMed]
125. Hanahan, D.; Weinberg, R.A. Hallmarks of Cancer: The Next Generation. *Cell* **2011**, *144*, 646–674. [CrossRef]
126. Saha, S.K.; Yin, Y.; Chae, H.S.; Cho, S.-G. Opposing Regulation of Cancer Properties via KRT19-Mediated Differential Modulation of Wnt/β-Catenin/Notch Signaling in Breast and Colon Cancers. *Cancers* **2019**, *11*, 99. [CrossRef] [PubMed]
127. Ju, J.-H.; Oh, S.; Lee, K.-M.; Yang, W.; Nam, K.S.; Moon, H.-G.; Noh, D.-Y.; Kim, C.G.; Park, G.; Park, J.B.; et al. Cytokeratin19 induced by HER2/ERK binds and stabilizes HER2 on cell membranes. *Cell Death Differ.* **2015**, *22*, 665–676. [CrossRef]
128. Ohtsuka, T.; Sakaguchi, M.; Yamamoto, H.; Tomida, S.; Takata, K.; Shien, K.; Hashida, S.; Miyata-Takata, T.; Watanabe, M.; Suzawa, K.; et al. Interaction of cytokeratin 19 head domain and HER2 in the cytoplasm leads to activation of HER2-Erk pathway. *Sci. Rep.* **2016**, *6*, 39557. [CrossRef]
129. Tanaka, S.; Kawano, S.; Hattori, T.; Matsubara, R.; Sakamoto, T.; Hashiguchi, Y.; Kaneko, N.; Mikami, Y.; Morioka, M.; Maruse, Y.; et al. Cytokeratin 19 as a biomarker of highly invasive oral squamous cell carcinoma with metastatic potential. *J. Oral Maxillofac. Surg. Med. Pathol.* **2020**, *32*, 1–7. [CrossRef]
130. Chan, J.K.; Yuen, D.; Too, P.H.-M.; Sun, Y.; Willard, B.; Man, D.; Tam, C. Keratin 6a reorganization for ubiquitin–proteasomal processing is a direct antimicrobial response. *J. Cell Biol.* **2017**, *217*, 731–744. [CrossRef]
131. Gu, L.-H.; Coulombe, P.A. Keratin function in skin epithelia: A broadening palette with surprising shades. *Curr. Opin. Cell Biol.* **2007**, *19*, 13–23. [CrossRef] [PubMed]
132. Jiang, R.; Gu, X.; Moore-Medlin, T.N.; Nathan, C.-A.; Hutt-Fletcher, L.M. Oral dysplasia and squamous cell carcinoma: Correlation between increased expression of CD21, Epstein-Barr virus and CK19. *Oral Oncol.* **2012**, *48*, 836–841. [CrossRef] [PubMed]
133. Takeda, T.; Sugihara, K.; Hirayama, Y.; Hirano, M.; Tanuma, J.-I.; Semba, I. Immunohistological evaluation of Ki-67, p63, CK19 and p53 expression in oral epithelial dysplasias. *J. Oral Pathol. Med.* **2006**, *35*, 369–375. [CrossRef] [PubMed]
134. Sharma, P.; Alsharif, S.; Fallatah, A.; Chung, B.M. Intermediate Filaments as Effectors of Cancer Development and Metastasis: A Focus on Keratins, Vimentin, and Nestin. *Cells* **2019**, *8*, 497. [CrossRef] [PubMed]
135. Kim, S.; Wong, P.; Coulombe, P.A. A keratin cytoskeletal protein regulates protein synthesis and epithelial cell growth. *Nat. Cell Biol.* **2006**, *441*, 362–365. [CrossRef] [PubMed]
136. Ernst, J.; Ikenberg, K.; Apel, B.; Schumann, D.; Huber, G.; Studer, G.; Rordorf, T.; Riesterer, O.; Rössle, M.; Korol, D.; et al. Expression of CK19 is an independent predictor of negative outcome for patients with squamous cell carcinoma of the tongue. *Oncotarget* **2016**, *7*, 76151–76158. [CrossRef]
137. Zhong, L.-P.; Chen, W.-T.; Zhang, C.-P.; Zhang, Z.-Y. Increased CK19 expression correlated with pathologic differentiation grade and prognosis in oral squamous cell carcinoma patients. *Oral Surgery Oral Med. Oral Pathol. Oral Radiol. Endodontology* **2007**, *104*, 377–384. [CrossRef]
138. Ram Prassad, V.V.; Nirmala, N.R.; Kotian, M.S. Immunohistochemical evaluation of expression of cytokeratin 19 in different histological grades of leukoplakia and oral squamous cell carcinoma. *Indian J. Dent. Res.* **2005**, *16*, 6–11.
139. Tada, H.; Takahashi, H.; Kuwabara-Yokobori, Y.; Shino, M.; Chikamatsu, K. Molecular profiling of circulating tumor cells predicts clinical outcome in head and neck squamous cell carcinoma. *Oral Oncol.* **2020**, *102*, 104558. [CrossRef]
140. Ravindranath, N.M.; Shuler, C. Cell-surface density of complement restriction factors (CD46, CD55, and CD59): Oral squamous cell carcinoma versus other solid tumors. *Oral Surg. Oral Med. Oral Pathol. Oral Radiol. Endodontology* **2007**, *103*, 231–239. [CrossRef]
141. Uhlén, M.; Zhang, C.; Lee, S.; Sjöstedt, E.; Fagerberg, L.; Bidkhori, G.; Benfeitas, R.; Arif, M.; Liu, Z.; Edfors, F.; et al. A pathology atlas of the human cancer transcriptome. *Science* **2017**, *357*, eaan2507. [CrossRef]
142. Roumenina, L.T.; Daugan, M.V.; Petitprez, F.; Sautès-Fridman, C.; Fridman, W.H. Context-dependent roles of complement in cancer. *Nat. Rev. Cancer* **2019**, *19*, 698–715. [CrossRef] [PubMed]
143. Hoadley, K.A.; Yau, C.; Hinoue, T.; Wolf, D.M.; Lazar, A.J.; Drill, E.; Shen, R.; Taylor, A.M.; Cherniack, A.D.; Thorsson, V.; et al. Cell-of-Origin Patterns Dominate the Molecular Classification of 10,000 Tumors from 33 Types of Cancer. *Cell* **2018**, *173*, 291–304.e6. [CrossRef] [PubMed]
144. Dakubo, G.D. *Cancer Biomarkers in Body Fluids: Biomarkers in Proximal Fluids*; Springer Nature: Cham, Switzerland, 2019; p. 296.

145. Csősz, É.; Lábiscsák, P.; Kalló, G.; Márkus, B.; Emri, M.; Szabó, A.; Tar, I.; Tőzsér, J.; Kiss, C.; Márton, I. Proteomics investigation of OSCC-specific salivary biomarkers in a Hungarian population highlights the importance of identification of population-tailored biomarkers. *PLoS ONE* **2017**, *12*, e0177282. [CrossRef]
146. Clayton, A.; Harris, C.L.; Court, J.; Mason, M.D.; Morgan, P. Antigen-presenting cell exosomes are protected from complement-mediated lysis by expression of CD55 and CD59. *Eur. J. Immunol.* **2003**, *33*, 522–531. [CrossRef]
147. Ludwig, S.; Sharma, P.; Theodoraki, M.-N.; Pietrowska, M.; Yerneni, S.S.; Lang, S.; Ferrone, S.; Whiteside, T.L. Molecular and Functional Profiles of Exosomes From HPV(+) and HPV(−) Head and Neck Cancer Cell Lines. *Front. Oncol.* **2018**, *8*. [CrossRef]

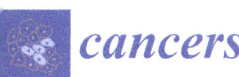

Article

Immune Cell Density Evaluation Improves the Prognostic Values of Staging and p16 in Oropharyngeal Cancer

Géraldine Descamps [1], Sonia Furgiuele [1], Nour Mhaidly [1], Fabrice Journe [1,2,†] and Sven Saussez [1,3,*,†]

1. Department of Human Anatomy and Experimental Oncology, Faculty of Medicine, Research Institute for Health Sciences and Technology, University of Mons (UMONS), Avenue du Champ de Mars, 8, B7000 Mons, Belgium
2. Laboratory of Clinical and Experimental Oncology, Institute Jules Bordet, Université Libre de Bruxelles (ULB), Rue Meylemeersch, 90, B1070 Anderlecht, Belgium
3. Department of Otolaryngology and Head and Neck Surgery, CHU Saint-Pierre, Rue aux Laines, 105, B1000 Brussels, Belgium
* Correspondence: sven.saussez@umons.ac.be; Tel.: +32-65-37-35-84
† These authors contributed equally to this work.

Simple Summary: Human papillomavirus (HPV) has become the major risk factor for the development of oropharyngeal squamous cell carcinomas (OPSCCs), the incidence of which continues to grow in Western countries. Their biological features, associated with a better prognosis as well as a greater response to treatment, has already led to their staging system reclassification and to the development of clinical trials to deintensify the therapeutic approaches. In this context, we proposed to evaluate the recruitment levels of immune cells to ameliorate the classification of some groups of OPSCCs that are always associated with poor outcomes. For this purpose, we scored the density of CD8 and FoxP3 lymphocytes, CD68 macrophages and CD1a Langerhans cells and associated the significant cells with either p16 status or TNM staging to create strong combinations that demonstrated powerful prognostic values in such patients. These results encourage the development of further studies based on the inclusion of immune criteria in the classification of OPSCCs.

Abstract: The incidence of oropharyngeal cancers (OPSCCs) has continued to rise over the years, mainly due to human papillomavirus (HPV) infection. Although they were newly reclassified in the last TNM staging system, some groups still relapse and have poor prognoses. Based on their implication in oncogenesis, we investigated the density of cytotoxic and regulatory T cells, macrophages, and Langerhans cells in relation to p16 status, staging and survival of patients. Biopsies from 194 OPSCCs were analyzed for HPV by RT-qPCR and for p16 by immunohistochemistry, while CD8, FoxP3, CD68 and CD1a immunolabeling was performed in stromal (ST) and intratumoral (IT) compartments to establish optimal cutoff values for overall survival (OS). High levels of FoxP3 IT and CD1a ST positively correlated with OS and were observed in p16-positive and low-stage patients, respectively. Then, their associations with p16 and TNM were more efficient than the clinical parameters alone in describing patient survival. Using multivariate analyses, we demonstrated that the respective combination of FoxP3 or CD1a with p16 status or staging was an independent prognostic marker improving the outcome of OPSCC patients. These two combinations are significant prognostic signatures that may eventually be included in the staging stratification system to develop personalized treatment approaches.

Keywords: oropharyngeal cancer; p16; staging; TNM; prognostic; T regulatory lymphocytes; FoxP3; Langerhans cells; CD1a; immune cells

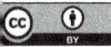

1. Introduction

Among head and neck squamous cell carcinomas (HNSCCs), those affecting the oropharynx arise due to human papillomavirus (HPV) infection or the influence of traditional risk factors [1]. Recently, HPV+ oropharyngeal cancers (OPSCCs) have been included in the 8th edition of the American Joint Committee on Cancer (AJCC) to re-evaluate their classification based on their better prognosis and unique treatment regimens [2]. The reasons for these longer survival times are mostly due to clinical and molecular factors. Indeed, the profile of affected patients corresponds to younger and nonsmoking males who better respond to conventional treatments. Additionally, these cancers can often originate from the epithelium of the tonsil crypts, which are rich in immune cells, favoring local immune activation and immune surveillance [3]. For several years, the involvement of the immune system in tumor progression has been well recognized, so it appears necessary to characterize this defense environment by specifying the expression profiles of immune biomarkers. This characterization will aim to improve the therapeutic efficacy and decrease the intensity of OPSCC treatments.

In this context, the most-studied immune type is undoubtedly CD8+ cytotoxic T lymphocytes, which are the major defensive elements against tumor cells. Their massive infiltration within the tumor generally predicts better survival [4–7]. Regarding HPV, some studies demonstrated that T-cell infiltration was associated with a good prognosis regardless of HPV status [8,9], while others demonstrated that higher CD8+ T-cell density was positively related to HPV status [10]. Regulatory T cells (Tregs) are also important actors in the immune tumor microenvironment (TME) of OPSCCs. They are characterized by the expression of the forkhead transcription factor (FoxP3), which is a key regulator of their functions and is used in most studies to distinguish Tregs from other immune cells [11–13]. Although they are physiologically involved in immune tolerance, their roles and impacts in the context of cancer are still quite controversial. Their involvement is demonstrated in the inhibition of antitumor responses leading to immune escape. In different types of cancers, such as gastric, hepatic, breast and melanomas, their high density is often reported to be associated with a poorer prognosis, whereas their presence in head and neck and colon cancers is synonymous with a better outcome [14]. Indeed, we have previously demonstrated that higher Treg infiltration correlated with longer overall survival (OS) and recurrence-free survival (RFS) in HNSCC patients [15,16].

Macrophages and particularly M2 tumor-associated macrophages (TAMs) with protumor effects are responsible for Treg differentiation and are able to create an immunosuppressive environment favoring tumor growth, notably through the secretion of cytokines (IL-10, TGFβ, TNFα) [17,18]. Since HNSCC is largely infiltrated by TAMs (up to 30%), their expression and abundance are often related to a poor prognosis and to the occurrence of recurrence [19–22]. In addition, our previous study demonstrated that the infiltration of CD68+ cells into the tumor increased during tumor progression and that a high infiltration of such macrophages correlated with shorter survival. In relation to HPV status, we previously observed that macrophage recruitment was higher in HPV+ tumors than in HPV- tumors [23]. Indeed, HPV is able to modulate the TME to promote tumor immune escape. In this respect, we also observed that the number of Tregs was increased in HPV+ HNSCCs and that, conversely, Langerhans cell (LC) infiltration was significantly decreased in these patients [15,24]. Of note, this population of dendritic cells specializes in presenting antigens to T cells, including viral antigens, to generate immune defenses against HPV. The modulation of the immune system by HPV has also been demonstrated by Nguyen et al., who reported a decrease in the number of LCs in the OPSCC stroma of infected patients [25]. Given the heterogeneity of OPSCC, some tumor regions are infiltrated by immune cells, reflecting different clinical outcomes. Indeed, intratumoral and stromal drivers may differentially influence the evolution of the cancer, leading either to tumor progression or regression, highlighting the importance of considering each compartment separately [26,27].

Currently, the OPSCC classification remains based on TNM clinical parameters assessing tumor extension, lymph node involvement and distant metastasis presence. In an era where immunoscores are becoming increasingly relevant and widespread, it appears that categorization based on HPV status or TNM alone is undervalued. Recently, an immunoscore assessing tumor-infiltrating lymphocytes (TILs) in colon cancer has been established as a new classification model, which has demonstrated better prognostic prediction than the classical TNM system [28,29]. Similarly, we recently identified a three-marker-based immunoscore that had a stronger prognostic performance than tumor stage [30]. Quantification of immune cells appears to be a promising approach but requires a comprehensive investigation of the immune landscape in OPSCCs. Therefore, in this study, we quantified the expression of CD8, FoxP3, CD68 and CD1a, compared their recruitment according to clinical characteristics and determined their prognostic value in a series of patients with oropharyngeal cancers. The aim of this study was to improve the classification system of OPSCC patients, regardless of HPV status, and to investigate the extent to which a combination of immune cells and clinical variables influence prognosis.

2. Materials and Methods

2.1. Patients and Clinical Characteristics

Patients with pathologist-confirmed oropharyngeal cancer were selected based on former cohorts and were diagnosed between 2001 and 2021. The 194 formalin-fixed, paraffin-embedded (FFPE) tumors were derived from patients who had undergone curative surgery at CHU Saint-Pierre (Bruxelles, Belgium), Jules Bordet Institute (Bruxelles, Belgium) and EpiCURA Baudour Hospital (Baudour, Belgium). Institutional research ethics board approvals were obtained, and written informed consent was signed by each patient enrolled in this retrospective study (Jules Bordet Institute, number CE2319). The cohort of patients and the clinicopathological data are summarized in Table 1.

Table 1. Clinical patient characteristics.

Variables	Number of OPSCC Cases
	n = 194
Age (years)	
Median (range)	59 (24–89)
Recurrence (RFS) (months)	
Median (range)	17 (1–188)
Yes	75
No	106
Unknown	13
Overall survival (OS) (months)	
Median (range)	23 (1–173)
Alive	104
Dead	76
Unknown	14
Gender	
Male	130
Female	64
Tumor stage 8th	
I–II	67
III–IV	107
Unknown	20
Histological grade	
Undifferentiated	50
Poorly differentiated	53
Moderately differentiated	9
Well differentiated	56
Unknown	26
Risk factors	
Tobacco	
Smoker	147
Non-Smoker	35
Unknown	12

Table 1. *Cont.*

Variables	Number of OPSCC Cases
Alcohol	
Drinker	132
Non-Drinker	50
Unknown	12
HPV detection	
Positive	27
Negative	49
Unknown	118
p16 staining	
Positive	52
Negative	142
p16 status	
p16+	52
p16+/HPV−	0
p16−/HPV+	9
p16−/HPV−	133

2.2. DNA Extraction

DNA extraction from FFPE specimens was performed as described in our previous publications [31]. Briefly, sections were deparaffinized and digested with proteinase K by overnight incubation at 56 °C. DNA was purified using the QIAmp FFPE tissue kit according to the manufacturer's protocol.

2.3. Detection of HPV by Polymerase Chain Reaction (PCR) Amplification

GP5+/GP6+ primers were used to amplify a consensus region located in the L1 region of the HPV genome. This PCR protocol chosen to detect HPV DNA has been fully described in a previous publication [31].

2.4. Real-Time PCR Amplification of HPV Type-Specific DNA

All DNA extracts were tested at the Algemeen Medisch Laboratorium (Antwerp, Belgium) for the presence of 18 different HPV genotypes using TaqMan-based real-time quantitative PCR that targeted type-specific sequences of the viral genes, as previously described [31].

2.5. p16 Immunohistochemistry

To determine the transcriptional activity of HPV, each HPV-positive case was further immunohistochemically evaluated for p16 expression using a mouse monoclonal antibody (CINtec p16, Ventana, Tucson, AZ, USA) and an automated immunostainer at the Jules Bordet Institute (Bond-Max, Leica Microsystems, Wetzlar, Germany). Briefly, after epitope retrieval (pH 6), sections were incubated with the p16 antibody for 30 min. Then, polymer detection was performed using Bond Polymer Refine Detection according to the manufacturer's protocol (Leica, Wetzlar, Germany), and the slides were counterstained with hematoxylin and Luxol fast blue. Tissue sections from cervical lesions were used as positive controls. A negative control was performed by omitting the primary antibody. Tumors were considered positive when strong and diffuse staining was scored both in the nucleus and the cytoplasm and in $\geq 70\%$ of the tumor.

2.6. Evaluation of Immune Cell Recruitment by Immunohistochemistry

Immunohistochemistry, targeting immune cells, was performed on 5 µm deparaffinized and alcohol-rehydrated tissue sections. The peroxidase activity was saturated with H_2O_2 for 10 min followed by antigen retrieval in $EDTA/H_2O$ or citrate buffer/H_2O (see Supplementary Table S1). Tissues were incubated with casein 0.5% for 1 h to block nonspecific epitopes and then with the specific primary antibody for 1 h at room temperature (RT) or overnight at 4 °C as described in Supplementary Table S1. Finally, the samples were incubated with BrightVision Poly-HRP–IgG (Klinipath, Duiven, Holland), and the antigens were visualized by the addition of a solution of 3–3′ diaminobenzidine and H_2O_2 buffer (Liquid DAB, San Ramon, CA, USA) before counterstaining with Mayer's hemalun and Luxol fast blue. Tonsil tissues from healthy patients were used as positive and negative controls. The number of each immune cell type was counted in 5 randomly selected fields at 400× magnification by three investigators (G.D., S.F., N.M.) in both stroma (ST) and intratumoral (IT) compartments. The mean was calculated for each patient and normalized to a 1-mm² area. Finally, optimal cutoffs allowing the best separation between low- and high-expressing groups of each immune cell type by compartment were calculated.

2.7. Statistical Analyses

Statistical analyses were performed using SPSS software version 21 (IBM, Portsmouth, UK). Univariate Cox regression analyses were performed to identify prognostic variables influencing OS as well as to calculate hazard ratios (HRs), 95% confidence intervals and significance. Multivariate analyses were applied to assess the independent contributions of immune cells to OS in the presence of other covariates, including p16 status and tumor stage. Kaplan–Meier curves were successively assessed for OS. The prognostic value of immune markers related to OS was evaluated based on the calculated optimal cutoffs. Immune cells expressed in different subgroups (p16− vs. p16+, low stages vs. high stages) were compared using the nonparametric Mann–Whitney U test. In all cases, two-sided p values < 0.05 were considered statistically significant.

3. Results

3.1. Immune Cell Density and Patient Survival

The typical immunohistochemical expression of cytotoxic T-lymphocytes, regulatory T-lymphocytes, Langerhans cells and macrophages was evaluated using specific antibodies against CD8, FoxP3, CD1a and CD68, respectively (Figure 1). Their quantitative expression was assessed in both stromal (ST) and intratumoral (IT) compartments by counting their number in five random fields, and their density was defined as low or high in each compartment based on optimal cutoffs evaluated regarding the p values for OS of patients. The cutoff values were 718 cells/mm² (CD8, ST), 110 cells/mm² (CD8, IT), 552 cells/mm² (FoxP3, ST), 83 cells/mm² (FoxP3, IT), 61 cells/mm² (CD1a, ST), 138 cells/mm² (CD1a, IT), 293 cells/mm² (CD68, ST) and 188 cells/mm² (CD68, IT).

Among the 194 surgical specimens of OPSCC, 44 could be analyzed for CD8 expression, 77 for CD68, 66 for CD1a and 69 for FoxP3 (Table 2). Their distribution was then compared between different subgroups of interest based on the median to display the variability of their density between p16-positive and p16-negative patients and between low- and high-stage tumors (Table 2).

Then, the associations between OS and the eight immune variables were also assessed to identify the immune type most likely to positively impact patient survival. Univariate Cox regression analysis revealed that three factors were significantly associated with OS, namely, CD68 IT, FoxP3 IT and CD1a ST (Table 3).

Moreover, to identify the best combination for improving p16 status and/or staging, a comparison of these two variables by Mann–Whitney tests according to immune cell density was performed. The results showed that CD68 infiltration in the ST is significantly associated with p16 status as well as IT Treg infiltration. Additionally, we observed that the density of Langerhans cells in the ST was significantly associated with the tumor stage of patients (Table 4).

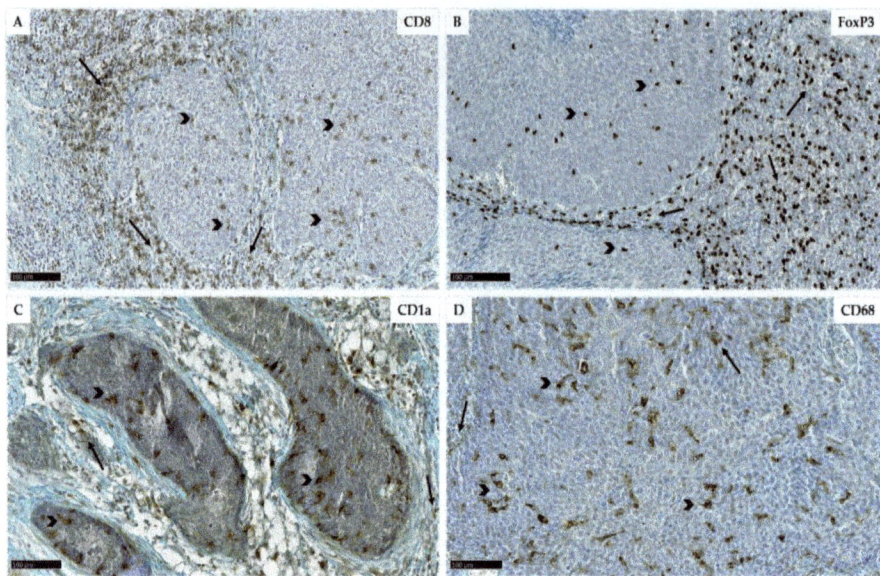

Figure 1. Immunohistochemical representation of CD8 (**A**), FoxP3 (**B**), CD1a (**C**) and CD68 (**D**) expression (scales = 100 μm) in stromal (arrows) and intratumoral (arrowheads) areas of oropharyngeal carcinomas. Bars = 100 μm.

Table 2. Descriptive table of immune cell density according to different subgroups including p16-negative, -positive, low-stage and high-stage patients.

Subgroups	Parameters	CD8 ST	CD8 IT	CD68 ST	CD68 IT	CD1a ST	CD1a IT	FoxP3 ST	FoxP3 IT
All data	n	44	44	77	77	66	66	69	69
	Median	90.6	14.4	55	16	8	55.5	92.5	12.6
	Min-Max	0–406.6	0–317.8	2.3–214	0–110	0–39	0–563	16–467	0–137
p16- tumors	n	24	24	49	49	52	52	45	45
	Median	90.6	13.35	60	14.1	8.35	53.5	88.2	7
	Min-Max	0–378.6	0–36.4	6.8–214	0–65	0–39	0–563	16–320	0–117
p16+ tumors	n	20	20	28	28	14	14	24	24
	Median	94.35	19.85	30.5	18	6	66	93.35	12.9
	Min-Max	3.3–406.6	0.2–317.8	2.3–182	0–110	0–27	0.8–180	17–467	2–137
Low stage patients	n	21	21	35	35	24	24	29	29
	Median	90.2	17.7	47	16	11.05	29.5	105	11
	Min-Max	3.3–406.6	0.2–317.8	2.3–182	0–110	0–27	0.3–199	16–467	0–137
High stage patients	n	12	12	29	29	29	29	25	25
	Median	106.45	13.65	58	22	6	56	84.5	13
	Min-Max	7.2–196.9	0.2–57.6	6.5–214	0–68.6	0–39	0.2–563	17–362	0–117

Representative box plots of significant Mann–Whitney tests comparing the cell density of CD68 and FoxP3 between p16+ and p16− patients revealed a lower density of macrophages in the ST ($p = 0.005$) along with a higher proportion of Tregs in the IT ($p = 0.02$) compartments of p16-positive tumors (Figure 2). Among these two immune cell types, only FoxP3+ cells correlated with patient survival (Table 3), supporting further investigation of the potential impact of their combination with p16 status. In the same manner, only CD1a ST had prognostic value (Table 3) and a correlation close to significance with patient staging (Table 4), leading to the examination of such a combination regarding OS.

Table 3. Univariate Cox regression analysis evaluating the influence of each immune cell type and their location (ST and IT) on OS. p values < 0.05 are highlighted in bold.

Univariate Analysis	Overall Survival	
	p Value	HR (95% CI)
CD8 ST	0.322	0.04 (0.0–25.7)
CD8 IT	0.173	0.35 (0.8–1.6)
CD68 ST	0.191	0.59 (0.3–1.3)
CD68 IT	**0.049**	**2.28 (1.0–5.2)**
FoxP3 ST	0.441	0.71 (0.30–1.68)
FoxP3 IT	**0.018**	**3.42 (0.10–0.81)**
CD1a ST	**0.029**	**2.91 (0.13–0.89)**
CD1a IT	0.183	0.54 (0.22–1.33)

Table 4. Mann–Whitney test between immune cell density in ST and IT compartments and p16 status or staging. p values < 0.05 are highlighted in bold.

Immune Cells	p Value versus p16	p Value versus Staging
CD8 ST	0.925	0.518
CD8 IT	0.071	0.868
CD68 ST	**0.005**	0.121
CD68 IT	0.155	0.761
FoxP3 ST	0.29	0.263
FoxP3 IT	**0.022**	0.627
CD1a ST	0.588	0.057
CD1a IT	0.451	0.335

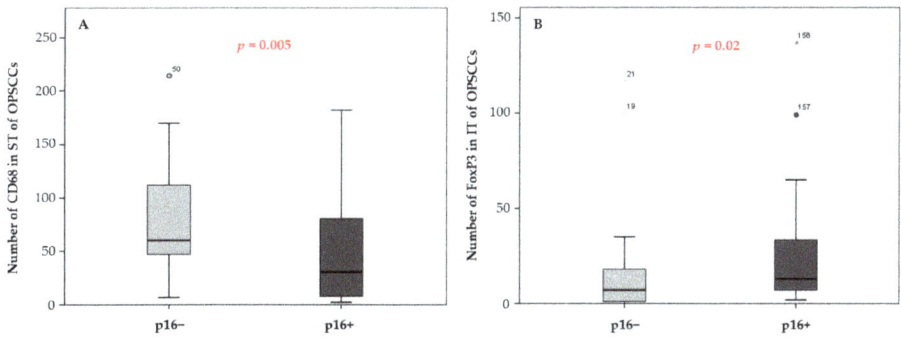

Figure 2. Evaluation of CD68 macrophage number in the ST compartment (**A**) and FoxP3 number in the IT area (**B**) of oropharyngeal tumors according to p16 status (Mann—Whitney U test, $p = 0.005$ and $p = 0.02$, respectively) (*) asterisk symbols correspond to extreme atypical values.

3.2. Combination of p16 Status and Regulatory T-Lymphocyte Density and Correlation with Patient Survival

Among the 194 patients included in this study, 52 had positive expression of p16 corresponding to a transcriptionally active infection. Regarding the relationship between p16 expression and the survival of OPSCC patients, p16-positive status predicted a significantly better prognosis ($p = 0.01$, Figure 3A). Next, we determined whether there may be a relationship between the density of FoxP3 in IT and the OS of OPSCCs, and the results showed that patients with high levels of FoxP3 had significantly longer survival than those with low numbers of FoxP3+ cells ($p = 0.018$, Figure 3B and Table 3).

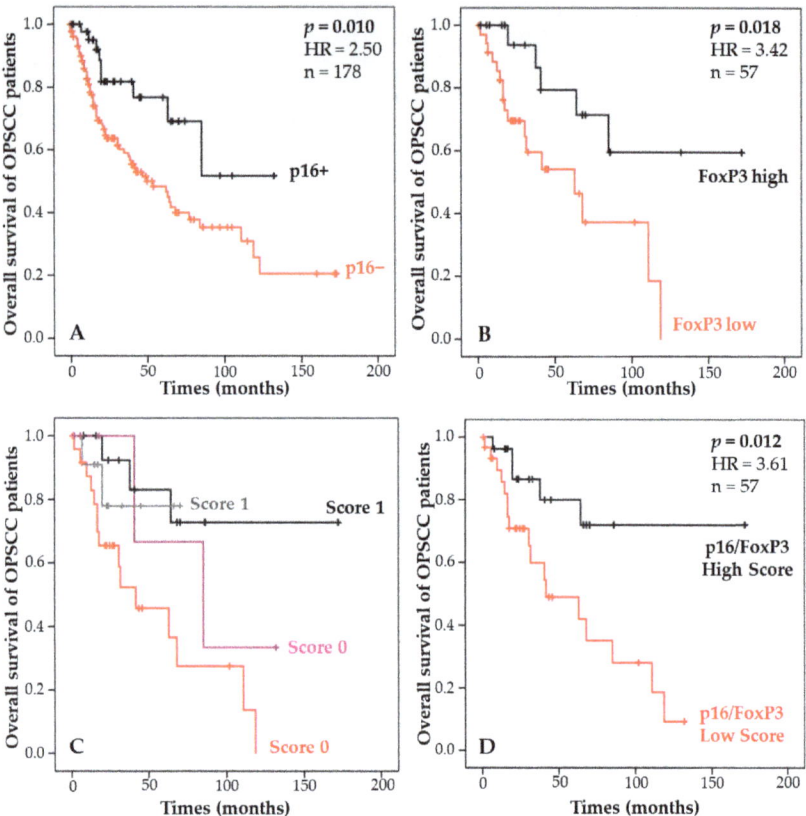

Figure 3. Kaplan-Meier curves of the OS of OPSCC patients according to p16 status (**A**), the number of FoxP3+ cells infiltrating the tumor (**B**), the combination of both parameters resulting in four groups (**C**), and the score combining p16 status and FoxP3 density (**D**).

Based on these significant correlations between OS and p16 status and OS and Treg infiltration, combinations of p16 and Treg were established, and four survival curves were plotted to determine the prognostic performance of each subgroup (Figure 3C), as summarized in Table 5. Finally, the two subgroups of patients who were associated with better survival were pooled to create a score (high versus low) based on p16 expression and Treg density. The results showed that OPSCC patients with a high score had significantly better survival than those with a low score ($p = 0.012$, Figure 3D). This score provides a stronger separation of patients than p16 and Treg status alone.

Table 5. Description of the prognostic performance of a score combining p16 status and FoxP3 infiltration in OPSCC patients.

Curves	p16	FoxP3 IT	Survival	Score
Red	Negative	Low	Poor − −	Low
Black	Negative	High	Good ++	High
Gray	Positive	Low	Good +	High
Purple	Positive	High	Poor −	Low

3.3. Combination of Staging and Langerhans Cell Density and Correlation with Patient Survival

Next, we investigated the relevance of the CD1a marker and staging, alone or in combination, regarding the survival of OPSCC patients. First, we evaluated the prognostic impact of staging alone, and as expected, stage I and II patients had a longer survival than stage III and IV patients ($p = 0.002$, Figure 4A). As previously demonstrated in Table 4, the density of Langerhans cells is associated with the tumor stage of patients. Boxplots illustrated that CD1a+ cells tended to be recruited more in the ST of low-stage patients ($p = 0.057$, Figure 2B). Correlation with patient survival demonstrates that a high infiltrate of Langerhans cells in the ST is significantly associated with a better prognosis compared with a low density ($p = 0.03$, Figure 4C and Table 3).

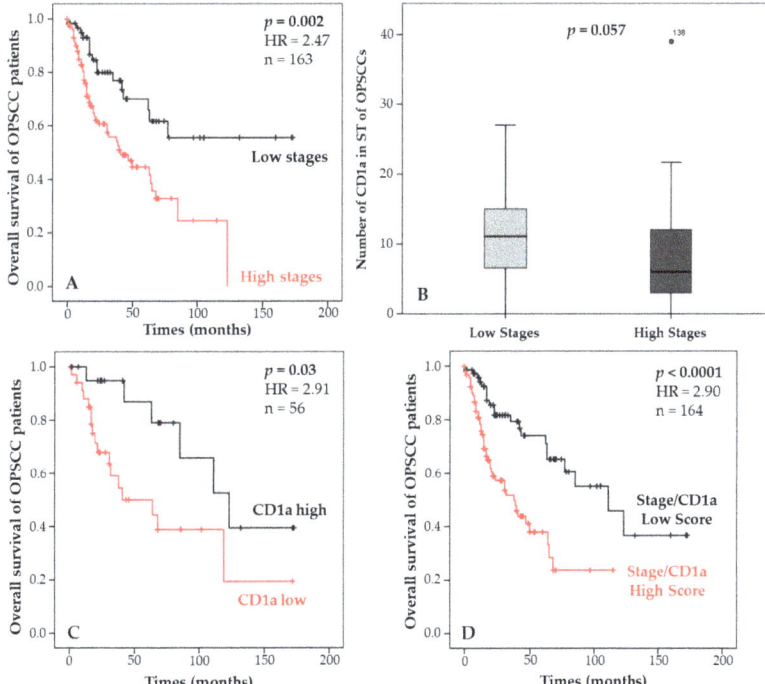

Figure 4. Kaplan–Meier curves of the OS of OPSCC patients according to staging (**A**), the number of CD1a+ cells infiltrating the ST (**C**), and the score combining the staging and CD1a density (**D**). Mann–Whitney test illustrating the number of CD1a cells in the ST of OPSCC patients according to the staging (low (I/II) versus high (III/IV) stages, as described in the TNM staging system 8) (**B**).

As described in Table 6, a combination was established between these two clinical and immune variables according to their prognostic performance. When the eighth version of the TNM was created, high-stage p16+ patients were downgraded from one group to another due to their favorable prognosis. In the same manner, we observed that high-stage patients with initially poor survival had a significantly improved prognosis when they had a high density of Langerhans cells. Based on this observation, these patients were grouped with low-stage patients to create a prognostic score (low versus high). This score was tested in relationship to OS and showed a significantly better survival for patients with a low score compared with those with a high score ($p < 0.0001$, Figure 4D). This result highlights a higher significance than stage or CD1a density used separately.

Table 6. Description of the prognostic performance of a score combining the staging and CD1a infiltration in OPSCC patients.

Stage	Survival Stage	CD1a ST	Survival CD1a ST	Survival Using Combination	Score
Low	Good	Low	Poor	Good	Low
Low	Good	High	Good	Good	Low
High	Poor	Low	Poor	Poor	High
High	Poor	High	Good	Good	Low

3.4. Development of a Model Improving the Prediction of Overall Survival in OPSCC Patients

Finally, a Cox multivariate analysis was performed including p16 status, staging, CD1a ST and FoxP3 IT densities to assess their independent contributions to OS. This result shows that the four factors are dependent on each other (Table 7). Indeed, p16 status is included in TNMv8, and as we have shown, there are correlations between Treg and p16 as well as between Langerhans cells and stage.

Table 7. Multivariate analysis evaluating the correlation between p16 positivity, staging, stromal CD1a, intratumoral FoxP3 and patient survival. p values < 0.05 are highlighted in bold.

Multivariate Analysis	Overall Survival	
	p Value	HR (95% CI)
p16	0.974	1.03 (0.19–5.50)
Staging	0.052	3.20 (0.98–10.40)
CD1a ST	0.376	1.70 (0.52–5.53)
FoxP3 IT	0.057	3.15 (0.96–10.31)

However, the combination of clinical factors with immune cells, as described above, allows these two scores to be independent. Multivariate analysis revealed that the two combinations were significant prognostic factors for OPSCCs, with better separations and prognostic values than each variable separately (Table 8). Therefore, such a signature provides the best prognostic information for OPSCC patients.

Table 8. Multivariate analysis evaluating the correlation between the p16/FoxP3 score, stage/CD1a score and patient survival. p values < 0.05 are highlighted in bold.

Multivariate Analysis	Overall Survival	
	p Value	HR (95% CI)
p16/FoxP3 score	**0.038**	3.24 (1.06–9.85)
Stage/CD1a score	**0.032**	2.92 (1.09–7.77)

4. Discussion

In recent years, it has been well accepted that the immune system plays a critical role in cancer development. Thus, many efforts have been intensified to identify new immune markers that could provide accurate predictive and prognostic information. In the TME, the active dialog between tumor and immune cells represents essential clinical information that should be integrated into the staging system of patients. Indeed, it has been recently demonstrated that the establishment of a new immune TNM based on TIL infiltration for low-stage tongue carcinoma patients provides additional prognostic information discriminating T1N0M0 from T2N0M0 patients and, therefore, improves their therapeutic management [32]. These combinations, commonly referred to as immunoscores, have been increasingly investigated for various cancers. The most accepted immune combination concerns colon cancers for which, in addition to the classical TNM, a clinical quantification of CD3+ and CD8+ cells is now routinely performed [28,33]. Furthermore, in breast cancers, an evaluation of TILs based on hematoxylin and eosin staining and morphology is highly recommended, as well as in non-small cell lung cancers where CD8+

and CD45RO+ lymphocyte markers appear to be promising candidates for improving TNM [5,34,35]. Indeed, it has been shown that their infiltration is a predictive factor of distant metastasis-free survival and OS [36]. This issue attracts increasing attention in head and neck cancers. Zhang et al., demonstrated that a scoring system evaluating the infiltration of CD3 and CD8 is of particular interest to ameliorate the TNM staging for HNSCCs [37]. Moreover, we recently proposed a new immunoscore combining CD68, CD8 and FoxP3 local distribution to identify patients with longer RFS and OS. Of note, this combination better discriminated HNSCC patients than the TNM classification [30].

In the current study, levels of CD8, FoxP3, CD68 and CD1a densities were assessed in both stromal and intratumoral compartments because it has been reported that their localization can result in different prognostic responses. As an example, Khoury et al., demonstrated that ST TILs can be distinguished from their IT counterparts regarding their biological behavior [27]. Hence, we determined immune cell density among a population of OPSCC patients, and based on the calculated cutoffs, we investigated their potential prognostic implications. Both IT CD68 and FoxP3 as well as ST CD1a correlated significantly with patient survival. Therefore, to identify differences in immune context between HPV-infected and -uninfected patients and between patients with low-stage and high-stage tumors, we compared the recruitment of immune cells between these four groups. Interestingly, we found that IT Treg infiltration was significantly different between p16+ and p16− patients, with greater infiltration observed in infected individuals. Similarly, stromal infiltrating Langerhans cells were also different between low- and high-stage patients, with a higher density of cells observed among low-stage tumors.

These four subgroups were specifically explored because they represent a challenge in terms of treatment. In fact, as the incidence of HPV+ OPSCC continues to rise, prognostic tools are sought to limit the deleterious side effects of surgery and radiotherapy techniques [38]. The aim of this principle of deintensification of treatments is to limit comorbidities and improve the quality of life and such approach is currently widely studied [39]. Although the eighth edition introduced a new classification for HPV+ tumors, we remain convinced that a method incorporating tumor biology, as represented by the immune system, would improve prognosis and patient management. Based on our promising results, we tested the prognostic performance of a score combining Treg density with tumor p16 status and demonstrated that this score provides a stronger discrimination than each parameter alone. Despite controversial findings in the literature, the prognostic role of Tregs remains frequently associated with improved survival in HNSCCs. Recently, a team made the same observations where FoxP3 was more highly expressed among HPV+ patients, and this high infiltration correlated with a better 5-year survival [40]. Moreover, we previously reported that FoxP3+ infiltration was associated with longer RFS and OS of patients suffering from HNSSC [15,16]. As we discussed previously, two populations of Tregs have been identified, one with immunosuppressive capabilities and the other with a proinflammatory role, both being associated with opposite prognoses [41]. Given the biological involvement of Tregs in HNSCCs and their positive prognostic impact, it seems relevant to consider this immune type in the risk stratification of such patients.

Quantification of the Langerhans cell number is not well documented for OPSCCs. They constitute a population of dendritic cells involved in antitumor immunity. Their main functions are to activate CD8+ lymphocytes, B lymphocytes and natural killer cells. These immature dendritic cells are characterized by the expression of the CD1a glycoprotein, the expression of which is reported to vary from one anatomical site to another. Indeed, we already reported that Langerhans cell infiltration was increased in HNSCCs compared with dysplastic lesions, whereas Gama-Cuellar et al., recently showed IT CD1a depletion in tonsillar carcinomas [24,42]. Moreover, other groups demonstrated in oral carcinomas that the decreased number of CD1a+ cells may be associated with cancer development [43,44]. Regarding their prognostic implications, the literature presents conflicting results. In the current study, we observed that high Langerhans cell density is synonymous with a better OS. This is in accordance with the findings of Karpathiou et al., who reported that high LC infiltration is associated with good prognostic values. Moreover, they demonstrated, like us, that a higher density of the dendritic cell marker S100 was associated with a lower T stage [45]. Additionally, a higher number of CD1a cells adjacent to the tumor improved the survival of tongue carcinoma patients [46]. In contrast, Minesaki et al., found that CD1a infiltration was an unfavorable prognostic factor for advanced laryngeal cancer [47].

Based on the reclassification performed on HPV+ OPSCC in 2018, we found with our score, combining staging with Langerhans cell density, that high-stage OPSCC highly infiltrated in ST had a better prognostic value than stage or LC infiltration alone. As proposed for p16 in the eighth edition of the AJCC, this group of high-stage patients could be downgraded when stromal-infiltrating CD1a+ cells are above the defined cutoff. Thus, we propose to clinically investigate their density in patients with T3 and T4 stages to better predict patient prognoses and to better guide the clinician in the treatment alternatives for these patients. However, a few limitations in our study need to be underlined, such as its retrospective design and the quantification of immune markers, which should be standardized based on digital scoring. Additionally, the number of cancer tissues that were used to examine immune cells should be increased. Nevertheless, even if they are low, the amount of immune information was strong enough to improve staging and p16 prognostic values, supporting the biological relevance of these combinations. Variables related to the TNM should also be collected in a comprehensive manner to accurately stratify low- and high-stage patients. Nevertheless, these encouraging results support the need for further studies focusing on FoxP3 and CD1a density and localization in OPSCC patients.

5. Conclusions

In conclusion, we have pointed out the importance of immune parameters as a part of the TNM staging system. The results reported in our work highlight the relevance of FoxP3 and CD1a densities in association with p16 positivity and TNM staging, respectively, to predict the prognosis of OPSCC patients with a greater accuracy. Indeed, these new combinations demonstrated a powerful prognostic value, outperforming p16 positivity and TNM systems alone. Ultimately, such new immune marker-containing scores should be implemented routinely to refine the prognostication and therapeutic management of these patients.

Supplementary Materials: The following supporting information can be downloaded at: https://www.mdpi.com/article/10.3390/cancers14225560/s1, Table S1: Description of immunostaining experimental conditions.

Author Contributions: Conceptualization, G.D., F.J. and S.S.; methodology, G.D., S.F. and N.M.; software, G.D. and F.J.; validation, G.D., F.J. and S.S.; formal analysis, G.D. and F.J.; investigation, G.D.; resources, G.D.; data curation, G.D. and F.J.; writing—original draft preparation, G.D.; writing—review and editing, G.D., F.J., S.F. and S.S.; visualization, S.F. and N.M.; supervision, F.J.; project administration, F.J. and S.S.; funding acquisition, S.S. All authors have read and agreed to the published version of the manuscript.

Funding: This research was funded by the Walloon Region via the ProtherWal society (Agreement 7289) (G.D.), the University of Mons and the EpiCURA Hospital (S.F.) and by the F.R.S-F.N.R.S. Télévie (N.M.).

Institutional Review Board Statement: This retrospective study has been reviewed and approved by the Ethics Committee of Jules Bordet Institute (number CE2319).

Informed Consent Statement: Informed consent was obtained from all subjects involved in the study.

Data Availability Statement: Data is contained within the article or supplementary material.

Acknowledgments: The authors thank Saint-Pierre Hospital (Brussels, Belgium), Jules Bordet Institute (Brussels, Belgium) and EpiCURA Baudour Hospital (Baudour, Belgium) for FFPE specimens and clinical data. The authors also thank UMONS, EpiCURA Hospital, ProtherWal and the fund for medical research in Hainaut (FRMH) for funding this work.

Conflicts of Interest: The authors declare no conflict of interest.

References

1. Oguejiofor, K.; Hall, J.; Slater, C.; Betts, G.; Hall, G.; Slevin, N.; Dovedi, S.; Stern, P.L.; West, C.M.L. Stromal Infiltration of CD8 T Cells Is Associated with Improved Clinical Outcome in HPV-Positive Oropharyngeal Squamous Carcinoma. *Br. J. Cancer* **2015**, *113*, 886–893. [CrossRef] [PubMed]
2. O'Sullivan, B.; Huang, S.H.; Su, J.; Garden, A.S.; Sturgis, E.M.; Dahlstrom, K.; Lee, N.; Riaz, N.; Pei, X.; Koyfman, S.A.; et al. Development and Validation of a Staging System for HPV-Related Oropharyngeal Cancer by the International Collaboration on Oropharyngeal Cancer Network for Staging (ICON-S): A Multicentre Cohort Study. *Lancet Oncol.* **2016**, *17*, 440–451. [CrossRef]
3. Taberna, M.; Mena, M.; Pavón, M.A.; Alemany, L.; Gillison, M.L.; Mesía, R. Human Papillomavirus-Related Oropharyngeal Cancer. *Ann. Oncol.* **2017**, *28*, 2386–2398. [CrossRef] [PubMed]
4. Balermpas, P.; Rödel, F.; Rödel, C.; Krause, M.; Linge, A.; Lohaus, F.; Baumann, M.; Tinhofer, I.; Budach, V.; Gkika, E.; et al. CD8+ Tumour-Infiltrating Lymphocytes in Relation to HPV Status and Clinical Outcome in Patients with Head and Neck Cancer after Postoperative Chemoradiotherapy: A Multicentre Study of the German Cancer Consortium Radiation Oncology Group (DKTK-ROG). *Int. J. Cancer* **2016**, *138*, 171–181. [CrossRef] [PubMed]
5. Donnem, T.; Hald, S.M.; Paulsen, E.-E.; Richardsen, E.; Al-Saad, S.; Kilvaer, T.K.; Brustugun, O.T.; Helland, A.; Lund-Iversen, M.; Poehl, M.; et al. Stromal CD8+ T-Cell Density—A Promising Supplement to TNM Staging in Non-Small Cell Lung Cancer. *Clin. Cancer Res.* **2015**, *21*, 2635–2643. [CrossRef]
6. Gabrielson, A.; Wu, Y.; Wang, H.; Jiang, J.; Kallakury, B.; Gatalica, Z.; Reddy, S.; Kleiner, D.; Fishbein, T.; Johnson, L.; et al. Intratumoral CD3 and CD8 T-Cell Densities Associated with Relapse-Free Survival in HCC. *Cancer Immunol. Res.* **2016**, *4*, 419–430. [CrossRef]
7. Ou, D.; Adam, J.; Garberis, I.; Blanchard, P.; Nguyen, F.; Levy, A.; Casiraghi, O.; Gorphe, P.; Breuskin, I.; Janot, F.; et al. Clinical Relevance of Tumor Infiltrating Lymphocytes, PD-L1 Expression and Correlation with HPV/P16 in Head and Neck Cancer Treated with Bio- or Chemo-Radiotherapy. *Oncoimmunology* **2017**, *6*, e1341030. [CrossRef]
8. Wansom, D.; Light, E.; Thomas, D.; Worden, F.; Prince, M.; Urba, S.; Chepeha, D.; Kumar, B.; Cordell, K.; Eisbruch, A.; et al. Infiltrating Lymphocytes and Human Papillomavirus-16—Associated Oropharyngeal Cancer. *Laryngoscope* **2012**, *122*, 121–127. [CrossRef]
9. Näsman, A.; Romanitan, M.; Nordfors, C.; Grün, N.; Johansson, H.; Hammarstedt, L.; Marklund, L.; Munck-Wikland, E.; Dalianis, T.; Ramqvist, T. Tumor Infiltrating CD8+ and Foxp3+ Lymphocytes Correlate to Clinical Outcome and Human Papillomavirus (HPV) Status in Tonsillar Cancer. *PLoS ONE* **2012**, *7*, e38711. [CrossRef]
10. Nordfors, C.; Grün, N.; Tertipis, N.; Ährlund-Richter, A.; Haeggblom, L.; Sivars, L.; Du, J.; Nyberg, T.; Marklund, L.; Munck-Wikland, E.; et al. CD8+ and CD4+ Tumour Infiltrating Lymphocytes in Relation to Human Papillomavirus Status and Clinical Outcome in Tonsillar and Base of Tongue Squamous Cell Carcinoma. *Eur. J. Cancer* **2013**, *49*, 2522–2530. [CrossRef]
11. Sakaguchi, S.; Yamaguchi, T.; Nomura, T.; Ono, M. Regulatory T Cells and Immune Tolerance. *Cell* **2008**, *133*, 775–787. [CrossRef]
12. Vignali, D.A.A.; Collison, L.W.; Workman, C.J. How Regulatory T Cells Work. *Nat. Rev. Immunol.* **2008**, *8*, 523–532. [CrossRef]
13. Weller, P.; Bankfalvi, A.; Gu, X.; Dominas, N.; Lehnerdt, G.F.; Zeidler, R.; Lang, S.; Brandau, S.; Dumitru, C.A. The Role of Tumour FoxP3 as Prognostic Marker in Different Subtypes of Head and Neck Cancer. *Eur. J. Cancer* **2014**, *50*, 1291–1300. [CrossRef]
14. Shang, B.; Liu, Y.; Jiang, S.; Liu, Y. Prognostic Value of Tumor-Infiltrating FoxP3+ Regulatory T Cells in Cancers: A Systematic Review and Meta-Analysis. *Sci. Rep.* **2015**, *5*, 15179. [CrossRef]
15. Kindt, N.; Descamps, G.; Seminerio, I.; Bellier, J.; Lechien, J.R.; Mat, Q.; Pottier, C.; Delvenne, P.; Journé, F.; Saussez, S. High Stromal Foxp3-Positive T Cell Number Combined to Tumor Stage Improved Prognosis in Head and Neck Squamous Cell Carcinoma. *Oral Oncol.* **2017**, *67*, 183–191. [CrossRef]
16. Seminerio, I.; Descamps, G.; Dupont, S.; de Marrez, L.; Laigle, J.-A.; Lechien, J.R.; Kindt, N.; Journe, F.; Saussez, S. Infiltration of FoxP3+ Regulatory T Cells Is a Strong and Independent Prognostic Factor in Head and Neck Squamous Cell Carcinoma. *Cancers* **2019**, *11*, 227. [CrossRef]
17. Evrard, D.; Szturz, P.; Tijeras-Raballand, A.; Astorgues-Xerri, L.; Abitbol, C.; Paradis, V.; Raymond, E.; Albert, S.; Barry, B.; Faivre, S. Macrophages in the Microenvironment of Head and Neck Cancer: Potential Targets for Cancer Therapy. *Oral Oncol.* **2019**, *88*, 29–38. [CrossRef]
18. Lechien, J.R.; Descamps, G.; Seminerio, I.; Furgiuele, S.; Dequanter, D.; Mouawad, F.; Badoual, C.; Journe, F.; Saussez, S. HPV Involvement in the Tumor Microenvironment and Immune Treatment in Head and Neck Squamous Cell Carcinomas. *Cancers* **2020**, *12*, 1060. [CrossRef]
19. Deng, R.; Lu, J.; Liu, X.; Peng, X.-H.; Wang, J.; Li, X.-P. PD-L1 Expression Is Highly Associated with Tumor-Associated Macrophage Infiltration in Nasopharyngeal Carcinoma. *Cancer Manag. Res.* **2020**, *12*, 11585–11596. [CrossRef]
20. Snietura, M.; Brewczynski, A.; Kopec, A.; Rutkowski, T. Infiltrates of M2-Like Tumour-Associated Macrophages Are Adverse Prognostic Factor in Patients with Human Papillomavirus-Negative but Not in Human Papillomavirus-Positive Oropharyngeal Squamous Cell Carcinoma. *Pathobiology* **2020**, *87*, 75–86. [CrossRef]
21. Troiano, G.; Caponio, V.C.A.; Adipietro, I.; Tepedino, M.; Santoro, R.; Laino, L.; Lo Russo, L.; Cirillo, N.; Lo Muzio, L. Prognostic Significance of CD68+ and CD163+ Tumor Associated Macrophages in Head and Neck Squamous Cell Carcinoma: A Systematic Review and Meta-Analysis. *Oral Oncol.* **2019**, *93*, 66–75. [CrossRef] [PubMed]

22. Costa, N.L.; Valadares, M.C.; Souza, P.P.C.; Mendonça, E.F.; Oliveira, J.C.; Silva, T.A.; Batista, A.C. Tumor-Associated Macrophages and the Profile of Inflammatory Cytokines in Oral Squamous Cell Carcinoma. *Oral Oncol.* **2013**, *49*, 216–223. [CrossRef] [PubMed]
23. Seminerio, I.; Kindt, N.; Descamps, G.; Bellier, J.; Lechien, J.R.; Mat, Q.; Pottier, C.; Journé, F.; Saussez, S. High Infiltration of CD68+ Macrophages Is Associated with Poor Prognoses of Head and Neck Squamous Cell Carcinoma Patients and Is Influenced by Human Papillomavirus. *Oncotarget* **2018**, *9*, 11046–11059. [CrossRef] [PubMed]
24. Kindt, N.; Descamps, G.; Seminerio, I.; Bellier, J.; Lechien, J.R.; Pottier, C.; Larsimont, D.; Journé, F.; Delvenne, P.; Saussez, S. Langerhans Cell Number Is a Strong and Independent Prognostic Factor for Head and Neck Squamous Cell Carcinomas. *Oral Oncol.* **2016**, *62*, 1–10. [CrossRef] [PubMed]
25. Nguyen, N.; Bellile, E.; Thomas, D.; McHugh, J.; Rozek, L.; Virani, S.; Peterson, L.; Carey, T.E.; Walline, H.; Moyer, J.; et al. Tumor Infiltrating Lymphocytes and Survival in Patients with Head and Neck Squamous Cell Carcinoma. *Head Neck* **2016**, *38*, 1074–1084. [CrossRef]
26. Galon, J.; Costes, A.; Sanchez-Cabo, F.; Kirilovsky, A.; Mlecnik, B.; Lagorce-Pagès, C.; Tosolini, M.; Camus, M.; Berger, A.; Wind, P.; et al. Type, Density, and Location of Immune Cells Within Human Colorectal Tumors Predict Clinical Outcome. *Science* **2006**, *313*, 1960–1964. [CrossRef]
27. Khoury, T.; Nagrale, V.; Opyrchal, M.; Peng, X.; Wang, D.; Yao, S. Prognostic Significance of Stromal Versus Intratumoral Infiltrating Lymphocytes in Different Subtypes of Breast Cancer Treated With Cytotoxic Neoadjuvant Chemotherapy. *Appl. Immunohistochem. Mol. Morphol.* **2018**, *26*, 523–532. [CrossRef]
28. Pagès, F.; Mlecnik, B.; Marliot, F.; Bindea, G.; Ou, F.-S.; Bifulco, C.; Lugli, A.; Zlobec, I.; Rau, T.T.; Berger, M.D.; et al. International Validation of the Consensus Immunoscore for the Classification of Colon Cancer: A Prognostic and Accuracy Study. *Lancet* **2018**, *391*, 2128–2139. [CrossRef]
29. Lanzi, A.; Pagès, F.; Lagorce-Pagès, C.; Galon, J. The Consensus Immunoscore: Toward a New Classification of Colorectal Cancer. *Oncoimmunology* **2020**, *9*, 1789032. [CrossRef]
30. Furgiuele, S.; Descamps, G.; Lechien, J.R.; Dequanter, D.; Journe, F.; Saussez, S. Immunoscore Combining CD8, FoxP3, and CD68-Positive Cells Density and Distribution Predicts the Prognosis of Head and Neck Cancer Patients. *Cells* **2022**, *11*, 2050. [CrossRef]
31. Duray, A.; Descamps, G.; Decaestecker, C.; Sirtaine, N.; Gilles, A.; Khalifé, M.; Chantrain, G.; Depuydt, C.E.; Delvenne, P.; Saussez, S. Human Papillomavirus Predicts the Outcome Following Concomitant Chemoradiotherapy in Patients with Head and Neck Squamous Cell Carcinomas. *Oncol. Rep.* **2013**, *30*, 371–376. [CrossRef]
32. Almangush, A.; Bello, I.O.; Heikkinen, I.; Hagström, J.; Haglund, C.; Kowalski, L.P.; Coletta, R.D.; Mäkitie, A.A.; Salo, T.; Leivo, I. Improving Risk Stratification of Early Oral Tongue Cancer with TNM-Immune (TNM-I) Staging System. *Cancers* **2021**, *13*, 3235. [CrossRef]
33. El Sissy, C.; Kirilovsky, A.; Zeitoun, G.; Marliot, F.; Haicheur, N.; Lagorce-Pagès, C.; Galon, J.; Pagès, F. Therapeutic Implications of the Immunoscore in Patients with Colorectal Cancer. *Cancers* **2021**, *13*, 1281. [CrossRef]
34. Salgado, R.; Denkert, C.; Demaria, S.; Sirtaine, N.; Klauschen, F.; Pruneri, G.; Wienert, S.; Van den Eynden, G.; Baehner, F.L.; Penault-Llorca, F.; et al. The Evaluation of Tumor-Infiltrating Lymphocytes (TILs) in Breast Cancer: Recommendations by an International TILs Working Group 2014. *Ann. Oncol.* **2015**, *26*, 259–271. [CrossRef]
35. Paulsen, E.-E.; Kilvaer, T.; Khanehkenari, M.R.; Maurseth, R.J.; Al-Saad, S.; Hald, S.M.; Al-Shibli, K.; Andersen, S.; Richardsen, E.; Busund, L.-T.; et al. CD45RO(+) Memory T Lymphocytes—A Candidate Marker for TNM-Immunoscore in Squamous Non-Small Cell Lung Cancer. *Neoplasia* **2015**, *17*, 839–848. [CrossRef]
36. Feng, W.; Li, Y.; Shen, L.; Zhang, Q.; Cai, X.-W.; Zhu, Z.-F.; Sun, M.-H.; Chen, H.-Q.; Fu, X.-L. Clinical Impact of the Tumor Immune Microenvironment in Completely Resected Stage IIIA(N2) Non-Small Cell Lung Cancer Based on an Immunoscore Approach. *Ther. Adv. Med. Oncol.* **2021**, *13*, 1758835920984975. [CrossRef]
37. Zhang, X.-M.; Song, L.-J.; Shen, J.; Yue, H.; Han, Y.-Q.; Yang, C.-L.; Liu, S.-Y.; Deng, J.-W.; Jiang, Y.; Fu, G.-H.; et al. Prognostic and Predictive Values of Immune Infiltrate in Patients with Head and Neck Squamous Cell Carcinoma. *Hum. Pathol.* **2018**, *82*, 104–112. [CrossRef]
38. Gillison, M.L.; Chaturvedi, A.K.; Anderson, W.F.; Fakhry, C. Epidemiology of Human Papillomavirus-Positive Head and Neck Squamous Cell Carcinoma. *J. Clin. Oncol.* **2015**, *33*, 3235–3242. [CrossRef]
39. Modesto, A.; Graff Cailleaud, P.; Blanchard, P.; Boisselier, P.; Pointreau, Y. Challenges and limits of therapeutic de-escalation for papillomavirus-related oropharyngeal cancer. *Cancer Radiother.* **2022**, *26*, 921–924. [CrossRef]
40. Ljokjel, B.; Haave, H.; Lybak, S.; Vintermyr, O.K.; Helgeland, L.; Aarstad, H.J. Tumor Infiltration Levels of CD3, Foxp3 (+) Lymphocytes and CD68 Macrophages at Diagnosis Predict 5-Year Disease-Specific Survival in Patients with Oropharynx Squamous Cell Carcinoma. *Cancers* **2022**, *14*, 1508. [CrossRef]
41. Saito, T.; Nishikawa, H.; Wada, H.; Nagano, Y.; Sugiyama, D.; Atarashi, K.; Maeda, Y.; Hamaguchi, M.; Ohkura, N.; Sato, E.; et al. Two FOXP3(+)CD4(+) T Cell Subpopulations Distinctly Control the Prognosis of Colorectal Cancers. *Nat. Med.* **2016**, *22*, 679–684. [CrossRef] [PubMed]
42. Gama-Cuellar, A.G.; Francisco, A.L.N.; Scarini, J.F.; Mariano, F.V.; Kowalski, L.P.; Gondak, R. Decreased CD1a + and CD83 + Cells in Tonsillar Squamous Cell Carcinoma Regardless of HPV Status. *J. Appl. Oral Sci.* **2022**, *30*, e20210702. [CrossRef] [PubMed]
43. Gomes, J.O.; de Vasconcelos Carvalho, M.; Fonseca, F.P.; Gondak, R.O.; Lopes, M.A.; Vargas, P.A. CD1a+ and CD83+ Langerhans Cells Are Reduced in Lower Lip Squamous Cell Carcinoma. *J. Oral Pathol. Med.* **2016**, *45*, 433–439. [CrossRef] [PubMed]

44. Silva, L.-C.; Fonseca, F.-P.; Almeida, O.-P.; Mariz, B.-A.; Lopes, M.-A.; Radhakrishnan, R.; Sharma, M.; Kowalski, L.-P.; Vargas, P.-A. CD1a+ and CD207+ Cells Are Reduced in Oral Submucous Fibrosis and Oral Squamous Cell Carcinoma. *Med. Oral Patol. Oral Cir. Bucal.* **2020**, *25*, e49–e55. [CrossRef]
45. Karpathiou, G.; Casteillo, F.; Giroult, J.-B.; Forest, F.; Fournel, P.; Monaya, A.; Froudarakis, M.; Dumollard, J.M.; Prades, J.M.; Peoc'h, M. Prognostic Impact of Immune Microenvironment in Laryngeal and Pharyngeal Squamous Cell Carcinoma: Immune Cell Subtypes, Immuno-Suppressive Pathways and Clinicopathologic Characteristics. *Oncotarget* **2016**, *8*, 19310–19322. [CrossRef]
46. Goldman, S.A.; Baker, E.; Weyant, R.J.; Clarke, M.R.; Myers, J.N.; Lotze, M.T. Peritumoral CD1a-Positive Dendritic Cells Are Associated with Improved Survival in Patients with Tongue Carcinoma. *Arch. Otolaryngol. Head Neck Surg.* **1998**, *124*, 641–646. [CrossRef]
47. Minesaki, A.; Kai, K.; Kuratomi, Y.; Aishima, S. Infiltration of CD1a-Positive Dendritic Cells in Advanced Laryngeal Cancer Correlates with Unfavorable Outcomes Post-Laryngectomy. *BMC Cancer* **2021**, *21*, 973. [CrossRef]

Article

Concordance of p16^{INK4a} and E6*I mRNA among HPV-DNA-Positive Oropharyngeal, Laryngeal, and Oral Cavity Carcinomas from the ICO International Study

Marisa Mena [1,2,*,†], Xin Wang [1,†], Sara Tous [1,2], Beatriz Quiros [1,2], Omar Clavero [1,2], Maria Alejo [3,4], Francisca Morey [1], Miren Taberna [5], Xavier Leon Vintro [6,7], Belén Lloveras Rubio [8], Llúcia Alos [9], Hisham Mehanna [10], Wim Quint [11], Michael Pawlita [12], Massimo Tommasino [13], Miguel Angel Pavón [1,2], Nubia Muñoz [14], Silvia De Sanjose [1,2,15], Francesc Xavier Bosch [1,2,16], Laia Alemany [1,2,*] and on behalf of the ICO International HPV in Head and Neck Cancer Study Group [‡]

1. Cancer Epidemiology Research Program, Catalan Institute of Oncology (ICO)-IDIBELL, L'Hospitalet de Llobregat, 08908 Barcelona, Spain
2. Centro de Investigación Biomédica en Red de Epidemiología y Salud Pública (CIBERESP), Instituto de Salud Carlos III, 28029 Madrid, Spain
3. Pathology Department, Hospital de Vic, 08500 Vic, Spain
4. Pathology Department, Hospital General de l'Hopitalet, L'Hospitalet de Llobregat, 08908 Barcelona, Spain
5. Oncology Department, Catalan Institute of Oncology (ICO)-IDIBELL, ONCOBELL, L'Hospitalet de Llobregat, 08908 Barcelona, Spain
6. Otorhinolaryngology Department, Hospital Sant Pau, 08026 Barcelona, Spain
7. Centro de Investigación Biomédica en Red de Bioingeniería, Biomateriales y Nanomedicina (CIBER-BBN), Instituto de Salud Carlos III, 28029 Madrid, Spain
8. Pathology Department, Hospital del Mar, 08003 Barcelona, Spain
9. Pathology Department, Hospital Clinic, 08036 Barcelona, Spain
10. Institute of Head and Neck Studies and Education, University of Birmingham, Birmingham B15 2TT, UK
11. DDL Diagnostic Laboratory, 2288 ER Rijswijk, The Netherlands
12. Division of Molecular Diagnostics of Oncogenic Infections, Research Program Infection, Inflammation and Cancer, German Cancer Research Center (DKFZ), 69120 Heidelberg, Germany
13. Infections and Cancer Biology Group, International Agency for Research on Cancer (IARC), 69372 Lyon, France
14. National Cancer Institute, Bogotá 111511, Colombia
15. ISGlobal, 08036 Barcelona, Spain
16. Universitat Oberta de Catalunya, 08035 Barcelona, Spain
* Correspondence: mmena@iconcologia.net (M.M.); lalemany@iconcologia.net (L.A.)
† These authors contributed equally to this work.
‡ A complete list of the investigators for the ICO International HPV in Head and Neck Cancer Study is provided in Supplementary Materials (available online).

Simple Summary: The utility of a diagnostic algorithm for the detection of HPV-driven oral cavity (OCC), oropharyngeal (OPC), and laryngeal (LC) carcinomas using HPV-DNA testing followed by p16^{INK4a} immunohistochemistry, taking E6*I mRNA detection as the reference standard, was assessed in HPV-DNA-positive formalin-fixed paraffin-embedded samples from 29 countries. The concordance of p16^{INK4a} and E6*I mRNA among 78, 257, and 51 HPV-DNA-positive OCC, OPC, and LC, respectively, was moderate to substantial in OCC and OPC but only fair in LC. A different p16^{INK4a} expression pattern was observed in those cases HPV-DNA-positive for types other than HPV16, as compared to HPV16-positive cases. We concluded that the diagnostic algorithm of HPV-DNA testing followed by p16^{INK4a} immunohistochemistry might be helpful in the diagnosis of HPV-driven OCC and OPC, but not LC. Our study provides new insights into the use HPV-DNA, p16^{INK4a}, and HPV-E6*I mRNA for diagnosing an HPV-driven head and neck carcinoma.

Abstract: Background: Tests or test algorithms for diagnosing HPV-driven oral cavity and laryngeal head and neck carcinomas (HNC) have not been yet validated, and the differences among oral cavity and laryngeal sites have not been comprehensively evaluated. We aimed to assess the utility of a diagnostic algorithm for the detection of HPV-driven oral cavity (OCC), oropharyngeal (OPC) and laryngeal (LC) carcinomas using HPV-DNA testing followed by p16^{INK4a} immunohistochemistry, taking E6*I mRNA detection as the reference standard. **Methods:** Formalin-fixed paraffin-embedded OCC, OPC, and LC carcinomas were collected from pathology archives in 29 countries. All samples were subjected to histopathological evaluation, DNA quality control, and HPV-DNA detection. All HPV-DNA-positive samples (including 78 OCC, 257 OPC, and 51 LC out of 3680 HNC with valid HPV-DNA results) were also tested for p16^{INK4a} immunohistochemistry and E6*I mRNA. Three different cutoffs of nuclear and cytoplasmic staining were evaluated for p16^{INK4a}: (a) >25%, (b) >50%, and (c) ≥70%. The concordance of p16^{INK4a} and E6*I mRNA among HPV-DNA-positive OCC, OPC, and LC cases was assessed. **Results:** A total of 78 OCC, 257 OPC, and 51 LC were HPV-DNA-positive and further tested for p16^{INK4a} and E6*I mRNA. The percentage of concordance between p16^{INK4a} (cutoff ≥ 70%) and E6*I mRNA among HPV-DNA-positive OCC, OPC, and LC cases was 79.5% (95% CI 69.9–89.1%), 82.1% (95% CI 77.2–87.0%), and 56.9% (95% CI 42.3–71.4%), respectively. A p16^{INK4a} cutoff of >50% improved the concordance although the improvement was not statistically significant. For most anatomical locations and p16^{INK4a} cutoffs, the percentage of discordant cases was higher for HPV16- than HPV-non16-positive cases. **Conclusions:** The diagnostic algorithm of HPV-DNA testing followed by p16^{INK4a} immunohistochemistry might be helpful in the diagnosis of HPV-driven OCC and OPC, but not LC. A different p16^{INK4a} expression pattern was observed in those cases HPV-DNA-positive for types other than HPV16, as compared to HPV16-positive cases. Our study provides new insights into the use HPV-DNA, p16^{INK4a}, and HPV-E6*I mRNA for diagnosing an HPV-driven HNC, including the optimal HPV test or p16^{INK4a} cutoffs to be used. More studies are warranted to clarify the role of p16^{INK4a} and HPV status in both OPC and non-OPC HNC.

Keywords: human papillomavirus; head and neck cancer; biomarkers

1. Introduction

Apart from oropharyngeal carcinomas (OPC), oral cavity (OCC) and laryngeal carcinomas (LC) are the predominant subtypes of head and neck carcinomas (HNC), where a fraction of cases are driven by human papillomavirus (HPV) [1]. However, HPV attributable fractions (AFs) in non-oropharyngeal HNC (OCC—2.1%, LC—2.3%) are much lower than in OPC (30%) [1]. On the other hand, since the number of incident OCC and LC exceeds that of OPC [2], even low HPV-AFs for these sites translate to high absolute numbers of HPV-driven OCC or LC. Worldwide, it is estimated that approximately 52,000 new HNC cases are caused by a persistent HPV infection every year. Of these, 42,000 correspond to OPC, 5900 correspond to OCC, and 4100 correspond to LC [3]. Thus, around 20% of new HPV-related HNC cases are oral cavity and laryngeal tumors.

The prognostic advantage of HPV-driven OPC versus non-HPV-driven OPC is well established. On the other hand, the clinical implications of HPV-status in OCC and LC are not clear [4]. Thus, while it is widely accepted to test all newly diagnosed OPC for HPV tumor status in the clinical setting, routine testing of non-oropharyngeal HNC for HPV is not currently recommended [5].

The WHO campaign for eliminating cervical cancer [6] raises the possibility of elimination of other HPV-related cancers. Therefore, from a public health perspective, estimating HPV-AFs in non-oropharyngeal HNC is relevant to help assess the possible protective effect of HPV vaccination. Therefore, country- and type-specific baseline estimations of HPV-AFs in all HPV-related cancers, including non-oropharyngeal HNC, are warranted.

The identification of p16^{INK4a}, a cell surrogate marker of HPV carcinogenic transformation, using immunohistochemistry is easy to implement and the most widely used standalone technique for HPV-driven OPC diagnosis in the clinical setting. A nuclear and cytoplasmatic 70% cutoff of stained cells is recommended [5].

However, to diagnose HPV-driven HNC at non-oropharyngeal sites, tests and test algorithms have not been validated so far, nor has there been an in-depth evaluation of the differences among non-oropharyngeal sites. While HPV E6/E7 mRNA detection is widely accepted as the reference standard test to elucidate the oncogenic role of HPV in the tumor, it is still challenging to implement in specific settings due to RNA fragmentation and degradation in paraffin-embedded tissue [7]. High-risk HPV RNA in situ hybridization is increasingly available as a clinical test on automated stainers and can detect highly fragmented RNA, but implementing the technique for HPV-driven HNC diagnosis is still under evaluation [7].

Moreover, despite the well-proven prognostic impact and clinical implications of HPV status in OPC and the wide use of $p16^{INK4a}$ immunohistochemistry alone to assess HPV status in OPC, a fraction of $p16^{INK4a}$-positive OPCs are HPV-DNA-negative, and HPV-DNA-negative/$p16^{INK4a}$-positive OPCs do not show a prognostic advantage with respect to HPV-DNA/$p16^{INK4a}$ double-negative cases [8,9]. These findings highlight the need for a test in addition to $p16^{INK4a}$ immunohistochemistry to confirm HPV causality in OPC tumors, but no consensus for HPV testing has been reached yet. Moreover, most studies analyzing the discordance between p16 and HPV used an HPV-DNA-based test rather than the reference standard, an mRNA-based test.

HPV-DNA/$p16^{INK4a}$ double testing is increasingly used for diagnosing HPV-driven OPC. In a meta-analysis of 11 studies [10], a sensitivity of 93% (95% CI 87–97%) and a specificity of 96% (95% CI 89–100%) for HPV-DNA/$p16^{INK4a}$ double positivity were estimated. Yet, there is still limited information about the accuracy and prognostic value of this combination of biomarkers in OPC, and even less in non-oropharyngeal HNC.

The ICO international study estimated the fraction of cases attributable to HPV in 3680 formalin-fixed paraffin-embedded (FFPE) HNC tissues collected from pathology archives in 29 countries [1]. Estimates of the fraction of cases attributable to HPV based on positivity for HPV-DNA and for either HPV E6*I mRNA or $p16^{INK4a}$ were 22.4%, 4.4%, and 3.5% for OPC, OCC, and LC, respectively [1,11].

Our aim in the present study was to assess the utility of a diagnostic algorithm for the detection of HPV-driven OCC, OPC, and LC of HPV-DNA testing followed by $p16^{INK4a}$ immunohistochemistry, taking E6*I mRNA detection as the reference standard. For that, we evaluated the concordance of $p16^{INK4a}$ and E6*I mRNA among HPV-DNA-positive OCC, OPC, and LC cases from the ICO international study.

2. Materials and Methods

2.1. Study Design

We conducted a statistical reanalysis of HNC cases positive for HPV-DNA, tested for $p16^{INK4a}$ immunohistochemistry and HPV E6*I-mRNA detection in the ICO international study, a large cross-sectional international study coordinated by the Catalan Institute of Oncology (ICO) (Barcelona, Spain) in collaboration with DDL Diagnostic Laboratory (Rijswijk, The Netherlands) [1,11]. The Ethics Committee of the Catalan Institute of Oncology-ICO (Comitè Ètic d'Investigació Clínica de l'Hospital Universitari de Bellvitge, L'Hospitalet de Llobregat, Barcelona, Spain) formally approved the study on 9 September 2010 (protocol code PR101/08).

2.2. FFPE Block Processing and Histopathological Evaluation

Details of the protocol were described elsewhere [1]. Briefly, the block processing and histopathological evaluation of FFPE were performed as follows: all specimen processing was centralized in the ICO. The samples were sectioned, and at least four sections were obtained. The first and last sections were stained with hematoxylin/eosin (HE) and were used for histopathological evaluation. Intermediate sections were used to determine viral DNA, E6*I mRNA, and $p16^{INK4a}$ detection.

2.3. HPV-DNA Detection and Genotyping

HPV determination was performed using PCR with the SPF-10 primer system followed by DEIA (DNA Enzyme Immuno Assay). DEIA-positive HPV-DNA samples were genotyped using the Line Probe Assay LiPA25 (Laboratory Biomedical Products, Rijswijk, The Netherlands); DNA quality was evaluated in all HPV-DNA-negative samples by testing for the tubulin-β gene. All DEIA and LiPA25 assays were performed at ICO.

2.4. HPV E6*I mRNA Detection

In all HPV-DNA-positive HNC, E6*I mRNA detection was performed by RT-PCR (real-time PCR). The E6*I mRNA assay targets 20 HPV types (HPVs 16/18/26/31/33/35/39/45/51/52/53/56/58/59/66/67/68/70/73/82). For each case, type-specific E6*I mRNA PCR was performed for all types detected by the SPF-10 PCR/DEIA/LiPA25 system that had at least one of the mRNA targeted types, in addition to HPV16. Quality control for mRNA detection was performed by detection of ubiquitin C mRNA. All E6*I mRNA assays were performed at DKFZ, Heidelberg, Germany.

2.5. $p16^{INK4a}$ Immunohistochemistry

All HPV-DNA-positive cases were evaluated for $p16^{INK4a}$ as previously described [1]. Three different nuclear and cytoplasmic staining cutoff values were considered: >25%, >50%, and ≥70%.

2.6. Statistical Analyses

Concordance percentage and kappa statistics were calculated to evaluate the agreement between $p16^{INK4a}$ and E6*I mRNA among OCC, OPC and LC cases that were HPV-DNA-positive, HPV16-DNA-positive, and HPV-DNA-positive for types other than HPV16. Concordance percentage was estimated according to whether the condition $np(1-p) > 5$ was met or not. If it was met, a normal distribution approximate method was applied [12]; if not, the estimates were obtained by the exact method based on binomial distribution [13]. The kappa statistic characterization was established as follows [14]: <0: poor; 0–0.20: slight; 0.21–0.40: fair; 0.41–0.60: moderate; 0.61–0.80: substantial; 0.81–1.0: almost perfect. The prevalence-adjusted bias-adjusted kappa (PABAK) statistic was explored when kappa was not valid (i.e., when the prevalence of a given response was very high or low, but low kappa values were observed in the 2 × 2 tables). The McNemar test p-value was also calculated to evaluate the distribution among the discordant cases. All statistical tests were two-sided, and statistical significance was set at a p-value of less than 0.05. All analyses were performed with STATA software, version 16.0 (Stata Corp, College Station, TX, USA).

3. Results

Figure 1 shows the disposition of cases included in the current analysis, in the context of the ICO international study. From the 3680 cases included in the main publication [1], 1264, 1090, and 1042 were OCC, OPC, and LC, respectively. Of those, a total of 78 (6.2%) OCC, 257 (23.6%) OPC, and 51 (4.9%) LC were HPV-DNA-positive and further tested for $p16^{INK4a}$ and E6*I mRNA. Most HPV-DNA-positive cases came from Europe (237) and Central and South America (121, see Supplementary Figure S1) and were males (71.5%) diagnosed between 2005 and 2009 (55.4%, see Supplementary Table S1). Mean age at diagnosis of HPV-DNA positive HNC cases was 58.5 years, being 60.2 for OCC, 58.5 for OPC, and 55.8 for LC. Conventional keratinizing squamous cell carcinoma was the most common histopathological diagnosis of HPV-DNA-positive OCC (55.1%) and LC (66.7%), whereas conventional non keratinizing squamous cell carcinoma was the most common histopathological diagnosis of HPV-DNA-positive OPC (42.4%).

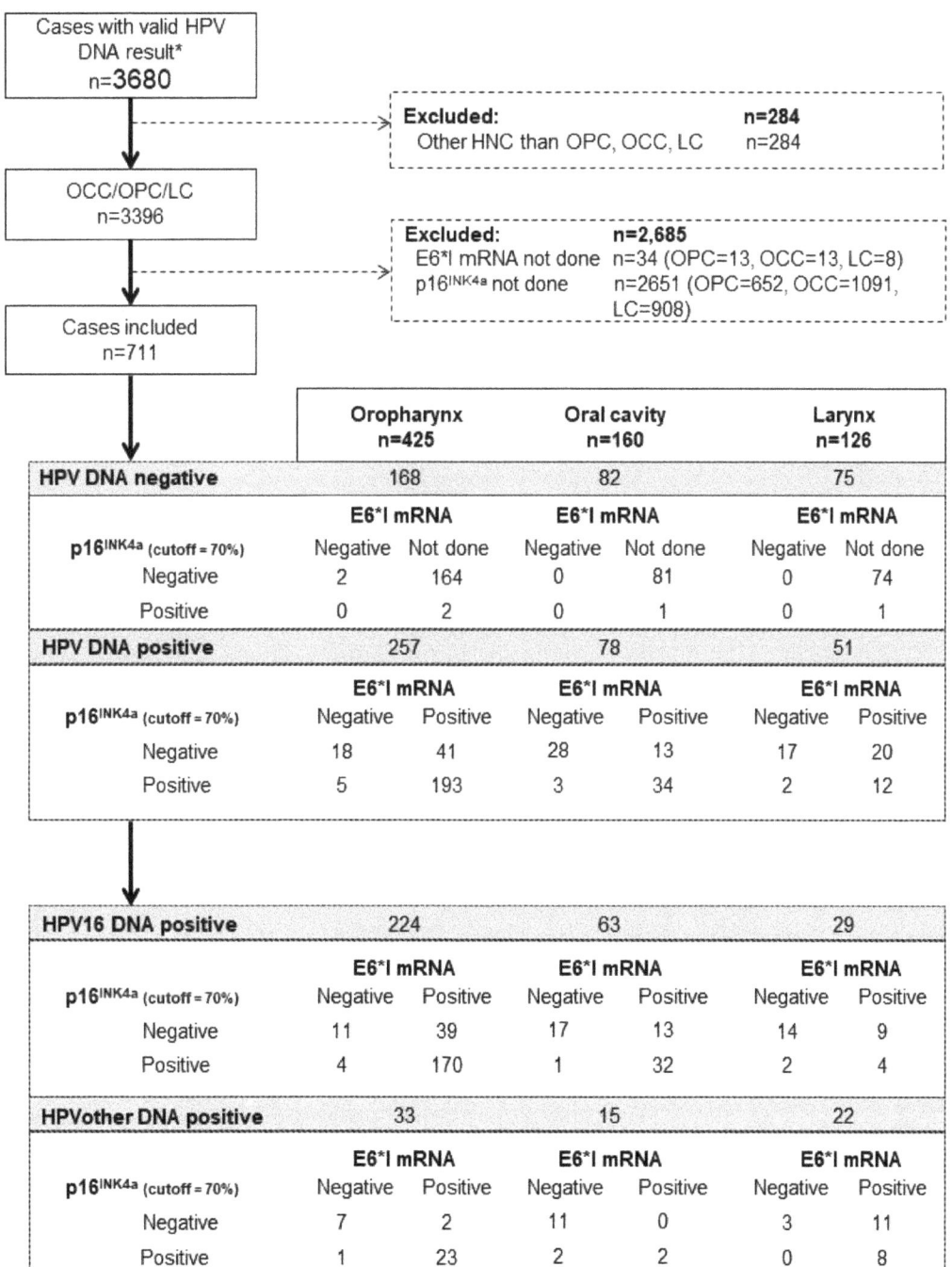

Figure 1. Flowchart of sample disposition and testing for HPV-related biomarkers. * Includes both cancers that were HPV-DNA positive and cancers that were HPV-DNA negative but tubulin positive.

The concordance between p16^{INK4a} at a cutoff ≥70% and E6*I mRNA was moderate among HPV-DNA-positive OCC (percentage of concordance 79.5% (95% CI 69.9–89.1%), kappa 0.59 (PABAK = 0.59)) and substantial among HPV-DNA-positive OPC (percentage of concordance 82.1% (95% CI 77.2–87.0%), kappa 0.36 (PABAK = 0.64)). Among LC cases, the concordance was only fair (percentage of concordance 56.9% (95% CI 42.3–71.4%), kappa 0.23 (PABAK = 0.14)) (Table 1). Lowering the p16^{INK4a} cutoff to >50% improved the concordance in all HN sites, although the improvement was not statistically significant (Table 1). The percentage of discordant cases (i.e., p16^{INK4a}+/E6*I mRNA− or p16^{INK4a}−/E6*I mRNA+) for HPV-DNA-positive LC was 42.1% when considering a p16^{INK4a} cutoff ≥70%, around two times higher than for HPV-DNA-positive OPC and OCC (17.9% and 20.5%, respectively). The same was also observed for p16^{INK4a} cutoffs of >25% and >50% (Table 1). For all anatomical locations and p16^{INK4a} cutoffs, the percentage of p16^{INK4a}−/E6*I mRNA+ cases was higher than the percentage of p16^{INK4a}+/E6*I mRNA− cases (Table 1).

Table 1. Concordance between p16^{INK4a} and E6*I mRNA among HPV-DNA-positive, HPV16-DNA-positive, and HPV-DNA-positive for types other than HPV16 by anatomical location of the head and neck tumors.

Head and Neck Carcinoma Cases	N	E6*I mRNA-Pos				E6*I mRNA-Neg				% Concordance (95% CI)**	Kappa (95% CI)	PABAK	McNemar Test p-Value
		p16^{INK4a}-Pos		p16^{INK4a}-Neg		p16^{INK4a}-Pos		p16^{INK4a}-Neg					
		n	%	n	%	n	%	n	%				
p16^{INK4a} Cutoff 70%													
OPC													
HPV-DNA-pos	257	193	75.1	41	16.0	5	1.9	18	7.0	82.1 (77.2, 87.0)	0.36 (0.22, 0.49)	0.64	**<0.001**
HPV16-DNA-pos	224	170	75.9	39	17.4	4	1.8	11	4.9	80.8 (75.4, 86.2)	0.26 (0.12, 0.41)	0.62	**<0.001**
HPVother-DNA-pos *	33	23	69.7	2	6.1	1	3.0	7	21.2	90.9 (75.7, 98.1)	0.76 (0.51, 1.00)	0.82	1.000
OCC													
HPV-DNA-pos	78	34	43.6	13	16.7	3	3.8	28	35.9	79.5 (69.9, 89.1)	0.59 (0.42, 0.77)	0.59	**0.021**
HPV16-DNA-pos	63	32	50.8	13	20.6	1	1.6	17	27.0	77.8 (66.7, 88.8)	0.55 (0.35, 0.74)	0.56	**<0.001**
HPVother-DNA-pos *	15	2	13.3	0	0.0	2	13.3	11	73.3	86.7 (59.5, 98.3)	0.59 (0.12, 1.00)	0.73	0.500
LC													
HPV-DNA-pos	51	12	23.5	20	39.2	2	3.9	17	33.3	56.9 (42.3, 71.4)	0.23 (0.03, 0.42)	0.14	**<0.001**
HPV16-DNA-pos	29	4	13.8	9	31.0	2	6.9	14	48.3	62.1 (42.7, 81.5)	0.19 (−0.12, 0.51)	0.24	**<0.001**
HPVother-DNA-pos *	22	8	36.4	11	50.0	0	0.0	3	13.6	50.0 (26.8, 73.2)	0.17 (−0.03, 0.36)	0.00	**0.001**
p16^{INK4a} Cutoff 50%													
OPC													
HPV-DNA-pos	257	200	77.8	34	13.2	6	2.3	17	6.6	84.4 (79.8, 89.1)	0.38 (0.24, 0.53)	0.69	**<0.001**
HPV16-DNA-pos	224	177	79.0	32	14.3	5	2.2	10	4.5	83.5 (78.4, 88.6)	0.28 (0.12, 0.44)	0.67	**<0.001**
HPVother-DNA-pos *	33	23	69.7	2	6.1	1	3.0	7	21.2	90.9 (75.7, 98.1)	0.76 (0.51, 1.00)	0.82	1.000
OCC													
HPV-DNA-pos	78	37	47.4	10	12.8	4	5.1	27	34.6	82.1 (72.9, 91.2)	0.64 (0.47, 0.81)	0.64	0.180
HPV16-DNA-pos	63	35	55.6	10	15.9	2	3.2	16	25.4	81.0 (70.5, 91.4)	0.59 (0.39, 0.79)	0.62	**<0.001**
HPVother-DNA-pos *	15	2	13.3	0	0.0	2	13.3	11	73.3	86.7 (59.5, 98.3)	0.59 (0.12, 1.00)	0.73	0.500
LC													
HPV-DNA-pos	51	16	31.4	16	31.4	4	7.8	15	29.4	60.8 (46.4, 75.2)	0.26 (0.02, 0.49)	0.22	**0.012**
HPV16-DNA-pos	29	5	17.2	8	27.6	4	13.8	12	41.4	58.6 (39.0, 78.3)	0.14 (−0.21, 0.49)	0.17	**<0.001**
HPVother-DNA-pos *	22	11	50.0	8	36.4	0	0.0	3	13.6	63.6 (41.3, 86.0)	0.27 (−0.003, 0.55)	0.27	**0.008**
p16^{INK4a} Cutoff 25%													
OPC													
HPV-DNA-pos	257	200	77.8	34	13.2	6	2.3	17	6.6	84.4 (79.8, 89.1)	0.38 (0.24, 0.53)	0.69	**<0.001**
HPV16-DNA-pos	224	177	79.0	32	14.3	5	2.2	10	4.5	83.5 (78.4, 88.6)	0.28 (0.12, 0.44)	0.67	**<0.001**
HPVother-DNA-pos *	33	23	69.7	2	6.1	1	3.0	7	21.2	90.9 (75.7, 88.6)	0.76 (0.51, 1.00)	0.82	1.000
OCC													
HPV-DNA-pos	78	38	48.7	9	11.5	5	6.4	26	33.3	82.1 (72.9, 91,2)	0.63 (0.46, 0.81)	0.64	0.424
HPV16-DNA-pos	63	36	57.1	9	14.3	3	4.8	15	23.8	81.0 (70.5, 91.4)	0.58 (0.37, 0.78)	0.62	**<0.001**
HPVother-DNA-pos *	15	2	13.3	0	0.0	2	13.3	11	73.3	86.7 (59.5, 98.3)	0.59 (0.12, 1.00)	0.73	0.500
LC													
HPV-DNA-pos	51	18	35.3	14	27.5	5	9.8	14	27.5	62.7 (59.5, 98.3)	0.27 (0.03, 0.52)	0.25	0.064
HPV16-DNA-pos	29	5	15.6	8	25.0	8	25.0	11	34.4	55.2 (35.3, 75.0)	−0.04 (−0.38, 0.31)	0.00	**<0.001**
HPVother-DNA-pos *	22	13	59.1	6	27.3	0	0.0	3	13.6	72.7 (49.8, 89.3)	0.37 (0.04, 0.71)	0.45	**0.031**

OPC: oropharyngeal carcinoma; OCC: oral cavity carcinoma; LC: laryngeal carcinoma; N: number of cases; Pos: positive; Neg: negative. * Cases DNA positive for types other than HPV16. ** Can be estimated in two different ways, see Section 2. Statistically significant values are shown in bold.

HPV16 was the most common type among HPV-DNA-positive cases for all HN sites, although with lower proportions in OCC (69.0%) and LC (51.0%) than in OPC (83.0%, Figure 2). The next most common HPV type was HPV18 for OCC (4.3%) and LC (8.5%), and HPV33 (3.3%) for OPC. When considering as HPV-positive those cases double-positive for HPV-DNA/HPV-E6*I mRNA or HPV-DNA/p16^{INK4a}, the percentage of HPV16-positive cases increased for OCC (96.0%, 85%) and OPC (89.0%, 87.0%) and decreased for LC (41.0%). These differences in HPV type distribution by HPV relatedness definition were statistically significant.

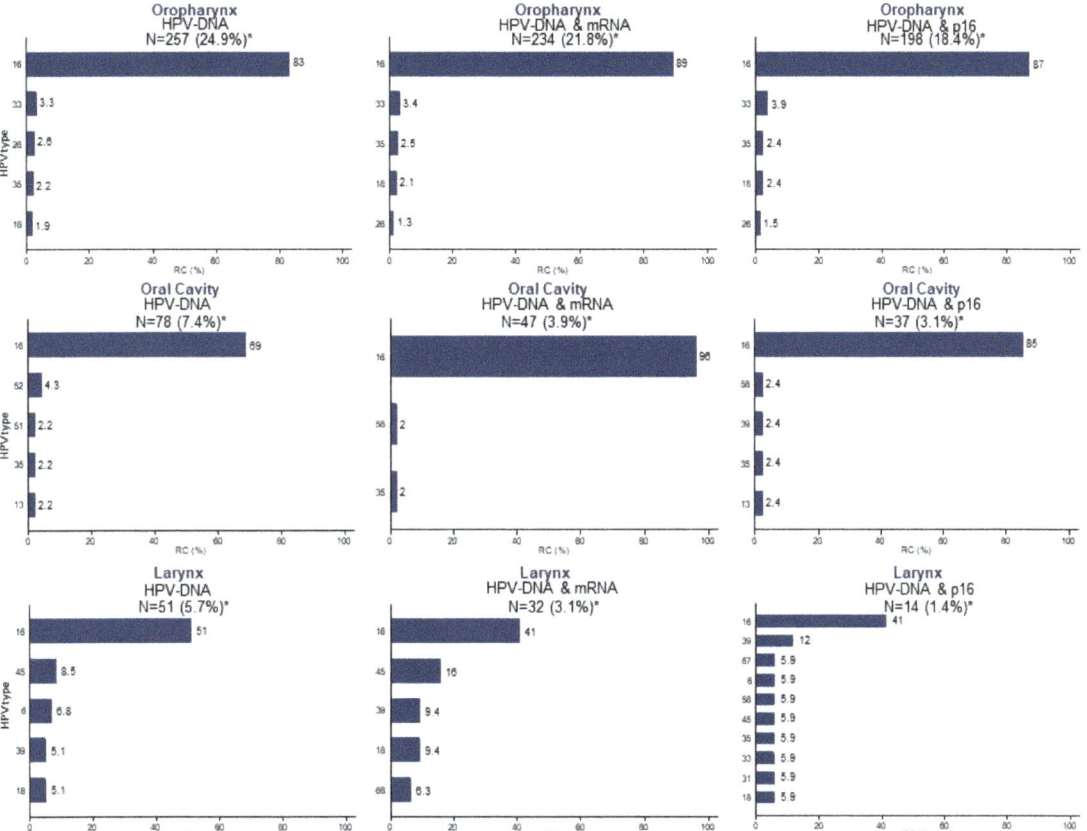

Figure 2. HPV type-specific relative contribution (RC) among HPV-positive cases when considering as HPV-positive HPV-DNA-, HPV-DNA/p16^{INK4a}-, and HPV-DNA/E6*I mRNA-positive cases by anatomical location of the head and neck tumors. RC: relative contribution; * HPV-attributable fractions considering the oral cavity, oropharyngeal, and laryngeal cancer cases included in the main study [1], and a p16^{INK4a} cutoff of 70%.

The concordance between p16^{INK4a} (all cutoffs) and E6*I mRNA decreased for all HN sites when only considering those cases that are HPV16-DNA-positive as compared to cases HPV-DNA-positive for any type, although this decrease was not statistically significant (Table 1). When only considering those cases HPV-DNA-positive for types other than HPV16, the concordance between p16^{INK4a} and E6*I mRNA was variable between HN sites and p16^{INK4a} cutoffs, albeit based on a very low number of cases. For most anatomical locations and p16^{INK4a} cutoffs, the percentage of discordant cases was higher for HPV16- than HPV-non16-positive cases. In particular, in OPC and OCC, p16^{INK4a}−/E6*I mRNA+ cases dropped from 17.4% and 20.6%, respectively, among HPV16-positive cases to 6.1% and 0% among HPV-non16-positive cases, whereas the percentage of double-negative cases increased in both locations. This pattern was not observed in LC where an increase of p16^{INK4a}+/E6*I mRNA+ and p16^{INK4a}−/E6*I mRNA+ cases was observed (Table 1).

4. Discussion

Despite the imperative need to accurately assign HPV status in OPC patients given its clinical implications and, to a lesser extent, in non-oropharyngeal HNC, there is not yet consensus for HPV testing in HNC. We aimed to evaluate the utility of a two-step diagnostic algorithm which is already used in some clinical settings for detection of HPV-driven OPC. This algorithm consists of HPV-DNA testing followed by p16^{INK4a} immunohistochemistry in HPV-DNA-positive OPC, OCC, and LC cases, collated from the ICO international study [1]. For that, we considered E6*I mRNA detection as the reference standard and evaluated the concordance of p16^{INK4a} and E6*I mRNA among HPV-DNA-positive cases.

Although evidence on the need of adding a second HPV test to p16^{INK4a} immunohistochemistry to accurately assign HPV status in OPC is accumulating and HPV-DNA/p16^{INK4a} double testing is increasingly used for this purpose, there is still limited information about this combination of biomarkers [8,9]. Some specific aspects such as the optimal HPV test or p16^{INK4a} cutoffs to be used when using the combination of biomarkers have not yet been comprehensively evaluated.

We found that the concordance between E6*I mRNA and p16^{INK4a} among HPV-DNA-positive cases was moderate to substantial for OCC and OPC cases but only fair for LC. Albeit similar in magnitude, the concordance pattern was substantially different between OCC and OPC: For OPC, the concordant cases were mainly (75.1%) triple-positive (i.e., HPV-DNA/p16^{INK4a}/E6*I mRNA-positive), whereas, for OCC, they decreased to 43.6%, and the percentage of HPV-DNA/p16^{INK4a}/E6*I mRNA triple-negative cases increased from 7.0% in OPC to 35.9% in OCC, meaning that a much lower proportion of OCC than OPC cases are truly HPV-driven. The reduction in p16^{INK4a} and E6*I mRNA concordance in LC was mainly due to a decrease in the triple positivity. Noteworthily, the proportion of cases HPV-DNA0positive/p16^{INK4a}0negative/E6*I mRNA0positive was much higher in LC than in OPC and OCC (39.2% vs. 16.0 % and 16.7%, respectively), strengthening the argument that p16^{INK4a} testing, even in combination with another HPV test, is not useful to diagnose an HPV-driven LC.

It has been previously reported that a higher proportion of both OCC and LC than OPC cases overexpress p16^{INK4a} but are HPV-negative [15,16]. In our study on HPV-DNA-positive HNC cases, p16^{INK4a} and E6*I mRNA discrepancies were substantially higher for LC than OCC. A possible higher misclassification of OPC cases as OCC than LC could partially account for those observed differences. Other aspects such as different type of tissue or different biology of the virus by anatomical site within the head and neck could also explain the observed differences [17]. The higher percentage of HPV-DNA-positive cases for types than other HPV16 in LC than in OPC and OCC could also explain our results, since a different p16^{INK4a} expression pattern was observed in those cases as compared to HPV16-positive or HPV-positive for any type.

Regarding studies comparing p16 performance for diagnosing an HPV-driven oral cavity, laryngeal, and oropharyngeal HNC, the group of Dr. Maura L. Gillison in the USA assessed the accuracy of two different criteria for p16 positivity in HPV-related OCC, OPC, and LC [18–20]. The two p16 criteria were (1) by the cutoff point of intense staining in >70% of the tumor, or (2) by H-score, derived from the cross product of the intensity of p16 staining (0–3) and percentage of tumor staining at a maximum intensity that was defined as positive if $\geq$60. The authors found that p16 immunohistochemistry as a standalone test, whether evaluated by the cutoff point of intense staining in >70% of the tumor or by H-score, had a high positive predictive value (PPV) for high-risk HPV E6/E7 mRNA in OPC [14]. In contrast, the assay had very poor PPV in LC and OCC [19,20]. A most recent study evaluated the characteristics and association of p16 and HPV in Thai patients with oropharyngeal and non-oropharyngeal HNC and found that discordance rates of HPV/p16 status were 23% and 7% for patients with oropharyngeal and non-oropharyngeal HNC, respectively [21].

We did not observe differences between p16^{INK4a} cutoffs for any site, although a non-statistically significant higher concordance between p16^{INK4a} and E6*I mRNA was observed for all HN sites when lowering the p16^{INK4a} cutoff from ≥70% to >50%. At the time the main study was published, the internationally agreed recommendations for testing all new OPC for high-risk HPV using a nuclear and cytoplasmatic 70% cutoff of stained cells [5] in the clinical setting were not yet published. A wide variety of definitions of a positive p16^{INK4a} immunohistochemistry test were used across studies [10]. Moreover, a 70% cutoff is not required in p16 testing in non-OPC HPV-related cancer sites [22]. A recent study examined and quantified p16 immunohistochemistry staining on cell blocks of cervical neck lymph nodes in OPC and used receiver operating characteristic (ROC) curve analysis to determine an optimal cutoff value with high sensitivity and specificity [23]. It found that a threshold of 15% p16 staining in cell block maximizes sensitivity and specificity. For the main study, a nuclear and cytoplasmatic 25% cutoff of stained cells was used [1], and differences in p16^{INK4a} accuracy by cutoff were not observed for any head and neck site. Thus, when considering HPV-DNA/p16^{INK4a} double test for diagnosis of HPV-driven OCC or LC, cutoffs other than 70% for p16 immunohistochemistry could be applied. Other authors have also pointed out that the 70% p16 cutoff used for HPV-OPC diagnosis may not be fully transferable to other HNC since the squamous epithelium is different within the HN area [24].

We found that, among HPV-DNA-positive HNC cases, the percentage of discordant cases was much higher for p16^{INK4a}−/E6*I mRNA+ cases than for p16^{INK4a}+/E6*I mRNA− cases. The observation was consistent for all HN sites and p16^{INK4a} cutoffs. Noteworthily, around 70%, 31%, and 52% of HPV-DNA+/p16^{INK4a}− OPC, OCC, and LC cases, respectively, were E6*I mRNA+ and 2.5%, 8.1%, and 14.3% of HPV-DNA+/p16^{INK4a}+ OPC, OCC, and LC cases, respectively, were E6*I mRNA−. These results may indicate the need for using and optimizing an mRNA-based test rather than a DNA-based test in combination with p16^{INK4a} for diagnosing an HPV-driven HNC, as also pointed out by other authors [9]. It would be important to evaluate if p16^{INK4a}−/E6*I mRNA+ cases have different survival outcomes than p16^{INK4a}+/E6*I mRNA− cases. A study from the US in OPC found that patients who were p16-negative but HPV mRNA-positive had a prognosis somewhat closer to double-positive patients, while those who were p16-positive, but HPV mRNA-negative had a prognosis closer to that of double-negative patients [9].

When considering only cases where HPV was the truly triggering carcinogenic agent (i.e., cases HPV-DNA/HPV-E6*I mRNA double-positive) or HPV-DNA/p16^{INK4a} double-positive cases, the percentage of HPV16-positive cases increased for OCC and OPC, but decreased for LC. Moreover, the percentage of discordant cases was higher for HPV16 than HPV-non16-positive cases. These results, if confirmed in other larger studies, may have implications when designing strategies of primary prevention of HPV-driven HNC with HPV vaccination. Moreover, current clinical practice algorithms for HPV testing make no effort to discern the impact of genotypes in HNC patients. A recent study found that HPV genotypes were unevenly distributed across anatomic sites of the head and neck, with an association of certain genotypes with small cell transformation [25].

The clinical significance of HPV status in OCC and LC is unclear, and previous studies have shown mixed results [4,26]. While some studies observed a prognostic advantage of HPV-positive cases in LC but not in OCC, others found the contrary or even worse survival outcomes for HPV-positive versus negative OCC [4]. However, most of the studies were not adequately powered to detect survival differences by HPV status, since HPV-AFs in LC and OCC were relatively small. Prospective, extensive studies assessing HPV status in LC and OCC are lacking. In addition to ours, research underway is currently delineating the role of HPV and p16 testing in non-oropharyngeal sites [24,27]. Noteworthily, Doll et al. [28] also considered three different p16 cutoffs (>25%, >50%, and ≥70%) when evaluating the prognostic significance of p16 in OCC.

In order to improve the diagnostic accuracy of the HPV-DNA/p16^{INK4a} double test, both in oropharyngeal and in non-oropharyngeal HNC sites, one could consider algorithms also involving tumor morphology [28], as already proposed for OPC [9]. However, it is important to keep in mind that HPV testing in non-oropharyngeal HNC is not currently recommended in the clinical setting.

Our study had several limitations. Not all cases were tested for $p16^{INK4a}$ and E6*I mRNA, and the limited sample size did not allow assessing differences between anatomical subsites within the oral cavity, oropharynx, and larynx or between histological diagnoses. Of note, the current clinical guidelines on HPV testing in HNC do not recommend HPV testing in non-oropharyngeal HNC or in non-squamous OPC [5]. Lastly, there was a difficulty for the pathologists to classify the "gray zone", i.e., cases with the percentage of cells overexpressing p16 between 25% and 70%.

In conclusion, the diagnostic algorithm of HPV-DNA testing followed by $p16^{INK4a}$ immunohistochemistry might be helpful in the diagnosis of HPV-driven OCC and OPC, but not LC. A different $p16^{INK4a}$ expression pattern in those cases HPV-DNA-positive for types other than HPV16, as compared to HPV16-positive cases, was observed. Our study provides new insights into the use HPV-DNA, $p16^{INK4a}$, and HPV-E6*I mRNA for diagnosing an HPV-driven HNC including which are the optimal HPV test or $p16^{INK4a}$ cutoffs to be used. More studies are warranted to clarify the role of $p16^{INK4a}$ and HPV status in both OPC and non-OPC HNC.

Supplementary Materials: The following supporting information can be downloaded at: https://www.mdpi.com/article/10.3390/cancers14153787/s1, Figure S1: Number of HPV-DNA positive head and neck cancer samples included in the study, by region. Table S1: Descriptive characteristics of HPV-DNA positive head and neck cancer patients included in the analysis. Members of the ICO International HPV in Head and Neck Cancer Study Group.

Author Contributions: Conceptualization, M.M., N.M., S.d.S., F.X.B. and L.A. (Laia Alemany); data curation and methodology, B.Q., M.M., L.A. (Laia Alemany), X.W., S.T. and F.M.; formal analysis, M.M., X.W., L.A. (Laia Alemany), S.T., B.Q. and F.M.; investigation and data curation, X.W., O.C., M.A., M.T. (Miren Taberna), X.L.V., B.L.R., L.A. (Llúcia Alos), H.M., W.Q., M.P., M.T. (Massimo Tomassino), M.A.P., N.M., S.d.S., F.X.B. and L.A. (Laia Alemany); writing—original draft, M.M., X.W. and L.A. (Laia Alemany); writing—review and editing, all authors. All authors have read and agreed to the published version of the manuscript.

Funding: We thank CERCA Programme/Generalitat de Catalunya for institutional support. This study was funded by Instituto de Salud Carlos III through the projects FIS PI081535, FIS PI1102096, FIS PI1102104, and CIBERESP CB06/02/007 (co-funded by European Regional Development Fund (ERDF), a way to build Europe), by the Agència de Gestió d'Ajuts Universitaris I de Recerca AGAUR (2017SGR1085), and by the AECC (Spanish Association Against Cancer). The research leading to these results received funding from the European Union's Seventh Framework Program (FP7/2007-2013) under grant agreement n° HEALTH-F2-2011-282562 HPV-AHEAD, from the Stichting Pathologie Ontwikkeling en Onderzoek (SPOO) foundation (The Netherlands), and from Sanofi Pasteur MSD and Merck & Co, Inc.

Institutional Review Board Statement: The study was conducted in accordance with the Declaration of Helsinki and approved by the Ethics Committee of the Catalan Institute of Oncology-ICO (Comitè Ètic d'Investigació Clínica de l'Hospital Universitari de Bellvitge, L'Hospitalet de Llobregat, Spain) on 9 September 2010 (protocol code PR101/08).

Informed Consent Statement: Patient consent was waived due to the characteristics of the study using archival tumor samples from 29 countries and its retrospective nature, since it represented an unreasonable effort (disproportionate time, work, and expenses).

Data Availability Statement: Data supporting reported results can be provided upon request to lalemany@iconcologia.net or mmena@iconcologia.net.

Conflicts of Interest: The study funders had no role in the design, analyses, interpretation and presentation of results, or the decision to submit for publication. Hisham Mehanna received research funding and speaker fees from GSK Biologicals and SPMSD. Nubia Muñoz is a member of the HPV Global Advisory Board of Merck. F. Xavier Bosch received institutional research funding from Merck, SPMSD, GSK Biologicals, Qiagen, Roche, Seegene, Hologic, and Genticel, occasional speaker fees from Merck, GSK, Roche, and SPMSD, and occasional travel grants from Merck, GSK, Roche,

Seegene, and SPMSD. Silvia de Sanjosé received institutional research funding from Merck, SPMSD, GSK Biologicals, and Qiagen and occasional travel assistance from Merck. Miren Taberna received scientific advisory board fees, speaker's fees, travel grants, or nonfinancial support from Merck, Astra Zeneca, Nanobiotics, MSD, and Bristol Meyers. The Cancer Epidemiology Research Program (Sara Tous, Beatriz Quiros, Xin Wang, Omar Clavero, Francisca Morey, Miquel Angel Pavón, Laia Alemany, and Marisa Mena) received sponsorship for grants from Merck and Co., Seegene, Hologic, and GSK. Michael Pawlita received institutional research funding from Roche and Qiagen. The remaining authors declare no conflicts of interest.

References

1. Castellsagué, X.; Alemany, L.; Quer, M.; Halec, G.; Quirós, B.; Tous, S.; Clavero, O.; Alòs, L.; Biegner, T.; Szafarowski, T.; et al. HPV Involvement in Head and Neck Cancers: Comprehensive Assessment of Biomarkers in 3680 Patients. *J. Natl. Cancer Inst.* **2016**, *108*, djv403. [CrossRef] [PubMed]
2. Ferlay, J.; Colombet, M.; Soerjomataram, I.; Mathers, C.; Parkin, D.M.; Znaor, A.; Bray, F. Estimating the global cancer incidence and mortality in 2018: GLOBOCAN sources and methods. *Int. J. Cancer* **2019**, *144*, 1941–1953. [CrossRef] [PubMed]
3. de Martel, C.; Georges, D.; Bray, F.; Ferlay, J.; Clifford, G.M. Global burden of cancer attributable to infections in 2018: A worldwide incidence analysis. *Lancet Glob. Health* **2020**, *8*, e180–e190. [CrossRef]
4. Schmitt, N.C. HPV in non-oropharyngeal head and neck cancer: Does it matter? *Ann. Transl. Med.* **2020**, *8*, 1120. [CrossRef]
5. Lewis, J.S., Jr.; Beadle, B.; Bishop, J.A.; Chernock, R.D.; Colasacco, C.; Lacchetti, C.; Moncur, J.T.; Rocco, J.W.; Schwartz, M.R.; Seethala, R.R.; et al. Human Papillomavirus Testing in Head and Neck Carcinomas: Guideline From the College of American Pathologists. *Arch. Pathol. Lab. Med.* **2018**, *142*, 559–597. [CrossRef]
6. Executive Board, 144. *Accelerating the Elimination of Cervical Cancer as a Global Public Health Problem: Draft Decision Proposed by Australia, Brazil, Canada, Colombia, Ecuador, India, Kenya, Monaco, Mozambique, New Zealand, Peru, Republic of Korea, South Africa, Sri Lanka, Ukraine, United States of America, Uruguay and the European Union and Its Member States*; World Health Organization: Geneva, Switzerland, 2019. Available online: https://apps.who.int/iris/handle/10665/327777 (accessed on 31 July 2022).
7. McMullen, C.; Chung, C.H.; Hernandez-Prera, J.C. Evolving role of human papillomavirus as a clinically significant biomarker in head and neck squamous cell carcinoma. *Expert Rev. Mol. Diagn.* **2019**, *19*, 63–70. [CrossRef]
8. Mena, M.; Taberna, M.; Tous, S.; Marquez, S.; Clavero, O.; Quiros, B.; Lloveras, B.; Alejo, M.; Leon, X.; Quer, M.; et al. Double positivity for HPV-DNA/p16(ink4a) is the biomarker with strongest diagnostic accuracy and prognostic value for human papillomavirus related oropharyngeal cancer patients. *Oral Oncol.* **2018**, *78*, 137–144. [CrossRef]
9. Shinn, J.R.; Davis, S.J.; Lang-Kuhs, K.A.; Rohde, S.; Wang, X.; Liu, P.; Dupont, W.D.; Plummer, D., Jr.; Thorstad, W.L.; Chernock, R.D.; et al. Oropharyngeal Squamous Cell Carcinoma With Discordant p16 and HPV mRNA Results: Incidence and Characterization in a Large, Contemporary United States Cohort. *Am. J. Surg. Pathol.* **2021**, *45*, 951–961. [CrossRef]
10. Prigge, E.S.; Arbyn, M.; von Knebel Doeberitz, M.; Reuschenbach, M. Diagnostic accuracy of p16 (INK4a) immunohistochemistry in oropharyngeal squamous cell carcinomas: A systematic review and meta-analysis. *Int. J. Cancer* **2017**, *140*, 1186–1198. [CrossRef]
11. de Sanjosé, S.; Serrano, B.; Tous, S.; Alejo, M.; Lloveras, B.; Quirós, B.; Clavero, O.; Vidal, A.; Ferrándiz-Pulido, C.; Pavón, M.A.; et al. Burden of Human Papillomavirus (HPV)-Related Cancers Attributable to HPVs 6/11/16/18/31/33/45/52 and 58. *JNCI Cancer Spectr.* **2018**, *2*, pky045. [CrossRef]
12. Fleiss, J.L. *Statistical Methods for Rates and Proportions*, 2nd ed.; John Wiley and Sons: Hoboken, NJ, USA, 1981.
13. Rosner, B. *Fundamentals of Biostatistics*, 5th ed.; Dubxury Press: Belmont, CA, USA, 2000.
14. Landi, J.R.; Koch, G.G. An Application of Hierarchical Kappa-Type Statistics in the Assessment of Majority Agreement among Multiple Observers. *Biometrics* **1977**, *33*, 363–374. [CrossRef]
15. Hernandez, B.Y.; Rahman, M.; Lynch, C.F.; Cozen, W.; Unger, E.R.; Steinau, M.; Thompson, T.; Saber, M.S.; Altekruse, S.F.; Goodman, M.T.; et al. p16(INK4A) expression in invasive laryngeal cancer. *Papillomavirus Res.* **2016**, *2*, 52–55. [CrossRef]
16. Palve, V.; Bagwan, J.; Krishnan, N.M.; Pareek, M.; Chandola, U.; Suresh, A.; Siddappa, G.; James, B.L.; Kekatpure, V.; Kuriakose, M.A.; et al. Detection of High-Risk Human Papillomavirus in Oral Cavity Squamous Cell Carcinoma Using Multiple Analytes and Their Role in Patient Survival. *J. Glob. Oncol.* **2018**, *4*, 1–33. [CrossRef]
17. Leemans, C.R.; Snijders, P.J.F.; Brakenhoff, R.H. The molecular landscape of head and neck cancer. *Nat. Rev.* **2018**, *18*, 269–282. [CrossRef]
18. Jordan, R.C.; Lingen, M.W.; Perez-Ordonez, B.; He, X.; Pickard, R.; Koluder, M.; Jiang, B.; Wakely, P.; Xiao, W.; Gillison, M.L. Validation of methods for oropharyngeal cancer HPV status determination in US cooperative group trials. *Am. J. Surg. Pathol.* **2012**, *36*, 945–954. [CrossRef]
19. Lingen, M.W.; Xiao, W.; Schmitt, A.; Jiang, B.; Pickard, R.; Kreinbrink, P.; Perez-Ordonez, B.; Jordan, R.C.; Gillison, M.L. Low etiologic fraction for high-risk human papillomavirus in oral cavity squamous cell carcinomas. *Oral Oncol.* **2013**, *49*, 1–8. [CrossRef]
20. Taberna, M.; Resteghini, C.; Swanson, B.; Pickard, R.K.; Jiang, B.; Xiao, W.; Mena, M.; Kreinbrink, P.; Chio, E.; Gillison, M.L. Low etiologic fraction for human papillomavirus in larynx squamous cell carcinoma. *Oral Oncol.* **2016**, *61*, 55–61. [CrossRef]

21. Arsa, L.; Siripoon, T.; Trachu, N.; Foyhirun, S.; Pangpunyakulchai, D.; Sanpapant, S.; Jinawath, N.; Pattaranutaporn, P.; Jinawath, A.; Ngamphaiboon, N. Discrepancy in p16 expression in patients with HPV-associated head and neck squamous cell carcinoma in Thailand: Clinical characteristics and survival outcomes. *BMC Cancer* **2021**, *21*, 504. [CrossRef]
22. WHO Classification of Tumours Editorial Board. *Female Genital Tumours*, 5th ed.; International Agency for Research on Cancer: Lyon, France, 2020; Available online: https://publications.iarc.fr/592 (accessed on 31 July 2022).
23. Wilson, B.L.; Israel, A.K.; Ettel, M.G.; Lott Limbach, A.A. ROC analysis of p16 expression in cell blocks of metastatic head and neck squamous cell carcinoma. *J. Am. Soc. Cytopathol.* **2021**, *10*, 423–428. [CrossRef]
24. Nauta, I.H.; Heideman, D.A.M.; Brink, A.; van der Steen, B.; Bloemena, E.; Koljenović, S.; de Jong, R.J.B.; Leemans, C.R.; Brakenhoff, R.H. The unveiled reality of human papillomavirus as risk factor for oral cavity squamous cell carcinoma. *Int. J. Cancer* **2021**, *149*, 420–430. [CrossRef]
25. Mashiana, S.S.; Navale, P.; Khandakar, B.; Sobotka, S.; Posner, M.R.; Miles, B.A.; Zhang, W.; Gitman, M.; Bakst, R.L.; Genden, E.; et al. Human papillomavirus genotype distribution in head and neck cancer: Informing developing strategies for cancer prevention, diagnosis, treatment and surveillance. *Oral Oncol.* **2021**, *113*, 105109. [CrossRef]
26. Sahovaler, A.; Kim, M.H.; Mendez, A.; Palma, D.; Fung, K.; Yoo, J.; Nichols, A.C.; MacNeil, S.D. Survival Outcomes in Human Papillomavirus-Associated Nonoropharyngeal Squamous Cell Carcinomas: A Systematic Review and Meta-analysis. *JAMA Otolaryngol. Head Neck Surg.* **2020**, *146*, 1158–1166. [CrossRef]
27. Doll, C.; Steffen, C.; Beck-Broichsitter, B.; Richter, M.; Neumann, K.; Pohrt, A.; Lohneis, P.; Lehmann, A.; Heiland, M.; Stromberger, C.; et al. The Prognostic Significance of p16 and its Role as a Surrogate Marker for Human Papilloma Virus in Oral Squamous Cell Carcinoma: An Analysis of 281 Cases. *Anticancer Res.* **2022**, *42*, 2405–2413. [CrossRef]
28. Rooper, L.M.; Windon, M.J.; Hernandez, T.; Miles, B.; Ha, P.K.; Ryan, W.R.; Van Zante, A.; Eisele, D.W.; D'Souza, G.; Fakhry, C.; et al. HPV-positive Squamous Cell Carcinoma of the Larynx, Oral Cavity, and Hypopharynx: Clinicopathologic Characterization with Recognition of a Novel Warty Variant. *Am. J. Surg. Pathol.* **2020**, *44*, 691–702. [CrossRef]

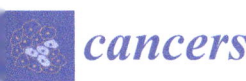

Review

Causes and Consequences of HPV Integration in Head and Neck Squamous Cell Carcinomas: State of the Art

Harini Balaji [1,2,*,†], Imke Demers [3,†], Nora Wuerdemann [1,2,4], Julia Schrijnder [3], Bernd Kremer [5], Jens Peter Klussmann [1,2,4], Christian Ulrich Huebbers [1,2,‡] and Ernst-Jan Maria Speel [3,‡]

1. Department of Otorhinolaryngology, Head and Neck Surgery, Faculty of Medicine, University of Cologne, Kerpener Strasse 62, 50931 Cologne, Germany; nora.wuerdemann@uk-koeln.de (N.W.); jens.klussmann@uk-koeln.de (J.P.K.); christian.huebbers@uk-koeln.de (C.U.H.)
2. Jean-Uhrmacher-Institute for Otorhinolaryngological Research, University of Cologne, Geibelstrasse 29–31, 50931 Cologne, Germany
3. Department of Pathology, GROW-School for Oncology and Developmental Biology, Maastricht University Medical Center, Universiteitssingel 40, 6229 ER Maastricht, The Netherlands; imke.demers@mumc.nl (I.D.); j.schrijnder@student.maastrichtuniversity.nl (J.S.); ernstjan.speel@mumc.nl (E.-J.M.S.)
4. Center for Molecular Medicine Cologne (CMMC), Faculty of Medicine, University of Cologne and University Hospital Cologne, Robert-Koch-Strasse 21, 50931 Cologne, Germany
5. Department of Otorhinolaryngology Head and Neck Surgery, GROW—School for Oncology and Developmental Biology, Maastricht University Medical Centre, P. Debyelaan 25, 6229 HX Maastricht, The Netherlands; bernd.kremer@mumc.nl
* Correspondence: harini.balaji@uk-koeln.de
† These authors contributed equally as first authors.
‡ These authors contributed equally as senior authors.

Simple Summary: In human papillomavirus (HPV) associated head and neck squamous cell carcinomas (HNSCC) s, the HPV genome is commonly found integrated in the human genome. The event of viral–human genome integration may act as a driver of carcinogenesis. Hence, it is vital to assess the viral integration status of a tumor. In this review, current and emerging techniques for integration detection are thoroughly discussed with their advantages and disadvantages. Additionally, the review also discusses the causes of HPV integration into the cellular genome, as well as its ramifications, impacting possible clinical implications.

Abstract: A constantly increasing incidence in high-risk Human Papillomaviruses (HPV)s driven head and neck squamous cell carcinomas (HNSCC)s, especially of oropharyngeal origin, is being observed. During persistent infections, viral DNA integration into the host genome may occur. Studies are examining if the physical status of the virus (episomal vs. integration) affects carcinogenesis and eventually has further-reaching consequences on disease progression and outcome. Here, we review the literature of the most recent five years focusing on the impact of HPV integration in HNSCCs, covering aspects of detection techniques used (from PCR up to NGS approaches), integration loci identified, and associations with genomic and clinical data. The consequences of HPV integration in the human genome, including the methylation status and deregulation of genes involved in cell signaling pathways, immune evasion, and response to therapy, are also summarized.

Keywords: high-risk human papillomaviruses; head and neck squamous cell carcinomas; viral DNA integration; PCR; DIPS-PCR; APOT-PCR; WGS; WES; capture-based assay; RNASeq; FISH; consequences of HPV integration

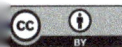

1. Introduction

Head and neck squamous cell carcinoma (HNSCC) is presently the sixth leading type of cancer worldwide, with 630,000 new patients resulting in over 350,000 deaths annually [1]. Generally, HNSCC originates from the mucosal linings of the upper aerodigestive tract. In more than 90% of the cases, HNSCCs arise in the oral cavity, oropharynx, and larynx [1,2], frequently due to the activation of oncogenes such as epidermal growth factor receptor (*EGFR*), as well as loss-of-function mutations in tumor-suppressor genes such as *TP53* and *CDKN2A* [3]. Treatment of early-stage HNSCC usually comprises surgery and/or radiotherapy. However, for patients with advanced HNSCC, multimodal treatment regimens such as surgery followed by radiation or definitive platinum-based chemoradiation are performed [2,3]. Additionally, in advanced and/or metastasized HNSCC, targeted therapy with the EGFR specific monoclonal antibody Cetuximab or immunotherapy using anti-PDL1 antibodies may be incorporated into the patient treatment regime [2,4–6]. Patient treatments unfortunately cause early and late toxicity which severely lower the quality of life [4]. Moreover, preneoplastic sites often persist after treatment, allowing the possibility of local recurrences and second primary tumors which are both responsible for a large proportion of deaths [2].

HNSCC carcinogenesis can be majorly classified into HNSCC mediated by high-risk human papilloma virus (HPV) infection and HPV-negative HNSCC that is primarily caused by tobacco and alcohol consumption [7]. Over the last decade, a striking increase in HPV-positive HNSCC incidences has been observed in the Western world [2], especially of oropharyngeal squamous cell carcinoma (OPSCC)s. Up to 90% of the OPSCCs have been associated with HPV [8]. Furthermore, it has been reported that, in the USA, the incidence of HPV-positive HNSCCs has surpassed that of HPV-positive cervical SCCs [9,10].

Despite the morphological (e.g., poorly differentiated), molecular (e.g., less chromosomal aberrations), and clinical characteristics (e.g., younger age, less tobacco and alcohol consumption) of HPV-positive tumors, patients with this type of HNSCC have a favorable prognosis, regardless of the treatment strategy applied [2,4,11]. This could be attributed to the fact that HPV-positive patients present with fewer genetic alterations, an impaired DNA double strand break repair response, and respond better to radiotherapy due to an intact apoptotic response [11]. The above are likely to be caused by single tumor-initiating events rather than field carcinogenesis. This is generally observed with younger and healthier age groups and hence they display fewer comorbidities. Moreover, radiotherapy and chemotherapy could trigger an immunological response against virus-specific antigens [12]. Nevertheless, additional risk factors such as smoking, EGFR overexpression, advanced nodal stage, and chromosomal instability can cause poor prognosis in patients with HPV-positive HNSCCs [8].

For a biologically relevant HPV infection, a couple of events are considered to be essential. Sites of infection involve stratified keratinocyte layers of epidermal origin. The virus particularly prefers functional epithelial appendages, such as salivary glands in the oral cavity and tonsillar crypts, as well as sites where stratified epithelium is adjacent to columnar epithelium, for instance in the uterine cervical transformation zone [13]. These sites are thought to be preferentially targeted because they lack the highly structured barrier function of the epithelium and have an increased occurrence of epithelial reserve cells/stem cells. To hijack these cells, wounds/microlesions are furthermore required to reach the basal cell layer so that it is ensured that actively proliferating cells become infected. At the sites of (micro)injury, an influx of serum containing Heparan sulfate proteoglycan (HSPGs), growth factors (GFs), and cytokines are produced to promote wound healing. Subsequently, HPV L1 capsid protein binds to exposed HSPGs [14]. In addition, virions binding to α6-integrins is required, initiating further intracellular signaling events. In turn, conformational changes induced in HSPGs result in L2 cleavage, binding of the exposed L2 N-terminus to an L2-specific receptor (annexin A2 heterotetramer), and subsequent clathrin-, caveolin-, lipid raft-, flotillin-, cholesterol-, and dynamin-independent endocytosis of HPV16 [15].

Starting from a transient HPV infection, the viral genome maintains as extra-chromosomal episomes. However, persistent infection by high-risk HPVs may lead to the integration of viral genome into the host genome. Viral integration requires both viral and host DNA breakage. Therefore, the rate of integration is expected to be related to the degree of DNA damage, which can be induced by a number of factors (Figure 1) [15,16]. In particular, excessive amounts of reactive nitrogen and oxygen species originating, for example, from inflammation caused by HPV infection itself (especially through the expression of E6 and E7) or from coinfection with other pathogens, as well as toxic agents originating from environmental or other sources, can cause DNA damage [17–19]. In addition, Apolipoprotein B mRNA-editing catalytic (APOBEC) polypeptides are recently identified as a source of DNA damage, as will be discussed later. Subsequently, there is accumulation of chromosomal alterations and activation of DNA damage repair mechanisms that could promote viral integration. Two possible mechanisms have been proposed by which integration occurs, namely direct insertion and looping integration (Figure 2).

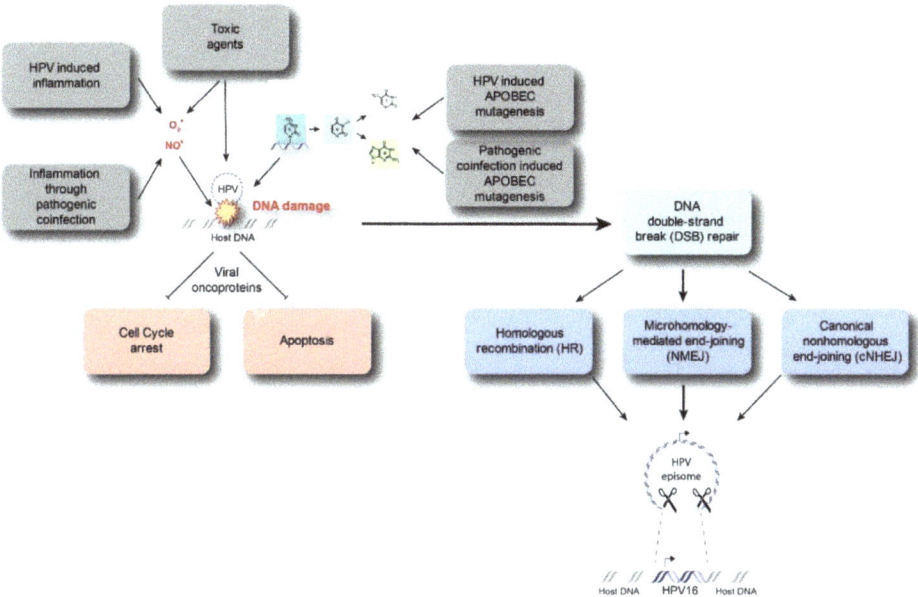

Figure 1. Discussed drivers of DNA damage and HPV integration. Intrinsic and extrinsic drivers such as inflammation, toxic agents, or APOBEC mutagenesis caused by HPV infection are able to instigate DNA damage. Subsequently, chromosomal aberrations and DNA damage repair mechanisms might promote viral integration. APOBEC = Apolipoprotein B mRNA-editing catalytic polypeptide.

Direct insertion is thought to occur by a process known as microhomology-mediated end-joining (MMEJ), which can be caused by the interference of HPV oncoproteins with the DNA double-strand break (DSB) repair pathway. MMEJ is highly error-prone and acts as a backup pathway for defects that occur in the homologous recombination (HR) pathways or major canonical non-homologous end-joining (cNHEJ) [20]. This can lead to repair events that are lethal. Interestingly, increased microhomology has been observed between HPV virus and viral integration genomic sites in oropharyngeal and cervical cancers, signifying a role of MMEJ. This is achieved when the broken viral genome exploits sequence homology, i.e., identical genomic nucleotide sequence, between the viral ends and the host genome. This is followed by deletion of these microhomologies from both genomes and insertion of the viral genome as a single genome or as concatemerized genomes into the host genome [21]. The DNA looping integration model proposes recurrent patterns of focal amplification and rearrangements, resulting in concatemers present downstream from the integration sites. This suggests that concatemers of the host and viral genomes become amplified in tandem and are reinserted back into the host genome [22]. Moreover, this may explain extrachromosomal virus-host fusion episomes that can arise when looping integration occurs without reinsertion [21].

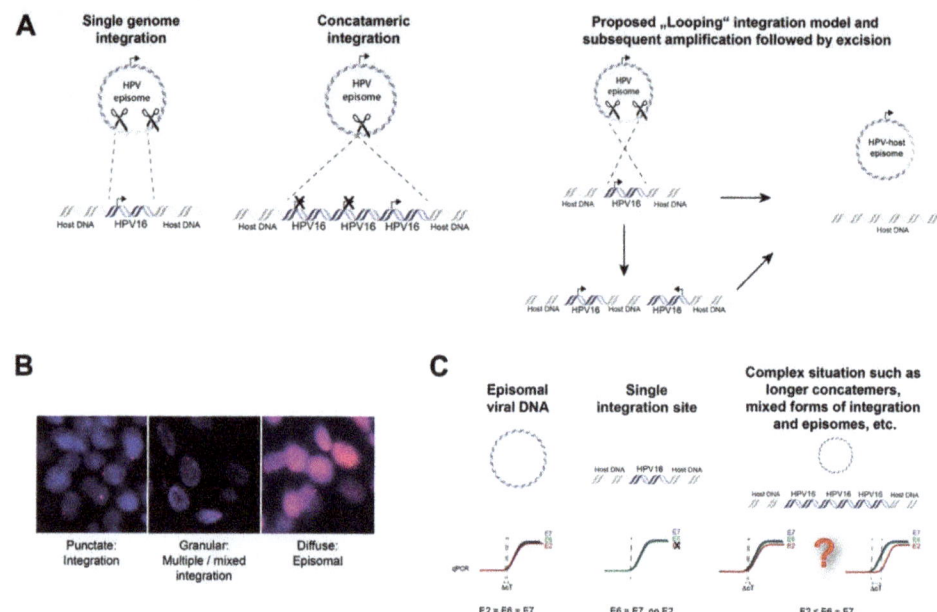

Figure 2. Mechanisms of episomal HPV-DNA integration into the human genome and non-sequencing based methods to prove integration. (**A**) Direct integration of a single viral genome into the host genome; direct integration of concatamerized viral genomes and proposed "Looping" integration of the viral genome with recurrent patterns of focal amplification and rearrangements next to the integration sites which finally may lead to excision and loss of viral DNA or viral-human fusion episomes; (**B**) fluorescence in situ hybridization with probes against HPV16 of tumor cells depicting integrated, mixed episomal and integrated and episomal status, magnification 100×; (**C**) qPCR strategy to analyze viral integration. An E2/E6 copy number ratio ≠ 1 may indicate disrupted E2 and viral integration. However, concatamerized HPV-genomes and/or additional HPV-episomes with several full-length E2 copies together with a single disrupted E2 gene will be challenging to detect.

Integration of the viral genome into the host genome often leads to deletion or truncation of the viral gene E2, resulting in loss of E2 transcript production. This in turn facilitates deregulated transcription of the viral E6 and E7 oncogenes, leading to ubiquitous expression of the corresponding E6 and E7 proteins [21]. Subsequently, this leads to deregulation of many cellular processes, including cell proliferation and apoptosis, for example by inactivation of the tumor-suppressors p53 and pRB [1–4,7–10]. Despite this knowledge, it is still unclear whether the integration of HPV into the human genome is associated with distinct biological consequences. Moreover, the association between HPV integration and poor patient outcomes is still debated, and results are controversial. Furthermore, tumors with a mixed viral physical status have been identified, posing the question whether or not these tumors show different biological behavior than tumors with solely integrated or episomal virus. This work aims to summarize the recent literature and adds to the knowledge of three reviews on HPV integration in HNSCC [15,21,23].

2. Materials and Methods

To find relevant literature on the causes and consequences of HPV integration in HNSCC, a detailed search was performed in the PubMed database (https://pubmed.ncbi.nlm.nih.gov, accessed 5 July 2021) using the search terms indicated in Appendix A. The timeframe of this analysis was fixed, by including papers published between January 2016 and April 2021. This systematic search resulted in a total of 101 papers, which were evaluated by reading the abstract followed by the full text (H.B. and I.D.). Thirty-six papers were eventually included in this study because they contained information about the physical status of HPV (episomal, integration) and HNSCC. One paper was included by screening references of the selected papers. To provide information, advantages and disadvantages of techniques to detect viral integration, 11 additional papers were included from PubMed database using search terms describing the different techniques

3. Results

3.1. Involvement of APOBEC Mediated Anti-Viral Defense in HPV Integration

Besides known mechanisms that can lead to DNA damage as represented in Figure 1, recent literature has provided evidence that Apolipoprotein B mRNA-editing catalytic (APOBEC) polypeptides are likely involved in HPV integration. APOBECs represent a family of 11 DNA cytosine deaminases that are a vital arm of the innate immune response. They potently inhibit retrovirus, transposon, and DNA virus replication. APOBECs catalyze the deamination of cytidine in both DNA and RNA. Inappropriate APOBEC expression has been identified as a genomic mutator that can eventually cause cancer [24]. Kondo et al., have reported that APOBECA3A (A3A) or A3B (A3B) expressions are involved in replication inhibition and increases the number of double strand breaks [24]. This in turn induces genomic instability and causes favorable circumstances for viral integration. Moreover, they found that A3A can catalyze the hypermutation of viral E2 and further state that A3A-induced deamination may increase the chance of viral integration Furthermore, supporting the results of Kondo et al., it was observed that the expression of A3B was found to be significantly higher in HPV-positive HNSCCs than in HPV-negative HNSCCs [25]. This additionally suggests that the high A3B expression in HPV-positive HNSCCs can cause beneficial genomic conditions allowing HPV integration. In conclusion, this association between APOBEC induced mutational signatures and HPV suggests that an impaired antiviral defense is a driving force in HPV-positive HNSCCs [25].

3.2. Approaches to Detect HPV Integration in Tumor Tissue

To date, several techniques have been used to detect HPV integration in tumor tissue. Initially, approaches included in situ hybridization (ISH) or fluorescence in situ hybridization (FISH), which could visualize HPV DNA or RNA as well as viral integration at the single cell level in cells and tissues (Figure 2B). Alternatively, PCR-based techniques have been developed, including quantitative PCR (qPCR), which determines E6/E7 copy numbers in relation to E2, Detection of Integrated Papillomavirus Sequences (DIPS) PCR which detects virus-human DNA sequences, and Amplification of Papillomavirus Oncogene Transcripts (APOT) PCR, which detects virus–human RNA transcripts (Figures 2C and 3).

In addition, Next Generation Sequencing (NGS) techniques have been coming of age, including Whole Genome Sequencing (WGS), Whole Exome Sequencing (WES), and RNASeq, all identifying HPV-human nucleic acid sequences (Figure 3).

Emerging techniques are being developed, investigating viral integration in combination with HPV sequences capturing utilizing HPV-specific custom-made RNA probes. This enables DNA enrichment for viral sequences, increasing the chance to find HPV integration. This enrichment step is followed by amplification and NGS [17–19]. Examples of emerging techniques to detect HPV integration are nanopore sequencing on DNA/RNA isolated from fresh frozen tissues, combining HPV capturing with long read sequencing, as well as Targeted Locus Amplification (TLA) on DNA isolated from FFPE tissues, combining HPV capturing with circularization of DNA fragments and amplification (Figure 3). An overview of all the currently used techniques to identify HPV integration, as well as their advantages and disadvantages, are given in Table 1.

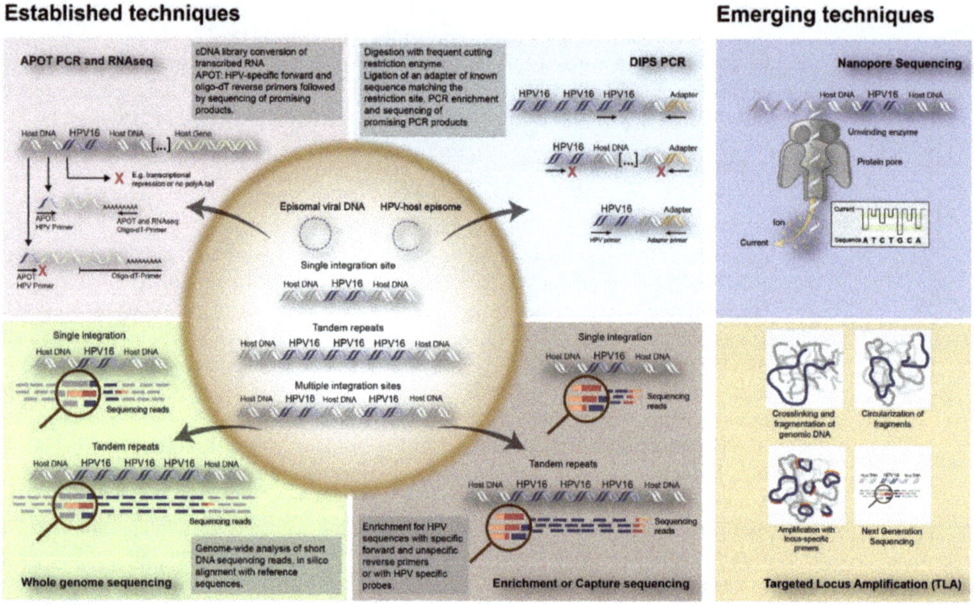

Figure 3. Overview of established and emerging techniques to detect HPV integration into the human genome. The established techniques to detect integration include RNA based techniques such as APOT PCR and RNAseq; DNA based techniques such as DIPS PCR, WGS, and Enrichment or Capture sequencing. Nanopore Sequencing and TLA are represented as emerging techniques for HPV integration detection. APOT = amplification of papilloma virus oncogene transcripts assay; DIPS-PCR = Detection of integrated papillomavirus sequences by ligation-mediated PCR; RNAseq = RNA sequencing.

Table 1. Advantages and disadvantages of techniques used to detect HPV integration.

Technique		Advantages	Disadvantages	Ref
In-situ hybridization (ISH)	(Fluorescence) in-situ hybridization ((F) ISH)	Highly sensitive Suitable for morphologically preserved isolated cells, histological tissue sections or chromosome preparations Relatively fast results within one day Relatively expensive with respect to PCR; relatively cheap with respect to sequencing Able to identify number of integration sites per nucleus Able to determine if integration site produces active transcripts (RNAse and DNAse pre-treatment)	Requires prior knowledge about sequence of interest, e.g., in case of human–virus colocalization Requires probe mixture to allow high-risk HPV detection, typing needs additional ISH experiment Cannot determine site of integration if only virus probe is used Cross-hybridization can occur when analyzing highly similar sequences (e.g., HPV6 and HPV11)	[26,27]
Polymerase Chain Reaction (PCR)	Quantitative or Real-Time PCR (qPCR, RT-PCR)	Highly specific Extremely sensitive Suitable for fresh frozen material Relatively cheap with respect to sequencing Able to detect viral load based on fluorescence timing	Less suitable for FFPE 1 material Cannot determine site of integration Cannot indicate physical status Cut-off for E2:E6/7-ratio is either less or strong discriminating Integration can occur in different genes: E2 is not always deleted, E1 can also be deleted	[28,29]

Table 1. Cont.

Technique		Advantages	Disadvantages	Ref
Polymerase Chain Reaction (PCR)	Detection of Integrated Papillomavirus Sequences PCR (DIPS-PCR)	Suitable for fresh frozen material Relatively cheap with respect to sequencing Able to indicate physical status Able to determine site of integration.	Less suitable for FFPE material Aimed only at fractures in E2 Restriction enzyme is a limiting factor, since the site of integration into the human genome is unknown Digested fragment needs to be at correct length: too long fragments make it difficult to be accurately detected by PCR, too short fragments ensures that integration site remains unknown	[30–33]
	Amplification of Papillomavirus Oncogene Transcripts PCR (APOT-PCR)	Suitable for fresh frozen material Relatively cheap with respect to sequencing Able to indicate physical status Able to determine site of integration if integration occurred in a gene Able to determine if integration site produces active transcripts Highly accurate Highly sensitive, even with large number of samples Able to determine site of integration and viral copy number Able to identify both 5′ and 3′ end breakpoints through hybrid reads Little to no bias due to nature of technique	Less suitable for FFPE material Requires stable RNA of good quality Requires expression of active transcripts Cannot determine site of integration if integration occurred in an intergenic region or an intron due to alternative splicing	[30–33]
Next Generation Sequencing (NGS)	RNASeq	Suitable for RNA from blood, fresh-frozen biopsy, FFPE, fine needle aspirates, core needle biopsies and single cells Able to deep profile the transcriptome Able to determine if integration site produces active transcripts Requires lower depth to find 3′ HPV breakpoints with respect to DNA-based NGS due to level of virus transcripts Unbiased approach to view entire RNA population	Cannot find 5′ ends of HPV breakpoints Cannot find HPV integrants that are transcriptionally repressed Can produce false 3′ calls with splice reads Depth may be reduced because of broadth of coverage	[21,26]
	Whole Genome Sequencing (WGS)	Suitable for genomic DNA (gDNA) from blood and fresh-frozen biopsy. Highly accurate Highly sensitive, even with large number of samples Able to determine site of integration and viral copy number Able to identify both 5′ and 3′ end breakpoints through hybrid reads Little to no bias due to nature of technique	Requires high read depth, deep sequencing and good coverage to find absolute integrant breakpoints Relatively expensive with respect to PCR and (F)ISH Relatively time consuming Cannot determine if HPV integrants are transcriptionally active	[21,34,35]

Table 1. *Cont.*

	Technique	Advantages	Disadvantages	Ref
Next-Generation Sequencing (NGS)	Whole Exome Sequencing (WES)	Suitable for genomic DNA (gDNA) from blood, fresh-frozen biopsy Highly accurate Extremely sensitive, even with large number of samples Relatively cheap with respect to WGS due to limited target Able to obtain higher depth with respect to WGS due to limited target Able to determine site of integration and viral copy number Able to identify both 5′ and 3′ end breakpoints through hybrid reads Little to no bias due to nature of technique	Less suitable for FFPE material Requires high read depth, deep sequencing and good coverage to find absolute integrant breakpoints. Cannot identify integration sites in non-coding regions. Cannot determine if HPV integrants are transcriptionally active	[21,34,35]
	Capture-based assay	Suitable for genomic DNA (gDNA) and/or RNA from blood, fresh-frozen biopsy, DNA and RNA from FFPE, fine needle aspirates, and core needle biopsies. Able to determine site of integration and viral copy number Able to identify both 5′ and 3′ end breakpoints through hybrid reads Increases chance of finding HPV integration sites due to sequence capture Little to no bias due to nature of technique Can be adapted for additional methods, such as chromosome conformation studies	Requires high read depth, deep sequencing and good coverage to find absolute integrant breakpoints Requires individual probes for each HPV type Cannot determine if HPV integrants are transcriptionally active Excludes majority of host sequence	[21,36]
Emerging Techniques	Nanopore Sequencing	Imaging equipment is not required; hence the system can be scaled down to portable level On comparison to other massively parallel sequencers, the device is of much lower cost The captured DNA can be sequenced rapidly Long reads of DNA can be sequenced Able to sequence long repetitive DNA sequences and structural variants	Less suitable for FFPE [1] material Not suitable for single nucleotide variation detection Extremely high molecular weight DNA needed for library preparation The sequencer has the drawback of having high error rate ranging from 5% to 20%, based on the sort of molecules and methods of library preparation	[37]
	Targeted Locus Amplification	Suitable for purified gDNA from fresh-frozen tissues, fresh tissues and FFPE material Does not require detailed knowledge on locus sequence information Able to determine site of integration and viral copy number Able to identify both 5′ and 3′ end breakpoints through hybrid reads Increases chance of finding HPV integration sites due to sequence capture	Requires high read depth, deep sequencing and good coverage to find absolute integrant breakpoints Complex and extensive integration profile may be challenging to map out completely. Integration sites could be missed in case of a large number of episomal HPV	[38]

Table 1. *Cont.*

Technique		Advantages	Disadvantages	Ref
Emerging Techniques	Targeted Locus Amplification	Relatively long reads of DNA can be sequenced (1 kb in FFPE up to 50–100 kb in fresh cells) surrounding a known/specific sequence/captured target enabling more robust analysis with respect to traditional/standard DNA-based NGS.	Requires individual probes for each HPV type Cannot determine if HPV integrants are transcriptionally active Excludes majority of host sequence	[38]

[1] FFPE = formalin fixed paraffin embedded.

As mentioned above, an increasing number of studies have employed NGS techniques to determine the presence and location of the HPV integration in the human host genome. Inherent to reliable NGS data is an optimal bioinformatic pipeline that ensures rapid and exclusive detection of the viral genome from the large-scale genome-wide DNA sequencing of the cancer genome, typically by detecting virus-host chimeric fusions or paired-end reads [21]. Various bioinformatical approaches to identify viral integration sites have been described in the literature, including VirusSeq, VirusFinder, SurVirus, VirTect, HIVID2, and HGT-ID, which have been used to detect integrated HPV genomes specifically [39–49]. The variety of viral integration detection software tools might at least partly explain the broad range in the number of reported HPV integration sites (0–600) in cervical cancers [22,50,51]. It has been suggested that these high integration rates are a result of a low-stringency bioinformatics approach [21]. When mapping integration sites, multiple aspects that may induce artifacts in bioinformatic data should be considered. For example, splicing from within the HPV genome into the distal host genome could result in a fusion transcript, which can be misidentified as a breakpoint. In addition, sequencing machine contamination could lead to overestimation of HPV integration sites and bioinformatic tools may not be able to differentiate between reads from circularized (episomal) sequences and linearized genome sequences. Furthermore, artifacts could be introduced due to microhomology sites, duplicate reads, mitochondrial genomes integrating in a highly similar manner as human genomic DNA, and mismatch bases. Hence, there is a necessity for quality control of the bioinformatics data and confirmation of integration sites by other established techniques [21,52].

As a consequence, newly developed bioinformatic tools have recently been described in the literature, of which some examples will be explained below. Viral integration and Fusion identification (ViFi) has been presented as a new tool in detecting viral integrations from WGS data and human–virus fusion mRNA from RNAseq data. Unlike other bioinformatic pipelines that only use reference-based alignment mapping to identify viral reads, ViFi combines this with a phylogenetic model of HPV families to better detect evolutionarily divergent viruses [53]. An approach that detects Virus integration sites through Reference Sequence customization (VERSE) was first described in 2015 and is designed to 'correct' human reference genomes to create a new 'personalized' human reference genome, which aims to improve alignment of short reads and thereby virus detection sensitivity through WGS, RNAseq, and targeted sequencing [25,54]. A number of capture-based sequencing methods have been reported with bioinformatics tools. For example, nanopore sequencing distinguishes itself from other sequencing techniques as it enables sequencing of extremely long DNA molecules. This is at the cost of less sequence accuracy and the inability to sequence relatively short DNA and RNA isolated from FFPE material (Table 1). Specifically designed bioinformatic methods are being developed to analyze the entire ultra-long sequencing reads and to perform error correction of the sequence data [36]. Furthermore, a novel pipeline, specifically for targeted capture sequencing data, has been generated, referred to as SearcHPV [55]. It has shown to operate in a more accurate and efficient manner than existing pipelines on capture sequencing data, something which has been lacking in the field. Another advantage of this software is that it performs local assembly of overlapping DNA segments around the junction site, which simplifies confirmation experiments.

Cameron et al. developed a virus-centric approach, called VIRUSBreakend. This tool uses single breakends, breakpoints in which only one side can be unambiguously placed to the reference genome, with the advantage that viral integration can be detected in regions of low mappability, such as centromeres and telomeres. VIRUSBreakend first identifies the viral genome within the host genome, compares this to viral NCBI taxonomy IDs, selects a viral reference genome based on sequence similarity, and aligns all read pairs with this viral reference genome. Subsequently, single breakends are assembled and host integration sites are identified [56].

3.3. Prevalence of HPV Integration

Uterine cervical SCCs are HPV-positive in 95–100% of the cases with varying frequencies of integration for different HPV subtypes. HPV16 tends to integrate in 50–80% of the cases and HPV18 in >90% [15,21,32]. In OPSCCs, HPV positivity ranges from 20–90% in different studies depending on geographical location, sample preparation, and detection method used, and, furthermore, 90–95% of virus-positive OPSCCs are infected with HPV16 [44,57].

Using FISH with whole virus genome probes, HPV integration percentages of 40–60% were described for OPSCCs [58]. An integration incidence of 40–100% was reported in tonsillar squamous cell carcinomas (TSCC)s using DIPS and APOT PCR techniques [32,59]. Recent literature describing E2, E6/E7 qPCR based HPV integration detection shows lower integration percentages (5–25%), dependent on anatomical tumor location, and a larger proportion of tumors containing both integrated and episomal HPV DNA (40–85%) [37,50–52,58,60,61]. Integration rates determined with NGS-based techniques range from 15% to 70% [60,62]. However, the number of included patients is often low and the majority of studies included tumors originating from multiple locations, also outside the oropharynx. In addition, often no distinction is made between solely integrated HPV and the mixed form, in which episomal DNA is also present. These aspects, among others, make it difficult to directly compare studies and observed integration rates. Furthermore, differences in applied bioinformatic pipelines to detect viral integration might also contribute to divergent integration rates, as mentioned before.

3.4. Low HPV Copy Numbers Are Associated with Integration in Liquid Biopsy

Recent research has shown that HPV DNA can also be efficiently detected in liquid biopsies (blood plasma, saliva), as part of the cell free DNA (cfDNA) fraction, and it is a promising biomarker for detection of early primary OPSCCs especially in groups of high risk patients [63]. cfDNA comprise DNA fragments of 160–180 base pairs, released in the blood by processes including apoptosis, necrosis, and secretion. Up to 0.1–1% of this cfDNA may consist of circulating tumor DNA. Plasma circulating tumor HPV-DNA (ctHPVDNA) can be measured over time to analyze the response of the tumor during cancer therapy using multianalyte digital PCR assays. Chera et al. investigated whether ctHPVDNA levels were associated with tumor HPV copy number and HPV physical state using digital droplet PCR [64]. In this study, the prevalence of HPV was observed in 44 patients from a total of 103 patients with OPSCC. HPV status was unknown in 49 patients though all tumors were p16^{INK4A} positive. Their results show that low baseline levels of ctHPVDNA ($\leq$200 copies/mL) were significantly associated with lower tumor HPV copy number (p = 0.04). In addition, low tumor HPV copy number ($\leq$5 copies/haploid genome) was significantly associated with HPV integration (p = 0.02). From this, it can be concluded that low base-line levels of ctHPVDNA are indicative for low tumor HPV copy number and a greater probability of HPV integration. However, in this study, only 8 out of 20 HPV16-positive patients showed viral integration. Further studies are required to investigate this correlation in a larger sample size and/or the possibility to detect HPV-human DNA fusions in plasma derived cfDNA by NGS.

Similarly, Tang et al. investigated whether HPV integration could be detected in saliva of OPSCC patients using qPCR analysis. They found a significant association between salivary HPV16 load (>10 copies/50 ng) and advanced disease stages [59]. Moreover, they identified mixed or fully integrated HPV in the saliva of 4 out of 127 OPSCC patients of which 74 patients harbored HPV16 DNA and 89 patients showed p16^{INK4A} staining. Even though this number is small and no correlation with disease stage was observed, the authors suggest that these results should be analyzed in a larger cohort.

3.5. Loci of HPV Integration in the Human Genome

Molecular studies have provided evidence that ≥1 integration site (s) can be detected in HPV-positive cancers, including HNSCC [15,65]. HPV integration sites are distributed all over the human genome and often lie within or close to fragile sites. HPV integration hotspots have been found in chromosome 2q22.3, 3p14.2, 3q28, 8q24.22, 9q22, 13q22.1, 14q24.1, 17p11.1, and 17q23.1–17q23.2 [65,66]. Interestingly, Walline et al., investigated if integration sites differed for oropharyngeal tumors comparing 10 HPV16 positive patients including five patients who responded well to therapy and five patients whose tumor persisted and recurred [67]. They found that, in responsive tumors, HPV often integrates in intergenic regions, whereas recurrent tumors exhibited complex HPV integration patterns in cancer-associated genes. HPV integration is most frequently detected in genic regions, most often cancer-related genes, such as oncogenes (e.g., *TP63*, *MYC*, *ERBB2*) or tumor suppressor genes (e.g., *BCL2*, *FANCC*, *HDAC2*, *RAD51B*, *CSMD1*) and to a lesser extent in miRNA regions [21,23]. For example, Parfenov et al. studied 279 HNSCC samples in which 35 patients were high risk HPV positive. They observed HPV integration in a known gene among 54% of HPV-positive OPSCC, and 17% within 20 kb of a gene [60]. Similarly, Olthof et al. analyzed 75 HPV16 OPSCC samples and identified 37 integration sites in 29 OPSCC, of which 27 were in known or predicted genes, including 17 with a known role in tumorigenesis [32]. Based on these data, amongst others, it is suggested that HPV integration is not simply a random event, but rather prefers less protected and more accessible chromosomal regions, including highly transcribed (cancer) genes [15].

An interesting finding using HPV integration detection for studying the clonal relationship between bilaterally developing TSCCs was reported by Pinatti et al. [68]. In a case study, six integration events were detected by DIPS-PCR, including two intragenic events in the genes *CD36*, involved in fatty acid import and *LAMA3*, involved in cell adhesion, migration and differentiation of keratinocytes. No identical integration sites were observed between the left and right TSCC. However, it is remarkable that both TSCCs contained HPV16 integration in *CD36*, although slightly different with respect to the genomic location, i.e., intron 5 vs. intron 6. Although the authors suggested this finding as one of the events pointing to a clonal relation between both TSCCs, further mutational profiling of cellular genes and transcripts and access to samples other than FFPE tissue with better quality DNA/RNA are required to provide more evidence for the clonal nature of both TSCCs.

3.6. Consequences of Viral Integration

3.6.1. Deregulated Viral Gene Expression

Based particularly on cell transfection studies, the general view is that, upon viral integration, the viral episome is most frequently opened in the E2 open reading frame. This often leads to deletion of E4 and E5 and part of E2 and L2 [13,14,66]. Deletion of E2 disrupts its transcriptional repressor function in the viral Long Control Region (LCR), leading to upregulation of E6 and E7 and subsequent deregulation of cell signaling pathways, increased cellular proliferation and inhibition of apoptosis [11,21]. Interestingly, Reuschenbach et al. found from a total of 57 patients with HPV-positive OPSCC that 16 samples with undisrupted E2 are associated with methylation of E2 binding sites (E2BS3 and E2BSx4) in the LCR, leading to loss of protein expression, pointing to the same effect as deletion of the E2 gene. In most of the latter cases, the LCR was not methylated [69].

More recent studies reported that viral genome methylation is not per se associated with HPV physical status. Although hypermethylation within the LCR was reported in two cell lines (UM-SCC-47 and CaSki), two other cell lines (UM-SCC-104 and SiHa) with a mixed physical status of the HPV genome contained a unmethylated LCR [70]. In this respect, Hatano et al. observed that the methylation status of the integrated HPV genome in three HNSCC cell lines (UPCI:SCC090, UPCI:SCC152, and UPCI:SCC154) correlated to the methylation status of the host genome flanking the integration breakpoints [71]. As a consequence, they suggested that viral (onco)gene expression might be dependent on the location of integration.

Nevertheless, multiple studies on primary tumors have shown that disruption of E2 upon viral integration will not per se lead to increased expression of E6 and E7 oncogenes, suggesting that constitutive rather than high-level expression of viral oncogene transcripts is required in HPV induced carcinogenesis. In tumors with episomal HPV, constitutive expression of E6 and E7 has also been reported [2,58,72–75].

3.6.2. Deregulated Human Gene Expression

Besides the effects on viral oncogene expression, HPV integration might also directly or indirectly affect the host genome. Direct involvement of viral integration on human gene expression may occur when the virus is integrating in or adjacent to a cancer gene, thereby (in) activating its expression. Integration in a tumor suppressor gene might result in loss of gene function, with loss of the wildtype gene on the other chromosome, or translation of truncated proteins. Integration adjacent to an oncogene could lead to gene amplification or enhanced expression from the viral promotor. Additionally, intra -or interchromosomal rearrangements followed by altered expression of genes in these regions might occur. Figure 4A–C shows a number of examples of reported genes directly affected by viral integrants [8,15,22,23,60]. Alternatively, human gene expression may be indirectly deregulated by ubiquitous E6 and E7 expression, independent of HPV physical status. Figure 4D shows reported examples and consequences of indirect deregulation of cellular pathways and processes by HPV infection. Below, examples from the recent literature are described.

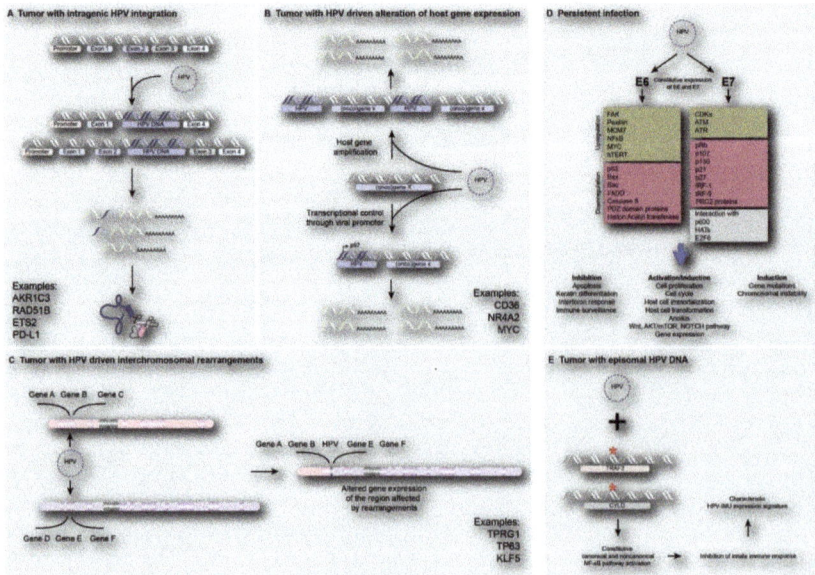

Figure 4. Direct and indirect consequences of HPV infection on human gene expression. (**A**) Integration of HPV in intragenic regions of the human genome causing loss of gene function and/or truncated

proteins e.g., *AKR1C3*, *RAD51B*, *ETS2* and *PD-L1* [22,32]; (**B**) integration of HPV near proto-oncogenes such as *CD36*, *NR4A2* and *MYC*, leading to oncogene activation, such as gene amplification or upregulation of gene expression [23]; (**C**) HPV integration may lead to interchromosomal rearrangements, amplification of genes and subsequent increase in expression of genes such as *TP63*, *TPRG1* and *KLF5* [22,32,60,76]; (**D**) The constitutive expression of E6 and E7 oncoproteins upon HPV infection (independent of physical status) will lead to deregulation of cell signaling pathways, inhibition of apoptosis, activation of cell proliferation and induction of gene mutations or chromosomal instability [11,77]; (**E**) Tumors harboring episomal HPV often show the presence of *TRAF3/CYLD* mutations leading to constitutive activation of NF-$\varkappa$B, resulting in inhibition of innate immune responses, which is a characteristic of HPV-immune response and mesenchymal cell differentiation (HPV-IMU) signature types [78].

3.6.3. Deregulated Expression of the Targeted Gene by HPV Integration

Hassounah et al. showed that HPV is able to integrate into the *CD274* gene encoding Programmed Death Ligand 1 (PD-L1), specifically in front of the sequence coding for the transmembrane domain of the protein (within the intron after exon 4) [79]. This results in transcription of a truncated isoform of PD-L1 that is unable to bind to the membrane but is rather secreted by the cell, as confirmed in vitro using cell lines and transfection experiments. The truncated isoform of PD-L1 maintains its ability to bind to PD-1, inducing a negative regulation of T cell function outside of the cell, which was confirmed by inhibition of IL-2 and IFN-γ secretion.

Additionally, Koneva et al., also identified three tumors in which *CD274* was used as an HPV integration site (integrations within intron 4 and two 'enhancer sites' upstream of *CD274*), which correlated with upregulated PD-L1 expression [80].

Broutian et al. observed HPV insertions flanking a 16-fold somatic amplification of the gene *PIM1* (Proviral insertion site for Moloney murine leukemia virus MuLV) in the HNSCC cell line UPCI:SCC090, in which more integration sites have been identified [8,22]. This amplification was accompanied by an increase of PIM1 transcripts [81]. PIM1 overexpression has been identified in HNSCCs and has been associated with poor survival [82–84]. PIM kinases are involved in cellular transformation and substrates of PIM kinase phosphorylation are involved in cell cycle progression, cell growth, and cell death. PIM1 activation causes phosphorylation of several substrates of the PIK3CA/AKT/mTOR pathway, which in turn promotes an increased activation of this pathway and allows increased cell metabolism and growth [81].

A case report published by Huebbers et al. describes a very rare malignant transformation of juvenile-onset recurrent respiratory papillomatosis of the larynx [85]. They reported that the tumor contained integration of low-risk HPV type 6 in the Aldo-Keto Reductase 1C3 (*AKR1C3*) gene, deletion of the corresponding chromosomal region 10p14–10p15.2, and loss of AKR1C3 protein expression [76].

3.6.4. Deregulated Expression of Human Genes by HPV Integration

Huebbers et al., investigated differences in human gene expression between oropharyngeal tumors with and without HPV integration (detected by APOT/DIPS PCR) [30]. They showed that AKR1C1 and AKR1C3 protein expression was upregulated in OPSCC with HPV integration. Upregulation of AKRs (compared to expression in the adjacent normal squamous epithelium) was also detected in HPV-negative OPSCC, most probably because of oxidative stress response, induced by mutations in the Keap1/Cul3/NRF2 system [30,86]. AKRs play a role in prostaglandin, steroid hormone, and retinoid metabolism. Furthermore, they are phase I detoxifying enzymes involved in the modification of chemotherapeutic drugs [76]. Interestingly, there are feedback loops between oxidative stress response and AKR1C expression with NRF2 binding to antioxidant response elements (ARE) in the promoter regions of the AKRCs increasing their expression [76]. Furthermore, the viral spliced isoform HPV16-E6*I was shown to interact with SP1-binding sites within the

AKR1C1 promoter regions also resulting in increased AKR1C1 expression [86]. On the other hand, an increase in AKR1C1 and AKR1C3 protein expression results in decreased concentrations of retinoic acids, known inhibitors of NRF2 function, which subsequently also lead to NRF2 activation [87]. The activation of NRF2 consequently activates PI3K-AKT signaling, metabolic reprogramming, cell proliferation, insufficiency in autophagy, chemotherapy resistance as well as impaired DNA damage response [30,88,89]. It was also demonstrated by Huebbers et al. and Zhang et al. that HPV16-E6*I expression was upregulated significantly in OPSCCs with integrated viral genome [30,88]. Furthermore, in both of these studies, viral integration and E6*I overexpression are correlated with keratinocyte differentiation signatures. Similarly, Paget-Bailly et al. reported that ectopic expression of HPV16 E6*I induced deregulation of cellular genes participating in ROS metabolism, promoting viral integration by inducing genome instability [90]. The presence of E6 partially counteracts the impact of E6*I. Additionally, the above is also supported by studying a clinical cohort, where the subgroup of tumors overexpressing E6*I was associated with key cancer pathways linked to ROS metabolism [91]. However, further studies should be performed to understand how E6*I regulates genes associated with oxidative stress and how this impacts HPV-driven tumorigenesis [90].

Pannone et al., showed an association between HPV integration (detected by ISH) and Toll like receptor (TLR) 4 downregulation [92]. TLRs are predominantly involved in the innate immune response to pathogens including HPV and recognize Pathogen-associated Molecular Patterns (PAMPs) such as nucleic acids or proteins of viral origin, which serve as TLR activating ligands. [93]. Ligand bound TLR4 then triggers lipid raft flowing, resulting in a conformational change. This in turn leads to aggregation of NADPH oxidase subunits on these lipid rafts resulting in ROS production and increased HIF1α expression adding to the hypoxic tumor conditions [93]. TLR4 furthermore activates signaling cascades including tumor necrosis factor receptor-associated factor 3 (TRAF3) and nuclear factor kappa-light-chain-enhancer of activated B cells (NF-κB), which regulate the production of interferons (INF), inflammatory cytokines, and chemokines. However, in uterine cervical carcinomas and HPV-positive OPSCCs, a decrease in the TLR4 expression compared to normal epithelium is observed [92]. The viral proteins E6 and E7 have the property to interfere with innate immunity, e.g., by interacting with interferon regulator factor 3 (IRF-3) (E6) or IRF-1 (E7). As a result, HPV gains the ability to escape both innate and adaptive immune response and further avoid being recognized by Antigen Presenting Cells (APC)s [92].

The presence of episomal HPV DNA also showed to correlate with deregulation of pathways involved in immune response and cell survival in an indirect manner. Hajek et al. discovered that 85% of tumors with mutations in the genes *TRAF3* and *CYLD* (Cylindromatosis Lysine 63 Deubiquitinase) contained episomal HPV (data from The Cancer Genome Atlas) [78]. *TRAF3* is one of the most frequently mutated genes in HPV-positive HNSCCs (25% of HPV-positive tumors), but, remarkably, is not usually found to be mutated in their HPV-negative counterparts (2%) [94]. In addition, the tumor suppressor gene *CYLD* was found to be mutated in 11% of HPV-positive tumors. Both TRAF3 and CYLD play a role in both negatively regulating NF-κB canonical and noncanonical pathways while simultaneously stimulating a potent and first-line antiviral response through type I IFN signaling. Mutations in these genes will therefore lead to constitutive activation of NF-κB, which promotes cell survival and an impaired innate immunity against viral infections [68,95,96]. Moreover, it is suggested that maintenance of episomal HPV even pressures cells to mutate *TRAF3/CYLD*. These mutations might provide support for an alternative mechanism of HPV tumorigenesis in HNSCCs, not depending on viral integration into the host cell genome, to provoke a malignant transformation [78].

3.7. Subgroups of HPV-Positive Tumors Associated with Viral Integration Status

Recent studies have shown that HPV-positive tumors represent a heterogeneous group with respect to mRNA expression signatures as well as HPV integration status, with biological and clinical relevance. Two main subgroups have been characterized based on mRNA expression signatures, namely HPV-IMU and HPV-KRT (HPV-keratinocyte differentiation and oxidative reduction process) [2,88,97]. Molecular analyses revealed that the HPV-KRT subgroup more frequently contains integrated HPV (70–78% of the cases), shows a lower expression of E2/E4/E5, and has a higher ratio of spliced E6 compared to full length E6, which is in agreement with observations described above. Furthermore, this group was enriched for chromosome 3q amplifications and PIK3CA mutations. HPV-IMU tumors showed less integration (25–36% of the cases) and were enriched for chromosome 16q losses (detected by RNA sequencing).

Another study of Locati et al. identified three main clusters of HPV-positive tumors; Cl1 (immune-related), Cl2 (epithelial-mesenchymal transition-related), and Cl3 (proliferation-related) [98]. Tumors classified as Cl1 showed viral integration in 45% of the cases, whereas tumors classified as Cl2 and Cl3 showed 100% and 77% integration, respectively. In addition, the three clusters have been observed to have prognostic relevance, with Cl1 correlating to the best survival rate, and Cl2 to the worst survival rate. Knowledge on subtypes within HPV-positive tumors might contribute to patient selection for either de-escalation or personalized therapeutic approaches [11].

3.8. HPV Integration in Relation to Prognosis

The association of HPV integration with patient prognosis has been a topic of debate for several years [15]. More recent studies indicate an association of viral integration with unfavorable prognosis.

Nulton et al., demonstrated, using the expression of E2 as a marker for integration in TCGA HNSCC samples, that patients with fully episomal or a mixed form of HPV16 showed better survival than patients with integrated HPV16 as well as patients with HPV-negative HNSCCs [99]. Similarly, Hajek et al. observed that the HPV-positive subset of HNSCC in the TCGA database with mutations in the genes TRAF3 and CYLD were associated with the maintenance of episomal HPV and improved survival of patients [78]. For this association, they used the NGS determined integration data from the study of Parfenov et al. [60]. Moreover, Veitía et al. evaluated 80 fresh biopsies of head and neck cancer, mostly oral cavity, larynx, and oropharynx tumors, using E2/E6 qPCR. Of the 28 HPV16 positive samples, 86% displayed integration, possessed low viral load and correlated to poor prognosis. [100]. Supporting these results, Koneva et al. showed that patients with (RNAseq determined) integration-positive oropharyngeal and oral cavity tumors had statistically significant worse survival than patients with integration-negative tumors and similar survival as patients with HPV-negative HNSCCs [80]. Moreover, patients with integrated HPV were significantly older than patients with episomal HPV and comparable to HPV-negative patients, suggesting that older age was associated with worse survival [80,99].

In addition, Huebbers et al. showed that HPV integration in oropharyngeal tumors (analyzed with APOT- and DIPS PCR) was associated with upregulation of AKR1C1 and AKR1C3 expression [30]. Upregulation of AKR1C1 and AKR1C3 correlated with negative outcomes for both chemo- and radiotherapy in both overall and disease-free survival. Contrastingly, low expression of AKR1C1 and/or AKR1C3 was significantly correlated with favorable outcomes in surgical treatment. Intriguingly, viral integration also seems to be associated with a more progressive and persistent disease [101–103].

In contrast, both Vojtechova et al. and Lim et al. showed that there were no significant differences in survival between patients with episomal, mixed or integrated HPV16 in oropharyngeal tumors (n = 186 and n = 179, respectively) [104,105]. Vojtechova used three different detection techniques (E2 transcript breakpoint analysis, APOT, and Southern blotting). Lim et al. observed a trend towards better survival in patients with mixed HPV compared to patients with either episomal or integrated HPV; however, they used E2/E6 qPCR, possibly leading to overestimation of mixed viral physical status, as discussed before.

Recently, Pinatti et al., showed, using DIPS-PCR analysis on 35 tumors, mainly of the oropharynx, that HPV integration was correlated with favorable disease-specific survival when compared to patients without integration [106].

Overall, studies reporting on the correlation of viral integration with patient prognosis of HPV-positive HNSCCs have shown inconsistent results. As mentioned before, the technique used to detect viral integration is important to consider when interpreting the results of these studies. As an example, PCR for E2 and E6/7 expression might overestimate mixed physical status of HPV. Furthermore, studies often include tumors from different anatomical locations and relatively small patient groups.

4. Conclusions

In conclusion, a number of different technologies (including FISH, PCR, and NGS) have been used to determine the physical status of HPV in HNSCC, predominantly HPV16 in oropharyngeal tumors. Dependent on the viral detection strategy, HPV integration prevalence may differ. Results indicate that HPV integration is not simply a random event but rather prefers less protected and more accessible chromosomal regions, including highly transcribed (cancer) genes. Besides known mechanisms that can lead to DNA damage and subsequent viral integration, for example ROS, toxic agents, and inflammation, recent literature has provided evidence that APOBEC expression, induced by antiviral response, is doing so. Recent studies show that HPV integration affects both the viral and host genome, leading to constitutive expression of viral oncoproteins and deregulation of cellular (cancer) genes, possibly conferring additional neoplastic pressure. HPV integration appears to upregulate genes involved in metabolic pathways and immune evasion and downregulate genes involved in inflammation, apoptosis, and immune responses. On the other hand, episomal HPV was associated with mutations in *TRAF3* and *CYLD*. Although new data suggest a correlation between HPV integration and unfavorable prognosis, more genome-wide studies with a larger sample size, especially of oropharyngeal origin, are required. Ideally, a uniform detection method utilizing NGS technology should be applied, and integration results should be validated using multiple techniques, to further investigate the biological and clinical implications of HPV integration in HNSCC.

Author Contributions: Conceptualization, H.B., I.D., J.S., C.U.H., and E.-J.M.S., methodology, H.B., I.D., J.S., C.U.H., and E.-J.M.S.; validation, H.B., I.D., J.S., C.U.H., and E.-J.M.S.; formal analysis, H.B., I.D., J.S., C.U.H., and E.-J.M.S.; investigation, H.B., I.D., J.S., C.U.H., and E.-J.M.S.; resources, B.K., J.P.K., C.U.H., and E.-J.M.S.; data curation, H.B., I.D., J.S., C.U.H., and E.-J.M.S.; writing—original draft preparation, H.B., I.D., and J.S., writing—review and editing, C.U.H. and E.-J.M.S.; visualization, H.B., I.D., J.S., C.U.H., and E.-J.M.S.; supervision, N.W., B.K., J.P.K., C.U.H., and E.-J.M.S.; project administration, H.B., I.D., J.S., C.U.H., and E.-J.M.S.; funding acquisition, B.K., J.P.K., and E.-J.M.S. All authors have read and agreed to the published version of the manuscript.

Funding: N.W. is supported by the Cologne Clinician Scientist Program (CCSP), funded by the German Research Council (FI 773/15-1).

Data Availability Statement: No new data were created or analyzed in this study. Data sharing is not applicable to this article.

Conflicts of Interest: H.B., I.D., J.S., and C.U.H. declare no conflict of interest. N.W. reports honoraria from BMS, MSD, and Merck. J.P.K. reports grants from MSD and honoraria from BMS, MSD, and Merck. B.K. reports grants from Pfizer and Novartis. E.-J.M.S. reports grants from Pfizer and Novartis and honoraria from BMS. The funders had no role in the design of the study; in the collection, analyses, or interpretation of data; in the writing of the manuscript, or in the decision to publish the results.

Appendix A. Search Terms Used for Systematic PubMed Search

- ((Head[Tiab] OR neck[Tiab] OR "head and neck" [Tiab] OR "head-neck" OR "head-and-neck" [Tiab] OR oral[Tiab] OR pharyn*[Tiab] OR OR laryn*[Tiab] OR oropharyn* [Tiab] OR nasopharyn*[Tiab] OR hypopharyn*[Tiab] OR throat[Tiab] OR glotti*[Tiab] OR mouth[Tiab] OR palate[Tiab] OR gingiva*[Tiab] OR lip[Tiab] OR cheek[Tiab] OR

- bucc*[Tiab] OR gum*[Tiab] OR tonsil*[Tiab] OR tongue[Tiab] OR nasal[Tiab] OR paranasal[Tiab] OR sinus[Tiab] OR saliv*[Tiab] OR ent[Tiab] OR aerodigestive[Tiab] OR "aero digestive" [Tiab] OR aero-digestive[Tiab])
- AND (cancer* OR carcinoma* OR neoplas* OR tumor* OR tumour* OR malignan* OR SCC OR "Neoplasms"[Mesh])) OR (hnscc[Tiab] OR scchn[Tiab] OR "Head and Neck Neoplasms"[Mesh])
- AND
- ("Human papilloma virus" [Tiab] OR "Human papilloma viruses" [Tiab] OR "Papillomavirus, Human" [Tiab] OR "Human papillomavirus" [Tiab] OR HPV [Tiab] OR HR-HPV [Tiab] OR "High-risk HPV" [Tiab] OR "HPV infection*" [Tiab] OR "Papillomavirus Infections/pathology" [Mesh])
- AND
- (integration [Tiab] OR "virus integration*" [Tiab] OR "virus integration" [Mesh] OR "Viral integration*" [Tiab] OR "human papillomavirus integration" [Tiab] OR "HPV integration" [Tiab] OR "genome integration" [Tiab] OR "viral DNA integration" [Tiab] OR "virus DNA integration" [Tiab] OR "HPV DNA integration" [Tiab] OR "HPV insertion*" [Tiab] OR "Human papillomavirus insertion*" [Tiab])

References

1. Vigneswaran, N.; Williams, M.D. Epidemiologic trends in head and neck cancer and aids in diagnosis. *Oral Maxillofac. Surg. Clin. N. Am.* **2014**, *26*, 123–141.
2. Leemans, C.R.; Braakhuis, B.J.M.; Brakenhoff, R.H. The molecular biology of head and neck cancer. *Nat. Rev. Cancer* **2010**, *11*, 9–22. [CrossRef] [PubMed]
3. Marur, S.; Forastiere, A.A. Head and Neck Squamous Cell Carcinoma: Update on Epidemiology, Diagnosis, and Treatment. *Mayo Clin. Proc.* **2016**, *91*, 386–396. [CrossRef] [PubMed]
4. Alsahafi, E.; Begg, K.; Amelio, I.; Raulf, N.; Lucarelli, P.; Sauter, T.; Tavassoli, M. Clinical update on head and neck cancer: Molecular biology and ongoing challenges. *Cell Death Dis.* **2019**, *10*, 1–17. [CrossRef]
5. Seiwert, T.Y.; Burtness, B.; Mehra, R.; Weiss, J.; Berger, R.; Eder, J.P.; Heath, K.; McClanahan, T.; Lunceford, J.; Gause, C.; et al. Safety and clinical activity of pembrolizumab for treatment of recurrent or metastatic squamous cell carcinoma of the head and neck (KEYNOTE-012): An open-label, multicentre, phase 1b trial. *Lancet Oncol.* **2016**, *17*, 956–965. [CrossRef]
6. Vermorken, J.B.; Trigo, J.; Hitt, R.; Koralewski, P.; Diaz-Rubio, E.; Rolland, F.; Knecht, R.; Amellal, N.; Schueler, A.; Baselga, J. Open-label, uncontrolled, multicenter phase II study to evaluate the efficacy and toxicity of cetuximab as a single agent in pa-tients with recurrent and/or metastatic squamous cell carcinoma of the head and neck who failed to respond to platinum-based therapy. *J. Clin. Oncol.* **2007**, *25*, 2171–2177.
7. Rietbergen, M.M.; Leemans, C.R.; Bloemena, E.; Heideman, D.A.; Braakhuis, B.J.; Hesselink, A.T.; Witte, B.I.; Baatenburg de Jong, R.J.; Meijer, C.J.; Snijders, P.J.; et al. Increasing prevalence rates of HPV attributable oropharyngeal squamous cell car-cinomas in the Netherlands as assessed by a validated test algorithm. *Int. J. Cancer* **2013**, *132*, 1565–1571. [CrossRef]
8. Olthof, N.C.; Huebbers, C.U.; Kolligs, J.; Henfling, M.; Ramaekers, F.C.; Cornet, I.; Van Lent-Albrechts, J.A.; Stegmann, A.P.; Silling, S.; Wieland, U.; et al. Viral load, gene expression and mapping of viral integration sites in HPV16-associated HNSCC cell lines. *Int. J. Cancer* **2014**, *136*, E207–E218. [CrossRef]
9. Faraji, F.; Zaidi, M.; Fakhry, C.; Gaykalova, D.A. Molecular mechanisms of human papillomavirus-related carcinogenesis in head and neck cancer. *Microbes Infect.* **2017**, *19*, 464–475. [CrossRef] [PubMed]
10. Pinatti, L.; Walline, H.; Carey, T. Human Papillomavirus Genome Integration and Head and Neck Cancer. *J. Dent. Res.* **2017**, *97*, 691–700. [CrossRef]
11. Olthof, N.C.; Straetmans, J.M.; Snoeck, R.; Ramaekers, F.C.; Kremer, B.; Speel, E.J. Next-generation treatment strategies for human papillomavirus-related head and neck squamous cell carcinoma: Where do we go? *Rev. Med. Virol.* **2012**, *22*, 88–105. [CrossRef]
12. Elrefaey, S.; Massaro, M.; Chiocca, S.; Chiesa, F.; Ansarin, M. HPV in oropharyngeal cancer: The basics to know in clinical practice. *Acta Otorhinolaryngol. Ital.* **2014**, *34*, 299–309.
13. Woodman, C.B.J.; Collins, S.I.; Young, L. The natural history of cervical HPV infection: Unresolved issues. *Nat. Rev. Cancer* **2007**, *7*, 11–22. [CrossRef]
14. Ozbun, M.A. Extracellular events impacting human papillomavirus infections: Epithelial wounding to cell signaling involved in virus entry. *Papillomavirus Res.* **2019**, *7*, 188–192. [CrossRef]
15. Speel, E.J.M. HPV Integration in Head and Neck Squamous Cell Carcinomas: Cause and Consequence. *HPV Infect. Head Neck Cancer* **2016**, *206*, 57–72. [CrossRef]
16. Williams, V.; Filippova, M.; Soto, U.; Duerksen-Hughes, P.J. HPV-DNA integration and carcinogenesis: Putative roles for inflammation and oxidative stress. *Futur. Virol.* **2011**, *6*, 45–57. [CrossRef]

17. Lace, M.J.; Anson, J.R.; Haugen, T.; Dierdorff, J.M.; Turek, L.P. Interferon treatment of human keratinocytes harboring extrachromosomal, persistent HPV-16 plasmid genomes induces de novo viral integration. *Carcinogenesis* **2014**, *36*, 151–159. [CrossRef] [PubMed]
18. Visalli, G.; Riso, R.; Facciolà, A.; Mondello, P.; Caruso, C.; Picerno, I.; Di Pietro, A.; Spataro, P.; Bertuccio, M.P. Higher levels of oxidative DNA damage in cervical cells are correlated with the grade of dysplasia and HPV infection. *J. Med. Virol.* **2015**, *88*, 336–344. [CrossRef] [PubMed]
19. Wei, L.; Gravitt, P.E.; Song, H.; Maldonado, A.M.; Ozbun, M.A. Nitric Oxide Induces Early Viral Transcription Coincident with Increased DNA Damage and Mutation Rates in Human Papillomavirus–Infected Cells. *Cancer Res.* **2009**, *69*, 4878–4884. [CrossRef] [PubMed]
20. Leeman, J.E.; Li, Y.; Bell, A.; Hussain, S.; Majumdar, R.; Rong-Mullins, X.; Blecua, P.; Damerla, R.; Narang, H.; Ravindran, P.; et al. Human papillomavirus 16 promotes microhomology-mediated end-joining. *Proc. Natl. Acad. Sci. USA* **2019**, *116*, 21573–21579. [CrossRef]
21. Groves, I.J.; Coleman, N. Human papillomavirus genome integration in squamous carcinogenesis: What have next-generation sequencing studies taught us? *J. Pathol.* **2018**, *245*, 9–18. [CrossRef] [PubMed]
22. Akagi, K.; Li, J.; Broutian, T.R.; Padilla-Nash, H.; Xiao, W.; Jiang, B.; Rocco, J.W.; Teknos, T.N.; Kumar, B.; Wangsa, D.; et al. Genome-wide analysis of HPV integration in human cancers reveals recurrent, focal genomic instability. *Genome Res.* **2013**, *24*, 185–199. [CrossRef]
23. Rusan, M.; Li, Y.Y.; Hammerman, P.S. Genomic Landscape of Human Papillomavirus–Associated Cancers. *Clin. Cancer Res.* **2015**, *21*, 2009–2019. [CrossRef] [PubMed]
24. Kondo, S.; Wakae, K.; Wakisaka, N.; Nakanishi, Y.; Ishikawa, K.; Komori, T.; Moriyama-Kita, M.; Endo, K.; Murono, S.; Wang, Z.; et al. APOBEC3A associates with human papillomavirus genome integration in oropharyngeal cancers. *Oncogene* **2016**, *36*, 1687–1697. [CrossRef]
25. Zapatka, M.; Pathogens, P.; Borozan, I.; Brewer, D.S.; Iskar, M.; Grundhoff, A.; Alawi, M.; Desai, N.; Sültmann, H.; Moch, H.; et al. The landscape of viral associations in human cancers. *Nat. Genet.* **2020**, *52*, 320–330. [CrossRef]
26. Kukurba, K.R.; Montgomery, S. RNA Sequencing and Analysis. *Cold Spring Harb. Protoc.* **2015**, *2015*, 951–969. [CrossRef]
27. Nouri-Aria, K.T. Allergy methods and protocols. In *Situ Hybridization*; Jones, M.G., Lympany, P., Eds.; Humana: Totowa, NJ, USA, 2008; Volume 138.
28. Abreu, A.L.P.; Souza, R.P.; Gimenes, F.; Consolaro, M.E.L. A review of methods for detect human Papillomavirus infection. *Virol. J.* **2012**, *9*, 262. [CrossRef]
29. Morgan, I.M.; DiNardo, L.J.; Windle, B. Integration of Human Papillomavirus Genomes in Head and Neck Cancer: Is It Time to Consider a Paradigm Shift? *Viruses* **2017**, *9*, 208. [CrossRef]
30. Huebbers, C.U.; Verhees, F.; Poluschkin, L.; Olthof, N.C.; Kolligs, J.; Siefer, O.G.; Henfling, M.; Ramaekers, F.C.; Preuss, S.F.; Beutner, D.; et al. Upregulation of AKR1C1 and AKR1C3 expression in OPSCC with integrated HPV16 and HPV-negative tumors is an indicator of poor prognosis. *Int. J. Cancer* **2019**, *144*, 2465–2477. [CrossRef]
31. Luft, F.; Klaes, R.; Nees, M.; Durst, M.; Heilmann, V.; Melsheimer, P.; von Knebel Doeberitz, M. Detection of integrated papillomavirus sequences by ligation-mediated PCR (DIPS-PCR) and molecular characterization in cervical cancer cells. *Int. J. Cancer* **2001**, *92*, 9–17. [CrossRef]
32. Olthof, N.C.; Speel, E.J.; Kolligs, J.; Haesevoets, A.; Henfling, M.; Ramaekers, F.C.; Preuss, S.F.; Drebber, U.; Wieland, U.; Silling, S.; et al. Comprehensive analysis of HPV16 integration in OSCC reveals no significant impact of physical status on viral on-cogene and virally disrupted human gene expression. *PLoS ONE* **2014**, *9*, e88718. [CrossRef]
33. Ziegert, C.; Wentzensen, N.; Vinokurova, S.; Kisseljov, F.; Einenkel, J.; Hoeckel, M.; Doeberitz, M.V.K. A comprehensive analysis of HPV integration loci in anogenital lesions combining transcript and genome-based amplification techniques. *Oncogene* **2003**, *22*, 3977–3984. [CrossRef] [PubMed]
34. Gradíssimo, A.; Burk, R.D. Molecular tests potentially improving HPV screening and genotyping for cervical cancer prevention. *Expert Rev. Mol. Diagn.* **2017**, *17*, 379–391. [CrossRef] [PubMed]
35. Petersen, B.-S.; Fredrich, B.; Hoeppner, M.P.; Ellinghaus, D.; Franke, A. Opportunities and challenges of whole-genome and -exome sequencing. *BMC Genet.* **2017**, *18*, 1–13. [CrossRef] [PubMed]
36. Harlé, A.; Guillet, J.; Thomas, J.; Demange, J.; Dolivet, G.; Peiffert, D.; Leroux, A.; Sastre-Garau, X. HPV insertional pattern as a personalized tumor marker for the optimized tumor diagnosis and follow-up of patients with HPV-associated carcinomas: A case report. *BMC Cancer* **2019**, *19*, 277. [CrossRef] [PubMed]
37. Kono, N.; Arakawa, K. Nanopore sequencing: Review of potential applications in functional genomics. *Dev. Growth Differ.* **2019**, *61*, 316–326. [CrossRef]
38. De Vree, P.J.P.; de Wit, E.; Yilmaz, M.; Van De Heijning, M.; Klous, P.; Verstegen, M.J.A.M.; Wan, Y.; Teunissen, H.; Krijger, P.; Geeven, G.; et al. Targeted sequencing by proximity ligation for comprehensive variant detection and local haplotyping. *Nat. Biotechnol.* **2014**, *32*, 1019–1025. [CrossRef]
39. Chen, Y.; Yao, H.; Thompson, E.J.; Tannir, N.M.; Weinstein, J.N.; Su, X. VirusSeq: Software to identify viruses and their inte-gration sites using next-generation sequencing of human cancer tissue. *Bioinformatics* **2013**, *29*, 266–267. [CrossRef]
40. Wang, Q.; Jia, P.; Zhao, Z. VirusFinder: Software for Efficient and Accurate Detection of Viruses and Their Integration Sites in Host Genomes through Next Generation Sequencing Data. *PLoS ONE* **2013**, *8*, e64465. [CrossRef]

41. Rajaby, R.; Zhou, Y.; Meng, Y.; Zeng, X.; Li, G.; Wu, P.; Sung, W.-K. SurVirus: A repeat-aware virus integration caller. *Nucleic Acids Res.* **2021**, *49*, e33. [CrossRef]
42. Khan, A.; Liu, Q.; Chen, X.; Stucky, A.; Sedghizadeh, P.; Adelpour, D.; Zhang, X.; Wang, K.; Zhong, J.F. Detection of human papillomavirus in cases of head and neck squamous cell carcinoma by RNA-seq and VirTect. *Mol. Oncol.* **2018**, *13*, 829–839. [CrossRef]
43. Li, W.; Tian, S.; Wang, P.; Zang, Y.; Chen, X.; Yao, Y.; Li, W. The characteristics of HPV integration in cervical intraepithelial cells. *J. Cancer* **2019**, *10*, 2783–2787. [CrossRef] [PubMed]
44. Baheti, S.; Tang, X.; O'Brien, D.R.; Chia, N.; Roberts, L.R.; Nelson, H.; Boughey, J.C.; Wang, L.; Goetz, M.P.; Kocher, J.-P.A.; et al. HGT-ID: An efficient and sensitive workflow to detect human-viral insertion sites using next-generation sequencing data. *BMC Bioinform.* **2018**, *19*, 271. [CrossRef]
45. Li, J.W.; Wan, R.; Yu, A.C.-S.; Na Co, N.; Wong, N.; Chan, T.-F. ViralFusionSeq: Accurately discover viral integration events and reconstruct fusion transcripts at single-base resolution. *Bioinformatics* **2013**, *29*, 649–651. [CrossRef] [PubMed]
46. Hawkins, T.B.; Dantzer, J.; Peters, B.; Dinauer, M.; Mockaitis, K.; Mooney, S.; Cornetta, K. Identifying viral integration sites using SeqMap 2.0. *Bioinformatics* **2011**, *27*, 720–722. [CrossRef] [PubMed]
47. Ho, D.W.; Sze, K.M.; Ng, I.O. Virus-Clip: A fast and memory-efficient viral integration site detection tool at single-base reso-lution with annotation capability. *Oncotarget* **2015**, *6*, 20959. [CrossRef] [PubMed]
48. Tennakoon, C.; Sung, W.K. BATVI: Fast, sensitive and accurate detection of virus integrations. *BMC Bioinform.* **2017**, *18*, 71–111. [CrossRef]
49. Forster, M.; Szymczak, S.; Ellinghaus, D.; Hemmrich, G.; Rühlemann, M.; Kraemer, L.; Mucha, S.; Wienbrandt, L.; Stanulla, M.; Franke, A. Vy-PER: Eliminating false positive detection of virus integration events in next generation sequencing data. *Sci. Rep.* **2015**, *5*, 1–13. [CrossRef] [PubMed]
50. Hu, Z.; Zhu, D.; Wang, W.; Li, W.; Jia, W.; Zeng, X.; Ding, W.; Yu, L.; Wang, X.; Ma, D.; et al. Genome-wide profiling of HPV integration in cervical cancer identifies clustered genomic hot spots and a potential microhomology-mediated integration mechanism. *Nat. Genet.* **2015**, *47*, 158–163. [CrossRef]
51. Liu, Y.; Zhang, C.; Gao, W.; Wang, L.; Pan, Y.; Gao, Y.; Lu, Z.; Ke, Y. Genome-wide profiling of the human papillomavirus DNA integration in cervical intraepithelial neoplasia and normal cervical epithelium by HPV capture technology. *Sci. Rep.* **2016**, *6*, 35427. [CrossRef] [PubMed]
52. Dyer, N.; Young, L.; Ott, S. Artifacts in the data of Hu et al. *Nat. Genet.* **2015**, *48*, 2–3. [CrossRef]
53. Nguyen, N.-P.; Deshpande, V.; Luebeck, J.; Mischel, P.S.; Bafna, V. ViFi: Accurate detection of viral integration and mRNA fusion reveals indiscriminate and unregulated transcription in proximal genomic regions in cervical cancer. *Nucleic Acids Res.* **2018**, *46*, 3309–3325. [CrossRef]
54. Wang, Q.; Jia, P.; Zhao, Z. VERSE: A novel approach to detect virus integration in host genomes through reference genome customization. *Genome Med.* **2015**, *7*, 1–9. [CrossRef] [PubMed]
55. Bs, L.M.P.; Gu, W.; Wang, Y.; Bs, A.E.; Ms, A.D.B.; Ba, C.V.B.; Carey, T.E.; Mills, R.E.; Brenner, J.C. SearcHPV: A novel approach to identify and assemble human papillomavirus–host genomic integration events in cancer. *Cancer* **2021**. [CrossRef]
56. Cameron, D.L.; Jacobs, N.; Roepman, P.; Priestley, P.; Cuppen, E.; Papenfuss, A.T. VIRUSBreakend: Viral Integration Recognition Using Single Breakends. *Bioinformatics* **2021**. [CrossRef]
57. Castellsagué, X.; Alemany, L.; Quer, M.; Halec, G.; Quirós, B.; Tous, S.; Clavero, O.; Alòs, L.; Biegner, T.; Szafarowski, T.; et al. HPV Involvement in Head and Neck Cancers: Comprehensive Assessment of Biomarkers in 3680 Patients. *J. Natl. Cancer Inst.* **2016**, *108*, djv403. [CrossRef] [PubMed]
58. Hafkamp, H.C.; Speel, E.J.; Haesevoets, A.; Bot, F.J.; Dinjens, W.N.; Ramaekers, F.C.; Hopman, A.H.; Manni, J.J. A subset of head and neck squamous cell carcinomas exhibits integration of HPV 16/18 DNA and overexpression of p16INK4A and p53 in the absence of mutations in p53 exons 5-8. *Int. J. Cancer* **2003**, *107*, 394–400. [CrossRef]
59. Tang, K.D.; Baeten, K.; Kenny, L.; Frazer, I.H.; Scheper, G.; Punyadeera, C. Unlocking the Potential of Saliva-Based Test to Detect HPV-16-Driven Oropharyngeal Cancer. *Cancers* **2019**, *11*, 473. [CrossRef]
60. Parfenov, M.; Pedamallu, C.S.; Gehlenborg, N.; Freeman, S.; Danilova, L.; Bristow, C.A.; Lee, S.; Hadjipanayis, A.G.; Ivanova, E.V.; Wilkerson, M.D.; et al. Characterization of HPV and host genome interactions in primary head and neck cancers. *Proc. Natl. Acad. Sci. USA* **2014**, *111*, 15544–15549. [CrossRef]
61. Deng, Z.; Hasegawa, M.; Kiyuna, A.; Matayoshi, S.; Uehara, T.; Agena, S.; Yamashita, Y.; Ogawa, K.; Maeda, H.; Suzuki, M. Viral load, physical status, and E6/E7 mRNA expression of human papillomavirus in head and neck squamous cell carcinoma. *Head Neck* **2013**, *35*, 800–808. [CrossRef]
62. Gao, G.; Wang, J.; Kasperbauer, J.L.; Tombers, N.M.; Teng, F.; Gou, H.; Zhao, Y.; Bao, Z.; Smith, D.I. Whole genome sequencing reveals complexity in both HPV sequences present and HPV integrations in HPV-positive oropharyngeal squamous cell car-cinomas. *BMC Cancer* **2019**, *19*, 352. [CrossRef]
63. Wuerdemann, N.; Jain, R.; Adams, A.; Speel, E.-J.M.; Wagner, S.; Joosse, S.A.; Klussmann, J.P. Cell-Free HPV-DNA as a Biomarker for Oropharyngeal Squamous Cell Carcinoma—A Step Towards Personalized Medicine? *Cancers* **2020**, *12*, 2997. [CrossRef]
64. Chera, B.S.; Kumar, S.; Beaty, B.T.; Marron, D.; Jefferys, S.; Green, R.; Goldman, E.C.; Amdur, R.; Sheets, N.; Dagan, R.; et al. Rapid Clearance Profile of Plasma Circulating Tumor HPV Type 16 DNA during Chemoradiotherapy Correlates with Disease Control in HPV-Associated Oropharyngeal Cancer. *Clin. Cancer Res.* **2019**, *25*, 4682–4690. [CrossRef]

65. Bodelon, C.; Untereiner, M.E.; Machiela, M.J.; Vinokurova, S.; Wentzensen, N. Genomic characterization of viral integration sites in HPV-related cancers. *Int. J. Cancer* **2016**, *139*, 2001–2011. [CrossRef] [PubMed]
66. Kelley, D.Z.; Flam, E.L.; Izumchenko, E.; Danilova, L.V.; Wulf, H.A.; Guo, T.; Singman, D.A.; Afsari, B.; Skaist, A.M.; Considine, M.; et al. Integrated Analysis of Whole-Genome ChIP-Seq and RNA-Seq Data of Primary Head and Neck Tumor Samples Associates HPV Integration Sites with Open Chromatin Marks. *Cancer Res.* **2017**, *77*, 6538–6550. [CrossRef] [PubMed]
67. Walline, H.M.; Komarck, C.M.; McHugh, J.B.; Bellile, E.L.; Brenner, J.C.; Prince, M.E.; McKean, E.L.; Chepeha, D.B.; Wolf, G.T.; Worden, F.P.; et al. Genomic Integration of High-Risk HPV Alters Gene Expression in Oropharyngeal Squamous Cell Carci-noma. *Mol. Cancer Res.* **2016**, *14*, 941–952. [CrossRef]
68. Pinatti, L.M.; Walline, H.M.; Carey, T.E.; Klussmann, J.P.; Huebbers, C.U. Viral Integration Analysis Reveals Likely Common Clonal Origin of Bilateral HPV16-Positive, p16-Positive Tonsil Tumors. *Arch. Clin. Med. Case Rep.* **2020**, *4*, 680–696. [CrossRef]
69. Reuschenbach, M.; Huebbers, C.; Prigge, E.-S.; Bermejo, J.L.; Kalteis, M.S.; Preuss, S.F.; Seuthe, I.M.C.; Kolligs, J.; Speel, E.-J.M.; Olthof, N.; et al. Methylation status of HPV16 E2-binding sites classifies subtypes of HPV-associated oropharyngeal cancers. *Cancer* **2015**, *121*, 1966–1976. [CrossRef]
70. Khanal, S.; Shumway, B.S.; Zahin, M.; Redman, R.A.; Strickley, J.D.; Trainor, P.J.; Rai, S.N.; Ghim, S.-J.; Jenson, A.B.; Joh, J. Viral DNA integration and methylation of human papillomavirus type 16 in high-grade oral epithelial dysplasia and head and neck squamous cell carcinoma. *Oncotarget* **2018**, *9*, 30419–30433. [CrossRef]
71. Hatano, T.; Sano, D.; Takahashi, H.; Hyakusoku, H.; Isono, Y.; Shimada, S.; Sawakuma, K.; Takada, K.; Oikawa, R.; Watanabe, Y.; et al. Identification of human papillomavirus (HPV) 16 DNA integration and the ensuing patterns of methylation in HPV-associated head and neck squamous cell carcinoma cell lines. *Int. J. Cancer* **2016**, *140*, 1571–1580. [CrossRef] [PubMed]
72. Hausen, H.Z. Papillomaviruses and cancer: From basic studies to clinical application. *Nat. Rev. Cancer* **2002**, *2*, 342–350. [CrossRef] [PubMed]
73. Pim, D.; Banks, L. Interaction of viral oncoproteins with cellular target molecules: Infection with high-risk vs low-risk human papillomaviruses. *APMIS* **2010**, *118*, 471–493. [CrossRef]
74. Arenz, R.N.A.; Ziemann, F.; Mayer, C.; Wittig, A.; Dreffke, K.; Preising, S.; Wagner, S.; Klussmann, J.-P.; Engenhart-Cabillic, R.; Wittekindt, C. Increased radiosensitivity of HPV-positive head and neck cancer cell lines due to cell cycle dysregulation and induction of apoptosis. *Strahlenther. Onkol.* **2014**, *190*, 839–846. [CrossRef]
75. Rieckmann, T.; Tribius, S.; Grob, T.J.; Meyer, F.; Busch, C.-J.; Petersen, C.; Dikomey, E.; Kriegs, M. HNSCC cell lines positive for HPV and p16 possess higher cellular radiosensitivity due to an impaired DSB repair capacity. *Radiother. Oncol.* **2013**, *107*, 242–246. [CrossRef] [PubMed]
76. Penning, T.M. Aldo-Keto Reductase Regulation by the Nrf2 System: Implications for Stress Response, Chemotherapy Drug Resistance, and Carcinogenesis. *Chem. Res. Toxicol.* **2016**, *30*, 162–176. [CrossRef] [PubMed]
77. Groves, I.J.; Coleman, N. Pathogenesis of human papillomavirus-associated mucosal disease. *J. Pathol.* **2015**, *235*, 527–538. [CrossRef]
78. Hajek, M.; Sewell, A.; Kaech, S.; Burtness, B.; Yarbrough, W.G.; Issaeva, N. TRAF3/CYLDmutations identify a distinct subset of human papillomavirus-associated head and neck squamous cell carcinoma. *Cancer* **2017**, *123*, 1778–1790. [CrossRef]
79. Hassounah, N.B.; Malladi, V.; Huang, Y.; Freeman, S.; Beauchamp, E.M.; Koyama, S.; Souders, N.; Martin, S.; Dranoff, G.; Wong, K.-K.; et al. Identification and characterization of an alternative cancer-derived PD-L1 splice variant. *Cancer Immunol. Immunother.* **2018**, *68*, 407–420. [CrossRef]
80. Koneva, L.A.; Zhang, Y.; Virani, S.; Hall, P.B.; McHugh, J.B.; Chepeha, D.; Wolf, G.T.; Carey, T.E.; Rozek, L.S.; Sartor, M.A. HPV Integration in HNSCC Correlates with Survival Outcomes, Immune Response Signatures, and Candidate Drivers. *Mol. Cancer Res.* **2017**, *16*, 90–102. [CrossRef]
81. Broutian, T.R.; Jiang, B.; Li, J.; Akagi, K.; Gui, S.; Zhou, Z.; Xiao, W.; Symer, D.E.; Gillison, M.L. Human papillomavirus inser-tions identify the PIM family of serine/threonine kinases as targetable driver genes in head and neck squamous cell carcinoma. *Cancer Lett.* **2020**, *476*, 23–33. [CrossRef] [PubMed]
82. Beier, U.H.; Weise, J.B.; Laudien, M.; Sauerwein, H.; Görögh, T. Overexpression of Pim-1 in head and neck squamous cell carcinomas. *Int. J. Oncol.* **2007**, *30*, 1381–1387. [CrossRef] [PubMed]
83. Peltola, K.; Hollmen, M.; Maula, S.-M.; Rainio, E.; Ristamäki, R.; Luukkaa, M.; Sandholm, J.; Sundvall, M.; Elenius, K.; Koskinen, P.J.; et al. Pim-1 Kinase Expression Predicts Radiation Response in Squamocellular Carcinoma of Head and Neck and Is under the Control of Epidermal Growth Factor Receptor. *Neoplasia* **2009**, *11*, 629–IN1. [CrossRef] [PubMed]
84. Chiang, W.-F.; Yen, C.-Y.; Lin, C.-N.; Liaw, G.-A.; Chiu, C.-T.; Hsia, Y.-J.; Liu, S.-Y. Up-regulation of a serine–threonine kinase proto-oncogene Pim-1 in oral squamous cell carcinoma. *Int. J. Oral Maxillofac. Surg.* **2006**, *35*, 740–745. [CrossRef]
85. Huebbers, C.U.; Preuss, S.F.; Kolligs, J.; Vent, J.; Stenner, M.; Wieland, U.; Silling, S.; Drebber, U.; Speel, E.-J.M.; Klussmann, J.P. Integration of HPV6 and downregulation of AKR1C3 expression mark malignant transformation in a patient with juve-nile-onset laryngeal papillomatosis. *PLoS ONE* **2013**, *8*, e57201. [CrossRef] [PubMed]
86. Wanichwatanadecha, P.; Sirisrimangkorn, S.; Kaewprag, J.; Ponglikitmongkol, M. Transactivation activity of human papil-lomavirus type 16 E6*I on aldo-keto reductase genes enhances chemoresistance in cervical cancer cells. *J. Gen. Virol.* **2012**, *93*, 1081–1092. [CrossRef]
87. Ruiz, F.X.; Porté, S.; Parés, X.; Farrés, J. Biological Role of Aldo–Keto Reductases in Retinoic Acid Biosynthesis and Signaling. *Front. Pharmacol.* **2012**, *3*, 58. [CrossRef]

88. Zhang, Y.; Koneva, L.A.; Virani, S.; Arthur, A.E.; Virani, A.; Hall, P.B.; Warden, C.D.; Carey, T.E.; Chepeha, D.; Prince, M.E.; et al. Subtypes of HPV-Positive Head and Neck Cancers Are Associated with HPV Characteristics, Copy Number Alterations, PIK3CA Mutation, and Pathway Signatures. *Clin. Cancer Res.* **2016**, *22*, 4735–4745. [CrossRef]
89. Smeets, S.J.; Hesselink, A.T.; Speel, E.-J.M.; Haesevoets, A.; Snijders, P.J.; Pawlita, M.; Meijer, C.J.; Braakhuis, B.J.; Leemans, C.R.; Brakenhoff, R.H. A novel algorithm for reliable detection of human papillomavirus in paraffin embedded head and neck cancer specimen. *Int. J. Cancer* **2007**, *121*, 2465–2472. [CrossRef]
90. Paget-Bailly, P.; Meznad, K.; Bruyère, D.; Perrard, J.; Herfs, M.; Jung, A.; Mougin, C.; Prétet, J.-L.; Baguet, A. Comparative RNA sequencing reveals that HPV16 E6 abrogates the effect of E6*I on ROS metabolism. *Sci. Rep.* **2019**, *9*, 1–15. [CrossRef]
91. Qin, T.; Koneva, L.A.; Liu, Y.; Zhang, Y.; Arthur, A.E.; Zarins, K.R.; Carey, T.E.; Chepeha, D.; Wolf, G.T.; Rozek, L.S. Significant association between host transcriptome-derived HPV oncogene E6* influence score and carcinogenic pathways, tumor size, and survival in head and neck cancer. *Head Neck* **2020**, *42*, 2375–2389. [CrossRef]
92. Pannone, G.; Bufo, P.; Pace, M.; Lepore, S.; Russo, G.M.; Rubini, C.; Franco, R.; Aquino, G.; Santoro, A.; Campisi, G.; et al. TLR4 down-regulation identifies high risk HPV infection and integration in head and neck squamous cell carcinomas. *Front. Biosci.* **2016**, *8*.
93. Yang, W.; Liu, Y.; Dong, R.; Liu, J.; Lang, J.; Yang, J.; Wang, W.; Li, J.; Meng, B.; Tian, G. Accurate Detection of HPV Integration Sites in Cervical Cancer Samples Using the Nanopore MinION Sequencer Without Error Correction. *Front. Genet.* **2020**, *11*, 660. [CrossRef]
94. Cancer Genome Atlas, N. Comprehensive genomic characterization of head and neck squamous cell carcinomas. *Nature* **2015**, *517*, 576–582. [CrossRef]
95. Häcker, H.; Tseng, P.-H.; Karin, M. Expanding TRAF function: TRAF3 as a tri-faced immune regulator. *Nat. Rev. Immunol.* **2011**, *11*, 457–468. [CrossRef]
96. Harhaj, E.W.; Dixit, V.M. Regulation of NF-kappaB by deubiquitinases. *Immunol. Rev.* **2012**, *246*, 107–124. [CrossRef]
97. Keck, M.K.; Zuo, Z.; Khattri, A.; Stricker, T.P.; Brown, C.D.; Imanguli, M.; Rieke, D.; Endhardt, K.; Fang, P.; Brägelmann, J.; et al. Integrative Analysis of Head and Neck Cancer Identifies Two Biologically Distinct HPV and Three Non-HPV Subtypes. *Clin. Cancer Res.* **2014**, *21*, 870–881. [CrossRef]
98. Locati, L.D.; Serafini, M.S.; Ianno', M.F.; Carenzo, A.; Orlandi, E.; Resteghini, C.; Cavalieri, S.; Bossi, P.; Canevari, S.; Licitra, L.; et al. Mining of Self-Organizing Map Gene-Expression Portraits Reveals Prognostic Stratification of HPV-Positive Head and Neck Squamous Cell Carcinoma. *Cancers* **2019**, *11*, 1057. [CrossRef]
99. Nulton, T.J.; Kim, N.-K.; DiNardo, L.J.; Morgan, I.M.; Windle, B. Patients with integrated HPV16 in head and neck cancer show poor survival. *Oral Oncol.* **2018**, *80*, 52–55. [CrossRef] [PubMed]
100. Veitía, D.; Liuzzi, J.; Ávila, M.; Rodriguez, I.; Toro, F.; Correnti, M. Association of viral load and physical status of HPV-16 with survival of patients with head and neck cancer. *ecancermedicalscience* **2020**, *14*. [CrossRef] [PubMed]
101. Niya, M.H.K.; Keyvani, H.; Tameshkel, F.S.; Salehi-Vaziri, M.; Teaghinezhad-S, S.; Salim, F.B.; Monavari, S.H.R.; Javanmard, D. Human Papillomavirus Type 16 Integration Analysis by Real-time PCR Assay in Associated Cancers. *Transl. Oncol.* **2018**, *11*, 593–598. [CrossRef] [PubMed]
102. Lorenzi, A.; Rautava, J.; Kero, K.; Syrjänen, K.; Longatto-Filho, A.; Grenman, S.; Syrjänen, S. Physical state and copy numbers of HPV16 in oral asymptomatic infections that persisted or cleared during the 6-year follow-up. *J. Gen. Virol.* **2017**, *98*, 681–689. [CrossRef]
103. Walline, H.M.; Bs, C.M.G.; McHugh, J.B.; Tang, A.L.; Owen, J.H.; Teh, B.T.; Mckean, E.; Glover, T.W.; Bs, M.P.G.; Prince, M.E.; et al. Integration of high-risk human papillomavirus into cellular cancer-related genes in head and neck cancer cell lines. *Head Neck* **2017**, *39*, 840–852. [CrossRef] [PubMed]
104. Vojtěchová, Z.; Sabol, I.; Saláková, M.; Turek, L.; Grega, M.; Šmahelová, J.; Vencalek, O.; Lukesova, E.; Klozar, J.; Tachezy, R. Analysis of the integration of human papillomaviruses in head and neck tumours in relation to patients' prognosis. *Int. J. Cancer* **2015**, *138*, 386–395. [CrossRef] [PubMed]
105. Lim, M.Y.; Dahlstrom, K.R.; Sturgis, E.M.; Li, G. Human papillomavirus integration pattern and demographic, clinical, and survival characteristics of patients with oropharyngeal squamous cell carcinoma. *Head Neck* **2016**, *38*, 1139–1144. [CrossRef] [PubMed]
106. Bs, L.M.P.; Sinha, H.N.; Ba, C.V.B.; Bs, C.M.G.; Bs, T.J.G.; Wilson, G.D.; Akervall, J.A.; Brenner, C.J.; Walline, H.M.; Carey, T.E. Association of human papillomavirus integration with better patient outcomes in oropharyngeal squamous cell carcinoma. *Head Neck* **2020**, *43*, 544–557. [CrossRef]

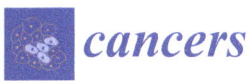

Review

Cancer Stem Cells in Oropharyngeal Cancer

Mehmet Gunduz [1,2], Esra Gunduz [3], Shunji Tamagawa [2], Keisuke Enomoto [2] and Muneki Hotomi [2,*]

1. Department of Otorhinolaryngology and Head and Neck Surgery, Shinmatsudo Central Hospital, Shinmatsudo 1-380, Matsudoshi 270-0034, Chiba, Japan; mgunduz@ims.gr.jp
2. Department of Otorhinolaryngology and Head and Neck Surgery, Wakayama Medical University, Kimiidera 811-1, Wakayamashi 641-8509, Wakayama, Japan; tamashun@wakayama-med.ac.jp (S.T.); kenomoto@wakayama-med.ac.jp (K.E.)
3. East Clinic Moriya Keiyu Corporation, Matsunami 1630-1, Moriya 302-0108, Ibaraki, Japan; gunduz.e@keiyu.or.jp
* Correspondence: mhotomi@wakayama-med.ac.jp; Tel.: +81-73-441-0651/5417; Fax: +81-73-446-3846

Simple Summary: Although there has been improvement in our understanding about cancer stem cells recently, we still don't know much about cancer stem cells of oropharyngeal cancer. Lack of knowledge solely on oropharyngeal cancer together with the information of human papilloma virus status, which is a specific factor of prognosis in oropharyngeal cancer, hardens to elucidate the distinction of the underlying mechanisms of cancer stem cell behavior. To proceed to an effective and durable therapy in oropharyngeal cancer it is necessary to reveal cancer stem cell function and related factors like its plasticity, niche, and pathways. Therefore in this review we aimed to contribute to this emerging area by focusing on the current literature and future prospects.

Abstract: Oropharyngeal cancer (OPC), which is a common type of head and neck squamous cell carcinoma (HNSCC), is associated with tobacco and alcohol use, and human papillomavirus (HPV) infection. Underlying mechanisms and as a result prognosis of the HPV-positive and HPV-negative OPC patients are different. Like stem cells, the ability of self-renewal and differentiate, cancer stem cells (CSCs) have roles in tumor invasion, metastasis, drug resistance, and recurrence after therapy. Research revealed their roles to some extent in all of these processes but there are still many unresolved points to connect to CSC-targeted therapy. In this review, we will focus on what we currently know about CSCs of OPC and limitations of our current knowledge. We will present perspectives that will broaden our understanding and recent literature which may connect to therapy.

Keywords: oropharyngeal cancer (OPC); human papillomavirus (HPV); cancer stem cells (CSCs); CSC markers; prognosis; tumor heterogeneity

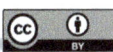

1. Introduction

Head and neck cancer is the sixth most common malignancy worldwide and includes tumors from the oral cavity, pharynx, larynx, nasal cavity, paranasal sinuses, thyroid, and major as well as minor salivary glands [1] The thyroid, nasal cavity as well as paranasal sinuses and salivary gland tumors are usually considered to be a different group and when the head and neck cancer is mentioned, mostly squamous cell carcinomas deriving from oral cavity, pharyngeal and laryngeal mucosa are taken into consideration. Most common risks for head and neck cancer are smoking, heavy drinking and virus contamination [2]. Within these groups, oral cavity and especially oropharyngeal cancer are related with human papilloma virus (HPV) infection. The identification of HPV especially in the USA and European countries in oropharyngeal cancer resulted in increased basic and clinical research and better outcomes for diagnosis and treatment of this head and neck cancer type.

Oropharyngeal cancer (OPC), a common subtype of head and neck squamous cell carcinoma (HNSCC), is mainly associated with tobacco as well as alcohol use and, HPV infection. Thus, oropharyngeal cancer has recently been categorized into HPV associated (positive) or unassociated (negative) subtypes, which show quite different etiologic as well as genetic backgrounds and therapeutic outcomes. Although high risk HPV subtypes are HPV16, 18, 31, 33, 35, 45, 51, 52, and 56 in relation to causing cancer of the head and neck, cervix, anus, vagina, vulva, and penis, HPV16 is the most common type in head and neck cancer [3]. Mechanism of HPV integration to the host genome is not clear yet but fusions through break-points of cellular and viral genome or the amplified segments of a genomic sequence flanked with HPV genome which is also found in patient samples as focal copy number elevation at sites of HPV integration are mainly suggested mechanisms [4]. While HPV-positive oropharyngeal cancer has low or no common genetic abnormalities, such as p53 mutation, and is directly associated with contamination of high risk HPV subtypes, HPV-negative oropharyngeal cancer is closely related with smoking and excessive alcohol consumption and demonstrates commonly activated mutation of oncogenes such as EGFR, RAS, PI3 kinase or functional loss of tumor suppressor genes such as p53, p16, and RB1 or both [2]. Thus, underlying mechanisms and as a result prognosis of the HPV-positive and HPV-negative OPC patients are quite different (Table 1). There are also conflicting reports about HPV status and HNSCC which may be due to not screening cancer of the oropharynx and the anterior oral cavity separately or different sampling techniques such as saliva, biopsies, and brushing and methods used to detect HPV status from those samples through polymerase chain reaction (PCR), dot-blot hybridization, and Southern blotting [5].

Table 1. Differences between HPV-positive and negative oropharyngeal cancer *.

Subjects	HPV-Positive	HPV-Negative
Age	Younger	Elder
Smoking/Alcohol	Less	Often
Radiochemotherapy response	Well	High resistant rate
Survival	Better	Worse
Genetic alterations		
P53 Mutation	3%	84%
CDKN2A Mutation	none	58%
CCND1 Mutation	3%	31%
FGFR1	none	10%

* Genetic alterations data are from Cancer Genome Atlas Network [6].

Cancer stem cells (CSCs) are a subgroup of cells in the heterogeneous tumor bulk, which have the ability of self-renewal and differentiation, like stem cells. They are supposed to have a role in tumor invasion, metastasis, drug resistance, and recurrence after therapy and therefore are accepted as one of the emerging targets for cancer therapy. Recently they have been studied by various researchers throughout the world and their roles in carcinogenesis, tumor invasion, metastasis, drug resistance, and recurrence after therapy have been shown but still more research and evidence are necessary to move forward to CSC-targeted therapy [7,8]. To be able to comprehend our knowledge of the CSC of OPC, in this study we will first present CSC origin and model followed by CSC markers of HNSCC. Then we will review the recent literature and our experience about CSC of OPC, and limitations of our current knowledge. We will discuss different perspectives, which may connect to better diagnostic as well as prognostic and therapeutic options. Lastly, we will comment on for further investigations that can be performed to connect CSC-targeted therapy for OPC.

CSC Model and Origin

CSCs were first identified in acute myeloid leukemia in 1997. The cells with $CD34^{++}$ $CD38^-$ cell-surface antigen were only 0.2% in the tumor but had the potential to form neoplasms in the immune-deficient mice. Conversely, even though $CD34^+$ $CD38^+$ cell-surface antigen cells were highly detected in the tumor they couldn't engraft new neoplasms [9]. In 2007, CSCs of head and neck squamous cell carcinoma were first identified. Prince et al.

defined CD44$^+$ cells comprising of lower than the 10% of HNSCC cells but could give rise to new tumors and the new tumors formed from CD44$^+$ purified cells could reproduce tumor heterogeneity and could be serially passaged like stem cells [10].

The hierarchic model of cancer which is also known as the CSC model implicates that only specific cells have the ability to form cancer cells. Although it is still unclear which cancers or which cancer stem cells expressing specific markers follow this model, increasing evidence supports this hypothesis. Contrary to the stochastic model of tumor growth in which all the tumor cells stochastically have the potential to self-renewal and differentiate, in CSC model CSCs are responsible for causing different lineages in the tumor that leads to tumor heterogeneity [11,12] (Figure 1).

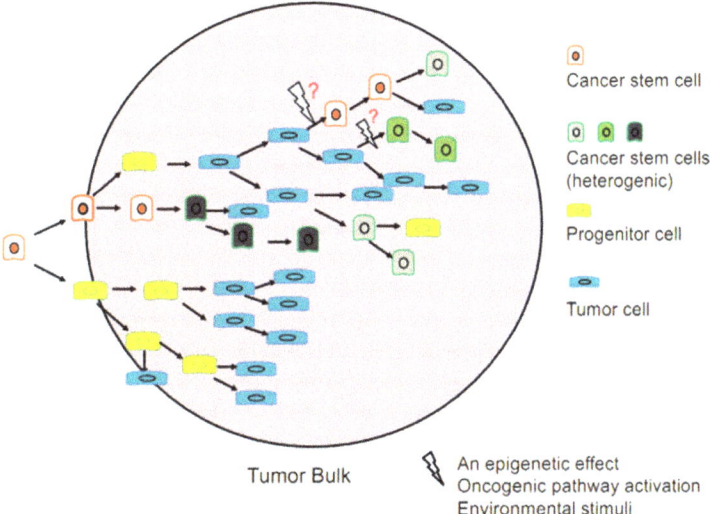

Figure 1. Origin and heterogeneity in cancer stem cell model; Cancer stem cells (CSCs) can form progenitor and cancer stem cells and can differentiate to cancer cells. When an appropriate epigenetic effect, oncogenic pathway activation or environmental stimuli event occur, differentiated cancer cells can transform to cancer stem cell.

The origin of CSCs is still under discussion. Three possibilities are raised that CSCs can be formed from: stem cells, progenitor cells or differentiated cells [13]. However, it is also possible that even some of differentiated cancer cells may gain CSC properties through oncogenic pathways and environmental stimuli. Therefore, it is questioned whether CSCs differentiate in a unidirectional hierarchic way like in the CSC model. Moreover, evidence supports that cancer cells have plasticity and can acquire CSC properties [14,15].

2. CSC Markers of HNSCC

In this part we will summarize widely used CSC markers in HNSCC studies (Table 2).

Table 2. Common Cancer Stem Cell Markers in Oropharyngeal Cancer *.

Cancer Stem Cell Marker	Chromosomal Location	Exon Count	Characteristics
ALDH1A1	9q21.13	13	major pathway of alcohol metabolism, most common CSC marker
CD44	11p13	21	cell-surface glycoprotein involved in cell-cell interactions, cell adhesion and migration

Table 2. *Cont.*

Cancer Stem Cell Marker	Chromosomal Location	Exon Count	Characteristics
BMI1	10p12.2	10	a proto-oncogene, a member of polycomb group complex 1 (PRC1) which is an epigenetic repressor of regulatory genes
OCT4	6p21.33	6	a transcription factor that plays role in embryonic development and stem cell pluripotency
SOX2	3q26.33	1(no introns)	SRY-box transcription factor 2
CD133	4p15.32	35	transmembrane glycoprotein expressed on adult stem cells, suppress differentiation to maintain stem cell properties

* https://www.ncbi.nlm.nih.gov/gene/ (accessed on 20 April 2021) data are used for Table 2.

2.1. ALDH1A1

Aldehyde dehydrogenase 1 (ALDH1A1) which is in the major pathway of alcohol metabolism is located at chromosome 9q21.13 with 13 exons [16]. ALDH1A1 is a valuable prognostic CSC marker. Chen et al. defined ALDH1A1 as a CSC marker in HNSCC, which was previously used as CSC marker in various cancers. They showed that ALDH1$^+$ cells displayed resistance to radiotherapy and had ability of generating tumors [17]. Likewise it was reported that ALDH1A1 is a highly selective marker for CSCs in HNSCC [18]. Qian et al. analyzed HNSCC specimens of which 80% was oropharyngeal cancer for ALDH1A1 expression and its relation to prognosis. Their results showed that HNSCC patients with ALDH1A1 expression displayed a significant p value ($p = 0.011$) for poor prognosis and those of oropharyngeal cancers with ALDH1A1 expression showed worse prognosis ($p = 0.001$) [19]. Similarly Szafarowski et al. compared CSC markers of HNSCC and their results revealed that ALDH1A1$^+$ patients showed 5.25 times worse overall survival (OS) than ALDH1A1$^-$ patients ($p = 0.01$) and only ALDH1A1 positivity had a significant effect on OS of HNSCC patients ($p = 0.02$) compared to other CSC markers of CD44, CD24 and CD133 [20]. In another study, it was confirmed that patients with ALDH1A1$^+$ had worse prognosis but also concluded that ALDH1A1 and CD44, alone or together, was not enough to identify CSC subpopulations [21]. Contradictory to this data we previously characterized CSCs of OPC and had been successful to isolate CSCs by ALDH1A1 marker and CSCs have the ability to form tumor spheres [22]. ALDH1A1 is one of the most specific markers that are used for HNSCC CSC research [23–26].

2.2. CD44

CD44 is a cell-surface glycoprotein involved in cell-cell interactions, cell adhesion and migration, which is located at chromosome 11p13 with 21 exons [27]. First defined by Prince et al., CD44 has been frequently used as a CSC marker in various HNSCC studies [10,28–30] and has been shown to play important role in HNSCC cancer stemness [31–33]. CD44 was also found to be related to angiogenesis, tumor aggressiveness, and worse prognosis in HNSCC [34–36]. In addition, a meta-analysis study displayed worse prognosis in pharyngeal and laryngeal cancer with CD44 expression but not in oral cancer [37].

2.3. BMI1

BMI1 is a proto-oncogene located at chromosome 10p12.2 with 10 exons. It is a member of polycomb group complex 1 (PRC1) which is an epigenetic repressor of regulatory genes in embryonic development and self-renewal of somatic stem cells via chromatin remodeling [38]. It was shown that inhibiting BMI1 sensitized tumors to cisplatin and eliminated lymph node metastasis in vivo, in vitro and primary human HNSCC samples contained highly tumorigenic, invasive, and cisplatin-resistant BMI1$^+$ CSCs [39,40]. Tumor growth was also suppressed by inhibiting BMI1 pharmacologically in HNSCC and targeting

BMI1 related CSC in oral squamous cell carcinoma (OSCC) has been shown as a clinically relevant anticancer therapy [41,42].

2.4. OCT4

OCT4 is located at chromosome 6p21.33 with six exons. It encodes a transcription factor that plays role in embryonic development and stem cell pluripotency [43]. It was reported as a CSC marker in HNSCC [32,44]. OCT4 was found to regulate epithelial-mesenchymal transition (EMT) in OSCC [45]. Because of its relation to poor prognosis it can be used as a predictive prognostic marker of HNSCC [46].

2.5. SOX2

SRY-box transcription factor 2 (SOX2) is located at chromosome 3q26.33 and it has no intron. It plays a role in the regulation of embryonic development and the determination of cell fate [47]. It has been shown to regulate CSC of HNSCC [48]. There are conflicting reports about its high expression related to prognosis [46,49,50].

2.6. CD133

CD133 is located at chromosome 4p15.32 with 35 exons. It is a transmembrane glycoprotein expressed on adult stem cells. It is supposed to suppress differentiation to maintain stem cell properties [51]. CD133 high expression was shown to increase cancer stemness and cause cell cycle arrest in HNSCC cell line resulting in chemoresistance [52]. Chen et al. proposed CD133/Src axis might be a potential therapeutic target in HNSCC because of being a regulatory switch to gain of EMT and of stemness properties in HNSCC [53]. It is also found to be a biomarker and predictor of prognosis [54].

3. OPC CSC Pathways

CSC markers ALDH1A1, CD44, BMI1, OCT4, SOX2, and CD133 and their effects on cancer stemness, metastasis, prognosis, chemo/radiotherapy resistance and recurrence have been studied in HNSCC by our group and other researchers [10,17,22,31–36,39–42,45,46,48–50,52–54]. Although there are conflicting reports about their expression and as being a prognostic marker in HNSCC, the differences may be due to factors such as use of cell lines in vitro vs primary tumor samples in vivo, the used isolation techniques such as fluorescence activated cell sorting (FACS) vs magnetic beads activated cell sorting (MACS), tumor sample/cell line kind e.g., pharyngeal cancer vs. oral cancer vs. laryngeal cancer, patient or sample size and, if primary tumors was used before chemo/radiotherapy vs after chemo/radiotherapy. Additionally, intratumor heterogeneity may also reflect different results.

CSC studies involving solely OPC are very limited. Moreover, underlying mechanisms are different due to the HPV status. Rietbergen et al. analyzed 711 oropharyngeal squamous cell carcinoma (OPSCC) patients from two Dutch university hospitals and showed that HPV-positive patients had lower CD44 and CD98 expression than HPV-negative patients. Moreover HPV-positive patients with high CD98 expression showed significantly worse overall survival (OS) and progression-free survival (PFS) rates compared to patients with low percentage of CD98 cells [55]. Likewise Näsman et al. presented that HPV-positive patients with CD44 absent/weak expression displayed significant favorable 3-year disease-free survival (DFS) and overall survival (OS) [36]. In a study, OPC patients who had undergone radiation therapy, it was shown that CD44 negative patients had significantly higher PFS and locoregional control (LRC) than CD44 positive patients. Furthermore, p16 protein positive (likely to be HPV-positive) and CD44 negative patients showed the best LRC while p16 protein negative (likely to be HPV-negative) and CD44 positive patients had the worst LCR [56]. These results indicate CD44 expression is low in HPV-positive cases while it is high in HPV-negative cases and if CD44 expression is high in HPV-positive cases, it results in a worse outcome. Our group isolated CSCs from HPV-negative cell line of UT-SCC 60A by CSC marker ALDH1A1 and showed that CSCs formed tumor spheres.

We also detected significantly high expression of OCT4, SOX2, KLF4 and BMI1 in the HPV-negative OPC CSCs as compared to the cancer cells, while CD133 expression was not different in the CSCs and the cancer cells. Those of the CSCs showed resistance to cisplatin treatment [22]. BMI1 was also found to be expressed more in HPV-negative OPC than HPV-positive OPC [57].

Orai1 was shown to be regulator of CSC phenotype by Lee et al. in oral/oropharyngeal cancer. According to their data Orai1 has been highly expressed in oral/oropharyngeal cancer and activates downstream molecule NFATc3 which proposes Orai1/NFAT axis to have importance on CSC in OPC [58]. In a later study Lee et al. introduced NFATc3 as a critical factor which affects cancer stemness through NFATc3-OCT4 axis in oral/oropharyngeal cancer. Their data included NFATc3 was highly expressed in CSC and required for self-renewal of CSC. Furthermore, their data indicated not only the gain of CSC phenotype but also gain of ALDH1A1$^+$ high cell population, morbidity and drug resistance when NFATc3 was ectopically expressed in immortalized oral epithelial cells as well [59].

Interestingly, Hufbauer et al. showed that HPV16 targets migratory and stationary stem cells and aberrantly expressed miR-3194-5p and miR-1281 in migratory CSCs, which might be the reason of OPC progression and metastasis [60]. Finding HPV16-positive HNSCC to have more CSC than HPV16-negative HNSCC, Zhang et al. discussed that rather than amount of CSC, CSC phenotype may be more important in the therapy resistance [61].

4. From the View of CSC Research to the Therapy of OPC

Possessing the ability of self-renewal and differentiate, CSCs are considered to be one of the emerging targets for cancer therapy. They are supposed to have roles in tumor invasion, metastasis, drug resistance, and recurrence after therapy. CSC, tumor microenvironment (TME), extracellular matrix (ECM) and epithelial-mesenchymal transition (EMT) all have cross-link and are affected from the stimuli one to each other. TME can alter ECM, and ECM can induce EMT while EMT, TME and ECM have effects on generation of cancer stem cells/malignant phenotype and enable invasion and metastasis [62–64]. Therefore each of these processes may be a part of the solution to cure cancer.

Together with technological developments drug delivery systems (DDSs) have been highly improved recent years but there are still many challenges to face to proceed for clinical implementation for CSC-targeted DDSs [65].

In this part we focus on the factors that have effects on the therapy of OPC through targeting CSC properties.

4.1. CSC Plasticity

Because of CSC plasticity, heterogeneity is an obstacle of targeting CSC. Recognizing that cancer cells have the possibility to gain CSC abilities, both genetically and phenotypically the complexity of tumor heterogeneity highly increases [8]. Regarding the same type of cancer, such as, here, oropharyngeal cancer, different populations in the same tumor complicates to proceed to a solution for therapy. As previously mentioned, we discussed ALDH1A1 as a valuable prognostic marker in HNSCC but there are reports displaying contradictory results. For example, in one study, ALDH1A1 was found to be uniquely expressed in a subset of suprabasal tonsillar crypt epithelium and was lost in HPV$^+$ and HPV$^-$ tumors suggesting ALDH1A1 positive cells not to be stem cell progenitors but a component of the crypt cellular microenvironment [66]. Additionally Xu et al. showed that ALDH1A1 may be a biomarker for predicting lymph node metastasis, but it is not an independent prognostic factor for survival in HNSCC patients [67]. These conflicts may be explained by sub-classification of CSCs according to their expression of marker proteins which may have different positions/roles in cancer as suggested by Geißler et al. Their data revealed that the amounts of CD44 and ALDH1A1 vary; while ALDH1A1 high tumor cells express low levels of CD44 and EGFR, ALDH1A1$^-$/CD44$^+$ high tumor cells express high levels of EGFR in HNSCC. They suggested that CSCs can also be sub-classified into migratory and stationary CSCs. They proposed that ALDH1A1 high/CD44 low/EGFR low tumor cells may be stationary and quiescent, while ALDH1A1$^-$/CD44 high/EGFR high cells may be invasive and migratory [68]. In a systematic review it was concluded that a single common CSC sorting marker may not even exist within identical types of tumor [69]. However, this raises the question instead of isolating CSCs with more than one marker would not be more enlightening to isolate CSCs with only one single marker but with the different CSC markers within the same sample to compare their roles in the carcinogenesis related processes, metastasis, resistance to therapy, therapy relapse tumor rather than grouping all CSC as one group. If there are different CSC markers in the identical types of tumor, do the CSCs expressing different markers have different roles in the carcinogenesis, invasion, metastasis, evading immune surveillance, resistance to therapy, therapy relapse? If there is more than one origin of CSC-like stem cells, progenitor cells and/or differentiated cells, is it possible that the origin of the CSC may cause differently expressed CSC markers in the same type of tumor? There are still a lot of questions to be answered. Many of the studies in HNSCC are focused on the prognosis of the patients comparing the expression of CSC markers or functional role of solely on one CSC marker. When differently expressed CSC markers and results are to be reported in the identical type of cancer in different research we can functionally and mechanistically (not only as the expression) compare the role of CSCs expressing different markers within the same tumor to have more precise results.

Not only for tumor heterogeneity but also for metastasis, CSCs are considered to have critical roles [70–72]. We do not know clearly yet whether a subgroup of CSCs metastasizes in OPC. Therefore studies revealing the role/function of different CSC subgroups are necessary for targeting CSC in OPC. These studies may have effect on preventing invasion, metastasis as well as curing OPC.

4.2. Resistance to Antitumor Therapies and Evade Immune Surveillance

CSCs are considered to be resistant to antitumor therapies and have the ability to escape immune surveillance [15,73–75]. For resistance to chemotherapy and radiation CSCs use mechanisms such as dormancy, DNA repair, multidrug-resistance-type membrane transporters, and escaping apoptosis [76]. Moreover, CSC markers such as CD44, ALDH1A1 have been reported to be intensely linked with EGFR and PI3K/AKT pathway. Coexistence of CD44v3 and ALDH1A1 in head and neck cancer cells provides escape from apoptosis, promotes survival and proliferation through activation of downstream effectors such as Sox2, Nanog, and Oct4 [77]. Not only resistance to therapeutics but recent therapies such as ionizing radiation therapy or cisplatin may even cause CSC characteristics of cancer cells is another challenging point [78,79]. Pützer et al. discussed that rather than unilateral anti-CSC approaches strengthening patient's immune defense and heading toward individualized therapies CSC treatment can be successful [80].

4.3. CSC Niche

Because of the difficulties in the way of cure, targeting CSC alone may not be a solution to cure oropharyngeal cancer. For example, the aforementioned CSC plasticity and additionally cancer cells' ability to gain CSC phenotype suggests complexity in targeting only one type of CSC. Additionally CSC niche, which is the tumor microenvironment in which CSC characteristics are regulated and supports self-renewal and survival of CSCs, can both be part of the problem and the solution. CD44 intracellular signaling in response to extracellular signals is reported as a mediator of the link between tumor-associated macrophages in the tumor microenvironment and CSCs [28]. Although we still do not know much about CSC niche, targeting CSC niche and crosstalk between CSCs may be an effective and durable way of cancer therapy [81]. Therefore studies that improve our understanding of the CSC niche are important for further developments.

4.4. CSC Mitochondria

CSC mitochondria are another target of the CSC research aiming at the therapy. In CSC, mitochondria have been shown to have a corresponding role like they serve in stem cells in the regulation of stem cell identity, differentiation and fate [82]. Not only these functions but also mitochondria can modify cell metabolism and can cause CSC evade apoptosis leading to survival of cancer cells as well [83]. In a clinical pilot study, CSCs were shown to be selectively eradicated through targeting mitochondria using doxycycline in early breast cancer patients [84]. There are also studies with promising results suggesting eradicating CSCs in cancer aiming mitochondria via antibiotics and vitamin C supplement [6,85,86].

5. Conclusions

After they were first defined in 1997 in leukemia, researchers around the world contributed to CSC research with valuable data that improved our understanding of CSCs. Now we can question more how to proceed for an effective therapy through CSC and CSC related factors. For HNSCC it has only been 14 years since CSCs were identified and accumulating information leads us to question the reason of controversial data. As we mentioned in prior parts these may be due to experimental related factors or may be due to different lineages and of their different role even in the same tumor type. Moreover, when considering OPC we not only face the same problems but lack of knowledge solely on OPC and different mechanisms for HPV-negative and HPV-positive cases. Therefore, there is still need for a vast number of further studies which would enlighten our understanding of CSC related characteristics and pathways of carcinogenesis, resistance to therapy and escaping immune surveillance, CSC plasticity, CSC niche and CSC mitochondria in OPC together with HPV status. To have an effective and a permanent therapy for OPC we believe all these factors have great importance and should be revealed. Targeting not only CSC but targeting cancer cells and CSC niche as well might be the preferable way to cure OPC (Figure 2).

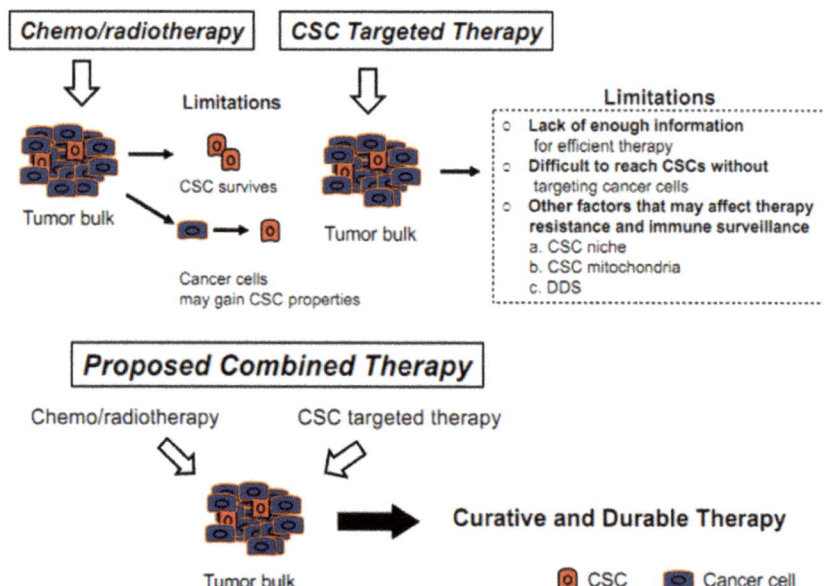

Figure 2. There are difficulties in each of conventional chemoradiotherapy and cancer stem cell (CSC) targeted therapy. While chemoradiotherapy leaves CSC untouched, CSC-targeted therapy leaves large tumor bulk with cancer cells, which may then gain CSC properties. Moreover, heterogeneity in various CSCs is another challenge to overcome.

Author Contributions: Writing—original draft preparation, M.G. and E.G.; Writing—review and editing, M.G., E.G., S.T., K.E. and M.H.; Supervision, M.H. All authors have read and agreed to the published version of the manuscript.

Funding: This research received no external funding.

Conflicts of Interest: The authors declare no conflict of interest.

References

1. Argiris, A.; Karamouzis, M.V.; Raben, D.; Ferris, R.L. Head and neck cancer. *Lancet* **2008**, *371*, 1695–1709. [CrossRef]
2. Johnson, D.E.; Burtness, B.; Leemans, C.R.; Lui, V.W.Y.; Bauman, J.E.; Grandis, J.R. Head and neck squamous cell carcinoma. *Nat. Rev. Dis. Primers* **2020**, *6*, 92. [CrossRef] [PubMed]
3. Spence, T.; Bruce, J.; Yip, K.W.; Liu, F.F. HPV Associated Head and Neck Cancer. *Cancers* **2016**, *8*, 75. [CrossRef]
4. Pinatti, L.M.; Walline, H.M.; Carey, T.E. Human Papillomavirus Genome Integration and Head and Neck Cancer. *J. Dent. Res.* **2018**, *97*, 691–700. [CrossRef]
5. Santacroce, L.; Di Cosola, M.; Bottalico, L.; Topi, S.; Charitos, I.A.; Ballini, A.; Inchingolo, F.; Cazzolla, A.P.; Dipalma, G. Focus on HPV Infection and the Molecular Mechanisms of Oral Carcinogenesis. *Viruses* **2021**, *13*, 559. [CrossRef] [PubMed]
6. Cancer Genome Atlas Network. Comprehensive genomic characterization of head and neck squamous cell carcinomas. *Nature* **2015**, *517*, 576–582. [CrossRef]
7. Sugihara, E.; Saya, H. Complexity of cancer stem cells. *Int. J. Cancer* **2013**, *132*, 1249–1259. [CrossRef]
8. Xie, X.; Teknos, T.N.; Pan, Q. Are all cancer stem cells created equal? *Stem Cells Transl. Med.* **2014**, *3*, 1111–1115. [CrossRef]
9. Bonnet, D.; Dick, J.E. Human acute myeloid leukemia is organized as a hierarchy that originates from a primitive hematopoietic cell. *Nat. Med.* **1997**, *3*, 730–737. [CrossRef]
10. Prince, M.E.; Sivanandan, R.; Kaczorowski, A.; Wolf, G.T.; Kaplan, M.J.; Dalerba, P.; Weissman, I.L.; Clarke, M.F.; Ailles, L.E. Identification of a subpopulation of cells with cancer stem cell properties in head and neck squamous cell carcinoma. *Proc. Natl. Acad. Sci. USA* **2007**, *104*, 973–978. [CrossRef]
11. Meacham, C.E.; Morrison, S.J. Tumour heterogeneity and cancer cell plasticity. *Nature* **2013**, *501*, 328–337. [CrossRef]
12. Beck, B.; Blanpain, C. Unravelling cancer stem cell potential. *Nat. Rev. Cancer* **2013**, *13*, 727–738. [CrossRef]
13. Moharil, R.B.; Dive, A.; Khandekar, S.; Bodhade, A. Cancer stem cells: An insight. *J. Oral Maxillofac. Pathol.* **2017**, *21*, 463. [CrossRef] [PubMed]
14. Vlashi, E.; Pajonk, F. Cancer stem cells, cancer cell plasticity and radiation therapy. *Semin. Cancer Biol.* **2015**, *31*, 28–35. [CrossRef]
15. Batlle, E.; Clevers, H. Cancer stem cells revisited. *Nat. Med.* **2017**, *23*, 1124–1134. [CrossRef] [PubMed]
16. ALDH1A1 Aldehyde Dehydrogenase 1 Family Member A1 [*Homo sapiens* (Human)]. Available online: https://www.ncbi.nlm.nih.gov/gene/216 (accessed on 20 April 2021).
17. Chen, Y.C.; Chen, Y.W.; Hsu, H.S.; Tseng, L.M.; Huang, P.I.; Lu, K.H.; Chen, D.T.; Tai, L.K.; Yung, M.C.; Chang, S.C.; et al. Aldehyde dehydrogenase 1 is a putative marker for cancer stem cells in head and neck squamous cancer. *Biochem. Biophys. Res. Commun.* **2009**, *385*, 307–313. [CrossRef] [PubMed]
18. Clay, M.R.; Tabor, M.; Owen, J.H.; Carey, T.E.; Bradford, C.R.; Wolf, G.T.; Wicha, M.S.; Prince, M.E. Single-marker identification of head and neck squamous cell carcinoma cancer stem cells with aldehyde dehydrogenase. *Head Neck* **2010**, *32*, 1195–1201. [CrossRef] [PubMed]
19. Qian, X.; Wagner, S.; Ma, C.; Coordes, A.; Gekeler, J.; Klussmann, J.P.; Hummel, M.; Kaufmann, A.M.; Albers, A.E. Prognostic significance of ALDH1A1-positive cancer stem cells in patients with locally advanced, metastasized head and neck squamous cell carcinoma. *J. Cancer Res. Clin. Oncol.* **2014**, *140*, 1151–1158. [CrossRef] [PubMed]
20. Szafarowski, T.; Sierdziński, J.; Ludwig, N.; Głuszko, A.; Filipowska, A.; Szczepański, M.J. Assessment of cancer stem cell marker expression in primary head and neck squamous cell carcinoma shows prognostic value for aldehyde dehydrogenase (ALDH1A1). *Eur. J. Pharm.* **2020**, *867*, 172837. [CrossRef]
21. Leinung, M.; Ernst, B.; Döring, C.; Wagenblast, J.; Tahtali, A.; Diensthuber, M.; Stöver, T.; Geissler, C. Expression of ALDH1A1 and CD44 in primary head and neck squamous cell carcinoma and their value for carcinogenesis, tumor progression and cancer stem cell identification. *Oncol. Lett.* **2015**, *10*, 2289–2294. [CrossRef] [PubMed]
22. Gunduz, M.; Gunduz, E.; Tamagawa, S.; Enomoto, K.; Hotomi, M. Identification and chemoresistance of cancer stem cells in HPV-negative oropharyngeal cancer. *Oncol. Lett.* **2020**, *19*, 965–971. [CrossRef] [PubMed]
23. Sterz, C.M.; Kulle, C.; Dakic, B.; Makarova, G.; Böttcher, M.C.; Bette, M.; Werner, J.A.; Mandic, R. A basal-cell-like compartment in head and neck squamous cell carcinomas represents the invasive front of the tumor and is expressing MMP-9. *Oral Oncol.* **2010**, *46*, 116–122. [CrossRef] [PubMed]
24. Duarte, S.; Loubat, A.; Momier, D.; Topi, M.; Faneca, H.; Pedroso de Lima, M.C.; Carle, G.F.; Pierrefite-Carle, V. Isolation of head and neck squamous carcinoma cancer stem-like cells in a syngeneic mouse model and analysis of hypoxia effect. *Oncol. Rep.* **2012**, *28*, 1057–1062. [CrossRef] [PubMed]
25. Chen, C.; Wei, Y.; Hummel, M.; Hoffmann, T.K.; Gross, M.; Kaufmann, A.M.; Albers, A.E. Evidence for epithelial-mesenchymal transition in cancer stem cells of head and neck squamous cell carcinoma. *PLoS ONE* **2011**, *6*, e16466. [CrossRef]

26. Liao, T.; Kaufmann, A.M.; Qian, X.; Sangvatanakul, V.; Chen, C.; Kube, T.; Zhang, G.; Albers, A.E. Susceptibility to cytotoxic T cell lysis of cancer stem cells derived from cervical and head and neck tumor cell lines. *J. Cancer. Res. Clin. Oncol.* **2013**, *139*, 159–170. [CrossRef] [PubMed]
27. CD44 CD44 Molecule (Indian Blood Group) [*Homo sapiens* (Human)]. Available online: https://www.ncbi.nlm.nih.gov/gene/960 (accessed on 20 April 2021).
28. Gomez, K.E.; Wu, F.; Keysar, S.B.; Morton, J.J.; Miller, B.; Chimed, T.S.; Le, P.N.; Nieto, C.; Chowdhury, F.N.; Tyagi, A.; et al. Cancer Cell CD44 Mediates Macrophage/Monocyte-Driven Regulation of Head and Neck Cancer Stem Cells. *Cancer Res.* **2020**, *80*, 4185–4198. [CrossRef]
29. Huang, C.; Yoon, C.; Zhou, X.H.; Zhou, Y.C.; Zhou, W.W.; Liu, H.; Yang, X.; Lu, J.; Lee, S.Y.; Huang, K. ERK1/2-Nanog signaling pathway enhances CD44(+) cancer stem-like cell phenotypes and epithelial-to-mesenchymal transition in head and neck squamous cell carcinomas. *Cell Death Dis.* **2020**, *11*, 266. [CrossRef] [PubMed]
30. Jakob, M.; Sharaf, K.; Schirmer, M.; Leu, M.; Küffer, S.; Bertlich, M.; Ihler, F.; Haubner, F.; Canis, M.; Kitz, J. Role of cancer stem cell markers ALDH1, BCL11B, BMI-1, and CD44 in the prognosis of advanced HNSCC. *Strahlenther. Onkol.* **2021**, *197*, 231–245. [CrossRef]
31. Chanmee, T.; Ontong, P.; Kimata, K.; Itano, N. Key Roles of Hyaluronan and Its CD44 Receptor in the Stemness and Survival of Cancer Stem Cells. *Front. Oncol.* **2015**, *5*, 180. [CrossRef] [PubMed]
32. Zhang, P.; Zhang, Y.; Mao, L.; Zhang, Z.; Chen, W. Side population in oral squamous cell carcinoma possesses tumor stem cell phenotypes. *Cancer Lett.* **2009**, *277*, 227–234. [CrossRef]
33. Pries, R.; Witrkopf, N.; Trenkle, T.; Nitsch, S.M.; Wollenberg, B. Potential stem cell marker CD44 is constitutively expressed in permanent cell lines of head and neck cancer. *In Vivo* **2008**, *22*, 89–92. [PubMed]
34. Ludwig, N.; Szczepanski, M.J.; Gluszko, A.; Szafarowski, T.; Azambuja, J.H.; Dolg, L.; Gellrich, N.C.; Kampmann, A.; Whiteside, T.L.; Zimmerer, R.M. CD44(+) tumor cells promote early angiogenesis in head and neck squamous cell carcinoma. *Cancer Lett.* **2019**, *467*, 85–95. [CrossRef] [PubMed]
35. Judd, N.P.; Winkler, A.E.; Murillo-Sauca, O.; Brotman, J.J.; Law, J.H.; Lewis, J.S., Jr.; Dunn, G.P.; Bui, J.D.; Sunwoo, J.B.; Uppaluri, R. ERK1/2 regulation of CD44 modulates oral cancer aggressiveness. *Cancer. Res.* **2012**, *72*, 365–374. [CrossRef] [PubMed]
36. Näsman, A.; Nordfors, C.; Grün, N.; Munck-Wikland, E.; Ramqvist, T.; Marklund, L.; Lindquist, D.; Dalianis, T. Absent/weak CD44 intensity and positive human papillomavirus (HPV) status in oropharyngeal squamous cell carcinoma indicates a very high survival. *Cancer Med.* **2013**, *2*, 507–518. [CrossRef] [PubMed]
37. Chen, J.; Zhou, J.; Lu, J.; Xiong, H.; Shi, X.; Gong, L. Significance of CD44 expression in head and neck cancer: A systemic review and meta-analysis. *BMC Cancer* **2014**, *14*, 15. [CrossRef]
38. BMI1 BMI1 Proto-Oncogene, Polycomb Ring Finger [*Homo sapiens* (Human)]. Available online: www.ncbi.nlm.nih.gov/gene/648 (accessed on 20 April 2021).
39. Chen, D.; Wu, M.; Li, Y.; Chang, I.; Yuan, Q.; Ekimyan-Salvo, M.; Deng, P.; Yu, B.; Yu, Y.; Dong, J.; et al. Targeting BMI1+ Cancer Stem Cells Overcomes Chemoresistance and Inhibits Metastases in Squamous Cell Carcinoma. *Cell Stem Cell* **2017**, *20*, 621–634.e6. [CrossRef]
40. Jia, L.; Zhang, W.; Wang, C.Y. BMI1 Inhibition Eliminates Residual Cancer Stem Cells after PD1 Blockade and Activates Antitumor Immunity to Prevent Metastasis and Relapse. *Cell Stem Cell* **2020**, *27*, 238–253. [CrossRef]
41. Wang, Q.; Li, Z.; Wu, Y.; Huang, R.; Zhu, Y.; Zhang, W.; Wang, Y.; Cheng, J. Pharmacological inhibition of Bmi1 by PTC-209 impaired tumor growth in head neck squamous cell carcinoma. *Cancer Cell Int.* **2017**, *17*, 107. [CrossRef]
42. Hu, J.; Mirshahidi, S.; Simental, A.; Lee, S.C.; De Andrade Filho, P.A.; Peterson, N.R.; Duerksen-Hughes, P.; Yuan, X. Cancer stem cell self-renewal as a therapeutic target in human oral cancer. *Oncogene* **2019**, *38*, 5440–5456. [CrossRef]
43. POU5F1 POU Class 5 Homeobox 1 [*Homo sapiens* (Human)]. Available online: www.ncbi.nlm.nih.gov/gene/5460 (accessed on 20 April 2021).
44. Koo, B.S.; Lee, S.H.; Kim, J.M.; Huang, S.; Kim, S.H.; Rho, Y.S.; Bae, W.J.; Kang, H.J.; Kim, Y.S.; Moon, J.H.; et al. Oct4 is a critical regulator of stemness in head and neck squamous carcinoma cells. *Oncogene* **2015**, *34*, 2317–2324. [CrossRef]
45. Tsai, L.L.; Hu, F.W.; Lee, S.S.; Yu, C.H.; Yu, C.C.; Chang, Y.C. Oct4 mediates tumor initiating properties in oral squamous cell carcinomas through the regulation of epithelial-mesenchymal transition. *PLoS ONE* **2014**, *9*, e87207. [CrossRef] [PubMed]
46. Fan, Z.; Li, M.; Chen, X.; Wang, J.; Liang, X.; Wang, H.; Wang, Z.; Cheng, B.; Xia, J. Prognostic Value of Cancer Stem Cell Markers in Head and Neck Squamous Cell Carcinoma: A Meta-analysis. *Sci. Rep.* **2017**, *7*, 43008. [CrossRef] [PubMed]
47. SOX2 SRY-Box Transcription Factor 2 [*Homo sapiens* (Human)]. Available online: www.ncbi.nlm.nih.gov/gene/6657 (accessed on 20 April 2021).
48. Keysar, S.B.; Le, P.N.; Miller, B.; Jackson, B.C.; Eagles, J.R.; Nieto, C.; Kim, J.; Tang, B.; Glogowska, M.J.; Morton, J.J.; et al. Regulation of Head and Neck Squamous Cancer Stem Cells by PI3K and SOX2. *J. Natl. Cancer Inst.* **2016**, *109*, djw189. [CrossRef] [PubMed]
49. Chung, J.H.; Jung, H.R.; Jung, A.R.; Lee, Y.C.; Kong, M.; Lee, J.S.; Eun, Y.G. SOX2 activation predicts prognosis in patients with head and neck squamous cell carcinoma. *Sci. Rep.* **2018**, *8*, 1677. [CrossRef]
50. Omori, H.; Sato, K.; Nakano, T.; Wakasaki, T.; Toh, S.; Taguchi, K.; Nakagawa, T.; Masuda, M. Stress-triggered YAP1/SOX2 activation transcriptionally reprograms head and neck squamous cell carcinoma for the acquisition of stemness. *J. Cancer Res. Clin. Oncol.* **2019**, *145*, 2433–2444. [CrossRef]

51. PROM1 Prominin 1 [Homo Sapiens (Human)]. Available online: www.ncbi.nlm.nih.gov/gene/8842 (accessed on 20 April 2021).
52. Lee, J.; Park, M.; Ko, Y.; Kim, B.; Kim, O.; Hyun, H.; Kim, D.; Sohn, H.; Moon, Y.L.; Lim, W. Ectopic overexpression of CD133 in HNSCC makes it resistant to commonly used chemotherapeutics. *Tumour Biol.* **2017**, *39*, 1010428317695534. [CrossRef] [PubMed]
53. Chen, Y.S.; Wu, M.J.; Huang, C.Y.; Lin, S.C.; Chuang, T.H.; Yu, C.C.; Lo, J.F. CD133/Src axis mediates tumor initiating property and epithelial-mesenchymal transition of head and neck cancer. *PLoS ONE* **2011**, *6*, e28053. [CrossRef]
54. Hu, Z.; Liu, H.; Zhang, X.; Hong, B.; Wu, Z.; Li, Q.; Zhou, C. Promoter hypermethylation of CD133/PROM1 is an independent poor prognosis factor for head and neck squamous cell carcinoma. *Medicine* **2020**, *99*, e19491. [CrossRef] [PubMed]
55. Rietbergen, M.M.; Martens-de Kemp, S.R.; Bloemena, E.; Witte, B.I.; Brink, A.; Baatenburg de Jong, R.J.; Leemans, C.R.; Braakhuis, B.J.; Brakenhoff, R.H. Cancer stem cell enrichment marker CD98: A prognostic factor for survival in patients with human papillomavirus-positive oropharyngeal cancer. *Eur. J. Cancer* **2014**, *50*, 765–773. [CrossRef]
56. Motegi, A.; Fujii, S.; Zenda, S.; Arahira, S.; Tahara, M.; Hayashi, R.; Akimoto, T. Impact of Expression of CD44, a Cancer Stem Cell Marker, on the Treatment Outcomes of Intensity Modulated Radiation Therapy in Patients with Oropharyngeal Squamous Cell Carcinoma. *Int. J. Radiat. Oncol. Biol. Phys.* **2016**, *94*, 461–468. [CrossRef]
57. Mohamed, H.; Hagström, J.; Jouhi, L.; Atula, T.; Almangush, A.; Mäkitie, A.; Haglund, C. The expression and prognostic value of stem cell markers Bmi-1, HESC5:3, and HES77 in human papillomavirus-positive and -negative oropharyngeal squamous cell carcinoma. *Tumour Biol.* **2019**, *41*, 1010428319840473. [CrossRef] [PubMed]
58. Lee, S.H.; Rigas, N.K.; Lee, C.R.; Bang, A.; Srikanth, S.; Gwack, Y.; Kang, M.K.; Kim, R.H.; Park, N.H.; Shin, K.H. Orai1 promotes tumor progression by enhancing cancer stemness via NFAT signaling in oral/oropharyngeal squamous cell carcinoma. *Oncotarget* **2016**, *7*, 43239–43255. [CrossRef]
59. Lee, S.H.; Kieu, C.; Martin, C.E.; Han, J.; Chen, W.; Kim, J.S.; Kang, M.K.; Kim, R.H.; Park, N.H.; Kim, Y.; et al. NFATc3 plays an oncogenic role in oral/oropharyngeal squamous cell carcinomas by promoting cancer stemness via expression of OCT4. *Oncotarget* **2019**, *10*, 2306–2319. [CrossRef]
60. Hufbauer, M.; Maltseva, M.; Meinrath, J.; Lechner, A.; Beutner, D.; Huebbers, C.U.; Akgül, B. HPV16 increases the number of migratory cancer stem cells and modulates their miRNA expression profile in oropharyngeal cancer. *Int. J. Cancer* **2018**, *143*, 1426–1439. [CrossRef]
61. Zhang, M.; Kumar, B.; Piao, L.; Xie, X.; Schmitt, A.; Arradaza, N.; Cippola, M.; Old, M.; Agrawal, A.; Ozer, E.; et al. Elevated intrinsic cancer stem cell population in human papillomavirus-associated head and neck squamous cell carcinoma. *Cancer* **2014**, *120*, 992–1001. [CrossRef]
62. Mani, S.A.; Guo, W.; Liao, M.J.; Eaton, E.N.; Ayyanan, A.; Zhou, A.Y.; Brooks, M.; Reinhard, F.; Zhang, C.C.; Shipitsin, M.; et al. The epithelial-mesenchymal transition generates cells with properties of stem cells. *Cell* **2008**, *133*, 704–715. [CrossRef] [PubMed]
63. Marcucci, F.; Stassi, G.; De Maria, R. Epithelial-mesenchymal transition: A new target in anticancer drug discovery. *Nat. Rev. Drug Discov.* **2016**, *15*, 311–325. [CrossRef] [PubMed]
64. Levental, K.R.; Yu, H.; Kass, L.; Lakins, J.N.; Egeblad, M.; Erler, J.T.; Fong, S.F.; Csiszar, K.; Giaccia, A.; Weninger, W.; et al. Matrix crosslinking forces tumor progression by enhancing integrin signaling. *Cell* **2009**, *139*, 891–906. [CrossRef] [PubMed]
65. Duan, H.; Liu, Y.; Gao, Z.; Huang, W. Recent advances in drug delivery systems for targeting cancer stem cells. *Acta Pharm. Sin. B.* **2021**, *11*, 55–70. [CrossRef] [PubMed]
66. Wu, V.; Auchman, M.; Mollica, P.A.; Sachs, P.C.; Bruno, R.D. ALDH1A1 positive cells are a unique component of the tonsillar crypt niche and are lost along with NGFR positive stem cells during tumourigenesis. *Pathology* **2018**, *50*, 524–529. [CrossRef] [PubMed]
67. Xu, J.; Müller, S.; Nannapaneni, S.; Pan, L.; Wang, Y.; Peng, X.; Wang, D.; Tighiouart, M.; Chen, Z.; Saba, N.F.; et al. Comparison of quantum dot technology with conventional immunohistochemistry in examining aldehyde dehydrogenase 1A1 as a potential biomarker for lymph node metastasis of head and neck cancer. *Eur. J. Cancer* **2012**, *48*, 1682–1691. [CrossRef] [PubMed]
68. Geißler, C.; Hambek, M.; Leinung, M.; Diensthuber, M.; Gassner, D.; Stöver, T.; Wagenblast, J. The challenge of tumor heterogeneity–different phenotypes of cancer stem cells in a head and neck squamous cell carcinoma xenograft mouse model. *In Vivo* **2012**, *26*, 593–598. [PubMed]
69. Yu, S.S.; Cirillo, N. The molecular markers of cancer stem cells in head and neck tumors. *J. Cell. Physiol.* **2020**, *235*, 65–73. [CrossRef]
70. Chaffer, C.L.; Weinberg, R.A. A perspective on cancer cell metastasis. *Science* **2011**, *331*, 1559–1564. [CrossRef]
71. Malanchi, I.; Santamaria-Martínez, A.; Susanto, E.; Peng, H.; Lehr, H.A.; Delaloye, J.F.; Huelsken, J. Interactions between cancer stem cells and their niche govern metastatic colonization. *Nature* **2011**, *481*, 85–89. [CrossRef]
72. Lawson, D.A.; Bhakta, N.R.; Kessenbrock, K.; Prummel, K.D.; Yu, Y.; Takai, K.; Zhou, A.; Eyob, H.; Balakrishnan, S.; Wang, C.Y.; et al. Single-cell analysis reveals a stem-cell program in human metastatic breast cancer cells. *Nature* **2015**, *526*, 131–135. [CrossRef]
73. Dawood, S.; Austin, L.; Cristofanilli, M. Cancer stem cells: Implications for cancer therapy. *Oncology* **2014**, *28*, 1101–1107.
74. Eun, K.; Ham, S.W.; Kim, H. Cancer stem cell heterogeneity: Origin and new perspectives on CSC targeting. *BMB Rep.* **2017**, *50*, 117–125. [CrossRef] [PubMed]
75. Miranda, A.; Hamilton, P.T.; Zhang, A.W.; Pattnaik, S.; Becht, E.; Mezheyeuski, A.; Bruun, J.; Micke, P.; de Reynies, A.; Nelson, B.H. Cancer stemness, intratumoral heterogeneity, and immune response across cancers. *Proc. Natl. Acad. Sci. USA* **2019**, *116*, 9020–9029. [CrossRef] [PubMed]

76. Morrison, R.; Schleicher, S.M.; Sun, Y.; Niermann, K.J.; Kim, S.; Spratt, D.E.; Chung, C.H.; Lu, B. Targeting the mechanisms of resistance to chemotherapy and radiotherapy with the cancer stem cell hypothesis. *J. Oncol.* **2011**, *2011*, 941876. [CrossRef] [PubMed]
77. Modur, V.; Thomas-Robbins, K.; Rao, K. HPV and CSC in HNSCC cisplatin resistance. *Front. Biosci.* **2015**, *7*, 58–66.
78. Ghisolfi, L.; Keates, A.C.; Hu, X.; Lee, D.K.; Li, C.J. Ionizing radiation induces stemness in cancer cells. *PLoS ONE* **2012**, *7*, e43628. [CrossRef]
79. Barr, M.P.; Gray, S.G.; Hoffmann, A.C.; Hilger, R.A.; Thomale, J.; O'Flaherty, J.D.; Fennell, D.A.; Richard, D.; O'Leary, J.J.; O'Byrne, K.J. Correction: Generation and Characterisation of Cisplatin-Resistant Non-Small Cell Lung Cancer Cell Lines Displaying a Stem-Like Signature. *PLoS ONE* **2020**, *15*, e0233739. [CrossRef] [PubMed]
80. Pützer, B.M.; Solanki, M.; Herchenröder, O. Advances in cancer stem cell targeting: How to strike the evil at its root. *Adv. Drug Deliv. Rev.* **2017**, *120*, 89–107. [CrossRef]
81. Oshimori, N. Cancer stem cells and their niche in the progression of squamous cell carcinoma. *Cancer Sci.* **2020**, *111*, 3985–3992. [CrossRef]
82. Skoda, J.; Borankova, K.; Jansson, P.J.; Huang, M.L.; Veselska, R.; Richardson, D.R. Pharmacological targeting of mitochondria in cancer stem cells: An ancient organelle at the crossroad of novel anti-cancer therapies. *Pharmacol. Res.* **2019**, *139*, 298–313. [CrossRef]
83. García-Heredia, J.M.; Carnero, A. Role of Mitochondria in Cancer Stem Cell Resistance. *Cells* **2020**, *9*, 1693. [CrossRef]
84. Scatena, C.; Roncella, M.; Di Paolo, A.; Aretini, P.; Menicagli, M.; Fanelli, G.; Marini, C.; Mazzanti, C.M.; Ghilli, M.; Sotgia, F.; et al. Doxycycline, an Inhibitor of Mitochondrial Biogenesis, Effectively Reduces Cancer Stem Cells (CSCs) in Early Breast Cancer Patients: A Clinical Pilot Study. *Front. Oncol.* **2018**, *8*, 452. [CrossRef]
85. Fiorillo, M.; Tóth, F.; Sotgia, F.; Lisanti, M.P. Doxycycline, Azithromycin and Vitamin C (DAV): A potent combination therapy for targeting mitochondria and eradicating cancer stem cells (CSCs). *Aging* **2019**, *11*, 2202–2216. [CrossRef]
86. De Francesco, E.M.; Ózsvári, B.; Sotgia, F.; Lisanti, M.P. Dodecyl-TPP Targets Mitochondria and Potently Eradicates Cancer Stem Cells (CSCs): Synergy with FDA-Approved Drugs and Natural Compounds (Vitamin C and Berberine). *Front. Oncol.* **2019**, *9*, 615. [CrossRef] [PubMed]

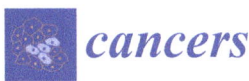

Review

Molecular Tumor Subtypes of HPV-Positive Head and Neck Cancers: Biological Characteristics and Implications for Clinical Outcomes

Tingting Qin [1,2,†], Shiting Li [1,†], Leanne E. Henry [1,3], Siyu Liu [1] and Maureen A. Sartor [1,2,*]

1. Department of Computational Medicine and Bioinformatics, Medical School, University of Michigan, Ann Arbor, MI 48109, USA; qinting@umich.edu (T.Q.); shitingl@umich.edu (S.L.); lechenry@umich.edu (L.E.H.); liusiyu@umich.edu (S.L.)
2. Rogel Comprehensive Cancer Center, University of Michigan, Ann Arbor, MI 48109, USA
3. Department of Computer Science, LS&A, University of Michigan, Ann Arbor, MI 48109, USA
* Correspondence: sartorma@umich.edu
† These authors contributed equally to this work.

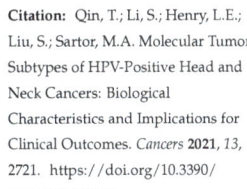

Citation: Qin, T.; Li, S.; Henry, L.E.; Liu, S.; Sartor, M.A. Molecular Tumor Subtypes of HPV-Positive Head and Neck Cancers: Biological Characteristics and Implications for Clinical Outcomes. *Cancers* **2021**, *13*, 2721. https://doi.org/10.3390/cancers13112721

Academic Editor: Frank Traub

Received: 30 April 2021
Accepted: 27 May 2021
Published: 31 May 2021

Publisher's Note: MDPI stays neutral with regard to jurisdictional claims in published maps and institutional affiliations.

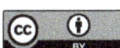

Copyright: © 2021 by the authors. Licensee MDPI, Basel, Switzerland. This article is an open access article distributed under the terms and conditions of the Creative Commons Attribution (CC BY) license (https://creativecommons.org/licenses/by/4.0/).

Simple Summary: Human papillomavirus (HPV) infections are responsible for a continually growing number of head and neck cancer (HNC) cases, with the incident rate overtaking that of HPV-related cervical cancers in the United States. Most HPV-related HNC cases arise in the oropharynx, and although they have a better 5-year survival rate than non-HPV-related HNC patients (80% compared to 50%), de-escalating treatment in all HPV(+) patients in an attempt to improve quality of life led to unacceptable results. Studying molecular subtypes of HPV(+) HNC can help to identify treatment regimens tailored to each patient's tumor characteristics. We synthesized information from several studies of HPV(+) HNC subtypes, and describe three main groups that differ by their immune cell content, level of keratinocyte differentiation, degree of epithelial-to-mesenchymal transition, probability of HPV integration, oxidoreductase activity and stromal cell (e.g., cancer-associated fibroblast) content. The differences have important implications for local or distant recurrence, treatment response and survival.

Abstract: Until recently, research on the molecular signatures of Human papillomavirus (HPV)-associated head and neck cancers mainly focused on their differences with respect to HPV-negative head and neck squamous cell carcinomas (HNSCCs). However, given the continuing high incidence level of HPV-related HNSCC, the time is ripe to characterize the heterogeneity that exists within these cancers. Here, we review research thus far on HPV-positive HNSCC molecular subtypes, and their relationship with clinical characteristics and HPV integration into the host genome. Different omics data including host transcriptomics and epigenomics, as well as HPV characteristics, can provide complementary viewpoints. Keratinization, mesenchymal differentiation, immune signatures, stromal cells and oxidoreductive processes all play important roles.

Keywords: human papillomavirus; head and neck cancer; cancer subtypes; gene expression; oropharynx; HPV integration; immune response; keratinization

1. Phenotypic, Clinical and Molecular Characteristics of HPV-Positive HNSCC, and Evidence That They Are Not a Homogenous Group

With an estimated 650,000 new cases and 330,000 deaths worldwide each year, head and neck cancer represents a surprisingly heterogeneous group of tumors, the great majority of which are head and neck squamous cell carcinomas (HNSCCs) [1]. High risk human papillomavirus (HPV) infections are responsible for a continually growing number of HNSCC cases, with the incident rate now overtaking that of HPV-related cervical cancers in the United States (https://www.cdc.gov/cancer/hpv/statistics/cases.htm, accessed on 25 January 2021). Most HPV-related head and neck cases arise in the oropharynx, however a smaller percent are in the oral cavity and larynx, with negligible numbers in the other sites [2]. Worldwide, there are approximately 93,000 new oropharynx cancers cases diagnosed each year, resulting in an expected 51,000 deaths [1]. In the US, HPV is associated with approximately 36,000 new cancer cases annually, with an estimated 14,000 of those in the oropharynx (https://www.cdc.gov/cancer/hpv/statistics/cases.htm, accessed on 25 January 2021).

There is consensus among researchers that HPV-associated head and neck tumors represent a distinct tumor entity, with patient demographic, clinical and molecular differences [3,4]. Demographically, HPV-positive HNSCC patients tend to be slightly younger (mode of 60–64 years) [5], less likely to smoke, and follow a healthier diet than HPV(−) HNSCC patients [6,7]. Clinically, HPV-positive HNSCC tumors tend to be poorly differentiated and more likely to have positive lymph node status [8]. In spite of these poor prognosis markers, they have a significant survival advantage over their HPV(−) HNSCC counterparts, with an approximate 80% 5-year survival rate compared to 50% for HPV(−) HNSCC. This difference can be attributed to higher response rates to induction chemotherapy and chemoradiation [9,10]. However, this survival advantage is observed mainly in HPV(+) oropharyngeal cancer cases, with much smaller HPV survival advantages in other sites [9,11,12]. Given the high rate of survival and severe adverse effects from standard treatment protocols that significantly reduce quality of life for survivors, interest has grown in treatment de-escalation for HPV(+) oropharyngeal cancer patients. Unfortunately, two clinical trials that de-escalated treatment for all HPV(+) oropharynx cases or all with minimal smoking history resulted in worse survival [13], with both trials testing the substitution of cisplatin with cetuximab. These results suggest the need to identify the subset of patients who are most likely to benefit from de-escalation.

At the molecular level, HPV elicits initial carcinogenic hits with its two main oncoproteins E6 and E7, which target *p53* and *Rb* for degradation, respectively [14]. Disabling these key tumor suppressor proteins alone, however, is not sufficient for malignancy; several other factors, including smoking or other tobacco use history, alcohol use, patient age, patient intrinsic immune function, genetics and epigenetics also contribute to carcinogenesis. Genetically, the most commonly mutated genes in HNSCC differ depending upon HPV status. For HPV(+) tumors, top driving gene mutations include the genes *PIK3CA*, *KMT2D*, *PTEN*, *TRAF3* and *FGFR3*, and the *APOBEC* mutation signature is strongly associated with patients' total mutational burdens [15,16]. In terms of DNA methylation, the most well-studied epigenetic mark, HPV(+) tumors tend to exhibit a hypermethylation phenotype compared to HPV(−) HNSCCs [17,18]. These factors also ultimately contribute to the heterogeneity observed within the group of HPV(+) HNSCC tumors and patient outcomes. This heterogeneity is not surprising, considering the many other important contributors to heterogeneity, including stage at diagnosis, tumor mutational profile, immune characteristics, effects of HPV integration and more.

However, despite the variations in molecular profiles and clinical outcomes of HPV(+) HNSCC patients, until recently the main research focus has been on the delineations of head and neck cancer by HPV(−)status. While many other works demonstrate the unique characteristics of HPV(+) tumors compared to HPV(−), e.g., [19], relatively few studies have examined the heterogeneity within HPV(+) tumors. As we and others have shown, such heterogeneity exists in terms of gene expression, genetics (driving mutations and copy number alterations), epigenetics (DNA methylation and 5-hydroxymethylation) and clinical outcomes, in some cases to the extent of differences by HPV(−)status. In other words, depending on the attribute studied, HPV(+) subtypes may be as different from each other as they are compared to HPV(−) tumors. Certain characteristics associated with HPV(+) tumors in general, may actually be attributable to only a subset of HPV(+) patients, and these characteristics may have important clinical effects.

Here, we review the literature on HPV(+) head and neck cancer subtypes, hoping that it will highlight the need to move the field forward from treating HPV(+) HNSCC as a homogeneous group to understanding HPV(+) HNSCC as a complex, multi-faceted group of heterogeneous cancers. We first review the early, initial recognitions of HPV(+) subtypes which were based on microarray gene expression data and thus limited in their discoveries. We then proceed to describe the defining characteristics of the main HPV(+) subtypes as fleshed out with next generation sequencing data and epigenomic assays. The HPV(+) HNSCC subtypes are then compared to HPV-associated cervical cancer subtypes, before reviewing the important role that HPV integration into the host genome plays in defining subtypes. Other mechanisms contributing to the subtypes are also discussed, before presenting what has been observed in terms of subtypes and HPV integration in relation to survival outcomes. Finally, the future potential for de-escalation treatment in a subset of HPV(+) oropharynx cancer patients is discussed, along with the potential of additional targeted therapies for subgroups with worse prognosis.

2. Early Research on HPV(+) Subtypes and Heterogeneity within HPV(+) HNSCCs

Studies as early as 2007 using microarray analysis were able to identify distinct subtypes in HPV(+) head and neck cancers using this gene expression data alone. In one study that included 42 head and neck cancer cases, 16 of which were HPV(+), two subgroups of HPV(+) cancers were identified after performing clustering techniques on differentially expressed genes between HPV(+) and HPV(−) cancers [20]. These two HPV(+) subgroups were consistently formulated regardless of clustering method and numbers of differentially expressed genes. Furthermore, the identified subgroups, referred to as α and β, did not significantly correlate with any particular clinical or demographic variables, such as anatomic site, age and clinical stage [20]. However, they were associated with unique pathways based on gene expression signatures. The α subgroup exhibited high up-regulation of B lymphocyte/lymphoma-related genes as well as genes expressed by endothelial cells. Genes related to small proline-rich proteins, structural cross-linking proteins of the cell envelope of keratinocytes, were down-regulated. Additionally, the α subgroup had an increased relative expression of *SYNPO2*, a gene important in regulating cell migration, which suggests that this subpopulation may have higher invasive potential [20]. The β subgroup expression pattern, conversely, suggested high keratinization (e.g., *KRT6B* and *KRT16*) and gap junction proteins for this subtype. Whether the differences in gene expression between these two subgroups reflect differences in biology and clinical outcomes remained to be determined.

A later study by Keck et al., using a microarray approach also identified two biologically distinct HPV(+) subtypes: inflamed/mesenchymal (IMS) and classical (CL) [21]. In contrast, HPV(−) head and neck cancers were molecularly categorized into three subgroups: IMS, CL and basal (BA). Despite some overlap in gene expression between HPV(+) and HPV(−) head and neck cancers within the same subgroup, many of the biological pathways associated with HPV(+) and (−) tumors remain distinct [21]. Tumors in the IMS group were characterized by expression of immune response, mesenchymal and proliferation gene signatures with downregulation of epithelial markers, and may therefore reflect tumors with CD8+ T lymphocyte infiltration, epithelial-to-mesenchymal transition (EMT) and high proliferation [21], similar to the α subgroup in Pyeon et al. This HPV subtype also had increased cell cycle pathway activities and histologically appeared poorly differentiated and non-keratinizing. Likewise, CL subtype HPV tumors also had upregulation of cell-cycle genes and proliferation signatures, but were characterized by activation of the polyamine degradation pathway [21]. However, CL subtype HPV tumors showed keratinization and were not as poorly differentiated morphologically as IMS subtype HPV tumors. Due to the use of microarray data, the relationship between HPV subtypes and characteristics of HPV itself could not be determined. However interestingly, the two molecular HPV subtypes were associated with prognosis. The IMS subtype demonstrated improved overall survival compared to the CL subtype, which may reflect the increased CD8 T cell infiltration in IMS tumors. These findings suggest that even within HPV(+) tumors, biological differences exist between tumor subtypes that may have implications on treatment and prognosis.

Studies of larger cohorts with higher resolution RNA-seq based data, genome-wide DNA methylation and HPV insertion sites into the host genome helped to further subclassify HPV(+) tumors and identify causal factors for the differing expression patterns. The first of these was from The Cancer Genome Atlas (TCGA) HNSC project. Using RNA-seq data for 36 HPV(+) and 243 HPV(−) head and neck cancer tumors, the TCGA HNSC project identified four gene expression subtypes: atypical, basal, classical and mesenchymal [16]. However, almost all HPV(+) samples were classified as atypical, which could be due to HPV(−) samples driving the subtype analysis, as there were many more HPV(−) samples than HPV(+). Overall, The TCGA analysis could not properly distinguish HPV(+) subtypes, but following their project, multiple RNA-seq based studies were able to identify subtypes within HPV(+) HNSCCs, often utilizing the HPV(+) TCGA samples which increased in number over time. Table 1 provides an overview of the main microarray and RNAseq studies used to define HPV(+) HNSCC subtypes.

Table 1. Gene Expression Studies that Defined HPV(+) HNSCC Subtypes.

Citation	HPV(+) Subtype Names	Figure Abbr	Data Used to Define Subtypes	Sample Size	Sites
Pyeon et al., 2007	α (B cell strong), β (highly keratinized)	-	Expression microarrays	16 HPV(+); 26 HPV(−)	Oropharynx; oral cavity
Keck et al., 2015	IMS (immune strong), BA (basal-like), CL (classical)	KECK	Expression microarrays	371 total; 55 HPV(+); 75 HPV(−) *	Oropharynx; oral cavity; larynx
TCGA 2015	Atypical, Basal, Classical, Mesenchymal	NAT	RNAseq	36 HPV(+); 243 HPV(−)	All HNSCC
Zhang et al., 2016	IMU (immune strong); KRT (highly keratinized)	CCR	RNAseq	84 HPV(+); 18 HPV(−)	Oropharynx; oral cavity
Lee et al., 2018	1 (cervical-like); 2 (HNSCC classical); 3 (lung-like)	ORA	RNAseq	1346 total; 514 HNSCC; 65 HPV(+)	HNSCC, esophageal, lung, cervical
Locati et al., 2019	Cl1 (immune strong, high stromal); Cl2 (highly keratinized; high stromal); Cl3 (highly keratinized; low stromal)	CAN	RNAseq and microarrays meta-analysis	346 HPV(+)	Oropharynx, oral cavity, larynx, hypopharynx

* For Keck et al., only 130 have known HPV status.

3. Defining Characteristics of the Main HPV(+) Subtypes

During the last five years, multiple studies have uncovered new evidence further characterizing the main HPV(+) HNSCC subtypes, the main ones being Zhang et al., Locati et al. and Lee et al. [22–24]. Based on gene expression profiles of a combination of 18 HPV(+) HNSCC from University of Michigan Hospital and 66 TCGA HPV(+) HNSCC samples, Zhang et al., revealed two HPV(+) subtypes, which were named IMU and KRT. Similar to the α and IMS subgroups described above, the IMU subtype was defined by a heightened immune response, mesenchymal differentiation and angiogenesis expression, whereas the KRT subtype was identified by stronger keratinization [22] (expression level shown as subtype.CCR in Figure 1A). By using RNAseq data, they were able to identify HPV integration breakpoints in the genome and predict HPV integration status. Studying this in relation to subtype led to the novel finding that the KRT subgroup was much more likely to harbor viral integration events than IMU (indicated by HPVint in Figure 1A). The study also linked the IMU subtype with stronger epithelial-to-mesenchymal transition (EMT) signatures and higher expression of *BCL2*, an anti-apoptotic regulator associated with resistance to chemotherapy and radiation. By retrieving gene expression from 11 HNSCC studies, Locati et al. characterized three distinct HPV(+) subtypes, defined as Cl1 (immune-related), Cl2 (highly keratinized, epithelial mesenchymal transition-related and hypoxia), and Cl3 (highly keratinized, proliferation-related) [23]. The Cl1 subtype was in agreement with the IMU subtype, while the KRT subtype was further stratified into Cl2 and Cl3 by their biological and prognostic characteristics (indicated as subtype.CAN in Figure 1A). A different approach to defining HPV(+) HNSCC subtypes was taken by comparing them to cervical, lung and esophageal tumors, which each have similarities to HNSCC. Instead of naming subtypes after their most distinguishing gene signatures, Lee et al., did so according to their similarity to other tumor types [24]. The three HPV(+) subtypes were called Subtype 1 (cervical-like; 22% HNSCC; activated Protein Kinase A signaling, Vascular endothelial growth factor (VEGF) signaling, mechanistic Target Of Rapamycin (mTOR) signaling and IL-8 signaling), Subtype 2 (HNSCC-classical; 91% HNSCC; activated RhoA, PI3K/AKT and NF-kB signaling pathway), and Subtype 3 (lung-like; 11% HNSCC; activated nicotine degradation, Notch signaling, Xenobiotic metabolism and Wnt/β-catenin signaling; basal cell active in cell cycle pathways), which are marked as subtype.ORA in Figure 1A. Even though most HPV(+) tumors (74%) fell into the cervical-like subtype, a significant fraction were designated as either lung or HNSCC-classical.

Together, these studies revealed several genetic subtype differences in HPV, copy number alterations and cancer gene mutations. In the classical subtypes, Keck et al., discovered frequent amplification of *E2F3* (6p22), which encodes a transcription factor important for cell-cycle regulation and DNA replication [21]. Consistent with the KRT subtype being more likely to have HPV genic integration than the IMU subtype, the KRT group also showed lower expression of the viral genes E2, E4 and E5, the expression of which is often lost upon integration. By analyzing tumor and blood single nucleotide polymorphism (SNP)-array data from the same cohorts, the authors were able to identify more amplifications in KRT tumors than IMU, especially at chromosomal arms, and being compared with the results from gene expression suggested that the gain and loss of copy numbers can partially drive the expression differences between the two subgroups. In terms of the differences in gene mutation frequencies between the two HPV(+) subtypes, analysis of non-synonymous mutations revealed only one gene with a difference of more than 20% between two groups, which occurred on oncogene *PIK3CA* in 37% of the KRT samples and only 16% of the IMU samples. *PIK3CA* activating mutations are able to enhance mTOR activity and inhibit autophagy in HPV(+) HNSCC, leading to the predisposition of these cancer cells to avoid autophagy, ferritinophagy and ferroptosis [25,26]. HPV(+) head and neck tumors with high mesenchymal expression, which includes the IMU/IMS subtype and a subset of the highly keratinized group (Cl2 subtype with high stromal and EMT), exhibit upregulation of lipid peroxidation [27], resulting in higher sensitivity to ferroptosis [26]. The *PIK3CA* activating mutations may therefore be a mechanism to avoid cell death by ferroptosis in these tumors, especially in the highly keratinized, high stromal and high EMT tumors which more often have *PIK3CA* mutations. The study by Lee et al. also characterized the mutation landscape of Subtype 1 (infrequent *TP53* mutation and *PIK3CA* amplification), Subtype 2 (*TP53* mutation, *CDKN2A* deletion and *NOTCH* alteration) and Subtype 3 (*TP53* mutation *CDKN2A* deletion, *PIK3CA* amplification and high mutation rate of *AJUBA*, *MUC17*, *KMT2D* and *NFE2L2*). The *PIK3CA* mutation status is also marked in Figure 1A.

Within HPV itself, the shorter isoforms of HPV 16 oncogene E6 (E6*) are known carcinogenic factors in HNSCC, and Zhang et al. identified that the HPV16-KRT subgroup is associated with higher E6* levels (defined as the percent of E6 expressed as E6*) than the IMU subtype [22]. Full length E6 and E6* were shown to bind to procaspase 8 at different domains, which has important implications for how they inhibit caspase 8 dependent apoptosis, necroptosis and caspase 8-E6 binding inhibitors to resensitize the tumor to apoptosis inducers [28]. In addition, a 2020 study developed an influence score of HPV16 E6* (the shorter isoforms of E6) and identified its significant association with carcinogenic pathways, tumor size and survival in HPV(+) HNSCC, suggesting that the E6* influence score can potentially serve as a prognostic factor for those patients [29]. This paper also found HPV integration (+) patients exhibited significantly higher E6* influence score than HPV integration(−) patients (Wilcoxon rank-sum test, $p = 0.02$), which is in line with the previous finding based on subtypes.

The HPV(+) subtypes also exhibit distinct epigenetic profiles. Differences between the two subtypes IMU and KRT were strikingly observed in a 2020 epigenetic study of the University of Michigan HNSCC cohort capturing the genome-wide 5-hydroxymethylation (5hmC) profiles [30]. The 5hmC epigenetic mark is the first step in the demethylation pathway and results in a loss of transcriptional repression in promoters and enhancers, often serving as a mechanism to activate differentiation and developmental programs [31]. In the above 5hmC HNSCC study, the IMU subtype was easily distinguished from the KRT HPV(+) and HPV(−) samples, whose 5hmC profiles overlapped with each other. Overall for HPV(+) tumors, global 5hmC levels were elevated in the KRT subtype compared to IMU, which is consistent with the more differentiated nature of KRT, and the 5hmC level on promoters alone was sufficient to distinguish these two subtypes [30]. These results should be interpreted in light of the fact that 5hmC is depleted in various cancer types [32–34], however higher 5hmC has been associated with aggressive tumors and worse survival outcomes specifically in oral cancers [35]. The epigenomic profiles in IMU and KRT highlighted extensive differences in regulatory marks at keratinocyte enhancer regions, and in the regulation of cell junction, migration and immune genes [30]. Based on previous evidence that DNA methylation patterns of HPV(+) HNSCC were involved in the activity of HPV oncoproteins (one of the key factors in identification of HPV(+) subtypes) [36], we hypothesize that the IMU and KRT subtypes could be differentiated by their DNA methylation profiles as well. Even though no published study has examined DNA methylation in HPV(+) subtypes directly, visualizing the TCGA methylation data from Infinium®450K BeadChip data (Illumina Inc, San Diego, CA, USA) (using the 1% most variable probes) reveals two main patient groups of approximately equal number distinguished by overall high vs low methylation levels. In relation to the previously-defined subtypes, these DNA methylation clusters demonstrate clear trends that the HPV(−)IMU (subtype.CCR), Subtype 1 (cervical-like in subtype.ORA), HPV integration-negative (HPVint-), Cl1 (immune strong in subtype.CAN) and "hot" tumors (hot and cold) are associated with higher methylation levels overall (Figure 2).

Deconvolution of tumor cell type composition can also be performed with genome-wide DNA methylation data, revealing patterns of immune cell infiltration. This type of analysis was conducted using the MethylCIBERSORT method on TCGA HNSCC samples, which were classified as either immune "hot" (more T-lymphocyte infiltration) or "cold" [37]. Even though most HPV(+) tumors were classified as "hot", nearly all of the "cold" HPV(+) tumors were of the KRT subtype and were HPV integration(+) (marked as hot and cold in Figures 1A and 2). These two or three HPV(+) subtypes described above may also carry implications for survival and prognosis, which is discussed in further detail below.

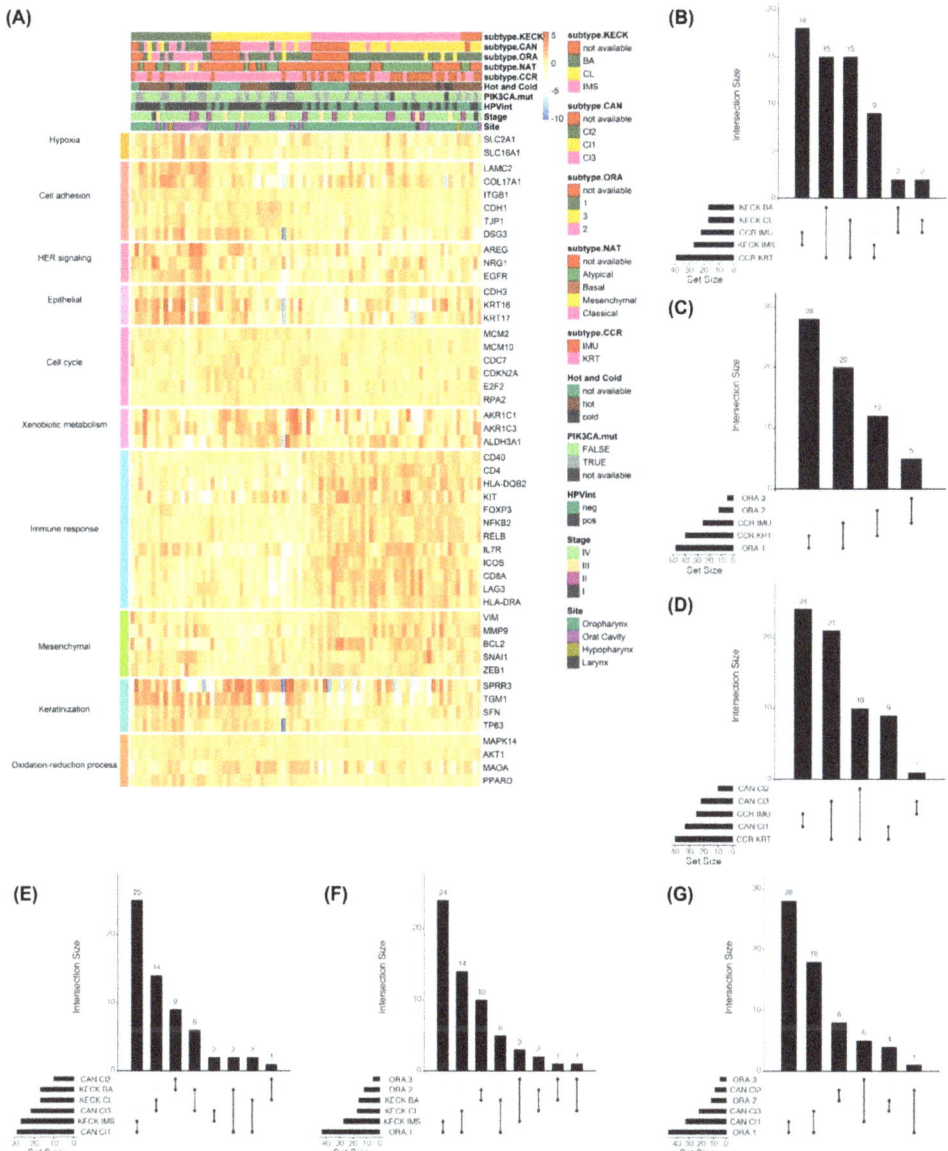

Figure 1. Comparison of the different definitions of HPV-positive head and neck subtypes: (**A**) Heatmap illustrating expression of genes and pathways previously identified as distinguishing HPV(+) subtypes; genes and pathways were combined from Keck et al. (KECK) and Zhang et al. (CCR) subtype findings, and visualized using log2FPKM values normalized (mean centered) by genes and samples. Additionally, shown are several annotations which indicate trends among subtypes and with tumor characteristics. KECK subtypes were re-designated for all 66 TCGA and 18 UM HPV(+) cases by applying their algorithm, while all other subtype definitions were obtained directly from the original publications. (**B–G**) Upset plots illustrating pairwise overlaps among subtype definitions: (**B**) KECK (BA/CL/IMS) vs. CCR (IMU/KRT), (**C**) ORA (1/2/3) vs. CCR (IMU/KRT), (**D**) CAN (Cl1/Cl2/Cl3) vs. CCR (IMU/KRT), (**E**) CAN (Cl1/Cl2/Cl3) vs. KECK (BA/CL/IMS), (**F**) ORA (1/2/3) vs. KECK (BA/CL/IMS) and (**G**) ORA (1/2/3) vs. CAN (Cl1/Cl2/Cl3).

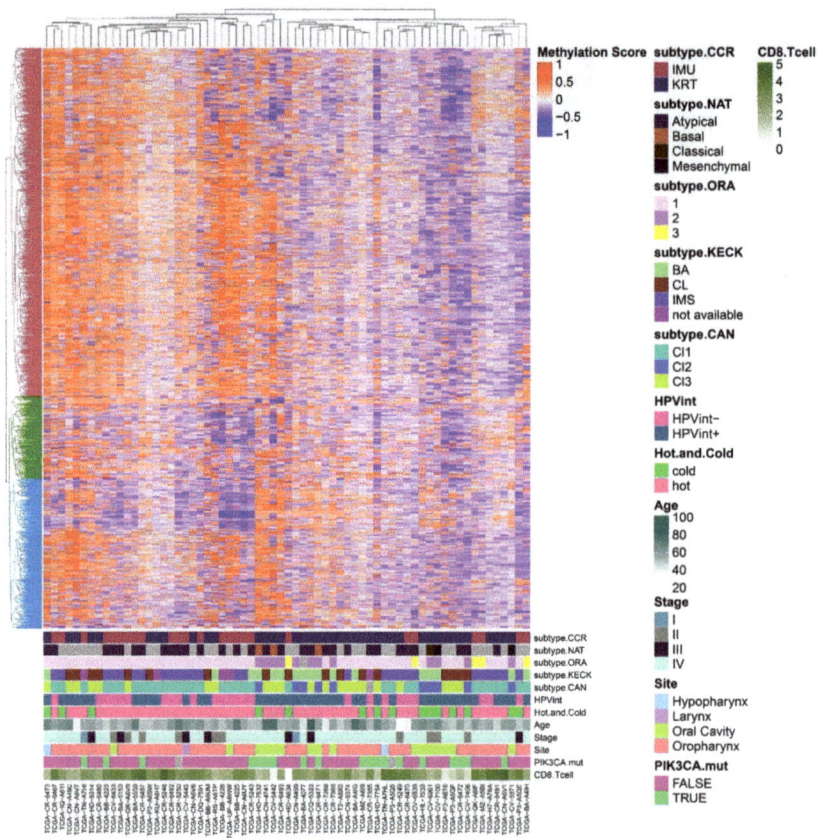

Figure 2. DNA methylation profiles associate with HPV(+) HNSCC subtype. Heatmap of DNA methylation data (normalized beta values) assessed by the Illumina 450K BeadChip for 66 HPV(+) HNSC TCGA samples, and annotated with subtypes and additional tumor characteristics. The top 1% most variable CpGs (probes) were used based on standard deviation. The distance matrix was calculated using Euclidean distance, and hierarchical clustering was performed using complete linkage. Cluster colors on left were determined by applying consensus clustering and selecting the optimal number of clusters.

4. Comparisons of the Identified Subtypes in HPV(+) HNSCC

Multiple studies have investigated HNSCC transcriptional profiles using the TCGA-HNSC cohort and identified varied subtypes by un-supervised clustering, including Atypical/Basal/Classical/Mesenchymal subgroups, referred to as "NAT" hereafter [16,38], BA/CL/IMS clusters, referred to as "KECK" [21], IMU/KRT HPV(+) subtypes, referred to as "CCR" [22], and clusters 1–3, referred to as "ORA" [24]. The five studies clustered different subsets of the TCGA expression data. In all studies except KECK subtypes, we used the original results published. For KECK subtypes, we reimplemented their algorithm on 84 HPV(+) HNSCC patients, including the TCGA HPV(+) HNSC cohort. Several tumors were classified as BA which differs from their original publication which had only HPV(−) samples belonging to the BA subtype (Figure 1A). By overlapping the identified subgroups of those HPV(+) samples, we found that ~83% (30/36) of HPV(+) samples were NAT Atypical [16], among which one half were CCR IMU (immune strong) and the other were CCR KRT (highly keratinized) subtypes. This suggests the TCGA clustering of the 279 TCGA-HNSC samples were driven by HPV(−) samples, and the HPV(+) samples mainly fall in the Atypical subgroup without preference to the IMU or KRT subtype.

As compared to the KECK subtypes, the majority of CCR IMU samples (18/22, ~82%) were assigned to the IMS cluster (immune strong), and the KRT samples were split between BA (basal-like) (15/39, ~38%) and CL (classical) (15/39, ~38%) clusters (Figure 1B). The ORA cluster 1 (cervical-like) subgroup contained the great majority of HPV(+) tumors and was a mixture of CCR IMU (28/48, ~58%) and KRT (20/48, ~42%) subtypes, however the 12 samples in ORA cluster 2 (HNSCC-classical) were all KRT, and the 5 in cluster 3 (lung-like) were all IMU (Figure 1C). The comparison between CCR and CAN subtypes showed that nearly all CCR IMU samples were in CAN Cl1 (immune strong; high stromal) (24/25, ~96%), and all of the 10 CAN Cl2 samples (highly keratinized; high stromal) and 21 out of the 22 (~95%) Cl3 (highly keratinized; low stromal) samples were CCR KRT subtype (Figure 1D). Moreover, the overlaps among KECK and CAN subgroups demonstrated that the KECK and CAN immune strong subtypes had high overlap (KECK IMS samples were mainly CAN Cl1 (25/27, ~93%)), and that KECK and CAN split the highly keratinized samples similarly: KECK CL were mainly CAN Cl3 (low stromal) (14/16, ~88%)) while nearly all CAN Cl2 (high stromal) were KECK BA (9/10 (90%)) (Figure 1E). The majority of KECK IMS and CL subtypes were ORA cluster 1 (cervical-like) (24/27 (~89%) and 14/26 (~88%), respectively), while over half of KECK BA was ORA cluster 2 (10/16, ~63%) (Figure 1F), and similarly, CAN Cl1 (28/31, ~90%) and Cl3 (18/22, ~82%) subtypes (both high stromal subtypes) were mostly ORA cluster 1 (cervical-like), and almost all CAN Cl2 (highly keratinized; high stromal subtype) (8/9, ~89%) was ORA cluster 2 (HNSCC classical) (Figure 1G).

These findings demonstrate that the subtypes identified by different studies although highly overlapping are not completely concordant, indicating how the input data and analysis pipeline impact the subtype definition by prioritizing different pathways. Of these five studies, only Locati et al., defined the subtypes using only HPV(+) samples, whereas the subgroups identified by TCGA and Lee et al., were mostly driven by HPV(−) samples. These differences in cohorts likely contributed to differences, partially confounding HPV(+) subtype definitions with HPV status tumor characteristics. Over 80% of basal (KECK BA: 16/19) and classical (KECK CL: 20/24) subtypes from Keck et al., were identified as HPV integration(+), and all highly keratinized/high stromal samples (CAN Cl2: 10/10) and ~77% of the high keratinized/low stromal subtype (CAN Cl3: 17/22) from Locati et al., were HPV integration(+). It is worth noting that out of the HPV(+) samples, over half of the BA cluster were oral cavity HNSCC (~56%), whereas CL (~83%) and IMS (~94%) samples were nearly all oropharynx (Fisher's exact test (FET), $p = 0.0002$); and over half of IMS (~67%) samples were HPV integration(−), a significantly lower percent than the other two subtypes (FET, $p = 2.86 \times 10^{-5}$) (Figure 1A). Similarly, the ~42% of CAN Cl1 (immune strong) samples that were HPV integration(+) is significantly lower than for the other two subtypes (FET, $p = 5.02 \times 10^{-4}$) (Figure 1A).

By synthesizing the findings of these studies, we arrive at three overall subtypes: (1) an immune strong subtype derived from mainly oropharynx tumors with no detected HPV integration, higher mesenchymal differentiation and high stromal content; (2) a highly keratinized, yet basal-like with high stromal content subtype that are most likely HPV integration(+) and more likely to be from oral cavity primary tumors, with more classical HNSCC expression signatures (as compared with lung or cervical); and (3) a highly keratinized subtype or oropharynx tumors with low stromal content also most likely to be HPV integration(+). However, a subset of immune strong tumors may have more lung cancer-like expression signatures with worse survival, as suggested by Lee et al.

5. Relationship to Cervical Cancer Subtypes

Since HPV(+) head and neck cancers have driving mutations and cancer pathways in common with cervical cancers, including *PIK3CA*, *FAT1*, *CASP8*, *PTEN*, etc. [39], comparing the subtypes of HPV(+) HNSCC with those of cervical cancer may reveal additional insights. Cervical tumors have histologically been characterized by adenocarcinoma (originating from glandular cells) and cervical squamous cell carcinoma (CSCC), in which CSCC accounts for ~80 to 90% of cases. Regardless of the histological subtypes, ~95% of cervical cancers are caused by persistent infection with carcinogenic HPV (mostly HPV16) [40], and substantial heterogeneity exists within HPV(+) CSCC. Lu et al., revealed two subtypes of HPV16(+) CSCC, HPV16-IMM and HPV16-KRT, by supervised clustering of immune signatures followed by pathway analysis to identify the keratinization in the weak immune group [41]. Similar to the IMU/IMS subtype in HPV(+) HNSCC, the HPV16-IMM exhibited a strong immune response and mesenchymal features, whereas HPV16-KRT was characterized by elevated expression of genes in keratinization, biological oxidation and Wnt signaling, which is comparable with KRT-HNSCC. Similarly, Wnt/β-catenin signaling was found to be upregulated in HNSCC cluster 3 by Lee et al. [24], which has been studied as a target pathway in many cancer treatments [42]. It is noted that the HPV16-IMM-CSCC demonstrated a significantly better overall survival (log-rank $p = 0.017$, HR = 0.3) and progression-free survival (log-rank $p = 0.035$, HR = 0.7) than HPV16-KRT-CSCC. A significant difference in overall survival was also observed in the HPV(+) HNSCC subtypes identified by Locati et al.,: Cl1 (immune strong) showed the best outcome, Cl2 the worst and Cl3 an intermediate survival rate (log-rank $p = 4.79 \times 10^{-9}$). Concordantly, both IMU-HNSCC and HPV16-IMM-CSCC have favorable prognosis, as compared to their KRT counterparts. However, Lu et al.. failed to identify a significant association of HPV integration status with a subtype, as shown for the KRT subgroup of Zhang et al. [22]. These findings indicate that HPV infection may induce similar mechanisms of malignant transformation in both HNSCC and CSCC, resulting in two different subtypes (IMU/KRT), although some distinct factors may exist in each entity.

6. Dominant Role of HPV Integration in Defining HPV(+) Tumor Characteristics and Subtypes

6.1. Approaches to Detect HPV Integration

One potential causative mechanism identified for explaining the differentiating characteristics of HPV(+) tumor subtypes is integration of the HPV oncogenes into the host genome. Multiple direct capturing integration event techniques and indirect computational algorithms for high-throughput sequencing data have been designed to detect or quantify HPV integration events and their insertional breakpoints. Which of these methods best correlate with HPV(+) tumor subtype and/or survival, however, is unknown. Amplification of papillomavirus oncogene transcripts (APOT) is a technique focusing on the detection of viral host fusion RNA transcripts, which is sensitive to distinguishing episome versus integration-derived HPV mRNAs [43]. An alternative approach to measure the integrated HPV gene transcript activity makes use of RNA-seq data, along with several software programs for sensitively capturing the specific insertion sites, and the associated genes [44,45]. However, a high-quality RNA requirement discourages those methods from being utilized with RNA retrieved from challenging, potentially highly-degraded specimens, such as from formalin-fixed and paraffin-embedded (FFPE) blocks [46].

Complementary to the RNA approach, and avoiding the difficulties of easily degradable RNA, is to measure DNA instead. Examples of this include the Detection of Integrated Papillomavirus Sequences (DIPS) assay, DNA FISH (Fluorescence in situ hybridization), quantitative and real time PCR, MLPA and DNA-seq [46–50]. Each DNA assay has its own limitations, for instance, DNA FISH is designed specifically for paraffin-embedded tissue, whereas quantitative PCR measures the relative E2 gene loss compared to E6, which may miss integration events that occur outside the E2 gene region. Nowadays, more studies focus on distinct DNA-seq techniques to capture HPV integration events, having shown to be more accurate and comprehensive [51,52]. However, whereas RNAseq methods may miss integration events that are transcribed but do not result in any viral-host fusion transcripts, the DNA approaches by their very nature cannot determine which integration events are transcribed. Even though DNA validation is sufficient to determine disruption of a gene function, RNA expression is needed if the goal is to understand the general, non-site-specific effects of HPV integration on cancer pathways, such as lymphocyte activation, keratinization, mesenchymal differentiation or oxidative phosphorylation. In summary, the most thorough way to study HPV integration is to combine RNA and DNA techniques, for example, Olthof examined HPV integration on 75 OSCC patients with both DIPS and APOT [53], and Ziegert et al., applied DIPS and APOT on anogenital lesions to study the integration loci [54]. Such designs allow both comprehensive DNA integration and transcriptional detection [55].

6.2. The Consequences of HPV Integration

In addition to its impact on viral gene expression, HPV integration has direct and indirect effects on host gene expression. The nonrandom appearance pattern of the integrated sites across the human genome discovered by many studies strongly indicate integration events influence HNC development [56,57]. Walline et al., used DIPS to identify HPV insertion sites and found that 7 of 9 HPV(+) cell lines exhibited integrations in cancer-related genes including *TP63, DCC, JAK1, TERT, ATR, ETV6, PGRP, PTPRN2* and *TMEM237*, which indicates integration is a potential carcinogenic driver [56]. Another study from 84 HPV(+) HNSCC RNA-seq revealed that integration events are overrepresented in genes often mutated in head and neck, lung, and urogenital (e.g., cervical) cancers, which included *CD274, FLJ37453, KLF12, RAD51B* and *TTC6* [57]. The discovery that insertion events are overrepresented in these cancer-related genes also indicates that there is a natural selection of tumor cells with breakpoints in or near HPV(−)associated HNSCC-relevant genes.

In addition to directly shifting host target gene expression, HPV integration also affects the DNA methylation of the host genome. Parfenov et al., revealed highly different DNA methylation profiles for samples with versus without HPV integration events, and reported four critical differentially methylated genes, two of which hypermethylated are tumor suppressors, *BARX2* and *IRX4*, and two others hypomethylated being related to tumorigenesis, *SIM2* and *CTSE* [58].

Since integration is not a normal process in the HPV replication cycle, it often results in partial deletion of the viral genome but maintains the main oncogenes E6 and E7 [59]. High E6 and E7 expression occurs in the early phase of normal HPV replication, which yields host cell growth, differentiation inhibition and chromosomal instability. Those effects contribute to carcinogenesis, and lead to the cells continuing in the basal or partially differentiated condition, which is also a distinguishing characteristic between the IMU and KRT subtypes [60–62]. Thus, HPV integration and loss of episomal HPV expression has strong indirect effects on expression of keratinocyte differentiation genes and could explain much of the differentiation differences observed between the IMU and highly keratinized subtypes.

The expression of important shorter isoforms of the E6 gene, collectively called E6* are also associated with HPV integration and have been found to correlate with HPV(+) tumor subtype classification, with higher relative E6* expression in the KRT subgroup. One study showed that higher E6* protein concentration increases the level of reactive oxygen species (ROS), inducing the oxidative stress mechanism resulting in heightened DNA damage [63]. Those two pathways have been shown as key factors separating IMU and KRT subtypes. In Qin et al., this DNA damage was further shown to be associated with a higher mutational burden [29], and a higher ratio of E6* to full length E6 impact score was associated with larger tumor size at diagnosis and worse overall survival, further suggesting unfavorable prognosis for HPV integration(+) patients.

A comprehensive network describing the relationship between E6, E6* and E7 oncoproteins with HPV integration remains to be fully understood based on the current studies. An increasing number of studies have verified that E7 suppresses the antitumor immune response by silencing important genes and pathways such as *CXCL14* and STING DNA-sensing [64–66], which is also a main differentiating factor between IMU and KRT, and KECK subtypes. A reasonable hypothesis for the HPV oncoproteins network is that HPV integration activates E6* expression, which has been shown to stimulate the translation of E7, resulting in increased immune suppression, oxidative phosphorylation and oxidative stress. Therefore, E6* may play a key role in leading to HPV (+) tumor subtypes.

7. Possible Contributors to Defining HPV(+) Tumor Subtypes Besides HPV Integration, and Potential for Defining Finer-Grained Subtypes

As described above, HPV integration is significantly associated with the identified subtypes in HPV(+) HNSCC, where the strongly keratinized subgroups (KRT, Cl2 and Cl3) tend to have more HPV integration events than the strong immune subgroups (IMU and Cl1) (Figure 3A) [22,24,57]. However, the subgroups still show heterogeneous HPV integration status: out of the 66 HPV(+) HNSCC in TCGA cohort, 36% (9/25) of IMU have HPV integration, and 22% (9/41) of KRT samples had no identified HPV integration events (Figure 3A). One possible explanation for this heterogeneity is that some integration events were incorrectly assigned, especially in samples with low E2 and/or E4 gene expression that were assigned as HPV integration negative. In these cases, an insertional site may have been missed; however, upon inspection we did not see any case with low E2 or E4 expression relative to E6 and E7 that was assigned to be HPV integration($-$). In addition, some samples classified as HPV integration positive may actually be mixed, having both episomal HPV copies and integrated expressed E6 and E7. To seek other possible contributors to the HPV(+) HNSCC subtypes, we visualized relevant supporting data together for each patient. Specifically, we calculated the pathway scores for the 84 HPV(+) HNSCC samples (18 UM SPORE and 66 TCGA) by summarizing the expression levels for the pre-defined gene sets (pathways) as described in [22], which measure the immune response ("Tcell.score", "CT8.Tcell", and scores for "Dendrite cell marker", "immune marker for hnscc" [67]) and cell differentiation ("keratinocyte.score", "Mesenchymal.score" and "EMT.score"), and correlated the scores with IMU/KRT, IMS/BA/CL, and other subtypes (Figure 3A). In line with the previous findings [22,57], overall IMUs showed lower keratinocyte but higher mesenchymal and immune scores, whereas KRTs showed lower mesenchymal but higher keratinocyte scores, independent of the HPV integration status (Figure 3A). The mesenchymal/EMT and immune scores in HPV integration(+) IMUs tend to be lower than those in HPV integration($-$) IMUs, although the difference is not statistically significant; what distinguishes them clearly from the KRTs is their overall lower keratinocyte score and higher mesenchymal/EMT. This reminds us that although HPV integration frees the tumor cells from the partial-differentiation program required to maintain the episomal HPV lifecycle, not all tumors with HPV integration become highly keratinized. To see why some HPV integration($-$) samples were classified as KRT, we first noted that the immune scores and the E2/E4 expression in HPV integration($-$) KRTs are actually comparable to those in IMU and significantly higher than those in HPV integration(+) KRTs (Figure 3A and Figure S1); what distinguishes these samples clearly from the IMU subtype is their overall higher keratinocyte score and lower mesenchymal/EMT. The findings suggest that the IMU/KRT subtypes are mainly directed by the cell differentiation status, and HPV integration attenuates the immune response and reduces the EMT in HPV integration(+) IMU HNSCC.

Fanconi Anemia (FA) is a known predisposition to HNSCC, and has been identified to be downregulated in sporadic HNSCC [68]. Qin et al., identified that HPV(+) patients had more Nonsynonymous, Rare and Damaging (NRD) expressed variants in FA genes than HPV($-$) patients [69]. We also found FA genes were significantly downregulated in KRT as compared to IMU (Wilcoxon test, $p = 0.002$), especially in HPV integration(+) KRT (Figure 3B, Figure S2A,B), and KRTs tended to have more mutations in FA genes (FET, $p = 0.06$). Interestingly, the distribution of the 4 HPV types (HPV16, 18, 33 and 35) was significantly different between IMU and KRT (FET, $p = 0.03$), with HPV16 in ~70% (23/33) of IMU and ~90% (46/51) of KRT, and all but one non-HPV16 type (HPV18) were in the IMU subtype, suggesting that HPV16 may be more successful at evading a host immune response. Age, stage and smoking status were not significantly different between IMU and KRT.

While KECK further divided the highly keratinized subgroup into basal (BA) and classical (CL) expression signatures, Locati, et al. divided this same group into high (Cl2) and low stromal (Cl3). These are associated with each other, as tumors having more basal features tend to have higher proportions of cancer-associated fibroblasts (CAFs), which constitute the majority of stromal cells [70]. This subset of KRT tumors may be more likely to exhibit a local invasion pattern, which enables the invading tumor cells to recruit CAFs, which evidence suggests can further promote invasion [71]. This may explain why high CAFs are associated with poor survival. With increasing data types and cohort sizes, more attributable factors will likely be identified to characterize the molecular subtypes in HPV(+) HNSCC, and finer-grained subtypes are expected to be defined.

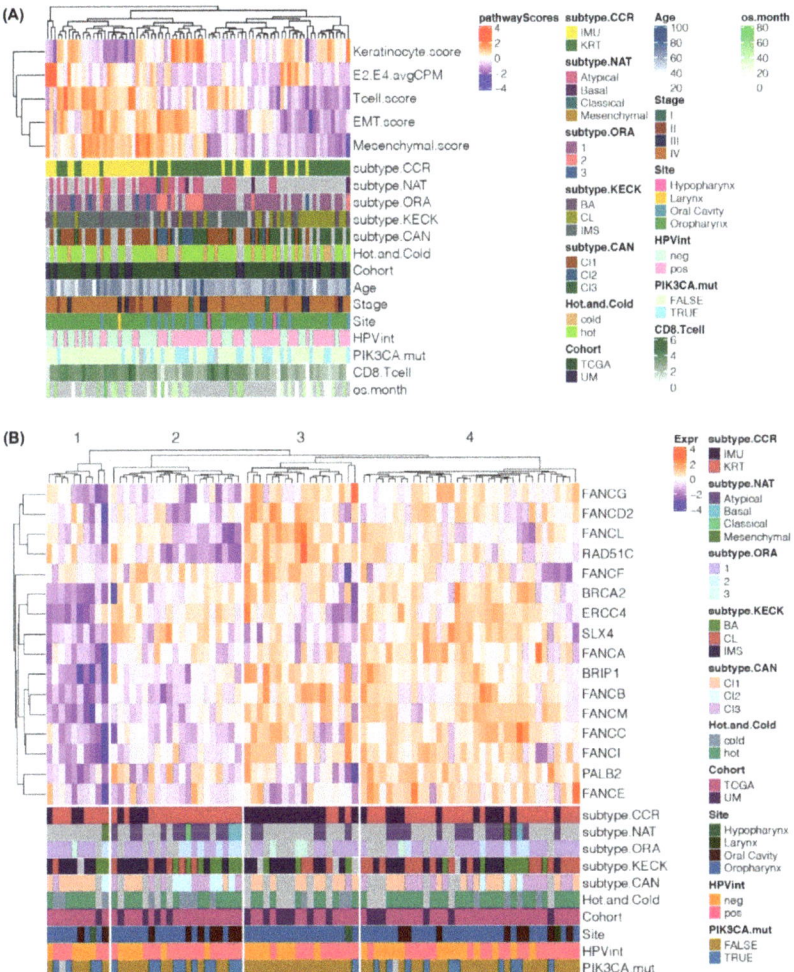

Figure 3. Clustering of the defining pathway scores and HPV scores visually distinguish the main HPV(+) subtypes. (**A**) Hierarchically clustered heatmap showing averaged HPV16 E2 and E4 expression (E2.E4.avgCPM) and pathway scores of keratinocyte differentiation (Keratinocyte.score:), T cell differentiation (Tcell.score), epithelial-mesenchymal transition (EMT.score) and mesenchymal cell differentiation (mesenchymal.score) among the 84 HPV(+) HNSCC samples from combined TCGA and UM cohorts. (**B**) Clustered heatmap based on genes in the Fanconi Anemia (FA) pathway. The 84 HPV(+) samples were clustered by K-means clustering (K = 4) based on the expression of 16 FA genes.

8. Survival in Relationship to Subtypes and HPV Integration Status

There is increasing evidence that HPV subtypes and integration impact patient outcomes. For example, Locati et al., examined the relationship between three biological HPV(+) HNSCC subtypes and HPV(−)integration [23]. As described above, they identified three biologically distinct HPV(+) HNSCC subtypes, Cl1, Cl2 and Cl3. Specifically, Cl1 had enrichment of immune-related pathways, Cl2 overexpressed genes relating to EMT and high stromal content, and Cl3 was tied to proliferation and low stromal content. Notably, these subtype classifications are consistent with the HPV(+) HNSCC subtypes defined by microarray gene signatures described above. Furthermore, these subtypes also had different survival rates, which appear to be correlated with HPV integration. This may be attributed to distinct biological properties associated with HPV integration. For example, subgroup Cl1, which had the best prognosis (80.9% 5 year survival rate), had the least number of HPV(−)integrated cases whereas Cl2 had the highest percent of HPV integration and the worst survival outcome (19.7% 5 year survival rate) [23].

Many studies have examined how HPV integration impacts prognosis and survival of HPV positive head and neck cancer patients, focusing in particular on survival differences in patients with episomal versus integrated HPV. Early studies did not detect a significant difference in survival based on HPV integration status. In particular, a study of 179 patients with HPV(+) oropharyngeal cancer classified patients as integrated, episomal or mixed using the E2/E6 DNA copy number ratio, and found no significant differences in 3-year overall survival for HPV episomal versus integrated oropharyngeal squamous cell carcinoma patients, although patients with both integrated and episomal HPV genomes (i.e., mixed HPV), alluded to having better overall survival [72]. Limitations of this study, however, were having only 22 and 42 episomal and integrated patients, respectively, and misclassifying HPV integration-positive patients who retained high levels of E2. Likewise, another study evaluated 186 head and neck cancer patients and determined HPV integration status by mapping E2 at the mRNA level. They also did not detect a significant difference in disease-specific survival between patients with integrated, mixed or episomal HPV [73], although there was a trend for patients with the mixed and episomal form of HPV to have a better prognosis. Despite these early observations, later studies have reported significant findings. Nulton et al. [74] analyzed 56 HPV16(+) head and neck cancer patients and found that patients with integrated HPV head and neck cancers, in which HPV integration was defined by E2 and E7 gene expression, had a statistically significant reduction in survival compared to episomal HPV patients. They compared the 5-year survival rate and saw episomal HPV head and neck cancer patients had a survival rate of 72% whereas integrated HPV patients had a lower survival rate of 30% [74]. Notably, the survival rate of the integrated HPV head and neck cancer patients was also worse than the survival for patients with HPV(−) head and neck cancer, who had a survival rate of 40% [74]. Another RNAseq-based study that evaluated the impact of HPV integration on 84 HPV(+) head and neck cancers showed similar results with better survival in integration-negative patients than integration-positive [57]. In particular, both univariate and multivariate analyses showed HPV integration was associated with worse overall survival, and it was suggested that differences in survival between HPV integration positive and negative head and neck cancers may explain the survival variability in HPV(+) head and neck cancer patients.

The differences in survival in HPV(+) patients based on integration status may be attributed to the biological effects resulting from HPV integration. For example, RNAseq analysis of integration(−) samples had higher expression of immune related genes, including genes related to T cell and B cell activation. In contrast, integration(+) samples had higher expression of genes related to keratinization and RNA metabolism and translation that had also been previously noted in specific HPV(+) molecular subtypes [57]. These studies are promising for using HPV integration status as an additional prognostic marker that may dictate treatment approach. However, these results are still controversial. Recently published results saw improved survival in patients who had HPV integration, conflicting previously published studies [75]. One possible reason for the discrepancies is differences in how HPV is detected, as the relationship with survival may heavily depend on how integration is defined. Regardless, additional studies will need to be performed with larger sample sizes.

Survival and treatment response may also be affected by keratinization, which has been shown to cause cell death pathway alterations. High keratin levels in tumor cells have multiple potential mechanisms to resist apoptosis. Raj et al., reported that the HPV E1^E4 isoform protein typically binds to keratins, but in their absence or low expression, E1^E4 instead binds to mitochondria which causes mitochondrial detachment from microtubules, and a large decrease in the mitochondrial membrane potential [76]. This in turn induces apoptosis, suggesting that high levels of cytokeratin inhibit this chain of events leading to apoptosis. Keratinization may also have a more direct effect on cell survival by altering the shape and function of mitochondria [77]. In this case, these alterations may protect the cells from oxidative damage and other stressors, reducing apoptosis [78]. In terms of metastasis, high expression of one keratin, K17, resulted in an approximate 6-fold increase in lymph node metastasis. However, when accounting for treatment response, the relationship between keratins and survival may be more complex, as low levels of K17 were shown to correlate with worse prognosis for patients treated with surgery or radiotherapy. Treatment response may also be associated with keratinization as observed for multiple cancer types [79,80], depending on the complex interplay between treatment and cellular structural integrity, angiogenesis (which may affect the ability of oxygen to permeate the tumor and thus cellular oxidative damage) and the DNA damage response. Indeed, the Cl2 subtype (highly keratinized and high hypoxia) in Locati et al., had the highest radiosensitivity (RSI) score indicating high radioresistance [23].In Gleber-Netto et al., E1^E4 was found to positively correlate with radiation sensitivity, potentially explained by its negative correlation with mitochondrial genes suggesting reduced ability to respond to oxidative stress. In this study, E1^E4 had only a modest negative association with HPV integration status [81].

9. Future for De-Escalation Treatment in HPV-Positive Oropharynx Cancer Patients

Despite markedly better 5-year survival rates of HPV(+) oropharyngeal cancer patients compared to HPV(−) (~80% vs. 50%, respectively), treatment toxicity and quality of life (QoL) remain diminished, because standard HNSCC therapy is unnecessarily aggressive for many HPV(+) patients [82]. QoL deteriorations include dry mouth with difficulty chewing and/or swallowing (dysphagia), and speech difficulties [83]. However, two clinical trials assessing de-escalation of treatment for HPV(+) oropharyngeal cancer patients resulted in worse survival compared to standard treatment protocols [84], underscoring the importance of classifying HPV(+) patients into high- and low- risk cohorts, as well as predicting which subgroup of patients would most likely benefit from immune checkpoint inhibitor (e.g., anti-PD1/PD-L1) therapies. Thus, uniform, non-personalized de-escalated therapy involves unacceptable risk. Biomarkers identifying poor prognosis and/or predicting targeted treatment response in HPV(+) patients are lacking [85], with the exception of an immune score estimating infiltrating cytotoxic CD8+ T cells, B cells and regulatory T cells in the tumor [86–88]. E6 and E7 have been reported to be involved in the PI3K/AKT/mTOR regulatory network in both normoxic and hypoxic HPV(+) cancer cells [89], and thus these pathways are potential target pathways for alternative cancer therapies. E6 activates AKT, inducing a signaling cascade involving NFkB and cytokine IL-6, resulting in phosphorylation of Signal Transducer and Activator Of Transcription 3 (STAT3) which leads to cell survival and proliferation. E6 also activates mTORC1 which may serve to reduce autophagy, suggesting the potential use of mTORC1 inhibitors such as rapamycin in a subset of HPV(+) patients [90,91]. The most well-known effect of E6, activating p53 protein degradation, further transactivates Survivin, because p53 normally inhibits survivin expression. Survivin as a member of (Inhibitors of Apoptosis) IAP gene family that is an essential regulator of cell division and protects cells from apoptosis [92,93], suggesting the possible use of IAP inhibitors (e.g., small molecular mimetics of SMAC) in a subset of HPV(+) patients with other indications of this pathway being overactivated [94].

While HPV(−)integration status has shown a tenuous relationship with survival, larger studies are needed, and biomarkers for the downstream effects will likely need to be taken into account in addition or in place of HPV integration status itself. This is due to the several carcinogenic pathways that are correlated, but not completely predictive, of HPV integration status. We conjecture that HPV(−)integration positive patients tend to have worse survival partly due to lower immunogenicity, and also potentially due to highly expressed keratins. In addition, the increased levels of the E6* spliced isoform observed in HPV(−)integration positive patients, which leads to higher E7 translation, may contribute to worse survival by altering the tumoral oxidative phosphorylation, oxidative stress and DNA damage. On the other hand, the higher EMT signatures in HPV(−)integration negative and IMU subgroup may lead to higher risk of distant metastasis, observed as the most common type of recurrence in HPV(+) oropharyngeal cancer [84]. Further investigations are necessary to disentangle the relative contributions of the various cancer pathway expression patterns to overall and disease-specific survival. Pathways likely to contribute and that differ by HPV(+) subtypes include tumor infiltrating lymphocyte levels, EMT and mesenchymal differentiation signatures, keratinization, cell cycle regulation and DNA damage response. This suggests the potential for using HPV(+) subtypes to identify patients at high risk and who are good candidates for alternative therapies including anti-PD-1 [95–97] or PI3K inhibitors [98]. Ultimately, classification of HPV(+) patients into two or three subgroups will remain an oversimplification of the complex, multi-dimensional signatures that together determine the prognosis and treatment response of each patient. Until the field reaches that advanced level of knowledge, however, understanding the characteristics of the major subtypes and their relationship with recurrence and survival will hopefully lead us to patient subgroups most likely to benefit from de-escalated therapy, ICI therapy or another targeted treatment.

Supplementary Materials: The following are available online at https://www.mdpi.com/article/10.3390/cancers13112721/s1, Figure S1: Comparisons of pathway scores among the 84 HPV(+) HNSCC samples, which were stratified by IMU/KRT subtypes and HPV integration status. Figure S2: Comparisons of average Fanconi Anemia (FA) genes among the 84 HPV(+) HNSCC samples.

Author Contributions: Conceptualization, M.A.S.; formal analysis, T.Q. and S.L. (Shiting Li); writing—original draft preparation, M.A.S., T.Q., S.L. (Shiting Li), S.L. (Siyu Liu) and L.E.H.; writing—review and editing, M.A.S., T.Q., S.L. (Shiting Li), S.L. (Siyu Liu) and L.E.H.; visualization, T.Q., S.L. (Shiting Li) and L.E.H.; funding acquisition, M.A.S. All authors have read and agreed to the published version of the manuscript.

Funding: This research was funded by the National Cancer Institute, National Institutes of Health Grants [R01-CA250214, P01-CA240239] and the University of Michigan Rogel Cancer Center Grant [P30-CA046592].

Institutional Review Board Statement: Not applicable.

Informed Consent Statement: Not applicable.

Data Availability Statement: The data presented in this study is openly available in reference numbers [21,23,24]. Publicly available datasets were analyzed in this study. This data can be found here: [https://portal.gdc.cancer.gov/, accessed on 30 April 2021, and Gene Expression Omnibus #GSE74956].

Conflicts of Interest: The authors declare no conflict of interest. The funders had no role in the design of the study; in the collection, analyses or interpretation of data; in the writing of the manuscript, or in the decision to publish the results.

References

1. Bray, F.; Ferlay, J.; Soerjomataram, I.; Siegel, R.L.; Torre, L.A.; Jemal, A. Global cancer statistics 2018: GLOBOCAN estimates of incidence and mortality worldwide for 36 cancers in 185 countries. *CA Cancer J. Clin.* **2018**, *68*, 394–424. [CrossRef] [PubMed]
2. Sathish, N.; Wang, X.; Yuan, Y. Human Papillomavirus (HPV)-associated oral cancers and treatment strategies. *J. Dent. Res.* **2014**, *93*, 29S–36S. [CrossRef] [PubMed]
3. Klussmann, J.P.; Gültekin, E.; Weissenborn, S.J.; Wieland, U.; Dries, V.; Dienes, H.P.; Eckel, H.E.; Pfister, H.J.; Fuchs, P.G. Expression of p16 protein identifies a distinct entity of tonsillar carcinomas associated with human papillomavirus. *Am. J. Pathol.* **2003**, *162*, 747–753. [CrossRef]
4. Gillison, M.L. Human papillomavirus-associated head and neck cancer is a distinct epidemiologic, clinical, and molecular entity. *Semin. Oncol.* **2004**, *31*, 744–754. [CrossRef]
5. Mahal, B.A.; Catalano, P.J.; Haddad, R.I.; Hanna, G.J.; Kass, J.I.; Schoenfeld, J.D.; Tishler, R.B.; Margalit, D.N. Incidence and Demographic Burden of HPV-Associated Oropharyngeal Head and Neck Cancers in the United States. *Cancer Epidemiol. Biomarkers Prev.* **2019**, *28*, 1660–1667. [CrossRef]
6. Hafkamp, H.C.; Manni, J.J.; Speel, E.J.M. Role of human papillomavirus in the development of head and neck squamous cell carcinomas. *Acta Otolaryngol.* **2004**, *124*, 520–526. [CrossRef]
7. Arthur, A.E.; Duffy, S.A.; Sanchez, G.I.; Gruber, S.B.; Terrell, J.E.; Hebert, J.R.; Light, E.; Bradford, C.R.; D'Silva, N.J.; Carey, T.E.; et al. Higher micronutrient intake is associated with human papillomavirus-positive head and neck cancer: A case-only analysis. *Nutr. Cancer* **2011**, *63*, 734–742. [CrossRef]
8. Syrjänen, S. The role of human papillomavirus infection in head and neck cancers. *Ann. Oncol.* **2010**, *21*, vii243–vii245. [CrossRef]
9. Fakhry, C.; Westra, W.H.; Li, S.; Cmelak, A.; Ridge, J.A.; Pinto, H.; Forastiere, A.; Gillison, M.L. Improved Survival of Patients With Human Papillomavirus-Positive Head and Neck Squamous Cell Carcinoma in a Prospective Clinical Trial. *J. Natl. Cancer Inst.* **2008**, *100*, 261–269. [CrossRef]
10. Perri, F.; Longo, F.; Caponigro, F.; Sandomenico, F.; Guida, A.; Della Vittoria Scarpati, G.; Ottaiano, A.; Muto, P.; Ionna, F. Management of HPV-Related Squamous Cell Carcinoma of the Head and Neck: Pitfalls and Caveat. *Cancers* **2020**, *12*, 975. [CrossRef]
11. Li, H.; Torabi, S.J.; Yarbrough, W.G.; Mehra, S.; Osborn, H.A.; Judson, B. Association of human Papillomavirus status at head and neck carcinoma subsites with overall survival. *JAMA Otolaryngol. Head Neck Surg.* **2018**, *144*, 519. [CrossRef]
12. Fakhry, C.; Westra, W.H.; Wang, S.J.; van Zante, A.; Zhang, Y.; Rettig, E.; Yin, L.X.; Ryan, W.R.; Ha, P.K.; Wentz, A.; et al. The prognostic role of sex, race, and human papillomavirus in oropharyngeal and nonoropharyngeal head and neck squamous cell cancer. *Cancer* **2017**, *123*, 1566–1575. [CrossRef]
13. Oosthuizen, J.C.; Doody, J. De-intensified treatment in human papillomavirus-positive oropharyngeal cancer. *Lancet* **2019**, *393*, 5–7. [CrossRef]
14. Chung, C.H.; Gillison, M.L. Human Papillomavirus in Head and Neck Cancer: Its Role in Pathogenesis and Clinical Implications. *Clin. Cancer Res.* **2009**, *15*, 6758–6762. [CrossRef]
15. Gillison, M.L.; Akagi, K.; Xiao, W.; Jiang, B.; Pickard, R.K.L.; Li, J.; Swanson, B.J.; Agrawal, A.D.; Zucker, M.; Stache-Crain, B.; et al. Human papillomavirus and the landscape of secondary genetic alterations in oral cancers. *Genome Res.* **2019**, *29*, 1–17. [CrossRef]
16. Network, T.C.G.A. The Cancer Genome Atlas Network Comprehensive genomic characterization of head and neck squamous cell carcinomas. *Nature* **2015**, *517*, 576–582. [CrossRef]
17. Lechner, M.; Fenton, T.; West, J.; Wilson, G.; Feber, A.; Henderson, S.; Thirlwell, C.; Dibra, H.K.; Jay, A.; Butcher, L.; et al. Identification and functional validation of HPV-mediated hypermethylation in head and neck squamous cell carcinoma. *Genome Med.* **2013**, *5*, 15. [CrossRef]
18. Sartor, M.A.; Dolinoy, D.C.; Jones, T.R.; Colacino, J.A.; Prince, M.E.P.; Carey, T.E.; Rozek, L.S. Genome-wide methylation and expression differences in HPV(+) and HPV(−) squamous cell carcinoma cell lines are consistent with divergent mechanisms of carcinogenesis. *Epigenetics* **2011**, *6*, 777–787. [CrossRef]
19. Carrero, I.; Liu, H.-C.; Sikora, A.G.; Milosavljevic, A. Histoepigenetic analysis of HPV- and tobacco-associated head and neck cancer identifies both subtype-specific and common therapeutic targets despite divergent microenvironments. *Oncogene* **2019**, *38*, 3551–3568. [CrossRef]
20. Pyeon, D.; Newton, M.A.; Lambert, P.F.; den Boon, J.A.; Sengupta, S.; Marsit, C.J.; Woodworth, C.D.; Connor, J.P.; Haugen, T.H.; Smith, E.M.; et al. Fundamental Differences in Cell Cycle Deregulation in Human Papillomavirus-Positive and Human Papillomavirus-Negative Head/Neck and Cervical Cancers. *Cancer Res.* **2007**, *67*, 4605–4619. [CrossRef]
21. Keck, M.K.; Zuo, Z.; Khattri, A.; Stricker, T.P.; Brown, C.D.; Imanguli, M.; Rieke, D.; Endhardt, K.; Fang, P.; Bragelmann, J.; et al. Integrative Analysis of Head and Neck Cancer Identifies Two Biologically Distinct HPV and Three Non-HPV Subtypes. *Clin. Cancer Res.* **2015**, *21*, 870–881. [CrossRef] [PubMed]
22. Zhang, Y.; Koneva, L.A.; Virani, S.; Arthur, A.E.; Virani, A.; Hall, P.B.; Warden, C.D.; Carey, T.E.; Chepeha, D.B.; Prince, M.E.; et al. Subtypes of HPV-Positive Head and Neck Cancers Are Associated with HPV Characteristics, Copy Number Alterations, PIK3CA Mutation, and Pathway Signatures. *Clin. Cancer Res.* **2016**, *22*, 4735–4745. [CrossRef] [PubMed]
23. Locati, L.D.; Serafini, M.S.; Iannò, M.F.; Carenzo, A.; Orlandi, E.; Resteghin, C.; Cavalieri, S.; Bossi, P.; Canevari, S.; Licitra, L.; et al. Mining of Self-Organizing Map Gene-Expression Portraits Reveals Prognostic Stratification of HPV-Positive Head and Neck Squamous Cell Carcinoma. *Cancers* **2019**, *11*, 1057. [CrossRef] [PubMed]

24. Lee, D.J.; Eun, Y.-G.; Rho, Y.S.; Kim, E.H.; Yim, S.Y.; Kang, S.H.; Sohn, B.H.; Kwon, G.H.; Lee, J.-S. Three distinct genomic subtypes of head and neck squamous cell carcinoma associated with clinical outcomes. *Oral Oncol.* **2018**, *85*, 44–51. [CrossRef] [PubMed]
25. Sewell, A.; Brown, B.; Biktasova, A.; Mills, G.B.; Lu, Y.; Tyson, D.R.; Issaeva, N.; Yarbrough, W.G. Reverse-phase protein array profiling of oropharyngeal cancer and significance of PIK3CA mutations in HPV-associated head and neck cancer. *Clin. Cancer Res.* **2014**, *20*, 2300–2311. [CrossRef] [PubMed]
26. Raudenská, M.; Balvan, J.; Masařík, M. Cell death in head and neck cancer pathogenesis and treatment. *Cell Death Dis.* **2021**, *12*, 192. [CrossRef] [PubMed]
27. Srivastava, S.; Natu, S.M.; Gupta, A.; Pal, K.A.; Singh, U.; Agarwal, G.G.; Singh, U.; Goel, M.M.; Srivastava, A.N. Lipid peroxidation and antioxidants in different stages of cervical cancer: Prognostic significance. *Indian J. Cancer* **2009**, *46*, 297–302. [CrossRef]
28. Tungteakkhun, S.S.; Filippova, M.; Fodor, N.; Duerksen-Hughes, P.J. The full-length isoform of human papillomavirus 16 E6 and its splice variant E6* bind to different sites on the procaspase 8 death effector domain. *J. Virol.* **2010**, *84*, 1453–1463. [CrossRef]
29. Qin, T.; Koneva, L.A.; Liu, Y.; Zhang, Y.; Arthur, A.E.; Zarins, K.R.; Carey, T.E.; Chepeha, D.; Wolf, G.T.; Rozek, L.S.; et al. Significant association between host transcriptome-derived HPV oncogene E6* influence score and carcinogenic pathways, tumor size, and survival in head and neck cancer. *Head Neck* **2020**, *42*, 2375–2389. [CrossRef]
30. Liu, S.; de Medeiros, M.C.; Fernandez, E.M.; Zarins, K.R.; Cavalcante, R.G.; Qin, T.; Wolf, G.T.; Figueroa, M.E.; D'Silva, N.J.; Rozek, L.S.; et al. 5-Hydroxymethylation highlights the heterogeneity in keratinization and cell junctions in head and neck cancers. *Clin. Epigenet.* **2020**, *12*, 175. [CrossRef]
31. Laird, A.; Thomson, J.P.; Harrison, D.J.; Meehan, R.R. 5-hydroxymethylcytosine profiling as an indicator of cellular state. *Epigenomics* **2013**, *5*, 655–669. [CrossRef]
32. Jin, S.-G.; Jiang, Y.; Qiu, R.; Rauch, T.A.; Wang, Y.; Schackert, G.; Krex, D.; Lu, Q.; Pfeifer, G.P. 5-Hydroxymethylcytosine Is Strongly Depleted in Human Cancers but Its Levels Do Not Correlate with IDH1 Mutations. *Cancer Res.* **2011**, *71*, 7360–7365. [CrossRef]
33. Yang, H.; Liu, Y.; Bai, F.; Zhang, J.-Y.; Ma, S.-H.; Liu, J.; Xu, Z.-D.; Zhu, H.-G.; Ling, Z.-Q.; Ye, D.; et al. Tumor development is associated with decrease of TET gene expression and 5-methylcytosine hydroxylation. *Oncogene* **2013**, *32*, 663–669. [CrossRef]
34. Jäwert, F.; Hasséus, B.; Kjeller, G.; Magnusson, B.; Sand, L.; Larsson, L. Loss of 5-hydroxymethylcytosine and TET2 in oral squamous cell carcinoma. *Anticancer Res.* **2013**, *33*, 4325–4328.
35. Wang, Y.; Hu, H.; Wang, Q.; Li, Z.; Zhu, Y.; Zhang, W.; Wang, Y.; Jiang, H.; Cheng, J. The level and clinical significance of 5-hydroxymethylcytosine in oral squamous cell carcinoma: An immunohistochemical study in 95 patients. *Pathol. Res. Pract.* **2017**, *213*, 969–974. [CrossRef]
36. Ekanayake Weeramange, C.; Tang, K.D.; Vasani, S.; Langton-Lockton, J.; Kenny, L.; Punyadeera, C. DNA Methylation Changes in Human Papillomavirus-Driven Head and Neck Cancers. *Cells* **2020**, *9*, 1359. [CrossRef]
37. Chakravarthy, A.; Furness, A.; Joshi, K.; Ghorani, E.; Ford, K.; Ward, M.J.; King, E.V.; Lechner, M.; Marafioti, T.; Quezada, S.A.; et al. Pan-cancer deconvolution of tumour composition using DNA methylation. *Nat. Commun.* **2018**, *9*, 3220. [CrossRef]
38. Chung, C.H.; Parker, J.S.; Karaca, G.; Wu, J.; Funkhouser, W.K.; Moore, D.; Butterfoss, D.; Xiang, D.; Zanation, A.; Yin, X.; et al. Molecular classification of head and neck squamous cell carcinomas using patterns of gene expression. *Cancer Cell* **2004**, *5*, 489–500. [CrossRef]
39. Cancer Genome Atlas Research Network; Albert Einstein College of Medicine; Analytical Biological Services; Barretos Cancer Hospital; Baylor College of Medicine; Beckman Research Institute of City of Hope; Buck Institute for Research on Aging; Canada's Michael Smith Genome Sciences Centre; Harvard Medical School; Helen, F. Graham Cancer Center\&Research Institute at Christiana Care Health Services; et al. Integrated genomic and molecular characterization of cervical cancer. *Nature* **2017**, *543*, 378–384. [CrossRef]
40. Schiffman, M.; Wentzensen, N.; Wacholder, S.; Kinney, W.; Gage, J.C.; Castle, P.E. Human Papillomavirus Testing in the Prevention of Cervical Cancer. *J. Natl. Cancer Inst.* **2011**, *103*, 368–383. [CrossRef]
41. Lu, X.; Jiang, L.; Zhang, L.; Zhu, Y.; Hu, W.; Wang, J.; Ruan, X.; Xu, Z.; Meng, X.; Gao, J.; et al. Immune Signature-Based Subtypes of Cervical Squamous Cell Carcinoma Tightly Associated with Human Papillomavirus Type 16 Expression, Molecular Features, and Clinical Outcome. *Neoplasia* **2019**, *21*, 591–601. [CrossRef] [PubMed]
42. Broglie, M.A.; Soltermann, A.; Haile, S.R.; Huber, G.F.; Stoeckli, S.J. Human papilloma virus and survival of oropharyngeal cancer patients treated with surgery and adjuvant radiotherapy. *Eur. Arch. Oto Rhino Laryngol.* **2015**, *272*, 1755–1762. [CrossRef] [PubMed]
43. Klaes, R.; Woerner, S.M.; Ridder, R.; Wentzensen, N.; Duerst, M.; Schneider, A.; Lotz, B.; Melsheimer, P.; von Knebel Doeberitz, M. Detection of high-risk cervical intraepithelial neoplasia and cervical cancer by amplification of transcripts derived from integrated papillomavirus oncogenes. *Cancer Res.* **1999**, *59*, 6132–6136. [PubMed]
44. Chen, Y.; Yao, H.; Thompson, E.J.; Tannir, N.M.; Weinstein, J.N.; Su, X. VirusSeq: Software to identify viruses and their integration sites using next-generation sequencing of human cancer tissue. *Bioinformatics* **2013**, *29*, 266–267. [CrossRef]
45. Schelhorn, S.-E.; Fischer, M.; Tolosi, L.; Altmüller, J.; Nürnberg, P.; Pfister, H.; Lengauer, T.; Berthold, F. Sensitive detection of viral transcripts in human tumor transcriptomes. *PLoS Comput. Biol.* **2013**, *9*, e1003228. [CrossRef]
46. Xu, B.; Chotewutmontri, S.; Wolf, S.; Klos, U.; Schmitz, M.; Dürst, M.; Schwarz, E. Multiplex Identification of Human Papillomavirus 16 DNA Integration Sites in Cervical Carcinomas. *PLoS ONE* **2013**, *8*, e66693.

47. Peitsaro, P.; Johansson, B.; Syrjänen, S. Integrated human papillomavirus type 16 is frequently found in cervical cancer precursors as demonstrated by a novel quantitative real-time PCR technique. *J. Clin. Microbiol.* **2002**, *40*, 886–891. [CrossRef]
48. Human papillomavirus multiplex ligation-dependent probe amplification assay for the assessment of viral load, integration, and gain of telomerase-related genes in cervical malignancies. *Hum. Pathol.* **2013**, *44*, 2410–2418. [CrossRef] [PubMed]
49. Luft, F.; Klaes, R.; Nees, M.; Dürst, M.; Heilmann, V.; Melsheimer, P.; von Knebel Doeberitz, M. Detection of integrated papillomavirus sequences by ligation-mediated PCR (DIPS-PCR) and molecular characterization in cervical cancer cells. *Int. J. Cancer* **2001**, *92*, 9–17. [CrossRef]
50. Hopman, A.H.N.; Kamps, M.A.; Smedts, F.; Speel, E.-J.M.; Herrington, C.S.; Ramaekers, F.C.S. HPV in situ hybridization: Impact of different protocols on the detection of integrated HPV. *Int. J. Cancer* **2005**, *115*, 419–428. [CrossRef]
51. Nkili-Meyong, A.A.; Moussavou-Boundzanga, P.; Labouba, I.; Koumakpayi, I.H.; Jeannot, E.; Descorps-Declère, S.; Sastre-Garau, X.; Leroy, E.M.; Belembaogo, E.; Berthet, N. Genome-wide profiling of human papillomavirus DNA integration in liquid-based cytology specimens from a Gabonese female population using HPV capture technology. *Sci. Rep.* **2019**, *9*, 1504. [CrossRef] [PubMed]
52. Yang, W.; Liu, Y.; Dong, R.; Liu, J.; Lang, J.; Yang, J.; Wang, W.; Li, J.; Meng, B.; Tian, G. Accurate Detection of HPV Integration Sites in Cervical Cancer Samples Using the Nanopore MinION Sequencer Without Error Correction. *Front. Genet.* **2020**, *11*, 660. [CrossRef] [PubMed]
53. Olthof, N.C.; Speel, E.-J.M.; Kolligs, J.; Haesevoets, A.; Henfling, M.; Ramaekers, F.C.S.; Preuss, S.F.; Drebber, U.; Wieland, U.; Silling, S.; et al. Comprehensive analysis of HPV16 integration in OSCC reveals no significant impact of physical status on viral oncogene and virally disrupted human gene expression. *PLoS ONE* **2014**, *9*, e88718. [CrossRef]
54. Ziegert, C.; Wentzensen, N.; Vinokurova, S.; Kisseljov, F.; Einenkel, J.; Hoeckel, M.; von Knebel Doeberitz, M. A comprehensive analysis of HPV integration loci in anogenital lesions combining transcript and genome-based amplification techniques. *Oncogene* **2003**, *22*, 3977–3984. [CrossRef]
55. Ojesina, A.I.; Lichtenstein, L.; Freeman, S.S.; Pedamallu, C.S.; Imaz-Rosshandler, I.; Pugh, T.J.; Cherniack, A.D.; Ambrogio, L.; Cibulskis, K.; Bertelsen, B.; et al. Landscape of genomic alterations in cervical carcinomas. *Nature* **2013**, *506*, 371–375. [CrossRef]
56. Walline, H.M.; Goudsmit, C.M.; McHugh, J.B.; Tang, A.L.; Owen, J.H.; Teh, B.T.; McKean, E.; Glover, T.W.; Graham, M.P.; Prince, M.E.; et al. Integration of high-risk human papillomavirus into cellular cancer-related genes in head and neck cancer cell lines. *Head Neck* **2017**, *39*, 840–852. [CrossRef]
57. Koneva, L.A.; Zhang, Y.; Virani, S.; Hall, P.B.; McHugh, J.B.; Chepeha, D.B.; Wolf, G.T.; Carey, T.E.; Rozek, L.S.; Sartor, M.A. HPV Integration in HNSCC Correlates with Survival Outcomes, Immune Response Signatures, and Candidate Drivers. *Mol. Cancer Res.* **2018**, *16*, 90–102. [CrossRef]
58. Parfenov, M.; Pedamallu, C.S.; Gehlenborg, N.; Freeman, S.S.; Danilova, L.; Bristow, C.A.; Lee, S.; Hadjipanayis, A.G.; Ivanova, E.V.; Wilkerson, M.D.; et al. Characterization of HPV and host genome interactions in primary head and neck cancers. *Proc. Natl. Acad. Sci. USA* **2014**, *111*, 15544–15549. [CrossRef]
59. Moody, C.A.; Laimins, L.A. Human papillomavirus oncoproteins: Pathways to transformation. *Nat. Rev. Cancer* **2010**, *10*, 550–560. [CrossRef]
60. Vande Pol, S.B.; Klingelhutz, A.J. Papillomavirus E6 oncoproteins. *Virology* **2013**, *445*, 115–137. [CrossRef]
61. McLaughlin-Drubin, M.E.; Münger, K. The human papillomavirus E7 oncoprotein. *Virology* **2009**, *384*, 335–344. [CrossRef]
62. Graham, S.V. The human papillomavirus replication cycle, and its links to cancer progression: A comprehensive review. *Clin. Sci.* **2017**, *131*, 2201–2221. [CrossRef]
63. Williams, V.M.; Filippova, M.; Filippov, V.; Payne, K.J.; Duerksen-Hughes, P. Human papillomavirus type 16 E6* induces oxidative stress and DNA damage. *J. Virol.* **2014**, *88*, 6751–6761. [CrossRef]
64. Westrich, J.A.; Warren, C.J.; Pyeon, D. Evasion of host immune defenses by human papillomavirus. *Virus Res.* **2017**, *231*, 21–33. [CrossRef]
65. Westrich, J.A.; Vermeer, D.W.; Silva, A.; Bonney, S.; Berger, J.N.; Cicchini, L.; Greer, R.O.; Song, J.I.; Raben, D.; Slansky, J.E.; et al. CXCL14 suppresses human papillomavirus-associated head and neck cancer through antigen-specific CD8 T-cell responses by upregulating MHC-I expression. *Oncogene* **2019**, *38*, 7166–7180. [CrossRef]
66. Luo, X.; Donnelly, C.R.; Gong, W.; Heath, B.R.; Hao, Y.; Donnelly, L.A.; Moghbeli, T.; Tan, Y.S.; Lin, X.; Bellile, E.; et al. HPV16 drives cancer immune escape via NLRX1-mediated degradation of STING. *J. Clin. Investig.* **2020**, *130*, 1635–1652. [CrossRef]
67. Li, H.; Chiappinelli, K.B.; Guzzetta, A.A.; Easwaran, H.; Yen, R.-W.C.; Vatapalli, R.; Topper, M.J.; Luo, J.; Connolly, R.M.; Azad, N.S.; et al. Immune regulation by low doses of the DNA methyltransferase inhibitor 5-azacitidine in common human epithelial cancers. *Oncotarget* **2014**, *5*, 587–598. [CrossRef]
68. Wreesmann, V.B.; Estilo, C.; Eisele, D.W.; Singh, B.; Wang, S.J. Downregulation of Fanconi anemia genes in sporadic head and neck squamous cell carcinoma. *ORL J. Otorhinolaryngol. Relat. Spec.* **2007**, *69*, 218–225. [CrossRef]
69. Qin, T.; Zhang, Y.; Zarins, K.R.; Jones, T.R.; Virani, S.; Peterson, L.A.; McHugh, J.B.; Chepeha, D.; Wolf, G.T.; Rozek, L.S.; et al. Expressed HNSCC variants by HPV-status in a well-characterized Michigan cohort. *Sci. Rep.* **2018**, *8*, 1–11. [CrossRef]
70. Rivera, C.; Venegas, B. Histological and molecular aspects of oral squamous cell carcinoma (Review). *Oncol. Lett.* **2014**, *8*, 7–11. [CrossRef]
71. Koontongkaew, S. The tumor microenvironment contribution to development, growth, invasion and metastasis of head and neck squamous cell carcinomas. *J. Cancer* **2013**, *4*, 66–83. [CrossRef] [PubMed]

72. Lim, M.Y.; Dahlstrom, K.R.; Sturgis, E.M.; Li, G. Human papillomavirus integration pattern and demographic, clinical, and survival characteristics of patients with oropharyngeal squamous cell carcinoma. *Head Neck* **2016**, *38*, 1139–1144. [CrossRef] [PubMed]
73. Vojtechova, Z.; Sabol, I.; Salakova, M.; Turek, L.; Grega, M.; Smahelova, J.; Vencalek, O.; Lukesova, E.; Klozar, J.; Tachezy, R. Analysis of the integration of human papillomaviruses in head and neck tumours in relation to patients' prognosis. *Int. J. Cancer* **2016**, *138*, 386–395. [CrossRef] [PubMed]
74. Nulton, T.J.; Kim, N.-K.; DiNardo, L.J.; Morgan, I.M.; Windle, B. Patients with integrated HPV16 in head and neck cancer show poor survival. *Oral Oncol.* **2018**, *80*, 52–55. [CrossRef]
75. Pinatti, L.M.; Sinha, H.N.; Brummel, C.V.; Goudsmit, C.M.; Geddes, T.J.; Wilson, G.D.; Akervall, J.A.; Brenner, C.J.; Walline, H.M.; Carey, T.E. Association of human papillomavirus integration with better patient outcomes in oropharyngeal squamous cell carcinoma. *Head Neck* **2021**, *43*, 544–557. [CrossRef]
76. Raj, K.; Berguerand, S.; Southern, S.; Doorbar, J.; Beard, P. E1 empty set E4 protein of human papillomavirus type 16 associates with mitochondria. *J. Virol.* **2004**, *78*, 7199–7207. [CrossRef]
77. Tao, G.-Z.; Looi, K.S.; Toivola, D.M.; Strnad, P.; Zhou, Q.; Liao, J.; Wei, Y.; Habtezion, A.; Omary, M.B. Keratins modulate the shape and function of hepatocyte mitochondria: A mechanism for protection from apoptosis. *J. Cell Sci.* **2009**, *122*, 3851–3855. [CrossRef]
78. Steen, K.; Chen, D.; Wang, F.; Majumdar, R.; Chen, S.; Kumar, S.; Lombard, D.B.; Weigert, R.; Zieman, A.G.; Parent, C.A.; et al. A role for keratins in supporting mitochondrial organization and function in skin keratinocytes. *Mol. Biol. Cell* **2020**, *31*, 1103–1111. [CrossRef]
79. Balakrishnan, A.; Koppaka, D.; Anand, A.; Deb, B.; Grenci, G.; Viasnoff, V.; Thompson, E.W.; Gowda, H.; Bhat, R.; Rangarajan, A.; et al. Circulating Tumor Cell cluster phenotype allows monitoring response to treatment and predicts survival. *Sci. Rep.* **2019**, *9*, 7933. [CrossRef]
80. Nagel, M.; Schulz, J.; Maderer, A.; Goepfert, K.; Gehrke, N.; Thomaidis, T.; Thuss-Patience, P.C.; Al-Batran, S.E.; Hegewisch-Becker, S.; Grimminger, P.; et al. Cytokeratin-18 fragments predict treatment response and overall survival in gastric cancer in a randomized controlled trial. *Tumour Biol.* **2018**, *40*, 1010428318764007. [CrossRef]
81. Gleber-Netto, F.O.; Rao, X.; Guo, T.; Xi, Y.; Gao, M.; Shen, L.; Erikson, K.; Kalu, N.N.; Ren, S.; Xu, G.; et al. Variations in HPV function are associated with survival in squamous cell carcinoma. *JCI Insight* **2019**, *4*, e124762. [CrossRef]
82. Posner, M.; Misiukiewicz, D.K.; Hwang, V.; Gupta, V.; Miles, B.; Bakst, R.L.; Genden, E.; Selkridge, I.; Surgeon, J.T.; Rainey, H.; et al. Survival and Quality of Life Analysis in a Randomized Deintensification Trial for Locally Advanced HPV Positive Oropharynx Cancer Patients. *Int. J. Radiat. Oncol.* **2020**, *106*, 1146. [CrossRef]
83. Høxbroe Michaelsen, S.; Grønhøj, C.; Høxbroe Michaelsen, J.; Friborg, J.; von Buchwald, C. Quality of life in survivors of oropharyngeal cancer: A systematic review and meta-analysis of 1366 patients. *Eur. J. Cancer* **2017**, *78*, 91–102. [CrossRef]
84. Gillison, M.L.; Trotti, A.M.; Harris, J.; Eisbruch, A.; Harari, P.M.; Adelstein, D.J.; Jordan, R.C.K.; Zhao, W.; Sturgis, E.M.; Burtness, B.; et al. Radiotherapy plus cetuximab or cisplatin in human papillomavirus-positive oropharyngeal cancer (NRG Oncology RTOG 1016): A randomised, multicentre, non-inferiority trial. *Lancet* **2019**, *393*, 40–50. [CrossRef]
85. Vainshtein, J.M.; Spector, M.E.; McHugh, J.B.; Wong, K.K.; Walline, H.M.; Byrd, S.A.; Komarck, C.M.; Ibrahim, M.; Stenmark, M.H.; Prince, M.E.; et al. Refining risk stratification for locoregional failure after chemoradiotherapy in human papillomavirus-associated oropharyngeal cancer. *Oral Oncol.* **2014**, *50*, 513–519. [CrossRef]
86. Economopoulou, P.; de Bree, R.; Kotsantis, I.; Psyrri, A. Diagnostic Tumor Markers in Head and Neck Squamous Cell Carcinoma (HNSCC) in the Clinical Setting. *Front. Oncol.* **2019**, *9*, 827. [CrossRef]
87. Ward, M.J.; Thirdborough, S.M.; Mellows, T.; Riley, C.; Harris, S.; Suchak, K.; Webb, A.; Hampton, C.; Patel, N.N.; Randall, C.J.; et al. Tumour-infiltrating lymphocytes predict for outcome in HPV-positive oropharyngeal cancer. *Br. J. Cancer* **2014**, *110*, 489–500. [CrossRef]
88. Ou, D.; Adam, J.; Garberis, I.; Blanchard, P.; Nguyen, F.; Levy, A.; Casiraghi, O.; Gorphe, P.; Breuskin, I.; Janot, F.; et al. Clinical relevance of tumor infiltrating lymphocytes, PD-L1 expression and correlation with HPV/p16 in head and neck cancer treated with bio- or chemo-radiotherapy. *OncoImmunology* **2017**, *6*, e1341030. [CrossRef]
89. Bossler, F.; Hoppe-Seyler, K.; Hoppe-Seyler, F. PI3K/AKT/mTOR signaling regulates the virus/host cell crosstalk in HPV-positive cervical cancer cells. *Int. J. Mol. Sci.* **2019**, *20*, 2188. [CrossRef]
90. Morgan, E.L.; Macdonald, A. Autocrine STAT3 activation in HPV positive cervical cancer through a virus-driven Rac1-NFκB-IL-6 signalling axis. *PLoS Pathog.* **2019**, *15*, e1007835. [CrossRef]
91. Spangle, J.M.; Münger, K. The human papillomavirus type 16 E6 oncoprotein activates mTORC1 signaling and increases protein synthesis. *J. Virol.* **2010**, *84*, 9398–9407. [CrossRef] [PubMed]
92. Borbély, Á.A.; Murvai, M.; Kónya, J.; Beck, Z.; Gergely, L.; Li, F.; Veress, G. Effects of human papillomavirus type 16 oncoproteins on survivin gene expression. *J. Gen. Virol.* **2006**, *87*, 287–294. [CrossRef] [PubMed]
93. Altieri, D.C. Survivin–the inconvenient IAP. *Semin. Cell Dev. Biol.* **2015**, *39*, 91–96. [CrossRef] [PubMed]
94. Eytan, D.F.; Snow, G.E.; Carlson, S.; Derakhshan, A.; Saleh, A.; Schiltz, S.; Cheng, H.; Mohan, S.; Cornelius, S.; Coupar, J.; et al. SMAC mimetic birinapant plus radiation eradicates human head and neck cancers with genomic amplifications of cell death genes FADD and BIRC2. *Cancer Res.* **2016**, *76*, 5442–5454. [CrossRef]

95. Canning, M.; Guo, G.; Yu, M.; Myint, C.; Groves, M.W.; Byrd, J.K.; Cui, Y. Heterogeneity of the Head and Neck Squamous Cell Carcinoma Immune Landscape and Its Impact on Immunotherapy. *Front. Cell Dev. Biol.* **2019**, *7*, 52. [CrossRef]
96. Hanna, G.J.; Liu, H.; Jones, R.E.; Bacay, A.F.; Lizotte, P.H.; Ivanova, E.V.; Bittinger, M.A.; Cavanaugh, M.E.; Rode, A.J.; Schoenfeld, J.D.; et al. Defining an inflamed tumor immunophenotype in recurrent, metastatic squamous cell carcinoma of the head and neck. *Oral Oncol.* **2017**, *67*, 61–69. [CrossRef]
97. Wang, J.; Sun, H.; Zeng, Q.; Guo, X.-J.; Wang, H.; Liu, H.-H.; Dong, Z.-Y. HPV-positive status associated with inflamed immune microenvironment and improved response to anti-PD-1 therapy in head and neck squamous cell carcinoma. *Sci. Rep.* **2019**, *9*, 13404. [CrossRef]
98. Jung, K.; Kang, H.; Mehra, R. Targeting phosphoinositide 3-kinase (PI3K) in head and neck squamous cell carcinoma (HNSCC). *Cancers Head Neck* **2018**, *3*, 3. [CrossRef]

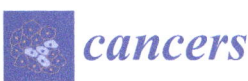

Article

Long-Term Survival and Recurrence in Oropharyngeal Squamous Cell Carcinoma in Relation to Subsites, HPV, and p16-Status

Malin Wendt [1,*], Lalle Hammarstedt-Nordenvall [1,2], Mark Zupancic [2,3], Signe Friesland [2,3], David Landin [1], Eva Munck-Wiklund [1,2], Tina Dalianis [2,3], Anders Näsman [3,4,†] and Linda Marklund [1,2,†]

1. Department of Clinical Science, Intervention and Technology—CLINTEC Division of Ear, Nose and Throat Diseases, Karolinska Institutet, Karolinska University Hospital, 171 64 Stockholm, Sweden; Lalle.Hammarstedt-Nordenvall@sll.se (L.H.-N.); David.Landin@ki.se (D.L.); Eva.Munck-Wiklund@ki.se (E.M.-W.); Linda.Marklund@ki.se (L.M.)
2. Medical Unit Head Neck, Lung and Skin Cancer, Karolinska University Hospital, 171 76 Stockholm, Sweden; Mark.Zupancic@ki.se (M.Z.); signe.friesland@sll.se (S.F.); Tina.Dalianis@ki.se (T.D.)
3. Department of Oncology-Pathology, Karolinska Institutet, Bioclinicum J6:20, Karolinska University Hospital, 171 64 Stockholm, Sweden; Anders.Nasman@ki.se
4. Department of Clinical Pathology, CCK R8:02, Karolinska University Hospital, 171 64 Stockholm, Sweden
* Correspondence: Anna.Malin.Wendt@ki.se
† Authors contributed equally to this work.

Simple Summary: Long-term survival in patients with oropharyngeal cancer is sparsely studied, but atypical recurrences in human papillomavirus-positive (HPV+) oropharyngeal cancer have been indicated. Furthermore, while the role of HPV is well established in tonsillar and base of tongue cancer, the dominant oropharyngeal subsites, its role in the minor oropharyngeal sites (the oropharyngeal walls, the uvula, and the soft palate) is not fully elucidated. The aim of this retrospective study was therefore to assess long-term outcome in relation to oropharyngeal sub-sites and HPV/p16 status. We confirm the prognostic role of p16+ in tonsillar and base of tongue cancer, but not the other sites. We find that combined HPV/p16-status gives better prognostic information than p16 alone. Lastly, we show that p16− cancer has more locoregional and late recurrences compared to p16+ cancer. Consequently, only combined HPV/p16 positivity in patients with tonsillar and tongue base cancer should be used in future treatment de-escalation trials.

Abstract: Long-term survival data in relation to sub-sites, human papillomavirus (HPV), and p16^{INK4a} (p16) for patients with oropharyngeal squamous cell carcinoma (OPSCC) is still sparse. Furthermore, reports have indicated atypical and late recurrences for patients with HPV and p16 positive OPSCC. Therefore, we assessed long-term survival and recurrence in relation to oropharyngeal subsite and HPV/p16 status. A total of 529 patients with OPSCC, diagnosed in the period 2000–2010, with known HPVDNA and p16-status, were included. HPV/p16 status and sub-sites were correlated to disease-free and overall survival (DFS and OS respectively). The overexpression of p16 (p16+) is associated with significantly better long-term OS and DFS in tonsillar and base of tongue carcinomas (TSCC/BOTSCC), but not in patients with other OPSCC. Patients with HPVDNA+/p16+ TSCC/BOTSCC presented better OS and DFS compared to those with HPVDNA−/p16− tumors, while those with HPVDNA−/p16+ cancer had an intermediate survival. Late recurrences were rare, and significantly more frequent in patients with p16− tumors, while the prognosis after relapse was poor independent of HPVDNA+/−/p16+/− status. In conclusion, patients with p16+ OPSCC do not have more late recurrences than p16−, and a clear prognostic value of p16+ was only observed in TSCC/BOTSCC. Finally, the combination of HPVDNA and p16 provided superior prognostic information compared to p16 alone in TSCC/BOTSCC.

Keywords: human papillomavirus; HPV; oropharyngeal cancer; OPSCC; tonsillar cancer; survival; OS; DFS; p16; recurrence

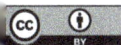

1. Introduction

Already in 1983, Syrjänen et al. suggested a possible correlation between human papillomavirus (HPV) infection and head and neck squamous cell carcinoma (HNSCC) [1]. In the following decades, extensive research, by ourselves and others, established high-risk HPV infection as a risk factor of oropharyngeal squamous cell carcinoma (OPSCC), and especially tonsillar and base of tongue cancer (TSCC and BOTSCC) [2–7]. Data also showed that patients with HPV positive OPSCC, more specifically HPV positive TSCC and BOTSCC, had a better clinical outcome, as well as a different epidemiological profile, when compared to patients with corresponding HPV negative cancer [8–10]. More specifically, the incidence of HPV positive TSCC and BOTSCC, and thereby OPSCC, has continuously increased in the Western world since the 1970's, and this increase has been described as an epidemic of viral induced OPSCC, or more specifically, TSCC and BOTSCC [5,11,12]. At the same time, the prevalence of smoking has decreased, resulting in a parallel decrease in the total incidence of HNSCC, but with a shift towards a larger proportion of HPV positive tumors in the oropharyngeal subsites [11].

The overexpression of $p16^{Ink4a}$ ($p16^+$) has, similar to the presence of HPV-DNA (HPVDNA$^+$), been shown to have a strong correlation to active HPV infection (i.e., expression of HPV E6 mRNA) in OPSCC, although the combined presence of both $p16^+$ and HPVDNA$^+$ is superior to using these markers separately [13]. Because $p16^+$ is easier to determine by immunohistochemistry (IHC), it was therefore suggested as a possible surrogate marker for HPV infection, and thereby also shown to be associated with a better prognosis in OPSCC [14,15]. In addition, $p16^+$ as a marker of HPV infection is now used in the 8th version of the American Joint Committee of Cancer (AJCC) AJCC Staging manual (TNM-8) to separate HPV-related from HPV-unrelated OPSCC [16].

However, recent studies, by ourselves and others, have suggested that the prevalence of HPV infection, its correlation to $p16^+$, and the impact of HPV infection on prognosis differs considerably between OPSCC sites. More specifically, the role of HPV on survival differs between tumors arising in lymphoepithelial oropharyngeal sites, i.e., TSCC and BOTSCC, and carcinomas arising in non-lymphoepithelial subsites of the oropharynx, i.e., carcinomas of the soft palate, uvula, and posterior pharyngeal wall (otherOPSCC) [17]. Therefore, while the prognostic role of HPV and the correlation between HPV infection and $p16^+$ is established in TSCC and BOTSCC, the role of HPV and its correlation to $p16^+$ in otherOPSCC is more ambiguous [18–24].

Irrespectively, roughly 10–20% of all patients with $p16^+$ or HPVDNA$^+$ OPSCC develop recurrent disease within 5 years after diagnosis [25,26]. Moreover, previous observations have proposed that patients with $p16^+$ or HPVDNA$^+$ OPSCC exhibit a different pattern of recurrence compared to those with corresponding $p16^-$ or HPVDNA$^-$ OPSCC [27,28]. It has specifically been indicated that the former group presents later recurrences and at different sites, compared to the latter, an issue that needs further study [29,30].

The aim of the present study was therefore to accumulate more knowledge regarding long-term survival, and recurrence in patients with OPSCC in relation to $p16^+$ and HPVDNA$^+$ status and OPSCC subsite.

2. Materials and Methods

2.1. Patients' Characteristics

All patients diagnosed in the period 2000–2010 with OPSCC, (TSCC: ICD-10 C09.0-9 and C02.4; BOTSCC C01.9; otherOPSCC: C10.0-9, C05.1-9), in the County of Stockholm/Gotland, Sweden were identified through the Swedish Cancer Registry. Patients treated with palliative intent were excluded from further studies. In addition, patients diagnosed with only cytology and/or with unknown p16 status, or there were no biopsies available, were also excluded (n = 25), and of these, 4 patients had a recurrence: 3 locoregional relapse (LRR) and 1 distant relapse (DR). Consequently, the study base consisted of 529 OPSCC patients, treated with the intention to cure and with known p16 and HPV DNA status (see below).

Patients' charts were assessed for TNM 7-stage, age, gender, smoking, WHO-status, type of treatment, recurrence, time to recurrence and location of recurrence, and survival. Treatment was classified as surgery, radiotherapy (including both external and brachytherapy), or chemoradiotherapy. Smoking data was obtained whenever noted in the charts, and was classified as "never" smoker or as "ever" smoker. The study was conducted according to ethical permissions 2005/431-31/4, 2005/1330-32 and 2009/1278-31/2 from the Stockholm Regional Ethical Review Board.

2.2. HPV-DNA and Overexpression of p16

Data on HPV DNA status and p16 status were obtained from previous studies [19,31]. Briefly, DNA was extracted from pre-treatment FFPE biopsies and analyzed for the presence of HPV DNA by PCR using broad-spectrum general primers bsGP5+/6+, and HPV-typing was performed utilizing a bead based multiplex assay (Luminex Magpix; Austin, TX, USA). For details, see [19,31].

Likewise, data on $p16^{Ink4a}$ overexpression by immunohistochemistry was obtained from previous studies [18,32]. Overexpression of p16 ($p16^+$) was defined as a strong nuclear and cytoplasmatic staining in more than 70% of tumor cells, as suggested by the College of American Pathologists [33].

2.3. Statistical and Survival Analysis

To evaluate differences in categorical data, we used a Chi^{-2} test; for the continuous variables we used an independent two-tailed t-test.

Overall survival (OS) was defined as time from diagnosis until death of any cause. Disease-free survival (DFS) was defined as time from diagnosis until recurrence of disease. A patient was considered to have recurrence of disease when treatment with curative intent was completed, patient was assessed as complete response at check-up, and then having a recurrence confirmed by radiology and/or histopathology. Recurrence was classified as LRR if in T- or N-position, and DR in M-position. Time-to recurrence was calculated as time from diagnosis until confirmed recurrence was noted in the patient chart. Patients who died tumor-free were censored at the time of death. Patients that never became tumor-free after treatment were censored at day 0. All patients had clinical controls every 3 months for the first 2 years, then every 6 months for a total of 5 years, and then if patients showed symptoms. In the case of recurrent disease, patients started clinical controls according to the same schedule after treatment.

OS and DFS was calculated for the whole OPSCC group, as well as for TSCC/BOTSCC and otherOPSCC separately, in relation to p16. Outcome was set as death of any cause or recurrence (LRR or DR). Results were presented in Kaplan–Meier curves, and survival was assessed with a log-rank test.

A sub-group analysis with univariate and multivariate analyzes was performed in patients with TSCC/BOTSCC and performance status (WHO/ECOG) (PS) 0 as a proxy for capacity to fulfill treatment. Here, hazard ratios (HR) for the combinations of $HPVDNA^{+/-}/p16^{+/-}$ status, age, stage, and smoking were estimated using the Cox proportional hazard model.

All analyses were made in SPSS (version 25 for Mac); p-values of <0.05 were considered significant.

3. Results

3.1. Patient and Tumor Characteristics

All patients at baseline, and their tumor characteristics, are depicted in Table 1. The largest proportion of primary tumors were TSCC (63%) and BOTSCC (22%), followed by otherOPSCC (15%). Patients with TSCC and BOTSCC (TSCC/BOTSCC) were younger at diagnosis compared to otherOPSCC (60.8 vs. 65.2 years, $p = 0.01$), and were diagnosed with a more advanced N-status (N0-1 vs. N2-3, $p = 0.01$).

Table 1. Patient and tumor characteristics.

		TSCC (%)	BOTSCC (%)	OtherOPSCC (%)	Total (%)
Number of patients		337	126	66	529
Age	Mean	60.4	62	65.2	61
	Median	59	62	65	61
	Range	29–90	30–84	46–88	29–90
Sex	Female	82 (24%)	39 (31%)	23 (35%)	144 (27%)
	Male	255 (76%)	87 (69%)	43 (65%)	385 (73%)
T (AJCC 7th Edition)	T1	78 (23%)	40 (32%)	8 (12%)	126 (24%)
	T2	129 (38%)	33 (26%)	24 (36%)	186 (35%)
	T3	70 (21%)	17 (13%)	25 (38%)	112 (21%)
	T4a	56 (17%)	36 (29%)	7 (11%)	99 (19%)
	T4b	4 (1%)	0 (0%)	2 (3%)	6 (1%)
N (AJCC 7th Edition)	N0	70 (21%)	28 (22%)	29 (44%)	127 (24%)
	N1	72 (21%)	16 (13%)	12 (18%)	100 (19%)
	N2a	49 (15%)	13 (10%)	4 (6%)	66 (12%)
	N2b	112 (33%)	32 (25%)	9 (14%)	153 (29%)
	N2c	21 (6%)	27 (21%)	11 (17%)	59 (11%)
	N3	13 (4%)	7 (6%)	1 (2%)	21 (4%)
	NX	0 (0%)	3 (2%)	1 (2%)	3 (1%)
M (AJCC 7th Edition)	M0	335 (99%)	120 (95%)	63 (95%)	518 (98%)
	M1	2 (1%)	2 (2%)	0 (0%)	4 (1%)
	MX	0 (0%)	4 (3%)	3 (5%)	7 (1%)
TNM Stage (AJCC 7th Edition)	I	10 (3%)	8 (6%)	3 (21%)	21 (4%)
	II	25 (7%)	7 (6%)	12 (21%)	44 (8%)
	III	83 (25%)	20 (16%)	23 (15%)	126 (24%)
	IVa	198 (59%)	82 (65%)	25 (33%)	305 (58%)
	IVb	19 (6%)	7 (6%)	3 (6%)	29 (5%)
	IVc	2 (1%)	2 (2%)	0 (4%)	4 (1%)
Smoking	Ever	237 (70%)	79 (63%)	51 (77%)	367 (69%)
	Never	92 (27%)	43 (34%)	7 (11%)	142 (27%)
	Not known	8 (2%)	4 (3%)	4 (6%)	20 (4%)
p16 overexpression	No	81 (24%)	41 (33%)	60 (91%)	182 (34%)
	Yes	256 (76%)	85 (67%)	6 (9%)	347 (66%)
HPV DNA status	Negative	78 (23%)	39 (31%)	47 (71%)	164 (31%)
	Positive	259 (77%)	87 (69%)	15 (23%)	361 (68%)
	Not known	0 (0%)	0 (0%)	4 (6%)	4 (1%)
Performance status (WHO/ECOG)	0	304 (90%)	102 (81%)	27 (41%)	433 (82%)
	1	20 (6%)	19 (15%)	20 (30%)	59 (11%)
	2	7 (2%)	5 (4%)	16 (24%)	28 (5%)
	3	5 (1%)	0 (0%)	3 (5%)	8 (2%)
	Not known	1 (0%)	0 (0%)	0 (0%)	1 (0%)
Treatment [1]	RT	234 (69%)	56 (44%)	48 (73%)	340 (64%)
	CRT	101 (30%)	70 (56%)	17 (26%)	183 (35%)
	Primary surgery	2 (1%)	0 (0%)	4 (6%)	6 (1%)
Recurrence	Yes	61 (18%)	30 (24%)	19 (29%)	110 (21%)
	No	276 (82%)	96 (76%)	47 (71%)	419 (79%)

[1] Neck dissection not included.

TSCC/BOTSCC were significantly more frequently p16$^+$ and HPV DNA$^+$, compared to otherOPSCC (70.4% p16$^+$ TSCC/BOTSCC vs. 22.2% p16$^+$ otherOPSCC, $p < 0.0001$, and 72.5% HPVDNA$^+$ TSCC/BOTSCC vs. 21% HPVDNA$^+$ otherOPSCC, $p < 0.0001$).

In the whole OPSCC cohort, 110/529 patients (20.8%), had recurrent disease, more specifically with 17.8% recurrences in TSCC, 24.2% in BOTSCC, and 28.8% in otherOPSCC (Table 1).

3.2. Long-Term Overall Survival and Disease-Free Survival in Relation to p16 and Subsites

Patients with p16$^+$ OPSCC had a significantly better OS and DFS, compared to patients with p16$^-$ OPSCC (log rank test <0.0001 and <0.0001, respectively). More specifically, 5-year OS and DFS were 76.4% and 84.9%, respectively, in patients with p16$^+$ OPSCC, and 42.4% and 64.7%, respectively, in patients with p16$^-$ OPSCC (Figure 1A,B). The 10-year OS and DFS were 65.4% and 83.7%, respectively, in patients with p16$^+$ OPSCC, and 22.9% and 59.6%, respectively, in patients with p16$^-$ OPSCC (Figure 1A,B).

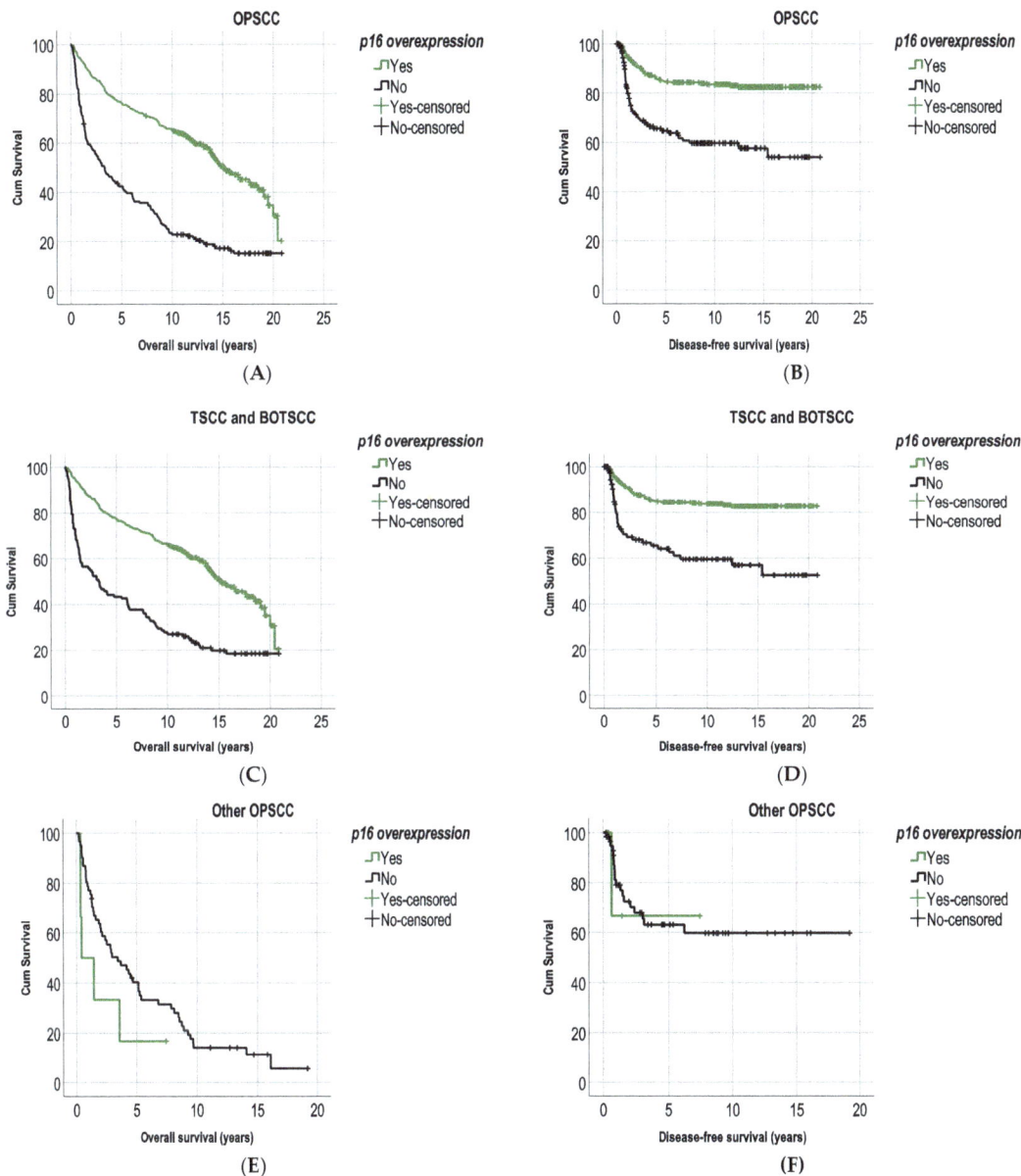

Figure 1. Kaplan–Meier figures with overall survival (OS) and disease-free survival (DFS) in patients with OPSCC (**A,B**) and separated on subsite with TSCC/BOTSCC (**C,D**) and otherOPSCC (**E,F**). (**A,B**) Patients with p16 positive OPSCC had a significantly better OS and DFS compared to patients with p16 negative OPSCC (log rank: $p < 0.0001$ and $p < 0.0001$, respectively). (**C,F**) Patients were separated into those with cancer in lymphoepithelial sub-sites (TSCC/BOTSCC) and non-lymphoepithelial subsites (otherOPSCC) and analyzed separately. (**C,D**) Patients with p16 positive TSCC/BOTSCC had a significantly better OS and DFS compared to patients with p16 negative TSCC/BOTSCC (log rank: $p < 0.0001$ and $p < 0.0001$, respectively). (**E,F**) No significant differences in OS and DFS between patients with p16 positive and p16 negative otherOPSCC were observed (log rank: $p = 0.13$ and $p = 0.9$, respectively).

When analyzing survival per subsite, patients with p16⁺ TSCC/BOTSCC had a significantly better OS and DFS compared to patients with p16⁻ TSCC/BOTSCC (log rank test < 0.0001 and <0.0001, respectively). More specifically, 5-year OS and DFS were 77.4% and 84.7%, respectively, in patients with p16⁺ TSCC/BOTSCC, compared to 43.4% and 65.4%, respectively, in patients with p16⁻ TSCC/BOTSCC. The 10-year OS and DFS were 66.3% and 83.8%, respectively, in patients with p16⁺ TSCC/BOTSCC, compared to 27% and 59.7%, respectively, in patients with p16⁻ TSCC/BOTSCC (Figure 1C,D). Notably, few late recurrences (>5 years after diagnosis) were observed in patients with p16⁺ TSCC/BOTSCC, which was not entirely the case in patients with p16⁻ TSCC/BOTSCC (Figure 1D). Patients with p16⁻ TSCC/BOTSCC had, in fact, a significantly higher risk of having a recurrent disease five years after diagnosis, compared to patients with p16⁺ TSCC/BOTSCC ($p < 0.001$, Figure 2).

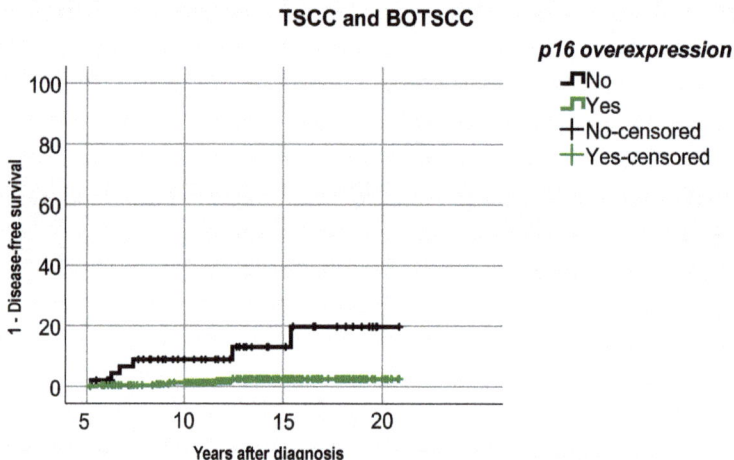

Figure 2. Kaplan–Meier figure with 1-disease-free survival (DFS) in patients with TSCC/BOTSCC five years after diagnosis. Patients with p16 positive TSCC/BOTSCC had a significantly better DFS compared to patients with p16 negative TSCC/BOTSCC (log rank: $p < 0.001$).

No differences in OS or DFS with regard to p16⁺/⁻ status were observed in patients with otherOPSCC (Figure 1E,F).

3.3. Localisation of Recurrence and Relation to Overexpression of p16 and Subsites

Of 112 recurrences, 74 (66%) were LRR and 38 (34%) were DR. In TSCC/BOTSCC, there was an equal distribution of LRR and DR, while most otherOPSCC had LRR (Figure 3). Notably, patients with p16⁺ OPSCC had a significantly higher proportion of DR, compared to those with p16⁻ OPSCC (p16⁺ OPSCC: Local relapse: $n = 16$; Regional relapse: $n = 15$; DR: $n = 24$; p16⁻ OPSCC: Local relapse: $n = 37$; Regional relapse: $n = 6$; DR: $n = 14$) ($p = 0.03$). Likewise, patients with p16⁺ TSCC/BOTSCC tended to have more DR compared to those with p16⁻ TSCC/BOTSCC, while the opposite was observed in patients with otherOPSCC; however, neither of these latter trends were significant.

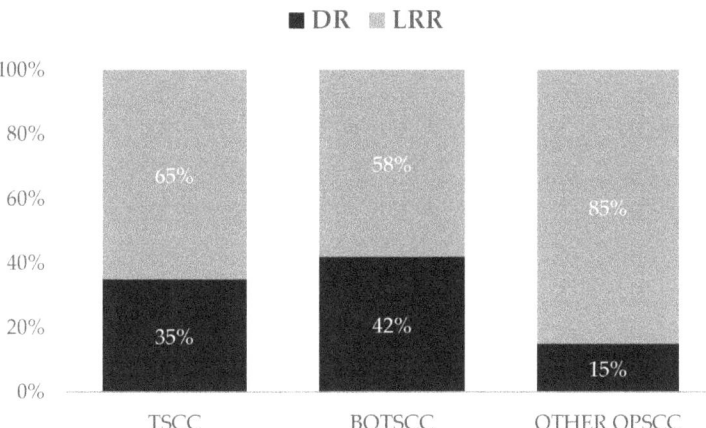

Figure 3. Distribution (percent) of loco-regional (LRR) and distant (DR) recurrencies separated per OPSCC sub-site. Patients with TSCC and BOTSCC had more often DR compared to otherOPSCC (*TSCC*: DR: $n = 21$, LRR: $n = 39$; *BOTSCC*: DR $n = 13$, LRR $n = 18$; otherOPSCC: DR $n = 3$, LRR $n = 17$).

3.4. Long-Term Overall and Disease-Free Survival in Relation to Both Overexpression of p16 and Presence of HPV DNA, in Patients with TSCC/BOTSCC

Because the prognostic role of p16$^+$ alone was only observed in patients with TSCC/BOTSCC, we continued our analysis by adding the presence of HPV DNA (HPVDNA$^+$) as an additional prognostic marker, only in these tumors.

Patients with combined HPVDNA$^+$/p16$^+$ TSCC/BOTSCC had a significantly better OS and DFS compared to patients with HPVDNA$^-$/p16$^-$ TSCC/BOTSCC (log rank: $p < 0.0001$ and $p < 0.0001$). However, patients with HPVDNA$^-$/p16$^+$ TSCC/BOTSCC presented an intermediate survival (Figure 4A,B). More explicitly, patients with HPVDNA$^-$/p16$^+$ TSCC/BOTSCC had a better OS and DFS compared to patients with HPVDNA$^-$/p16$^-$ cancer (log rank test: $p = 0.001$ and $p = 0.05$, respectively), but a worse OS compared to patients with HPVDNA$^+$/p16$^+$ cancer (OS: log rank test: $p = 0.047$), and the trend was similar for DFS (log rank test: $p = 0.1$). Similarly, patients with HPVDNA$^+$/p16$^-$ TSCC/BOTSCC ($n = 42$) also presented an intermediate survival.

In more detail, 5-year OS and DFS were 78.8% and 85.9%, respectively, in patients with HPVDNA$^+$/p16$^+$ TSCC/BOTSCC and 37.9% and 57.5%, respectively, in patients with HPVDNA$^-$/p16$^-$ cancer. Patients with discordant HPV and p16 status presented an intermediate survival, with 63.3% 5-year OS and 74.1% 5-year DFS in those with HPVDNA$^-$/p16$^+$ TSCC/BOTSCC, while corresponding figures for those with HPVDNA$^+$/p16$^-$ cancers were 57.1% and 85.4% for OS and DFS, respectively. Moreover, 10-year OS and DFS were 67.8% and 85.6%, respectively, in patients with HPVDNA$^+$/p16$^+$ TSCC/BOTSCC and 11.5% and 50.9%, respectively, in patients with HPVDNA$^-$/p16$^-$ cancer. Patients with discordant HPV and p16 status presented an intermediate survival, with 36.5% 10-year OS and 74.1% DFS in those with HPVDNA$^-$/p16$^+$ TSCC/BOTSCC, while corresponding figures for those with HPVDNA$^+$/p16$^-$ cancers were 42.9% and 80.9% for OS and DFS, respectively.

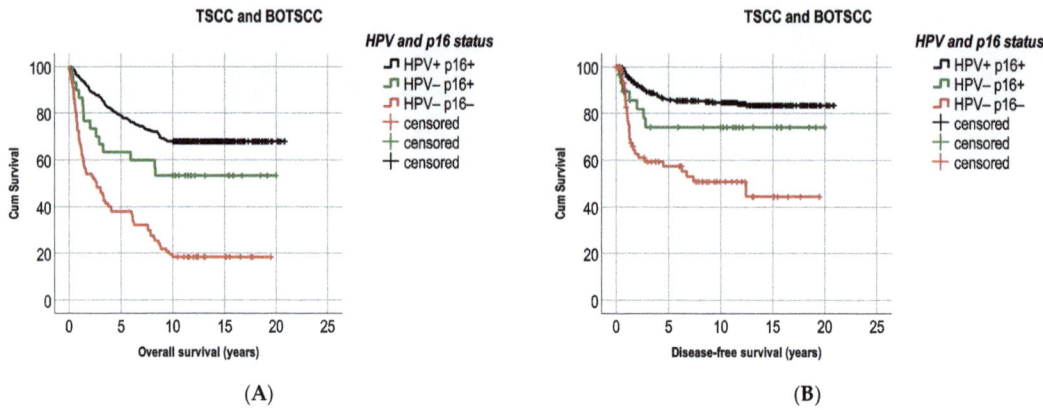

Figure 4. Kaplan–Meier figures with overall survival (OS) and disease-free survival (DFS) in patients with TSCC/BOTSCC (**A,B**). Patients with HPV DNA positive and p16 positive (HPV+/p16+) TSCC/BOTSCC had a significantly better OS and DFS, respectively (**A,B**, respectively), as compared to patients with HPV DNA negative and p16 negative TSCC/BOTSCC (log rank: $p < 0.0001$ and $p < 0.0001$, respectively). However, patients with p16 positive but HPV negative (HPV−/p16+) TSCC/BOTSCC presented an intermediate OS and DFS compared to patients with double positive or double negative HPV/p16 status. (HPV+p16+ vs. HPV−p16+ (log rank test): OS: $p = 0.047$; DFS: $p = 0.1$, and HPV−p16+ vs. HPV−p16− (log rank test): OS: $p = 0.001$; DFS: $p = 0.05$).

3.5. HPV, p16 Status and Other Prognostic Factors in Patients with TSCC/BOTSCC

A univariate and multivariate subgroup analysis, including patients with TSCC/BOTSCC and performance status (WHO/ECOG) (PS) 0, as a surrogate marker for completion of intended treatment, was performed and included 87.7% of all TSCC/BOTSCC patients. Uni- and multi-variate analyses for OS and DFS were performed for HPVDNA$^{+/-}$/p16$^{+/-}$ status, age, dichotomized smoking status (Ever vs. Never), and dichotomized TNM-7 stage (1–2 vs. 3–4) (Table 2).

Table 2. Uni- and multivariable analysis of OS and DFS in patients with TSCC/BOTSCC and PS 0.

		Overall Survival (OS)						Disease-Free Survival (DFS)					
			Univariable			Multivariable			Univariable			Multivariable	
		HR	95% CI	p-Value	HR	95% CI	p-Value	HR	95% CI	p	HR	95% CI	p
HPV/p16 status	HPV−p16−	1			1			1			1		
	HPV−p16+	0.31	0.15–0.66	0.002	0.49	0.23–1.05	0.07	0.34	0.12–0.98	0.05	0.43	0.15–1.3	0.1
	HPV+p16+	0.23	0.17–0.34	<0.0001	0.30	0.21–0.44	<0.0001	0.25	0.15–0.42	<0.0001	0.29	0.17–0.50	<0.0001
Age		1.06	1.05–1.09	<0.0001	1.1	1.04–1.08	<0.0001	1.04	1.02–1.06	0.001	1.03	1.008–1.06	0.009
Smoking	Ever	1			1			1			1		
	Never	0.46	0.30–0.68	<0.0001	0.58	0.38–0.88	0.01	0.54	0.31–0.93	0.03	0.69	0.39–1.3	0.2
Stage (TNM-7)	I/II	1			1			1			1		
	III/IV	1.12	0.66–1.9	0.7	1.6	0.93–2.8	0.09	1.36	0.59–3.1	0.5	1.8	0.78–4.3	0.2

Notably, patients with HPVDNA$^+$/p16$^+$ TSCC/BOTSCC had a clearly better OS and DFS than those with HPVDNA$^-$/p16$^-$ TSCC/BOTSCC, both in the uni- and in the multivariate analysis, while those with HPVDNA$^-$/p16$^+$ TSCC/BOTSCC only had a significantly better OS compared to those with HPVDNA$^-$/p16$^-$ cancer in the univariate analysis (Table 2). Moreover, irrespective of HPVDNA and p16, age was also significantly correlated to both OS and DFS in the univariate and multivariate analysis. For the dichotomized stage (1–2 vs. 3–4), no significant differences were observed for either OS or DFS (Table 2).

3.6. Survival after Recurrence TSCC/BOTSCC in Relation to HPV and Overexpression of p16

Survival after recurrence (LRR or DR) in patients with TSCC/BOTSCC was also assessed in correlation to HPVDNA$^{+/-}$ and p16$^{+/-}$ status. Survival was generally low (5.9%) after LRR/DR and did not differ significantly between patients with HPVDNA$^+$/p16$^+$, HPVDNA$^-$/p16$^-$, and HPVDNA$^-$/p16$^+$ TSCC/BOTSCC (Figure 5).

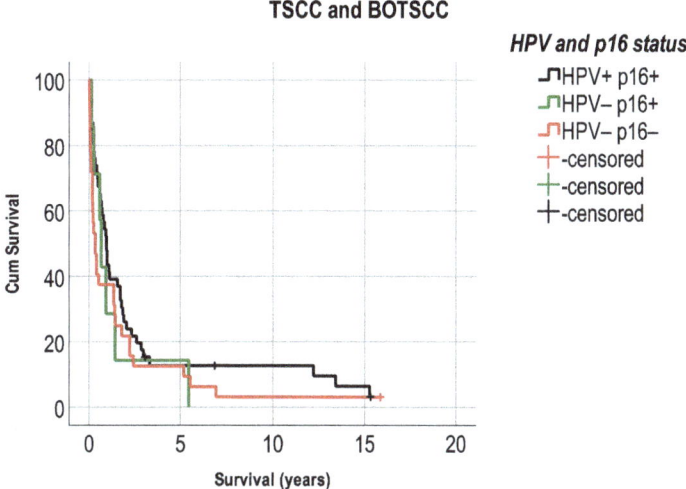

Figure 5. Kaplan–Meier figures with survival after a loco-regional or distant recurrence (LRR/DR) separated for HPV and p16 status. No significant differences were observed in survival between patients with TSCC/BOTSCC after recurrent disease independent of HPV and p16 status. (HPV+p16+ vs. HPV−p16−) (log rank test): $p = 0.17$.

4. Discussion

In this large, long term follow-up cohort study of OPSCC and its subsites, we disclosed that p16$^+$ was correlated to a favorable OS and DFS in patients with TSCC/BOTSCC as compared to those with corresponding p16$^-$ cancer, while in patients with otherOPSCC, no such analogy was observed. Likewise, patients with HPVDNA$^+$/p16$^+$ TSCC/BOTSCC presented a better OS and DFS compared to those with HPVDNA$^-$/p16$^-$ tumors, while notably, those with HPVDNA$^-$/p16$^+$ carcinomas presented an intermediate survival. Finally, late recurrences were rare, but were significantly more frequent in patients with p16$^-$ tumors, but nevertheless, the prognosis for recurrent disease was poor independent of the HPVDNA$^{+/-}$/p16$^{+/-}$ status of the tumor.

Consequently, in this report, we confirm previous results by ourselves and others that patient and tumor characteristics differ significantly between OPSCC arising in a lymphoepithelial context (TSCC/BOTSCC) and those arising in a non-lymphoepithelial context (otherOPSCC) [17–24]. In a previous study, we found that p16-status was poorly correlated to 5-year OS and DFS in patients with otherOPSCC, and that p16$^+$ was not a reliable surrogate marker for active HPV infection in this tumor type [32]. In addition, we have earlier shown that patients with p16$^+$ otherOPSCC at a low stage have a significantly worse OS compared to patients with TSCC/BOTSCC at the same stage [18]. Taken together, the data suggest that survival and pattern of recurrence for p16$^+$ otherOPSCC, instead resembles p16$^-$ TSCC/BOTSCC/otherOPSCC. Consequently, p16$^+$ status is not suitable to determine stage or choices of treatment in patients with otherOPSCC.

In addition, we also demonstrated in a subgroup analysis of TSCC/BOTSCC patients that patients with discordant (HPVDNA$^-$/p16$^+$) have a worse survival, compared to those with HPVDNA$^+$/p16$^+$ TSCC/BOTSCC. Moreover, patients with discordant HPV and p16 status had a more ambiguous survival benefit over patients with HPVDNA$^-$/p16$^-$ cancer, compared to those with HPVDNA$^+$/p16$^+$ TSCC/BOTSCC. Our data imply that there may be a risk of future undertreatment of patients with HPVDNA$^-$/p16$^+$ tumors, and possibly the opposite upon treatment of patients with HPVDNA$^+$/p16$^-$ tumors when patients are classified only based on p16$^{+/-}$ status with the new TNM- 8 staging system. These data suggest that the prognostic value of p16 is inferior to the combination of p16 and HPVDNA [13].

Although the above data need to be confirmed, they still suggest that some caution is necessary when conducting novel treatment strategies based on the new TNM-8 staging system [20].

Finally, we could not confirm earlier findings from smaller studies that patients with p16$^+$ TSCC/BOTSCC have a higher incidence of late relapses compared to patients with p16$^-$ TSCC/BOTSCC [32,33]. In general, only few cases relapsed after 5 years, and these tended to originate from p16$^-$ tumors. In addition, we did not observe any difference in survival between patients with p16$^+$ and p16$^-$ TSCC/BOTSCC-patients upon recurrence, which also differs from some earlier reports [34,35].

Of note, in most countries, the current first line of treatment in OPSCC is radiotherapy or chemoradiotherapy, with fairly good results in patients with p16$^+$ TSCC/BOTSCC, but with less favorable outcome in patients with p16$^-$ TSCC/BOTSCC and with otherOPSCC, regardless of p16 status. This calls for further studies on how to improve survival for patients with p16$^-$ TSCC/BOTSCC. As for otherOPSCC, it is not unlikely that the tumors within this group may better resemble oral cancer and benefit from primary surgery regardless of p16$^{+/-}$ status. In fact, one report demonstrated better recurrence free survival in patients with p16$^-$ OPSCC when they were treated with upfront surgery instead of radiotherapy and chemotherapy; however, surgery did not have an impact on OS [36].

This study has several limitations. Firstly, although the study population is relatively large, it is a retrospective single-center study with clinical data collected prospectively from patients' records. Secondly, we have not adjusted data for treatment modalities or for changes in treatment regimens over time. However, at our center, treatment has been consistent within and between the subsites over time, irrespective of p16$^{+/-}$ and HPVDNA$^{+/-}$ status, implying accuracy in the results. Finally, the group of otherOPSCC was relatively small, resulting in limited numbers of p16$^+$ tumors in that group. To confirm our findings, we encourage larger multicenter studies.

5. Conclusions

In conclusion, this study of long-term outcome and recurrence shows that patients with p16$^+$ TSCC/BOTSCC have better long-term OS and DFS than patients with corresponding p16$^-$ cancer. However, the combination of HPVDNA$^+$ and p16$^+$ status presented more accurate and detailed prognostic information than p16$^{+/-}$ status alone in patients with TSCC/BOTSCC. We therefore recommend the use of combined HPVDNA$^+$/p16$^+$ analysis for TSCC/BOTSCC when conducting treatment decisions and future tailored trials. In addition, importantly, p16$^+$ status did not affect long-term outcome in patients with otherOPSCC. However, larger studies will be required to confirm these results. Finally, late recurrences were rare in OPSCC, and patients with p16$^+$ TSCC/BOTSCC did not have a higher frequency of late metastasis compared to those with corresponding p16$^-$ carcinomas, nor did p16$^+$ status in their carcinomas affect outcome after recurrence.

Author Contributions: Conceptualization, M.W., L.H.-N., S.F., E.M.-W., T.D., A.N. and L.M.; methodology, M.W., L.H.-N., T.D., A.N. and L.M.; software, A.N.; validation, M.W., L.H.-N., M.Z., D.L., A.N. and L.M.; formal analysis, M.W., L.H.-N., A.N. and L.M.; investigation, M.W., D.L. and M.Z.; resources, E.M.-W., T.D. and A.N.; data curation, M.W., L.H.-N., M.Z., D.L. and L.M.; writing—original draft preparation, M.W., A.N. and L.M.; writing—review and editing M.W., L.H.-N., M.Z., S.F., D.L., E.M.-W., T.D., A.N. and L.M.; visualization, M.W., A.N. and L.M.; supervision, T.D., A.N. and L.M.; project administration, T.D., A.N. and L.M.; funding acquisition, T.D., L.M. and A.N. All authors have read and agreed to the published version of the manuscript.

Funding: This research was funded by THE SWEDISH CANCER SOCIETY, grant numbers 200778P, 200704P, 200764Fk, and 210292JCIA; STOCKHOLMS LÄNS LANDSTING (ALF), grant number 20200059; THE CANCER AND ALLERGY FOUNDATION, grant numbers 10127 and 10137; MAGNUS BERGVALLS STIFTELSE, grant number 2020-03737; TORNSPIRAN, grant number 2020; THE STOCKHOLM CANCER SOCIETY, grant numbers 201242 and 201092; and SVENSKA LÄKARESÄLLSKAPET, grant number SLS-935256.

Institutional Review Board Statement: The study was conducted according to the guidelines of the Declaration of Helsinki and approved by the Institutional Review Board of Karolinska Institutet (2005/431-31/4; 2009/1278-31/4; 2017/1035-31/2).

Informed Consent Statement: Informed consent was obtained from all subjects involved in the study according to the ethical permissions stated above.

Data Availability Statement: The data presented in this study are available on request from the corresponding author. The data are not publicly available due to Swedish laws on personal confidential information.

Conflicts of Interest: The authors declare no conflict of interest.

References

1. Syrjänen, K.J.; Syrjänen, S.M.; Lamberg, M.A.; Pyrhönen, S. Human papillomavirus (HPV) involvement in squamous cell lesions of the oral cavity. *Proc. Finn. Dent. Soc.* **1983**, *79*, 1–8.
2. Chaturvedi, A.K.; Engels, E.A.; Pfeiffer, R.M.; Hernandez, B.Y.; Xiao, W.; Kim, E.; Jiang, B.; Goodman, M.T.; Sibug-Saber, M.; Cozen, W.; et al. Human papillomavirus and rising oropharyngeal cancer incidence in the United States. *J. Clin. Oncol.* **2011**, *29*, 4294–4301. [CrossRef] [PubMed]
3. Marklund, L.; Hammarstedt, L. Impact of HPV in Oropharyngeal Cancer. *J. Oncol.* **2011**, *2011*, 509036. [CrossRef]
4. Mork, J.; Lie, A.K.; Glattre, E.; Hallmans, G.; Jellum, E.; Koskela, P.; Møller, B.; Pukkala, E.; Schiller, J.T.; Youngman, L.; et al. Human papillomavirus infection as a risk factor for squamous-cell carcinoma of the head and neck. *N. Engl. J. Med.* **2001**, *344*, 1125–1131. [CrossRef] [PubMed]
5. Nasman, A.; Attner, P.; Hammarstedt, L.; Du, J.; Eriksson, M.; Giraud, G.; Ahrlund-Richter, S.; Marklund, L.; Romanitan, M.; Lindquist, D.; et al. Incidence of human papillomavirus (HPV) positive tonsillar carcinoma in Stockholm, Sweden: An epidemic of viral-induced carcinoma? *Int. J. Cancer* **2009**, *125*, 362–366. [CrossRef]
6. Dahlgren, L.; Dahlstrand, H.M.; Lindquist, D.; Hogmo, A.; Bjornestal, L.; Lindholm, J.; Lundberg, B.; Dalianis, T.; Munck-Wikland, E. Human papillomavirus is more common in base of tongue than in mobile tongue cancer and is a favorable prognostic factor in base of tongue cancer patients. *Int. J. Cancer* **2004**, *112*, 1015–1019. [CrossRef]
7. Rietbergen, M.M.; Leemans, C.R.; Bloemena, E.; Heideman, D.A.; Braakhuis, B.J.; Hesselink, A.T.; Witte, B.I.; de Jong, R.J.B.; Meijer, C.J.; Snijders, P.J.; et al. Increasing prevalence rates of HPV attributable oropharyngeal squamous cell carcinomas in the Netherlands as assessed by a validated test algorithm. *Int. J. Cancer* **2013**, *132*, 1565–1571. [CrossRef]
8. Fakhry, C.; Westra, W.H.; Li, S.; Cmelak, A.; Ridge, J.A.; Pinto, H.; Forastiere, A.; Gillison, M.L. Improved survival of patients with human papillomavirus-positive head and neck squamous cell carcinoma in a prospective clinical trial. *J. Natl. Cancer Inst.* **2008**, *100*, 261–269. [CrossRef]
9. Dahlstrand, H.; Näsman, A.; Romanitan, M.; Lindquist, D.; Ramqvist, T.; Dalianis, T. Human papillomavirus accounts both for increased incidence and better prognosis in tonsillar cancer. *Anticancer Res.* **2008**, *28*, 1133–1138.
10. Nygård, M.; Aagnes, B.; Bray, F.; Møller, B.; Mork, J. Population-based evidence of increased survival in human papillomavirus-related head and neck cancer. *Eur. J. Cancer* **2012**, *48*, 1341–1346. [CrossRef]
11. Sturgis, E.M.; Cinciripini, P.M. Trends in head and neck cancer incidence in relation to smoking prevalence: An emerging epidemic of human papillomavirus-associated cancers? *Cancer* **2007**, *110*, 1429–1435. [CrossRef] [PubMed]
12. Marur, S.; D'Souza, G.; Westra, W.H.; Forastiere, A.A. HPV-associated head and neck cancer: A virus-related cancer epidemic. *Lancet Oncol.* **2010**, *11*, 781–789. [CrossRef]
13. Smeets, S.J.; Hesselink, A.T.; Speel, E.J.; Haesevoets, A.; Snijders, P.J.; Pawlita, M.; Meijer, C.J.; Braakhuis, B.J.; Leemans, C.R.; Brakenhoff, R.H. A novel algorithm for reliable detection of human papillomavirus in paraffin embedded head and neck cancer specimen. *Int. J. Cancer* **2007**, *121*, 2465–2472. [CrossRef] [PubMed]
14. Wagner, S.; Prigge, E.S.; Wuerdemann, N.; Reder, H.; Bushnak, A.; Sharma, S.J.; Obermueller, T.; von Knebel Doeberitz, M.; Dreyer, T.; Gattenlöhner, S.; et al. Evaluation of p16(INK4a) expression as a single marker to select patients with HPV-driven oropharyngeal cancers for treatment de-escalation. *Br. J. Cancer* **2020**, *123*, 1114–1122. [CrossRef]
15. Dahlstrand, H.M.; Lindquist, D.; Björnestål, L.; Ohlsson, A.; Dalianis, T.; Munck-Wikland, E.; Elmberger, G. P16(INK4a) correlates to human papillomavirus presence, response to radiotherapy and clinical outcome in tonsillar carcinoma. *Anticancer Res.* **2005**, *25*, 4375–4383.
16. Amin, M.B.; Edge, S.B.; Greene, F.; Byrd, D.R.; Brookland, R.K.; Washington, M.K.; Gershenwald, J.E.; Compton, C.C.; Hess, K.R.; Sullivan, D.C.; et al. *AJCC Cancer Staging Manual*, 8th ed.; Springer: Chicago, IL, USA, 2017.

17. Haeggblom, L.; Ramqvist, T.; Tommasino, M.; Dalianis, T.; Nasman, A. Time to change perspectives on HPV in oropharyngeal cancer. A systematic review of HPV prevalence per oropharyngeal sub-site the last 3 years. *Papillomavirus Res.* **2017**, *4*, 1–11. [CrossRef]
18. Marklund, L.; Holzhauser, S.; de Flon, C.; Zupancic, M.; Landin, D.; Kolev, A.; Haeggblom, L.; Munck-Wikland, E.; Hammarstedt-Nordenvall, L.; Dalianis, T.; et al. Survival of patients with oropharyngeal squamous cell carcinomas (OPSCC) in relation to TNM 8—Risk of incorrect downstaging of HPV-mediated non-tonsillar, non-base of tongue carcinomas. *Eur. J. Cancer* **2020**, *139*, 192–200. [CrossRef]
19. Hammarstedt, L.; Holzhauser, S.; Zupancic, M.; Kapoulitsa, F.; Ursu, R.G.; Ramqvist, T.; Haeggblom, L.; Näsman, A.; Dalianis, T.; Marklund, L. The value of p16 and HPV DNA in non-tonsillar, non-base of tongue oropharyngeal cancer. *Acta Otolaryngol.* **2021**, *141*, 89–94. [CrossRef]
20. Tham, T.; Wotman, M.; Roche, A.; Kraus, D.; Costantino, P. The prognostic effect of anatomic subsite in HPV-positive oropharyngeal squamous cell carcinoma. *Am. J. Otolaryngol.* **2019**, *40*, 567–572. [CrossRef]
21. Gelwan, E.; Malm, I.J.; Khararjian, A.; Fakhry, C.; Bishop, J.A.; Westra, W.H. Nonuniform Distribution of High-risk Human Papillomavirus in Squamous Cell Carcinomas of the Oropharynx: Rethinking the Anatomic Boundaries of Oral and Oropharyngeal Carcinoma from an Oncologic HPV Perspective. *Am. J. Surg. Pathol.* **2017**, *41*, 1722–1728. [CrossRef]
22. Ljokjel, B.; Lybak, S.; Haave, H.; Olofsson, J.; Vintermyr, O.K.; Aarstad, H.J. The impact of HPV infection on survival in a geographically defined cohort of oropharynx squamous cell carcinoma (OPSCC) patients in whom surgical treatment has been one main treatment. *Acta Otolaryngol.* **2014**, *134*, 636–645. [CrossRef] [PubMed]
23. Garnaes, E.; Kiss, K.; Andersen, L.; Therkildsen, M.H.; Franzmann, M.B.; Filtenborg-Barnkob, B.; Hoegdall, E.; Krenk, L.; Josiassen, M.; Lajer, C.B.; et al. A high and increasing HPV prevalence in tonsillar cancers in Eastern Denmark, 2000–2010: The largest registry-based study to date. *Int. J. Cancer* **2015**, *136*, 2196–2203. [CrossRef] [PubMed]
24. Haeggblom, L.; Attoff, T.; Hammarstedt-Nordenvall, L.; Nasman, A. Human papillomavirus and survival of patients per histological subsite of tonsillar squamous cell carcinoma. *Cancer Med.* **2018**, *7*, 1717–1722. [CrossRef] [PubMed]
25. Gillison, M.L.; Trotti, A.M.; Harris, J.; Eisbruch, A.; Harari, P.M.; Adelstein, D.J.; Jordan, R.C.K.; Zhao, W.; Sturgis, E.M.; Burtness, B.; et al. Radiotherapy plus cetuximab or cisplatin in human papillomavirus-positive oropharyngeal cancer (NRG Oncology RTOG 1016): A randomised, multicentre, non-inferiority trial. *Lancet* **2019**, *393*, 40–50. [CrossRef]
26. Christopherson, K.M.; Moreno, A.C.; Elgohari, B.; Gross, N.; Ferrarotto, R.; Mohamed, A.S.R.; Gunn, G.B.; Goepfert, R.P.; Mott, F.E.; Shah, J.; et al. Outcomes after salvage for HPV-positive recurrent oropharyngeal cancer treated with primary radiation. *Oral Oncol.* **2020**, *113*, 105125. [CrossRef] [PubMed]
27. Trosman, S.J.; Koyfman, S.A.; Ward, M.C.; Al-Khudari, S.; Nwizu, T.; Greskovich, J.F.; Lamarre, E.D.; Scharpf, J.; Khan, M.J.; Lorenz, R.R.; et al. Effect of human papillomavirus on patterns of distant metastatic failure in oropharyngeal squamous cell carcinoma treated with chemoradiotherapy. *JAMA Otolaryngol. Head Neck Surg.* **2015**, *141*, 457–462. [CrossRef]
28. Huang, S.H.; Perez-Ordonez, B.; Weinreb, I.; Hope, A.; Massey, C.; Waldron, J.N.; Kim, J.; Bayley, A.J.; Cummings, B.; Cho, B.C.; et al. Natural course of distant metastases following radiotherapy or chemoradiotherapy in HPV-related oropharyngeal cancer. *Oral Oncol.* **2013**, *49*, 79–85. [CrossRef]
29. Guo, T.; Rettig, E.; Fakhry, C. Understanding the impact of survival and human papillomavirus tumor status on timing of recurrence in oropharyngeal squamous cell carcinoma. *Oral Oncol.* **2016**, *52*, 97–103. [CrossRef]
30. O'Sullivan, B.; Adelstein, D.L.; Huang, S.H.; Koyfman, S.A.; Thorstad, W.; Hope, A.J.; Lewis, J.S., Jr.; Nussenbaum, B. First Site of Failure Analysis Incompletely Addresses Issues of Late and Unexpected Metastases in p16-Positive Oropharyngeal Cancer. *J. Clin. Oncol.* **2015**, *33*, 1707–1708. [CrossRef]
31. Nasman, A.; Nordfors, C.; Holzhauser, S.; Vlastos, A.; Tertipis, N.; Hammar, U.; Hammarstedt-Nordenvall, L.; Marklund, L.; Munck-Wikland, E.; Ramqvist, T.; et al. Incidence of human papillomavirus positive tonsillar and base of tongue carcinoma: A stabilisation of an epidemic of viral induced carcinoma? *Eur. J. Cancer* **2015**, *51*, 55–61. [CrossRef]
32. Marklund, L.; Näsman, A.; Ramqvist, T.; Dalianis, T.; Munck-Wikland, E.; Hammarstedt, L. Prevalence of human papillomavirus and survival in oropharyngeal cancer other than tonsil or base of tongue cancer. *Cancer Med.* **2012**, *1*, 82–88. [CrossRef] [PubMed]
33. Lewis, J.S., Jr.; Beadle, B.; Bishop, J.A.; Chernock, R.D.; Colasacco, C.; Lacchetti, C.; Moncur, J.T.; Rocco, J.W.; Schwartz, M.R.; Seethala, R.R.; et al. Human Papillomavirus Testing in Head and Neck Carcinomas: Guideline from the College of American Pathologists. *Arch. Pathol. Lab. Med.* **2018**, *142*, 559–597. [CrossRef] [PubMed]
34. Fakhry, C.; Zhang, Q.; Nguyen-Tan, P.F.; Rosenthal, D.; El-Naggar, A.; Garden, A.S.; Soulieres, D.; Trotti, A.; Avizonis, V.; Ridge, J.A.; et al. Human papillomavirus and overall survival after progression of oropharyngeal squamous cell carcinoma. *J. Clin. Oncol.* **2014**, *32*, 3365–3373. [CrossRef] [PubMed]
35. Argiris, A.; Li, S.; Ghebremichael, M.; Egloff, A.M.; Wang, L.; Forastiere, A.A.; Burtness, B.; Mehra, R. Prognostic significance of human papillomavirus in recurrent or metastatic head and neck cancer: An analysis of Eastern Cooperative Oncology Group trials. *Ann. Oncol.* **2014**, *25*, 1410–1416. [CrossRef] [PubMed]
36. Culié, D.; Viotti, J.; Modesto, A.; Schiappa, R.; Chamorey, E.; Dassonville, O.; Poissonnet, G.; Guelfucci, B.; Bizeau, A.; Vergez, S.; et al. Upfront surgery or definitive radiotherapy for patients with p16-negative oropharyngeal squamous cell carcinoma. A GETTEC multicentric study. *Eur. J. Surg. Oncol.* **2021**, *47*, 367–374. [CrossRef]

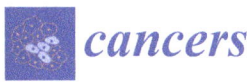

Article

Metabolic Plasticity and Combinatorial Radiosensitisation Strategies in Human Papillomavirus-Positive Squamous Cell Carcinoma of the Head and Neck Cell Lines

Mark D. Wilkie [1,2,*], Emad A. Anaam [1], Andrew S. Lau [1,2], Carlos P. Rubbi [1], Nikolina Vlatkovic [1], Terence M. Jones [1,2] and Mark T. Boyd [1]

[1] Cancer Research Centre, Department of Molecular & Clinical Cancer Medicine, The University of Liverpool, 200 London Road, Liverpool L3 9TA, UK; E.Anaam@liverpool.ac.uk (E.A.A.); andrew.lau@liverpool.ac.uk (A.S.L.); C.Rubbi@liverpool.ac.uk (C.P.R.); Vlatko@liverpool.ac.uk (N.V.); T.M.Jones@liverpool.ac.uk (T.M.J.); mboyd@liverpool.ac.uk (M.T.B.)

[2] Department of Otorhinolaryngology–Head & Neck Surgery, University Hospital Aintree, Lower Lane, Liverpool L9 7AL, UK

* Correspondence: mdwilkie@doctors.org.uk

Citation: Wilkie, M.D.; Anaam, E.A.; Lau, A.S.; Rubbi, C.P.; Vlatkovic, N.; Jones, T.M.; Boyd, M.T. Metabolic Plasticity and Combinatorial Radiosensitisation Strategies in Human Papillomavirus-Positive Squamous Cell Carcinoma of the Head and Neck Cell Lines. *Cancers* **2021**, *13*, 4836. https://doi.org/10.3390/cancers13194836

Academic Editor: Heather Walline

Received: 6 September 2021
Accepted: 14 September 2021
Published: 28 September 2021

Publisher's Note: MDPI stays neutral with regard to jurisdictional claims in published maps and institutional affiliations.

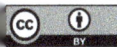

Copyright: © 2021 by the authors. Licensee MDPI, Basel, Switzerland. This article is an open access article distributed under the terms and conditions of the Creative Commons Attribution (CC BY) license (https://creativecommons.org/licenses/by/4.0/).

Simple Summary: A subset of head and neck cancers (SCCHN) are caused by human papillomavirus (HPV). As these tumours tend to affect younger patients and are associated with favourable survival, there is a pressing need to find ways to reduce long-term treatment toxicity while maintaining oncological efficacy. We studied utilisation of metabolic pathways in HPV-positive SCCHN cells with the aim of exploiting such for potential therapeutic benefit. We found that these tumours maintained metabolic diversity, in contrast to what we have observed in traditional SCCHN cells associated with mutations in the *TP53* gene. This, in turn, correlated with susceptibility to metabolic inhibitors, insofar as a combination of these agents acting on different metabolic pathways was required to augment the effects of ionising radiation (a mainstay of treatment for SCCHN). Notionally, this may provide a means of treatment de-intensification by facilitating radiation dose reduction to minimise the impact of treatment on long-term function.

Abstract: Background: A major objective in the management of human papillomavirus (HPV)-positive squamous cell carcinoma of the head and neck (SCCHN) is to reduce long-term functional ramifications while maintaining oncological outcomes. This study examined the metabolic profile of HPV-positive SCCHN and the potential role of anti-metabolic therapeutics to achieve radiosensitisation as a potential means to de-escalate radiation therapy. Methods: Three established HPV-positive SCCHN cell lines were studied (UM-SCC-104, UPCI:SCC154, and VU-SCC-147), together with a typical *TP53* mutant HPV-negative SCCHN cell line (UM-SCC-81B) for comparison. Metabolic profiling was performed using extracellular flux analysis during specifically designed mitochondrial and glycolytic stress tests. Sensitivity to ionising radiation (IR) was evaluated using clonogenic assays following no treatment, or treatment with: 25 mM 2-deoxy-D-glucose (glycolytic inhibitor) alone; 20 mM metformin (electron transport chain inhibitor) alone; or 25 mM 2-deoxy-D-glucose and 20 mM metformin combined. Expression levels of p53 and reporters of p53 function (MDM2, p53, Phospho-p53 [Ser15], TIGAR and p21 [CDKN1A]) were examined by western blotting. Results: HPV-positive SCCHN cell lines exhibited a diverse metabolic phenotype, displaying robust mitochondrial and glycolytic reserve capacities. This metabolic profile, in turn, correlated with IR response following administration of anti-metabolic agents, in that both 2-deoxy-D-glucose and metformin were required to significantly potentiate the effects of IR in these cell lines. Conclusions: In contrast to our recently published data on HPV-negative SCCHN cells, which display relative glycolytic dependence, HPV-positive SCCHN cells can only be sensitised to IR using a complex anti-metabolic approach targeting both mitochondrial respiration and glycolysis, reflecting their metabolically diverse phenotype. Notionally, this may provide an attractive platform for treatment de-intensification in the clinical setting by facilitating IR dose reduction to minimise the impact of treatment on long-term function.

Keywords: p53; cancer; glycolysis; oxidative phosphorylation; metabolism; head and neck cancer; human papillomavirus

1. Introduction

Squamous cell carcinoma of the head and neck (SCCHN) is the sixth most common cancer globally, with an estimated incidence of 750,000 cases per year [1]. Whilst tobacco and alcohol consumption are traditional risk factors [2], there is also now a considerable body of evidence implicating human papillomavirus (HPV) as a cause of SCCHN, in particular of oropharyngeal SCC affecting the base of tongue and tonsils [3].

Although rates of oral and laryngeal cancers are stable or decreasing slightly in developed countries, primarily because the population is smoking less, there has been a dramatic upsurge in the incidence of oropharyngeal cancer in the developed world in recent years. In the United States (US), the incidence of oropharyngeal SCC increased by 22% between 1999 and 2006, after no change between 1975 and 1999 [4], and the United Kingdom (UK) has seen a doubling in incidence from 1/100,000 population to 2.3/100,000 in just over a decade [5]. This rapid increase has been widely attributed to an exponential rise in the incidence of HPV-related disease, a consensus corroborated by several prevalence studies [6,7].

HPV-positive SCCHN is associated with favourable survival outcomes irrespective of the treatment modality employed [8,9]. This, together with the fact that HPV-driven disease tends to affect younger and generally medically fitter patients, who are therefore likely to experience the functional ramifications of their treatment long-term, has led many to propose treatment de-intensification [10]. Consequently, a key objective in translational research is to identify ways of sensitising these tumours to the effects of current treatments, not only to improve efficacy, but also to minimise the substantial toxic effects. Fundamental to this is to elucidate the cellular processes that may determine radio- and/or chemo-sensitivity to facilitate therapeutic targeting of the key pathways that may impinge on these processes.

Alteration of cellular metabolism is now widely considered to be a hallmark of the cancer phenotype, intrinsic to malignant transformation [11], and as such presents a potentially attractive therapeutic target. However, whilst disruption of metabolic circuitry may occur to some degree in all tumours, there is undoubtedly heterogeneity, which may reflect both tissue-specific effects and distinct oncogenic events driving tumorigenesis in different tumour types [12]. Detailed study and consideration of the metabolic phenotype of individual cancers is paramount, therefore, if effective therapeutic strategies targeting metabolism are to be developed and effectively deployed.

In the context of HPV-negative SCCHN, we and others have shown previously that metabolic phenotype and associated therapeutic opportunities are dictated by *TP53* status, with mutational loss of wild-type p53 function conferring a metabolic switch away from oxidative phosphorylation and towards glycolytic dependence [13–15]. Whilst HPV-positive tumours rarely harbour *TP53* mutations (2–3% of cases [16]), the importance of the HPV E6 oncoprotein in targeting p53 for proteasomal degradation in HPV oncogenesis [17,18], invites scrutiny of metabolism in HPV-positive disease, particularly given the dearth of previously published data. The aims of this study, therefore, were to examine the metabolic profile in HPV-positive SCCHN and to determine whether anti-metabolic therapy might be employed to potentiate the effects of ionising radiation (IR).

2. Methods

2.1. Cell Lines and Culture Conditions

The following established immortalised cell lines were used in this study: UM-SCC-1, UM-SCC-81B, and UM-SCC-104 (kindly provided by Professor T.E. Carey, University of Michigan, Ann Arbor, MI, USA); UPCI:SCC154 (kindly provided by Professor S. Gollin,

University of Pittsburgh, Pittsburgh, PA, USA); and VU-SCC-147 (kindly provided by Dr Josephine Dorsman, VU University Medical Centre, Amsterdam, The Netherlands). UM-SCC-104, UPCI:SCC154, and VU-SCC-147 are all SCCHN cell lines reported to be HPV-positive [19,20]. UM-SCC-1, a SCCHN cell line known to be p53 null [21], was used as a negative control in p53 Western blot analysis, while UM-SCC-81B, an HPV-negative oropharyngeal SCC cell line known to harbour a *TP53* mutation (H193R) [22], was used for comparative purposes in metabolic profiling and clonogenic survival experiments being typical of the lines we recently described [15]. All cell lines were confirmed as identical to their published genotype [23–25] via short tandem repeat (STR) analysis with GenePrint® 10 System (Promega, Southampton, UK) and screened and confirmed negative for mycoplasma contamination using the e-Myco™ mycoplasma PCR detection kit (ChemBio, Luton, UK). Cells lines were grown in Nunc™ cell culture treated flasks with filter caps (Thermo Fisher Scientific, Paisley, UK) in a humidified cell incubator at 37 °C with 5% CO_2 and, with the exception of UPCI:SCC154, were maintained in Dulbecco's modified Eagle's media (DMEM, Sigma-Aldrich, Gillingham, UK) supplemented with 10% fetal bovine serum (FBS), 1% penicillin/streptomycin, 1% L-glutamine, and 1% non-essential amino acids. UPCI:SCC154 was maintained in Eagle's minimum essential medium supplemented with 15% FBS, with additional supplements as above.

2.2. Western Blotting

Cells were harvested either untreated or 8 h after irradiation at a dose of 6Gy. Proteins extracted as described previously [26]. Typically, 50 μg samples of total protein were separated by SDS–PAGE and transferred to Immun-Blot® PVDF Membrane (Bio-Rad, Hercules, CA, USA). Western blotting was performed as described previously [23]. Mouse monoclonal antibodies against MDM2 (IF-2) (Calbiochem, San Diego, CA, USA), p53 (DO-1) (Calbiochem), TIGAR (E-2) (Santa Cruz, Dallas, TX, USA), p21 (*CDKN1A*) (F-5) (Santa Cruz), and a rabbit polyclonal antibody against Phospho-p53 (Ser15) (#9284) (Cell Signaling Technology, Danvers, MA, USA) were used to probe the expression of those proteins. Detection of Vinculin, using a mouse monoclonal antibody (V9131) (Sigma-Aldrich), was included as a loading control. Secondary antibodies were sheep anti-mouse (RPN4201) and donkey anti-rabbit (NA934) (GE Healthcare, Little Chalfont, UK) used at dilutions of 1:2500 and 1:5000 respectively. Membranes were washed with PBS-0.1% (v/v) Tween®-20 for all proteins except for phospho-p53 (Ser15) where the membrane was washed with TBS-0.1% (v/v) Tween®-20. Bio-Rad EveryBlot Blocking Buffer was used to suppress non-specific antibody binding. Signals were detected by chemiluminescence using Clarity Western ECL Substrate (Bio-Rad) and recorded using ChemiDoc MP imaging system (Bio-Rad).

2.3. Metabolic Profiling Studies

Metabolic studies were performed using an XF24 analyser (Seahorse Bioscience, Copenhagen, Denmark) to undertake either mitochondrial or glycolytic stress tests, essentially according to the manufacturer's instructions. Experimental readouts are oxygen consumption rate (OCR) in pmol/min and extracellular acidification rate (ECAR) in mPH/min, to provide surrogate measures of oxidative phosphorylation and glycolysis respectively. Data were analysed using Wave software (Seahorse Bioscience). During mitochondrial stress tests, inhibitors were injected sequentially as follows: oligomycin 1.25 μM, FCCP 1.5 μM, and lastly a combination of rotenone and antimycin-A 1 μM. During glycolytic stress tests, inhibitors were injected sequentially as follows: glucose 10 mM, oligomycin 1.25 μM, and finally 2-DG 50 mM. ECAR was measured in mPH/min.

To enable quantification and for comparison of OCR and ECAR metabolic measurements between cell lines, normalisation to sample DNA content was employed. The DNA content of samples following completion of mitochondrial and glycolytic stress tests was determined in Corning® 96-well black bottom plates (Sigma-Aldrich) and then DNA content was measured using a CyQUANT® cell proliferation assay kit (Invitrogen, Paisley,

UK), according to the manufacturer's instructions. Fluorescence was measured at 520 nm following excitation at 508 nm using a POLARstar Omega plate reader (BMG LABTECH, Ortenberg, Germany).

When analysing data between different cell lines non-parametric statistics were used due to the number of samples in each group (<30) as per central limit theorem. Specifically, Mann-Whitney U tests were utilised and the significance level for all tests was set at 0.05. For the purposes of meaningful and valid comparison analysis of metabolic parameters derived from mitochondrial and glycolytic stress tests was performed for the HPV-positive cell lines grouped together and compared with the *TP53* mutant HPV-negative cell line (UM-SCC-81B).

2.4. Clonogenic Survival Assays

Clonogenic survival assays were performed using a "plating after treatment" method as described previously [27]. Data were analysed as follows: the plating efficiency (PE) was calculated from the 0 Gy condition by dividing the number of colonies formed by the number of cells seeded. The number of colonies formed after treatment was then used to calculate the surviving fraction (SF) for each treatment condition, accounting for the plating efficiency: SF = (number of colonies formed/number of cells seeded) × PE. Survival parameters to generate treatment-dose survival curves for treatment conditions were then derived from fitting the data by weighted, stratified, linear regression according to the linear–quadratic formula $S(D) = \exp(\alpha D + \beta D^2)$, where S is survival following a given dose (D) of IR, which also allowed comparison between treatment conditions as described by Franken et al. [27] Specifically, the model summary examined whether the data scatter across two treatment-dose survival curves was described best with one modelled survival curve (null hypothesis) or was best described by two distinct modelled curves (test hypothesis) (i.e., a statistically significant difference [$p < 0.05$] between the compared treatment-dose survival curves) [27].

3. Results

3.1. HPV-Positive SCCHN Cells Maintain Metabolic Diversity

Metabolic profiling of the HPV-positive SCCHN cell lines (UM-SCC-104, UPCI:SCC 154, VU-SCC-147) demonstrated that these cells exhibit a diverse metabolic phenotype, displaying both robust mitochondrial and robust glycolytic reserve capacities (Figure 1). In contrast, and in accordance with what we and others have shown previously [13–15], the HPV-negative SCCHN mutant *TP53* SCCHN cell line (UM-SCC-81B) displayed markedly reduced mitochondrial and glycolytic reserves, functioning near or at capacity under basal conditions (Figure 1). FCCP doses were also titrated to ensure the reduced mitochondrial reserve was not related to suboptimal FCCP dosing (Supplementary Figure S1).

To allow for a clearer interpretation of the overall metabolic picture comparison of normalised absolute values for the metabolic parameters generated from the mitchondrial and glyolcytic stress tests was also performed and are depicted in Figure 2. In keeping with the clear patterns shown in the relative stress test plots in Figure 1, the absolute values for maximal respiration, spare respiratory capacity, maximal glycolysis, and glycolytic reserve were significantly greater in the HPV-positive cell lines compared with HPV-negative mutant *TP53* cell line (Figure 2A,B). Interestingly, however, capturing absolute OCR and ECAR values revealed that HPV-positive cells exhibited discernibly higher rates of mitochondrial respiration and lower rates of glycolysis under basal conditions, findings which were borne out more definitively when analysing the relative basal utilisation of mitochondrial respiration and glycolysis (Figure 2C).

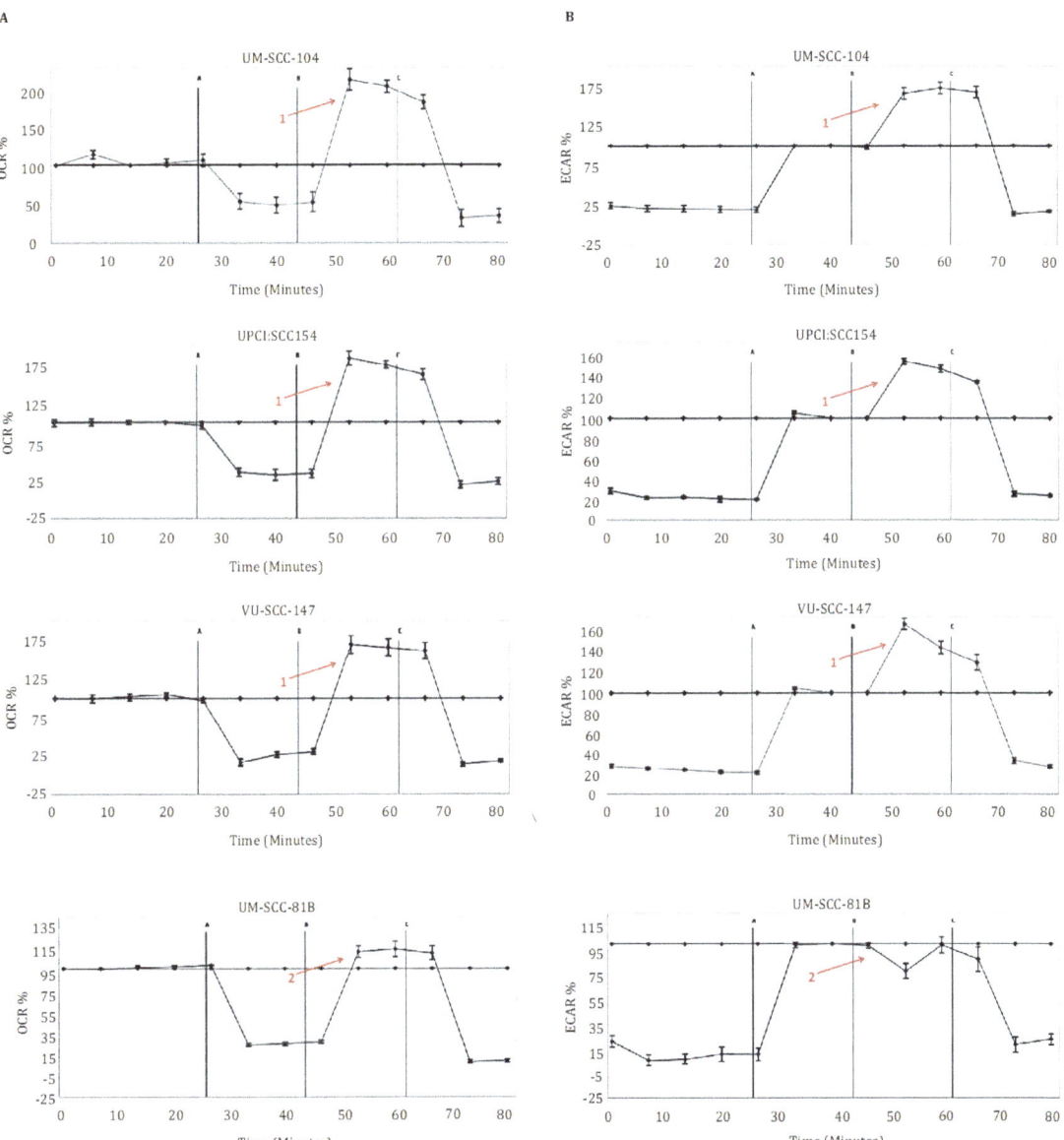

Figure 1. Metabolic profiling in HPV-positive SCCHN cell lines and for comparison, a typical *TP53* mutant HPV-negative line (UM-SCC-81B). Cells were subjected to mitochondrial and glycolytic stress tests (panels (**A**,**B**) respectively). During mitochondrial stress tests, oligomycin 1.25 µM (point A), FCCP 1.5 µM (point B), and rotenone and antimycin-A 1 µM (point C) were sequentially injected, and OCR (pmol/min) measured. During glycolytic stress tests, glucose 10 mM (point A), oligomycin 1.25 µM (point B), and 2-DG 50 mM (point C) were sequentially injected, and ECAR (mpH/min) measured. Data is presented as percentage increases or decreases in OCR and ECAR relative to baseline measurements. The baseline is shown as the black line on the graphs. HPV-positive SCCHN cell lines maintained marked spare respiratory capacities and glycolytic reserves, in contrast to UM-SCC-81B, which exhibited reduced spare respiratory capacity and reduced glycolytic reserved (contrast arrows labelled 1 and 2). Error bars represent standard error of the mean (SEM).

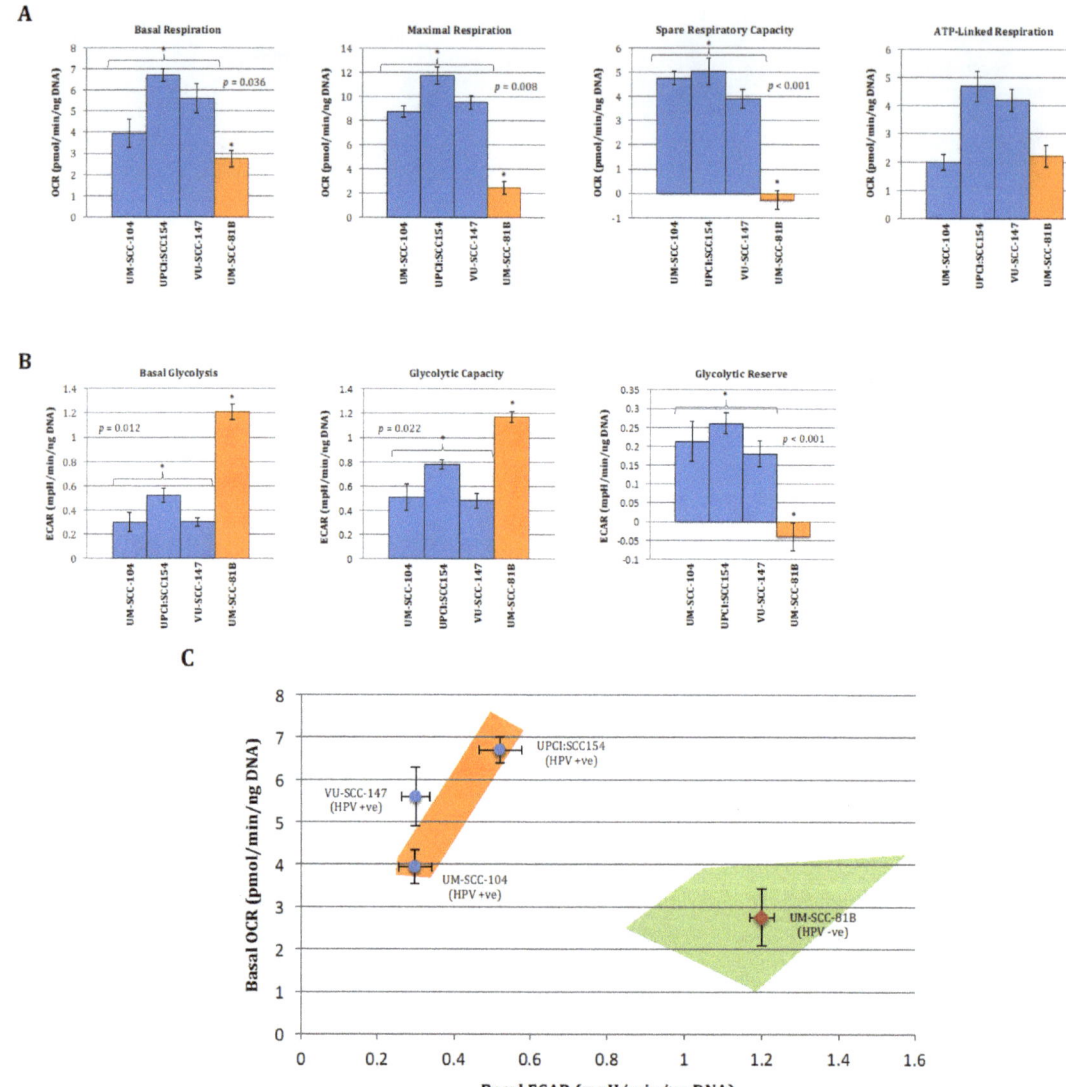

Figure 2. Quantitative OCR and ECAR data, normalised to DNA content for HPV-positive SCCHN cell lines and for comparison, a typical *TP53* mutant HPV-negative line (UM-SCC-81B). As stated in the methods, statistical comparison of absolute values for metabolic parameters was performed for the HPV-positive cell lines grouped together and compared with the *TP53* mutant HPV-negative cell line. (**A**) displays data from mitochondrial stress tests with statistical analysis as follows: basal respiration * $p = 0.036$; maximal respiration * $p = 0.008$; spare respiratory capacity * $p < 0.001$; ATP-linked respiration p = non-significant. (**B**) displays data from glycolytic stress tests with statistical analysis as follows: basal glycolysis * $p = 0.012$; glycolytic capacity * $p = 0.022$; glycolytic reserve * $p < 0.001$. (**C**) Plot of relative basal utilisation of mitochondrial respiration and glycolysis. Normalised basal values from glycolytic and mitochondrial stress tests for all cell lines plotted against each other. There is clear grouping of the HPV-positive SCCHN cell lines and the mutant *TP53* cell line, with the former displaying high levels of mitochondrial respiration relative to glycolysis and the latter the opposite. Blue diamonds represent HPV-positive SCCHN cell lines and the red diamond represents the mutant *TP53* cell line. The green and orange shaded areas represent the respective distributions of mutant *TP53* and wild-type SCCHN cell lines as we have demonstrated previously [15]. For all panels error bars represent SEM for each measurement.

Taken together, these findings suggest that HPV-positive SCCHN (and by association p53 wild-type [16]) cells predominantly catabolise glucose through oxidative phosphorylation under basal conditions and maintain robust mitochondrial function, enabling these cells to mount a maximal increase in ETC activity when exposed to mitochondrial stressors. In contrast, in the context of mutational inactivation of wild-type p53 function mitochondrial function appears to be compromised as cells display reduced oxidative phosphorylation under basal conditions and are unable to mount an increase in activity in response to mitochondrial stressors. Glycolysis seemingly predominates with significantly heightened basal levels, which are elevated to maximal cellular capacity leaving little or no glycolytic reserve. This is again consistent with what we and others have shown previously in HPV-negative SCCHN cell lines divergent on TP53 status [13–15].

3.2. HPV-Positive SCCHN Metabolic Diversity May Be Related to Residual Wild-Type p53 Function

That HPV-positive SCCHN cells maintain metabolic diversity was perhaps surprising given that previous data has shown loss of wild-type p53 function to be associated with a metabolic switch away from mitochondrial respiration and towards glycolytic dependence [13–15], and that targeting p53 for proteasomal degradation is key to HPV oncogenesis [17,18]. This prompted us to examine expression of p53 and reporters of p53 function (MDM2, p53, Phospho-p53 [Ser15], TIGAR and p21 [CDKN1A]) in the HPV-positive SCCHN cell lines, with the hypothesis that there may be residual wild-type p53 function sufficient to prevent metabolic re-programming.

Accordingly, western blotting revealed VU-SCC-147 to express p53 under basal conditions, and more importantly exposure to p53-activating genotoxic stress (6Gy IR) induced p53 stabilisation and activation of p53 reporters in this cell line (Figure 3 [original western bots are shown in Supplementary Figure S2]). This, however, was not demonstrated convincingly for the other HPV-positive SCCHN cell lines (UM-SCC-104 and UPCI:SCC 154). Consistent with this, such expression patterns have also been reported previously for these HPV-positive SCCHN cell lines [28,29].

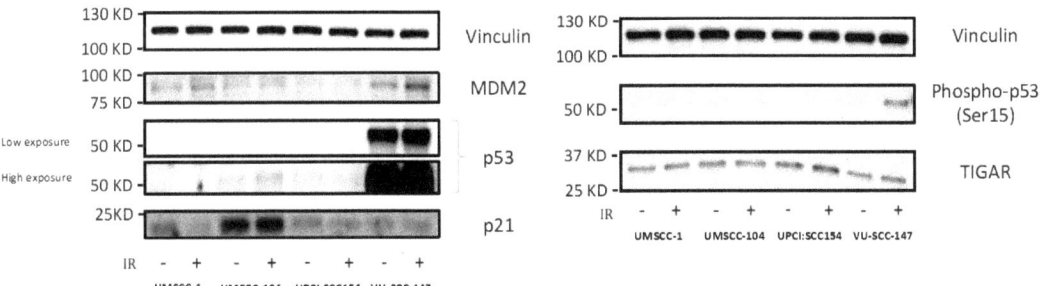

Figure 3. Expression levels of p53 and reporters of p53 function in HPV-positive SCCHN cell lines and for comparison, an endogenously p53-null SCCHN cell line. Western blotting revealed VU-SCC-147 to express p53 under basal conditions, but not so in the cases of UM-SCC-104 and UPCI:SCC 154. As VU-SCC-147 was observed to express high levels of p53 both high and low exposure blots are shown for clarity. Exposure to p53-activating genotoxic stress (6Gy IR [denoted by +]) also induced p53 stabilisation and activation of p53 reporters (specifically Phospho-p53 [Ser15]) in VU-SCC-147. Again, this was not demonstrated convincingly for UM-SCC-104 and UPCI:SCC 154. UM-SCC-1, a SCCHN cell line known to be endogenously p53 null, was included for comparison.

3.3. HPV-Positive SCCHN Cells Require a Combinatorial Anti-Metabolic Therapeutic Approach

Having shown that HPV-positive SCCHN cell lines exhibit a diverse metabolic phenotype in keeping with functional wild-type p53, we sought to evaluate the potential of anti-metabolic approaches that could be used therapeutically. Cells were exposed to IR following no treatment, 2-DG alone, metformin alone, or combined 2-DG and metformin treatment. 2-DG is a stable glucose analogue and a well-recognised glycolytic inhibitor that interferes with glycolysis by inhibiting the glycolytic enzymes phosphoglucose isomerase and hexokinase [30,31]. Metformin has demonstrated activity against mitochondrial respiration, specifically against electron transport chain (ETC) complex I [32], and thus represents an appropriate choice to combine with 2-DG to enable targeting of both glycolysis and mitochondrial respiration.

Accordingly, we predicted that HPV-positive SCCHN cells would display unaltered sensitivity to IR if only glycolysis or the ETC were inhibited, since the cells retain the metabolic flexibility to adapt to these inhibitors, in contrast to our recent findings in *TP53* mutant HPV-negative SCCHN cells, in which metabolic restriction allowed for radiosensitisation by 2-DG alone [15]. Moreover, we hypothesised that the drug combination might radiosensitise these metabolically more flexible cells. As expected, whilst 2-DG or metformin alone failed to have any effect on IR response, the combination of 2-DG and metformin resulted in significant potentiation of IR effects (Figure 4). Again, for comparative purposes anti-metabolic therapeutic approaches were evaluated in UM-SCC-81B as a typical representative *TP53* mutant line. Consistent with what others and we have reported previously [13–15], in this HPV-negative cell line IR effects were potentiated significantly by glycolytic inhibition alone (Figure 4).

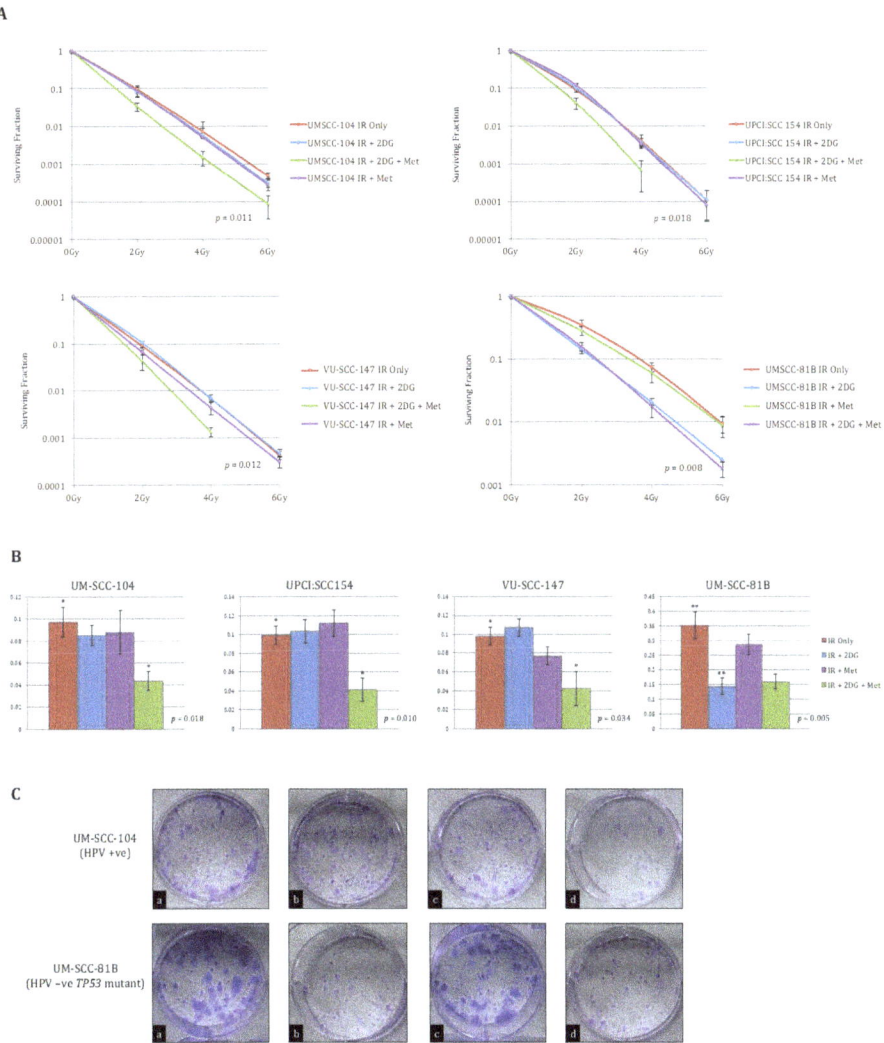

Figure 4. Clonogenic survival data for HPV-positive SCCHN cell lines and for comparison, a typical *TP53* mutant HPV-negative line (UM-SCC-81B). A stated in the methods, clonogenic assays were performed on the indicated SCCHN cell lines exposed to the indicated doses of IR. Cells were either left untreated or pre-treated with 25 mM 2-DG, 20 mM metformin (met), or combined treatment for one hour prior to irradiation. (**A**) displays clonogenic survival curves for each of the SCCHN cell lines and (**B**) the survival fractions at 2 Gy for each indicated treatment condition. Whilst 2-DG or metformin alone failed to have any significant effect on radiation response in any of the HPV-positive cell lines, the combination of 2-DG and metformin resulted in a significant reduction in clonogenic survival (in the case of the HPV-positive cell lines *p*-values represent the difference between the survival curves for the untreated condition and when combined pre-treatment with 2-DG and metformin was administered). In contrast, the addition of 2-DG alone consistently potentiated the effects of IR in UM-SCC-81B cells, while the addition of metformin has no discernible effect on clonogenic survival (the *p*-value in this case represents the difference between the survival curves for the untreated condition and when pre-treatment with 2-DG alone was administered). The results shown represent the mean values obtained from at least three separate experiments and error bars represent the SEMs. * $p < 0.05$, ** $p < 0.005$. (**C**) depicts representative example images of colony formation at 2 Gy for each treatment condition (a = IR alone; b = IR +2-DG; c = IR + 2-DG + Metformin; d = IR + Metformin) for the indicated cell lines.

4. Discussion

In recent years cancer cell metabolism has come to the forefront of cancer research because of increasing links between tumour metabolism and the causal changes determining the cancer phenotype (reviewed in [33]), yet has received relatively little attention in the context of SCCHN generally, and in particular with respect to HPV-positive disease. Renewed interest in this field in cancer research more generally has led to the development of new drugs and re-purposing of existing drugs that target cellular metabolism, which, when combined with standard therapies can offer a selective therapeutic gain (reviewed in [34]). However, the specific nature and extent of the metabolic perturbations can differ significantly between cancers, depending both on genotype and tissue of origin [12]. For instance, although aerobic glycolysis is the best-documented metabolic phenotype, glutaminolysis has been shown to predominate in cervical cancer and glioblastoma [35,36], while enhanced rather than reduced oxidative phosphorylation is a feature of both breast cancer [37] and chronic lymphocytic leukaemia [38], findings that highlight the importance of detailed study of metabolism in cancer site-specific experimental systems.

Until relatively recently metabolic studies in SCCHN were lacking, and for the most part had focused on isolated or limited transporter/enzyme expression, rather than characterising dynamic metabolic flux and presenting a clear picture of the metabolic phenotype (reviewed in [39]). More recent and comprehensive metabolic studies, undertaken in our laboratory and by the Myers' laboratory, have revealed *TP53* status as a determinant of the metabolic phenotype and therapeutic response in HPV-negative SCCHN [13,15]. These studies, which utilised a similar experimental platform to the present study, demonstrated that cells with compromised p53 function displayed a distinct metabolic phenotype to that retained by wild-type p53 cells. Specifically, wild-type p53 cells displayed robust spare mitochondrial respiratory capacity, while those with compromised p53 function, (regardless of whether this is due to *TP53* mutation or as a consequence of RNAi-mediated down-regulation of wild-type p53), displayed markedly reduced respiratory reserve, functioning near maximal capacity under basal conditions [13,15]. Importantly, this was associated with altered IR response following glycolytic inhibition with 2-DG, which potentiated IR effects in mutant and in cells with RNAi-mediated knock-down of p53 but not in wild-type *TP53* cells [13,15]. Furthermore, these results were reproducible in isogenic cell lines divergent on *TP53* functional status, corroborating a functional dependence on p53 [13,15].

Cognisant of this causal link between loss of p53 function and a less flexible "Warburg" metabolic phenotype, results from the present study are somewhat surprising. It is well documented that HPV, specifically via the viral E6 oncoprotein, inactivates p53 [40], and that as a result *TP53* mutations are highly unusual in HPV-driven tumours of the cervix and also oropharynx (2–3% of cases [16]). Since there is ample evidence that p53 function is compromised in HPV-driven tumours, we might expect that HPV-positive tumour cells would display a similarly inflexible metabolic profile to that observed in SCCHN cells with compromised p53 function. On the contrary, we have found that HPV-positive SCCHN cells display greater metabolic diversity than cells in which p53 function is compromised (either through genetic mutation or experimentally by RNAi), indeed comparable to that observed in p53 wild-type cells [15], and by extension require a combinatorial anti-metabolic approach targeting both mitochondrial respiration and glycolysis to be sensitised to the effects of IR. Although unexpected, these results are broadly consistent with the limited published data on metabolism in HPV-positive SCCHN. In a 2014 study examining metabolic protein expression, increased levels of proteins indicative of oxidative phosphorylation and lower levels of extracellular lactate accumulation were observed in both HPV-positive SCCHN resection specimens and an HPV-positive SCCHN cell line relative to HPV-negative SCCHN models [41]. Similarly, a more recent and robust analysis, including RNA sequencing, gene ontology analysis, and extracellular flux analysis, revealed increased expression of glycolytic genes and higher rates of glycolysis and glycolytic capacity in HPV-negative tumours and cell lines respectively, albeit on a background of a globally altered metabolic profile in HPV-negative disease (including elevated mitochondrial respiration) [42]. Unlike the present study, however, neither of these previous studies examined associated pharmacological manipulation specific to HPV-positive SCCHN.

A highly interesting implication of these data is the suggestion that HPV-positive SCCHN cells display evidence of only partial inhibition of p53. It may be the case that E6-mediated inactivation of p53 is incomplete, leaving sufficient functional wild-type p53 to maintain a balanced and diversified metabolic phenotype. If correct, this raises the intriguing prospect of distinguishing between functions of p53 that are sensitive to E6-mediated inactivation from those that are resistant to this. This could have significant implications for the future management of HPV-positive tumours insofar as treatment strategies may be targeted towards the residual p53 function that we have detected. Consistent with this, genome-wide microarray data from a recent study examining radiation response in HPV-positive and HPV-negative SCCHN cell lines suggested that low levels of wild-type p53 remain in HPV-positive cell lines, that this p53 can be activated by exogenous stress such as IR, and that this effect can be overcome by more complete knockdown of p53 using shRNA [43]. However, whilst our findings of p53 stabilisation and activation of p53 reporters in response to genotoxic stress in one HPV-positive SCCHN cell line (VU-SCC-147) are supportive of this notion, this was not observed convincingly in the other HPV-positive cell lines. Moreover, perhaps the most likely explanation for the observed protein levels relates to the fact that VU-SCC-147 cells harbour a *TP53* mutation leading to a substitution (L257R) [25], which also renders the mutant transcriptionally inactive for, inter alia, MDM2. p53 L257R would be expected to bind to MDM2 but fail to result in upregulation, leading to a potential failure of the auto-regulatory feedback loop. Additionally, specific mutations in the p53 DNA binding domain have been shown to inhibit E6 binding [44,45], and thus the L257R mutation might similarly lead to protein stabilisation, and may indicate another site in this region that alters binding, either indirectly or directly. Whilst this raises the possibility that naturally occurring p53 variants, related to single nucleotide polymorphisms (SNPs), may impact on E6 binding and subsequent p53 degradation, we suggest this is unlikely to be the case. If SNPs, such as the codon 73 Arg/Pro polymorphism, were responsible for differential binding to, and consequently inactivation of, p53, this would be expected to manifest as differential oncogenicity of HPV in individuals with different haplotypes, something for which no reliable association has been detected to date.

We acknowledge several limitations of the work presented here, principally related to the fact that experiments have been conducted exclusively using homotypic, monolayer cell culture of immortalised cell lines derived from SCCHN tumours. Although such cultured cancer cell lines are the most widely used model systems and have formed the basis for much of our current understanding of cancer biology, the clinical relevance of these models has been questioned [46]. One of the major concerns is that of clonal evolution, whereby cells adapt to the culture environment in vitro as they grow and may develop genetic and phenotypic differences from the original tumour [46]. Genetic and molecular cytogenetic data for SCCHN cells lines in culture, however, has shown a close resemblance to those in the primary tumours [22]. In addition, to counteract clonal evolution as best possible, our experiments were performed with cells at relatively early times after thawing from cryopreserved stocks. Nonetheless, to mitigate against this issue more definitively, future pre-clinical experiments could be conducted using short-term, fresh, primary cell cultures. Isolating and propagating such cell lines from HPV-positive SCCHN tumours, however, has proven notoriously difficult. Indeed, whilst there are now thousands of HPV-positive SCCHN and biopsy specimens available, there are only a handful of documented HPV-related SCCHN cell lines available worldwide and there is currently a scarcity of established cell lines with such characteristics, which raises an important question over the validity of the cell lines that do exist, and specifically those used in this study. Recent comprehensive characterisation of these cell lines, however, has revealed integrated and/or episomal viral DNA that is transcriptionally active providing convincing evidence of a persisting viral oncogenic driver [19,20]. However, until E6/7 manipulation of cells is accomplished there will not be a truly reliable link to HPV and functional studies, and this is part of on-going work by other researchers in our laboratory.

A further potential limitation of the work presented here relates to the specificity of the mechanisms of actions of the metabolic inhibitors used. 2-DG is a stable glucose analogue that is taken up by glucose transporters and phosphorylated. 2-DG, however, cannot be fully metabolised and 2-DG-6-phosphate accumulates in the cell and interferes with glycolysis by inhibiting the glycolytic enzymes phosphoglucose isomerase and hexokinase [30,31]. The general assumption, therefore, is that the biological effects of 2-DG are the consequence of this block in carbohydrate catabolism. This assumption, however, has been challenged and any observed effects of 2-DG may not be simply the result of a catabolic block [47]. Nonetheless, the specificity of 2-DG anti-glycolytic effects in suppressing cellular proliferation and anchorage-independent growth in SCCHN cell lines has been demonstrated previously, with effects reproduced under conditions of glucose deprivation [14]. Furthermore, differential sensitivity to halogenated 2-DG analogues consistent with their underlying chemical structure has been reported, and quantitative, broad-based analysis of changes in intracellular metabolite levels in response to 2-DG revealed time-dependent reductions in lactate production and levels of upstream glycolytic and tricarboxylic acid cycle intermediates [14]. Similarly, whilst metformin has well demonstrated activity against electron transport chain complex I [32], multiple other mechanisms of action have been identified including both AMPK-dependent and independent inhibition of mitochondrial respiration, altered fat metabolism, and direct inhibition of fructose-1,6-bisphosphatase [48].

It is widely acknowledged that there is a need for more selective and personalised therapeutic approaches in the wider field of cancer research, and currently much research effort is focused on this key strategy. Such molecularly targeted therapies, however, have as yet had limited translation into the treatment of SCCHN patients and it remains a major challenge to develop such treatments. Novel therapeutic approaches are generally predicated on a discernible therapeutic index of the chosen agent, either in isolation or in combination with other treatment regimes. In contrast to traditional cytotoxic agents, which largely rely on the inherently more incessant proliferative rate of cancer cells rather than true tumour cell specificity, metabolic targeting can exploit the fact that tumour cells become dependent on particular metabolic pathways, providing a selective therapeutic gain while sparing most normal cells. To this end, the findings presented here proffer the opportunity for a tailored anti-metabolic approach to the treatment of HPV-positive SCCHN, whereby these tumours can be sensitised to IR using a combinatorial anti-metabolic approach targeting both mitochondrial respiration and glycolysis. We believe this targeted radiosensitising approach is particularly attractive given the key role of IR as a treatment modality in HPV-positive disease, either as a primary treatment with or without concurrent chemotherapy or as an adjuvant treatment following surgery [49]. Furthermore, this may provide an attractive platform for treatment de-intensification in carefully selected cases by facilitating IR dose reduction to minimise the impact of treatment on long-term function in this ever-increasing patient group.

As alluded to previously, these findings will require further evaluation in the preclinical setting prior to translation into clinical practice but do provide rationale for initiating clinical trials. Although no previous clinical studies have been conducted using 2-DG in SCCHN patients, 2-DG in combination with IR has been evaluated more extensively in patients with cerebral gliomas and has been well tolerated with a relatively minor, predictable, and reversible side-effect profile akin to that of hypoglycaemia (reviewed in [50]). Therefore, this data could be extrapolated to inform dosing schedules and safety profiles in SCCHN patients, potentially obviating the need for phase I/II trials before proceeding to phase II/III trials. Similarly, metformin is commonly used in clinical practice as a first line of treatment for type II diabetes with minimal toxicity. Although more specific mitochondrial inhibitors, such as rotenone and cyanide, are available, their associated toxicity makes them unlikely therapeutic options. Indeed, there has been an ever-increasing interest in re-purposing metformin as a therapeutic agent in the context of cancer treatment [51], an interest which stems from several epidemiological studies demonstrating a lower cancer incidence in diabetic patients taking metformin than in the general diabetic population [52], and retrospective data indicating that metformin users have higher rates of disease control when treated with neoadjuvant chemotherapy for breast cancer [53].

Supplementary Materials: The following are available online at https://www.mdpi.com/article/10.3390/cancers13194836/s1, Figure S1: FCCP dose titration for UM-SCC-81B to ensure the reduced mitochondrial reserve was not related to suboptimal FCCP dosing, Figure S2: Original western blots.

Author Contributions: M.D.W.—study conception, design and execution of experiments, data analysis, and writing of manuscript. E.A.A.—design and execution of experiments, and critical revisions to manuscript. A.S.L.—design and execution of experiments, and critical revisions to manuscript. C.P.R.—data analysis, and critical revisions to manuscript. N.V.—study conception, design of experiments, and critical revisions to manuscript. T.M.J.—study conception, design of experiments, and critical revisions to manuscript. M.T.B.—study conception, design of experiments, and critical revisions to manuscript. All authors have read and agreed to the published version of the manuscript.

Funding: This work was funded by Cancer Research UK (PhD Studentship support for MDW); the Royal College of Surgeons of England; the University of Liverpool Northwest Cancer Research Centre; and the Isle of Man Anti-Cancer Association.

Institutional Review Board Statement: Not applicable.

Informed Consent Statement: Not applicable.

Data Availability Statement: As there are no relevant publicly available data repositories for this work any data is available upon request from the authors.

Acknowledgments: These studies would not have been possible without the generous provision of cell lines by Thomas Carey at the University of Michigan and S. Gollin at the University of Pittsburgh. At the University of Liverpool, we thank Andy Birss and Lakis Liloglou for confirming cell line identification by STR profiling, and Robert Sutton and Jane Armstrong for providing expert assistance with the Seahorse XF24 analyser.

Conflicts of Interest: The authors declare no conflict of interest.

References

1. Ferlay, J.S.I.; Ervik, M.; Dikshit, R.; Eser, S.; Mathers, C.; Rebelo, M.; Parkin, D.M.; Forman, D.; Bray, F. GLOBOCAN 2012 v1.0, Cancer Incidence and Mortality Worldwide. Available online: http://globocan.iarc.fr (accessed on 1 February 2021).
2. Lewin, F.; Norell, S.E.; Johansson, H.; Gustavsson, P.; Wennerberg, J.; Biörklund, A.; Rutqvist, L.E. Smoking tobacco, oral snuff, and alcohol in the etiology of squamous cell carcinoma of the head and neck: A population-based case-referent study in Sweden. *Cancer* **1998**, *82*, 1367–1375. [CrossRef]
3. IARC Working Group on the Evaluation of Carcinogenic Risks to Humans. Human papillomaviruses. In *IARC Monographs on the Evaluation of Carcinogenic Risks to Humans*; IARC (International Agency for Research on Cancer): Lyon, France, 2007; Volume 90, pp. 1–670.
4. National Cancer Institute. Surveillance Epidemiology and End Results. Available online: http://seer.cancer.gov/faststats/selections.php-Output (accessed on 1 February 2021).
5. National Cancer Institute Network. Profile of Head and Neck Cancers. Available online: http://library.ncin.org.uk/docs/100504-OCIUHead_and_Neck_Profi-les.pdf (accessed on 1 February 2021).
6. Ramqvist, T.; Dalianis, T. An epidemic of oropharyngeal squamous cell carcinoma (OSCC) due to human papillomavirus (HPV) infection and aspects of treatment and prevention. *Anticancer Res.* **2011**, *31*, 1515–1519.
7. Mehanna, H.; Beech, T.; Nicholson, T.; El-Hariry, I.; McConkey, C.; Paleri, V.; Roberts, S. Prevalence of human papillomavirus in oropharyngeal and nonoropharyngeal head and neck cancer–systematic review and meta-analysis of trends by time and region. *Head Neck* **2013**, *35*, 747–755. [CrossRef] [PubMed]
8. Ang, K.K.; Harris, J.; Wheeler, R.; Weber, R.; Rosenthal, D.I.; Nguyen-Tân, P.F.; Westra, W.H.; Chung, C.H.; Jordan, R.C.; Lu, C.; et al. Human papillomavirus and survival of patients with oropharyngeal cancer. *N. Engl. J. Med.* **2010**, *363*, 24–35. [CrossRef] [PubMed]
9. Licitra, L.; Perrone, F.; Bossi, P.; Suardi, S.; Mariani, L.; Artusi, R.; Oggionni, M.; Rossini, C.; Cantù, G.; Squadrelli, M.; et al. High-risk human papillomavirus affects prognosis in patients with surgically treated oropharyngeal squamous cell carcinoma. *J. Clin. Oncol. Off. J. Am. Soc. Clin. Oncol. J. Clin. Oncol.* **2006**, *24*, 5630–5636. [CrossRef]

10. Mehanna, H.; Olaleye, O.; Licitra, L. Oropharyngeal cancer—Is it time to change management according to human papilloma virus status? *Curr. Opin. Otolaryngol. Head Neck Surg.* **2012**, *20*, 120–124. [CrossRef]
11. Hanahan, D.; Weinberg, R.A. Hallmarks of cancer: The next generation. *Cell* **2011**, *144*, 646–674. [CrossRef]
12. Yuneva, M.O.; Fan, T.W.M.; Allen, T.D.; Higashi, R.M.; Ferraris, D.V.; Tsukamoto, T.; Matés, J.M.; Alonso, F.J.; Wang, C.; Seo, Y.; et al. The metabolic profile of tumors depends on both the responsible genetic lesion and tissue type. *Cell Metab.* **2012**, *15*, 157–170. [CrossRef] [PubMed]
13. Sandulache, V.C.; Skinner, H.D.; Ow, T.J.; Zhang, A.; Xia, X.; Luchak, J.M.; Wong, L.C.; Pickering, C.R.; Zhou, G.; Myers, J.N. Individualizing antimetabolic treatment strategies for head and neck squamous cell carcinoma based on TP53 mutational status. *Cancer* **2012**, *118*, 711–721. [CrossRef] [PubMed]
14. Sandulache, V.C.; Ow, T.J.; Pickering, C.R.; Frederick, M.J.; Zhou, G.; Fokt, I.; Davis-Malesevich, M.; Priebe, W.; Myers, J.N. Glucose, not glutamine, is the dominant energy source required for proliferation and survival of head and neck squamous carcinoma cells. *Cancer* **2011**, *117*, 2926–2938. [CrossRef]
15. Wilkie, M.D.; Anaam, E.A.; Lau, A.S.; Rubbi, C.P.; Jones, T.M.; Boyd, M.T.; Vlatković, N. TP53 mutations in head and neck cancer cells determine the Warburg phenotypic switch creating metabolic vulnerabilities and therapeutic opportunities for stratified therapies. *Cancer Lett.* **2020**, *478*, 107–121. [CrossRef]
16. Cancer Genome Atlas Network. Comprehensive genomic characterization of head and neck squamous cell carcinomas. *Nature* **2015**, *517*, 576–582. [CrossRef] [PubMed]
17. Miller, D.L.; Puricelli, M.D.; Stack, M.S. Virology and molecular pathogenesis of HPV (human papillomavirus)-associated oropharyngeal squamous cell carcinoma. *Biochem. J.* **2012**, *443*, 339–353. [CrossRef] [PubMed]
18. Scheffner, M.; Werness, B.A.; Huibregtse, J.M.; Levine, A.J.; Howley, P.M. The E6 oncoprotein encoded by human papillomavirus types 16 and 18 promotes the degradation of p53. *Cell* **1990**, *63*, 1129–1136. [CrossRef]
19. Olthof, N.C.; Huebbers, C.U.; Kolligs, J.; Henfling, M.; Ramaekers, F.C.S.; Cornet, I.; van Lent-Albrechts, J.A.; Stegmann, A.P.A.; Silling, S.; Wieland, U.; et al. Viral load, gene expression and mapping of viral integration sites in HPV16-associated HNSCC cell lines. *Int. J. Cancer* **2015**, *136*, E207–E218. [CrossRef]
20. Greaney-Davies, F.S.T.; Risk, J.M.; Robinson, M.; Liloglou, T.; Shaw, R.J.; Schache, A.G. Essential characterisation of human papillomavirus positive head and neck cancer cell lines. *Oral. Oncol.* **2020**, *103*, 104613. [CrossRef]
21. Bradford, C.R.; Zhu, S.; Ogawa, H.; Ogawa, T.; Ubell, M.; Narayan, A.; Johnson, G.; Wolf, G.T.; Fisher, S.G.; Carey, T.E. p53 mutation correlates with cisplatin sensitivity in head and neck squamous cell carcinoma lines. *Head Neck* **2003**, *25*, 654–661. [CrossRef]
22. Lin, C.J.; Grandis, J.R.; Carey, T.E.; Gollin, S.M.; Whiteside, T.L.; Koch, W.M.; Ferris, R.L.; Lai, S.Y. Head and neck squamous cell carcinoma cell lines: Established models and rationale for selection. *Head Neck* **2007**, *29*, 163–188. [CrossRef]
23. Tang, A.L.; Hauff, S.J.; Owen, J.H.; Graham, M.P.; Czerwinski, M.J.; Je Park, J.; Walline, H.; Papagerakis, S.; Stoerker, J.; McHugh, J.B.; et al. UM-SCC-104: A new human papillomavirus-16-positive cancer stem cell-containing head and neck squamous cell carcinoma cell line. *Head Neck* **2012**, *34*, 1480–1491. [CrossRef]
24. White, J.S.; Weissfeld, J.L.; Ragin, C.C.R.; Rossie, K.M.; Martin, C.L.; Shuster, M.; Ishwad, C.S.; Law, J.C.; Myers, E.N.; Johnson, J.T.; et al. The influence of clinical and demographic risk factors on the establishment of head and neck squamous cell carcinoma cell lines. *Oral. Oncol.* **2007**, *43*, 701–712. [CrossRef] [PubMed]
25. Steenbergen, R.D.; Hermsen, M.A.; Walboomers, J.M.; Joenje, H.; Arwert, F.; Meijer, C.J.; Snijders, P.J. Integrated human papillomavirus type 16 and loss of heterozygosity at 11q22 and 18q21 in an oral carcinoma and its derivative cell line. *Cancer Res.* **1995**, *55*, 5465–5471.
26. Brady, M.; Vlatkovic, N.; Boyd, M.T. Regulation of p53 and MDM2 activity by MTBP. *Mol. Cell. Biol.* **2005**, *25*, 545–553. [CrossRef]
27. Franken, N.A.; Rodermond, H.M.; Stap, J.; Haveman, J.; van Bree, C. Clonogenic assay of cells in vitro. *Nat. Protoc.* **2006**, *1*, 2315–2319. [CrossRef]
28. Nair, T.S.; Thomas, T.B.; Yang, L.; Kakaraparthi, B.N.; Morris, A.C.; Clark, A.M.; Campredon, L.P.; Brouwer, A.F.; Eisenberg, M.C.; Meza, R.; et al. Characteristics of head and neck squamous cell carcinoma cell Lines reflect human tumor biology independent of primary etiologies and HPV status. *Transl. Oncol.* **2020**, *13*, 100808. [CrossRef]
29. Bullenkamp, J.; Raulf, N.; Ayaz, B.; Walczak, H.; Kulms, D.; Odell, E.; Thavaraj, S.; Tavassoli, M. Bortezomib sensitises TRAIL-resistant HPV-positive head and neck cancer cells to TRAIL through a caspase-dependent, E6-independent mechanism. *Cell Death Dis.* **2014**, *5*, e1489. [CrossRef] [PubMed]
30. Wick, A.N.; Drury, D.R.; Nakada, H.I.; Wolfe, J.B. Localization of the primary metabolic block produced by 2-deoxyglucose. *J. Biol. Chem.* **1957**, *224*, 963–969. [CrossRef]
31. Chen, W.; Gueron, M. The inhibition of bovine heart hexokinase by 2-deoxy-D-glucose-6-phosphate: Characterization by 31P NMR and metabolic implications. *Biochimie* **1992**, *74*, 867–873. [CrossRef]
32. El-Mir, M.Y.; Nogueira, V.; Fontaine, E.; Avéret, N.; Rigoulet, M.; Leverve, X. Dimethylbiguanide inhibits cell respiration via an indirect effect targeted on the respiratory chain complex I. *J. Biol. Chem.* **2000**, *275*, 223–228. [CrossRef] [PubMed]
33. Levine, A.J.; Puzio-Kuter, A.M. The control of the metabolic switch in cancers by oncogenes and tumor suppressor genes. *Science* **2010**, *330*, 1340–1344. [CrossRef]
34. Galluzzi, L.; Kepp, O.; Vander Heiden, M.G.; Kroemer, G. Metabolic targets for cancer therapy. *Nat. Rev. Drug Discov.* **2013**, *12*, 829–846. [CrossRef]

35. De Berardinis, R.J.; Mancuso, A.; Daikhin, E.; Nissim, I.; Yudkoff, M.; Wehrli, S.; Thompson, C.B. Beyond aerobic glycolysis: Transformed cells can engage in glutamine metabolism that exceeds the requirement for protein and nucleotide synthesis. *Proc. Natl. Acad. Sci. USA* **2007**, *104*, 19345–19350. [CrossRef] [PubMed]
36. Reitzer, L.J.; Wice, B.M.; Kennell, D. Evidence that glutamine, not sugar, is the major energy source for cultured HeLa cells. *J. Biol. Chem.* **1979**, *254*, 2669–2676. [CrossRef]
37. Bonuccelli, G.; Tsirigos, A.; Whitaker-Menezes, D.; Pavlides, S.; Pestell, R.G.; Chiavarina, B.; Frank, P.G.; Flomenberg, N.; Howell, A.; Martinez-Outschoorn, U.E.; et al. Ketones and lactate "fuel" tumor growth and metastasis: Evidence that epithelial cancer cells use oxidative mitochondrial metabolism. *Cell Cycle* **2010**, *9*, 3506–3514. [CrossRef] [PubMed]
38. Jitschin, R.; Hofmann, A.D.; Bruns, H.; Giessl, A.; Bricks, J.; Berger, J.; Saul, D.; Eckart, M.J.; Mackensen, A.; Mougiakakos, D. Mitochondrial metabolism contributes to oxidative stress and reveals therapeutic targets in chronic lymphocytic leukemia. *Blood* **2014**, *123*, 2663–2672. [CrossRef] [PubMed]
39. Wilkie, M.D.; Lau, A.S.; Vlatkovic, N.; Jones, T.M.; Boyd, M.T. Metabolic signature of squamous cell carcinoma of the head and neck: Consequences of *TP53* mutation and therapeutic perspectives. *Oral. Oncol.* **2018**, *83*, 1–10. [CrossRef] [PubMed]
40. Huibregtse, J.M.; Scheffner, M.; Howley, P.M. A cellular protein mediates association of p53 with the E6 oncoprotein of human papillomavirus types 16 or 18. *EMBO J.* **1991**, *10*, 4129–4135. [CrossRef]
41. Krupar, R.; Robold, K.; Gaag, D.; Spanier, G.; Kreutz, M.; Renner, K.; Hellerbrand, C.; Hofstaedter, F.; Bosserhoff, A.K. Immunologic and metabolic characteristics of HPV-negative and HPV-positive head and neck squamous cell carcinomas are strikingly different. *Virchows Arch.* **2014**, *465*, 299–312. [CrossRef] [PubMed]
42. Fleming, J.C.; Woo, J.; Moutasim, K.; Mellone, M.; Frampton, S.J.; Mead, A.; Ahmed, W.; Wood, O.; Robinson, H.; Ward, M.; et al. HPV, tumour metabolism and novel target identification in head and neck squamous cell carcinoma. *Br. J. Cancer* **2019**, *120*, 356–367. [CrossRef]
43. Kimple, R.J.; Smith, M.A.; Blitzer, G.C.; Torres, A.D.; Martin, J.A.; Yang, R.Z.; Peet, C.R.; Lorenz, L.D.; Nickel, K.P.; Klingelhutz, A.J.; et al. Enhanced radiation sensitivity in HPV-positive head and neck cancer. *Cancer Res.* **2013**, *73*, 4791–4800. [CrossRef]
44. Bernard, X.; Robinson, P.; Nomine, Y.; Masson, M.; Charbonnier, S.; Ramirez-Ramos, J.R.; Deryckere, F.; Trave, G.; Orfanoudakis, G. Proteasomal Degradation of p53 by Human Papillomavirus E6 Oncoprotein Relies on the Structural Integrity of p53 Core Domain. *PLoS ONE* **2011**, *6*, e25981. [CrossRef]
45. Martinez-Zapien, D.; Ruiz, F.X.; Poirson, J.; Mitschler, A.; Ramirez, J.; Forster, A.; Cousido-Siah, A.; Masson, M.; Pol, S.V.; Podjarny, A.; et al. Structure of the E6/E6AP/p53 complex required for HPV-mediated degradation of p53. *Nature* **2016**, *529*, 541–545. [CrossRef]
46. Gillet, J.P.; Varma, S.; Gottesman, M.M. The clinical relevance of cancer cell lines. *J. Natl. Cancer Inst.* **2013**, *105*, 452–458. [CrossRef] [PubMed]
47. Ralser, M.; Wamelink, M.M.; Struys, E.A.; Joppich, C.; Krobitsch, S.; Jakobs, C.; Lehrach, H. A catabolic block does not sufficiently explain how 2-deoxy-D-glucose inhibits cell growth. *Proc. Natl. Acad. Sci. USA* **2008**, *105*, 17807–17811. [CrossRef] [PubMed]
48. Rena, G.; Hardie, D.G.; Pearson, E.R. The mechanisms of action of metformin. *Diabetologia* **2017**, *60*, 1577–1585. [CrossRef]
49. Mehanna, H.; Evans, M.; Beasley, M.; Chatterjee, S.; Dilkes, M.; Homer, J.; O'Hara, J.; Robinson, M.; Shaw, R.; Sloan, P. Oropharyngeal cancer: United Kingdom National Multidisciplinary Guidelines. *J. Laryngol. Otol.* **2016**, *130*, S90–S96. [CrossRef] [PubMed]
50. Dwarakanath, B.S.; Singh, D.; Banerji, A.K.; Sarin, R.; Venkataramana, N.K.; Jalali, R.; Vishwanath, P.N.; Mohanti, B.K.; Tripathi, R.P.; Kalia, V.K.; et al. Clinical studies for improving radiotherapy with 2-deoxy-D-glucose: Present status and future prospects. *J. Cancer Res. Ther.* **2009**, *5* (Suppl. 1), S21–S26. [CrossRef]
51. Pollak, M.N. Investigating metformin for cancer prevention and treatment: The end of the beginning. *Cancer Discov.* **2012**, *2*, 778–790. [CrossRef]
52. Noto, H.; Goto, A.; Tsujimoto, T.; Noda, M. Cancer risk in diabetic patients treated with metformin: A systematic review and meta-analysis. *PLoS ONE* **2012**, *7*, e33411. [CrossRef]
53. Jiralerspong, S.; Palla, S.L.; Giordano, S.H.; Meric-Bernstam, F.; Liedtke, C.; Barnett, C.M.; Hsu, L.; Hung, M.C.; Hortobagyi, G.N.; Gonzalez-Angulo, A.M. Metformin and pathologic complete responses to neoadjuvant chemotherapy in diabetic patients with breast cancer. *J. Clin. Oncol. Off. J. Am. Soc. Clin. Oncol.* **2009**, *27*, 3297–3302. [CrossRef]

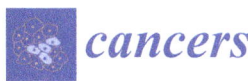

Article

Application of Community Detection Algorithm to Investigate the Correlation between Imaging Biomarkers of Tumor Metabolism, Hypoxia, Cellularity, and Perfusion for Precision Radiotherapy in Head and Neck Squamous Cell Carcinomas

Ramesh Paudyal [1,†], Milan Grkovski [1,†], Jung Hun Oh [1], Heiko Schöder [2], David Aramburu Nunez [1], Vaios Hatzoglou [2], Joseph O. Deasy [1], John L. Humm [1], Nancy Y. Lee [3,‡] and Amita Shukla-Dave [1,2,*,‡]

[1] Department of Medical Physics, Memorial Sloan Kettering Cancer Center, New York, NY 10065, USA; paudyalr@mskcc.org (R.P.); grkovskm@mskcc.org (M.G.); OhJ@mskcc.org (J.H.O.); aramburd@mskcc.org (D.A.N.); DeasyJ@mskcc.org (J.O.D.); hummj@mskcc.org (J.L.H.)
[2] Department of Radiology, Memorial Sloan Kettering Cancer Center, New York, NY 10065, USA; schoderh@mskcc.org (H.S.); HatzoglV@mskcc.org (V.H.)
[3] Department of Radiation Oncology, Memorial Sloan Kettering Cancer Center, New York, NY 10065, USA; leen2@mskcc.org
* Correspondence: davea@mskcc.org; Tel.: +1-212-639-3184
† Contributed equally to this study as co-first authors.
‡ Contributed equally to this study as co-senior authors.

Citation: Paudyal, R.; Grkovski, M.; Oh, J.H.; Schöder, H.; Nunez, D.A.; Hatzoglou, V.; Deasy, J.O.; Humm, J.L.; Lee, N.Y.; Shukla-Dave, A. Application of Community Detection Algorithm to Investigate the Correlation between Imaging Biomarkers of Tumor Metabolism, Hypoxia, Cellularity, and Perfusion for Precision Radiotherapy in Head and Neck Squamous Cell Carcinomas. Cancers 2021, 13, 3908. https://doi.org/10.3390/cancers13153908

Academic Editor: Heather Walline

Received: 29 May 2021
Accepted: 30 July 2021
Published: 3 August 2021

Publisher's Note: MDPI stays neutral with regard to jurisdictional claims in published maps and institutional affiliations.

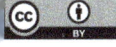

Copyright: © 2021 by the authors. Licensee MDPI, Basel, Switzerland. This article is an open access article distributed under the terms and conditions of the Creative Commons Attribution (CC BY) license (https://creativecommons.org/licenses/by/4.0/).

Simple Summary: Integration of multimodality imaging (MMI) methods in head and neck squamous cell carcinomas (HNSCC) provides complementary information of the tumor and its microenvironment. Quantitative positron emission tomography (PET)/computed tomography (CT), DW- and DCE-MRI provide the functional information of tumor tissue based on metabolic process, diffusion of water molecules, and enhancement of water proton relaxation with a contrast agent, respectively. The present study aimed to investigate correlations at pre-treatment between quantitative imaging metrics derived from FDG-PET/CT(SUL), FMISO-PET/CT (K_1, k_3, TBR, and DV), DW-MRI (ADC, IVIM [D, D*, and f]), and FXR DCE-MRI [K^{trans}, v_e, and τ_i]) using a community detection algorithm (CDA) based on the "spin-glass model" and Spearman rank analysis in patients with HNSCC. Correlations between MMI-derived quantitative metrics evaluated using a CDA in addition to the Spearman analysis in a larger population may enable the identification of potential biomarkers for prognostication and management of patients with HNSCC.

Abstract: The present study aimed to investigate the correlation at pre-treatment (TX) between quantitative metrics derived from multimodality imaging (MMI), including ^{18}F-FDG-PET/CT, ^{18}F-FMISO-PET/CT, DW- and DCE-MRI, using a community detection algorithm (CDA) in head and neck squamous cell carcinoma (HNSCC) patients. Twenty-three HNSCC patients with 27 metastatic lymph nodes underwent a total of 69 MMI exams at pre-TX. Correlations among quantitative metrics derived from FDG-PET/CT (SUL), FMISO-PET/CT (K_1, k_3, TBR, and DV), DW-MRI (ADC, IVIM [D, D*, and f]), and FXR DCE-MRI [K^{trans}, v_e, and τ_i]) were investigated using the CDA based on a "spin-glass model" coupled with the Spearman's rank, ρ, analysis. Mean MRI T_2 weighted tumor volumes and SUL_{mean} values were moderately positively correlated (ρ = 0.48, p = 0.01). ADC and D exhibited a moderate negative correlation with SUL_{mean} (ρ ≤ −0.42, p < 0.03 for both). K_1 and K^{trans} were positively correlated (ρ = 0.48, p = 0.01). In contrast, K^{trans} and k_{3max} were negatively correlated (ρ = −0.41, p = 0.03). CDA revealed four communities for 16 metrics interconnected with 33 edges in the network. DV, K^{trans}, and K_1 had 8, 7, and 6 edges in the network, respectively. After validation in a larger population, the CDA approach may aid in identifying useful biomarkers for developing individual patient care in HNSCC.

Keywords: positron emission tomography; diffusion-weighted; dynamic contrast-enhanced; kinetic modeling; fast exchange regime model; community detection algorithm; spin-glass model

1. Introduction

Head and neck squamous cell carcinoma (HNSCC) is a complex disease with remarkable intratumoral heterogeneity resulting in different treatment responses and outcomes [1]. HNSCC arises from the mucosa lining of the aerodigestive tract, including the oropharyngeal axis. Human papillomavirus (HPV)-related oropharyngeal cancers (OPCs) have molecular features and etiology distinct from those of smoking- and alcohol-related HNSCC [2,3]. Both qualitative and quantitative imaging, including computed tomography (CT), T_1-weighted and T_2-weighted magnetic resonance imaging (MRI), positron emission tomography (PET)/CT, diffusion-weighted (DW-), and dynamic contrast-enhanced (DCE)-MRI, have shown potential in staging, predicting treatment (TX) response, and post-TX follow-up of patients with HNSCC [4–8].

Quantitative analysis of multimodality imaging (MMI), including ^{18}F-Fluorodeoxyglucose (FDG) PET/CT, ^{18}F-Fluoromisonidazole (FMISO) PET/CT, DW- and DCE-MRI, data provide imaging metrics, reflecting the tumor metabolism, hypoxia, cellularity, and vessel permeability in HNSCC [6,9–12]. Therefore, the measurement of MMI-derived quantitative imaging (QI) metrics at pre-TX is vital for evaluating and planning precision radiotherapy in HNSCC. The standardized uptake value (SUV) from ^{18}F-FDG-PET/CT assesses the changes in glucose uptake as a measure of response to radiotherapy (RT) [13]. Pharmacokinetic modeling of FMISO yields a metric, a biomarker of cell oxygenation (hypoxia), reflecting malignant tissue radiosensitivity [14]. Previous studies have reported that pre-TX ^{18}F-FMISO-PET/CT could aid in predicting RT outcome and survival prognosis in HNSCC [9,15]. Riaz et al. recently demonstrated that dose de-escalation of radiotherapy to 30 Gy based on intra-treatment hypoxia using imaging response utilizing ^{18}F-FMISO-PET/CT was feasible, safe, and associated with minimal toxicity [16].

The measurement of diffusion of water molecules in malignant tissue can reveal abnormalities of the tissue cellular organization and microstructure [17]. The ADC derived from monoexponential modeling of diffusion-weighted (DW) signal data with at least two b-values, a surrogate marker of tumor cellularity, has shown promise in predicting and detecting early response to chemo-RT HNSCC in metastatic lymph nodes (LNs) [18,19]. Quantitative imaging (QI) metrics derived from the intravoxel incoherent motion (IVIM) model [20] without contrast agent (CA), including perfusion fraction (f) and true diffusion coefficient (D), exhibited potential markers for early prediction of chemo-RT response in HNSCC patients [21–23]. Paudyal et al. further reported subtypes within human papillomavirus-positive (HVP+) patients with HNSCC treated with 70 Gy chemo-RT. This finding raises the question of whether every individual should be treated with the same dose of radiation [23].

DCE-MRI pharmacokinetics modeling estimates perfusion/permeability and volume fractions of the CA distribution spaces based on the changes in the time course of signal intensity from target tissue after a bolus administration of CA [24]. The post-TX DCE-MRI showed potential for identifying residual masses, both in primary tumors and in metastatic LNs, that had failed [25]. The extended Tofts model [24], assuming an infinitesimally fast water exchange kinetics between the tissue compartments, derived volume transfer constant (K^{trans}), extravascular extracellular volume fraction [EES] (v_e), and plasma volume fraction (v_p) from primary tumors and metastatic LNs have shown promise in differentiating responders from non-responders [26]. Shukla-Dave et al. reported that the skewness of pre-TX K^{trans} values was the strongest predictor of progression-free survival and overall survival in Stage IV HNSCC patients with the nodal disease [27]. Kim et al. implemented the fast exchange (FXR) model, accounting for the finite rate of transcytolemmal water exchange, and reported that the pre-TX K^{trans} exhibited a potential to predict metastatic

LNs treatment response to chemo-RT in HNSCC cancer patients [28]. The poor pre-TX tumor perfusion may be a common mechanism associated with radioresistance and the development of the distant metastatic phenotype [29]. Recent preclinical and clinical studies suggested that the FXR model-derived intracellular water molecule's mean lifetime (τ_i) can be a surrogate marker of tumor cell metabolic activity [30,31]. Chawla et al. reported that the metric τ_i could be a prognostic marker in HNSCC patients [32].

Previous studies explored the correlation between metastatic LN tumor volume and ^{18}F-FDG-PET/CT and ^{18}F-FMISO-PET/CT derived QI metrics [15,33,34]. The correlations between ADC and ^{18}F-FDG SUV results were inconsistent in HNSCC [33–35]. The mean K^{trans} and SUV_{max} showed a trend towards a significant positive correlation in 28 primary tumors of HNSCC [11]. Jansen reported significantly lower median K^{trans} and the rate constant of CA from the EES back into the plasma space, k_{ep}, values in hypoxic than in non-hypoxic nodes in HNSCC [36]. Wiedenmann demonstrated that the multiple parameters' values differ significantly between hypoxic and non-hypoxic tumor regions, defined on FMISO-PET/CT in HNSCC [37].

A Spearman correlation analysis between MMI-derived QI metrics measures the strength of a monotonic relationship. Still, it does not explicitly show how and to what extent these metrics are interconnected within a group. These QI metrics can be represented as a network in which nodes (metrics) with similar characteristics are clustered to form sub-networks (communities) [38]. Herein, the community detection algorithm (CDA) based on a "spin-glass model" was employed to create a community for MMI-derived metrics [39]. In the network, nodes within the same groups are densely coupled. In contrast, nodes between the group's nodes are sparsely connected, indicating the CDA approach can be helpful to identify the cancer biomarkers for understanding solid tumor biology. To our knowledge, this is the first study that introduces a CDA-based "spin-glass model" approach in patients with HNSCC.

Despite the significant advances in MMI methods, identifying useful QI metrics that can assess the effectiveness of RT response in patients with HNSCC is still a challenging task. We hypothesize that the CDA approach could help identify robust biomarkers in developing cutting-edge strategies for precision therapy in HNSCC patients. The present study aimed to investigate correlations between QI metrics derived from MMI methods using a CDA based on the "spin-glass model" in HNSCC patients.

2. Materials and Methods

2.1. Patient Selection

Our institutional review board approved this prospective study compliant with the Health Insurance Portability and Accountability Act. We obtained written informed consent from all eligible patients who had a biopsy-proven, newly diagnosed HN cancer; diagnostic biopsies were tested for human papillomavirus (HPV) status before the CT and MRI study. Patients with previous chemotherapy or radiation therapy planned for upfront surgery and other primaries than HNSCC were excluded from the study. Between December 2013 and November 2015, a total of twenty-three (N = 23) HPV (21 HPV positive [+] and 2 HPV negative [−]) HN cancer patients (median age = 58 years, range = 45–82 years; Male/Female = 21/2) enrolled in the study and underwent a total of 69 pre-TX examinations, including ^{18}F-FDG-PET/CT (N = 23), ^{18}F-FMISO dynamic PET/CT (N = 23), and MRI (combined DW- and DCE-MRI; N = 23). Of the 23 patients included with HNSCC, 15 patients had tumor sites in the base of the tongue, seven patients with tumors in a tonsil, one patient had an unknown primary tumor site, and four patients had bilateral metastatic LNs. The patients were categorized according to the American Joint Committee on Cancer (AJCC) tumor, node, metastasis (TNM) system. The majority of patients had T2 (65%), N2 nodal mass was found in all 23 patients, and none had M0. Patients were treated with concurrent chemotherapy and radiotherapy (70 Gy).

2.2. PET Data Acquisition

Baseline FDG-PET scans on HNSCC patients were performed for radiotherapy planning purposes.

Patients were positioned on a flat-top couch wearing a customized radiotherapy treatment immobilization mask, which allows for accurate repositioning. The same immobilization mask was subsequently used for FMISO dynamic PET scans as detailed elsewhere [10,40]. Patients were administered an intravenous bolus injection of 390 ± 16 MBq of FMISO. Approximately 300–450MBq of FDG was administered after a fasting period of ≥6 h through intravenous lines inserted in antecubital veins. The PET acquisition commenced at 70–80 min post-injection on the General Electric Discovery ST scanner (GE Health Care Inc., Chicago, IL, USA) with an imaging time of 5 min per bed position. The corresponding x-ray computed tomography (CT) images were acquired immediately prior to commencement of the PET scan and with the following settings: 140 kVp, 250 mAs, and 3.8-mm slice thickness. Each FMISO dynamic PET acquisition consisted of 3 segments: (i) at time t = 0, a 30 min dynamic acquisition binned into 6 × 5-sec, 3 × 10-sec, 4 × 60-sec, 2 × 150-sec, 2 × 300-sec, and 1 × 600-sec frames; (ii) a 10 min static acquisition, starting at ~90 min, and; (iii) a 10 min static acquisition starting at ~160 min post-injection. Between scans, patients rested in quiet waiting rooms.

2.3. PET/CT Data Analysis

All PET data were corrected for attenuation, scatter, and random events, and were iteratively reconstructed into a 256 × 256 × 47 matrix (voxel dimensions: 1.95 × 1.95 × 3.27 mm^3) using the ordered subset expectation maximization algorithm provided by the manufacturer. ^{18}F-FDG-PET and three ^{18}F-FMISO-PET scans were spatially co-registered using the rigid-body transformation calculated with the General Co-Registration TM tool applied to their corresponding CT scans (Advantage Workstation v4.7; GE Healthcare, Chicago, IL, USA). Lesions were segmented using the adaptive threshold algorithm in PET VCAR^{TM} (Advantage Workstation 4.7; GE Healthcare, Chicago, IL, USA) semi-automated software based on the companion CT as a fiduciary marker and a count-based edge recognition algorithm.

FDG uptake was calculated as the standard uptake value (SUV) corrected by lean body mass (SUL). SUV normalized by total body weight overestimates metabolic activity in all patients. Thus, the SUL is recommended for more accurate SUV results for quantitative assessment of clinical PET [20]. Tumor lesions were delineated on the FDG PET/CT images, using the adaptive threshold algorithm in the PET VCAR^{TM} (Volume Computer-Assisted Reading; General Electric Advantage Workstation v4.7) semi-automated software, based on the companion CT as a fiduciary marker and a count-based edge recognition algorithm. The resulting segmented lesson was used to calculate the metastatic LN volumes (V_{t-PET}) for PET/CT [41]. Pharmacokinetic modeling of FMISO dynamic PET data was conducted in PMOD v3.604 (PMOD Software, RRID: SCR_016547) as reported previously [10,40]. Briefly, an irreversible one-plasma two-tissue compartment model with a blood volume component was utilized to calculate surrogate biomarkers of tumor hypoxia (k_3, tumor-to-blood ratio [TBR]), perfusion (K_1), and total ^{18}F-FMISO distribution volume (DV), i.e., the overall concentration of unbound FMISO relative to blood. Image-based input function (IF) was derived from the dynamic FMISO-PET images by segmenting the jugular vein on the early frame with the highest image intensity and fitting the time-activity curves with a triphasic exponential function.

2.4. MRI Data Acquisition

HNSCC patients underwent MRI examinations on a 3 Tesla (T) MRI scanner (Philips Ingenia; Philips Healthcare, Eindhoven, Netherlands) using a neurovascular phased-array coil. The standard MR multiplanar (axial, coronal, and sagittal) T$_2$-weighted (T$_2$w) and T$_1$-weighted images were acquired as detailed elsewhere [23,42]. DW- and DCE-MRI acquisitions followed standard T_1w and T_2w imaging. The total MR acquisition time was approximately 30 min for the whole examination.

DW-MRI data were acquired using a single-shot echo-planar imaging (SS-EPI) sequence with the following MR parameters: repletion time (TR)/echo time (TE) = 4000/minimum (80) ms, NA = 2, matrix = 128 × 128, FOV = 20–24 cm, slices = 8–10, slice thickness = 5 mm, and ten b-values (i.e., b = 0, 20, 50, 80, 200, 300, 500, 800, 1500, and 2000 s/mm²). The spatial saturation bands were graphically prescribed on scout images by the technologist prior to DW-MRI scanning. Their angulation, center, and width were adjusted, depending on the neck anatomy of the patients. The total acquisition time was 5 min.

The T_1w images for both pre-contrast (T_{10}) and dynamic (i.e., before, during, and after an injection of CA) were acquired using a fast 3D T1w spoiled gradient recalled echo sequence. The pre-contrast T_1 images were acquired with the multiple flip angles (FA) of 5°, 15°, and 30° with TR/TE = 7/2.7 ms; acquisition matrix = 256 ×1 28, FOV = 20–24 cm, slice thickness = 5 mm, and slices = 8–10. Dynamic series images were acquired using FA = 15° and other acquisition MR parameters, as mentioned above. A bolus of 0.1 mmol/kg Gd-based CA was injected through an antecubital vein catheter at two cc/s, followed by a 20-mL saline flush after acquiring 5–6 images as detailed elsewhere. A total of 40 dynamic images were obtained with a temporal resolution ranging from 7.20–8.96.0 s/image.

2.5. MRI Data Analysis

2.5.1. DWI Analysis

DW signal intensity data from multiple b-values were fitted to (i) a monoexponential (Equation (1)) and (ii) bi-exponential equation of the IVIM model (Equation (2)) [20]:

$$S(b) = S_0 \, e^{-b \times ADC} \quad (1)$$

$$S(b) = S_0\left[f e^{-b \times D^*} + (1-f)e^{-b \times D}\right] \quad (2)$$

where S_0 and S_b are the signal intensities without and with diffusion weighting, b is the diffusion weighting factor (s/mm²), D (mm²/s) is the true diffusion coefficient, D^* (mm²/s) is the pseudo-diffusion coefficient (mm²/s), and f is the perfusion fraction.

2.5.2. Fast Exchange Regime DCE-MRI Analysis

The longitudinal relaxation rate constant-with time course for tissue R_{1t} ($R_{1t} = 1/T_{1t}$) and EES R_{1e} in the fast exchange limit is given by Equations (3) and (4) as follows [43]:

$$R_{1t}(t) = R_{10} + r_1(t)C_t(t) \quad (3)$$

$$R_{1e}(t) = R_{10e} + r_1(t)C_e(t) \quad (4)$$

where R_{10} and R_{10e} are the precontrast longitudinal relation rate constants for tissue and EES, respectively, $C_t(t)$ and $C_e(t)$ are the CA concentration with time in tissue and EES. The r_1 is the longitudinal relaxivity of CA.

The CA concentration with time in tissue is given by the standard Toft model (Equation (5)) [24].

$$C_t(t) = K^{trans}\int_0^t e^{-k_{ep}(t-\tau)}C_p(\tau)\,d\tau \quad (5)$$

where K^{trans} is the volume transfer constant, C_p is the plasma CA concentration (called arterial input function [AIF]), and k_{ep} ($k_{ep} = K^{trans}/v_e$) is the CA transfer rate constant from the EES to vascular space. The CA concentration in EES is given by $C_e(t) = C_t(t))/v_e$.

The two-site water exchange (2SX) model (i.e., between the intracellular space [ICS] and EES) is derived from the three-site-two water exchange model formulated based on Bloch-McConnell's, assuming a negligible vascular space [44,45]. The solution of Bloch-

McConnell's 2SX system yields two eigenvalues [46]. One of the eigenvalues represents the observable longitudinal relaxation rate R_1 of the FXR model given by Equation (6) [16].

$$R_{1t}(t) = \frac{1}{2}\left[(R_{1i} + k_{ie} + R_{1e} + k_{ei}) - \sqrt{(R_{1i} + k_{ie} - R_{1e} - k_{ei})^2 + 4 k_{ie}k_{ei}}\right] \quad (6)$$

where R_{1i} and R_{1e} are the ICS and EES longitudinal relaxation rate constants. The k_{ie} ($k_{ie} = 1/\tau_i$) and k_{ei} are the water exchange rates between ICS and EES and vice versa. The k_{ie} is related to P (A/v_i), where P is the cell membrane water permeability coefficient, and A/v_i is the ratio of surface area to volume of a cell. For DCE data analysis, the R_{1i} value was set equal to that of R_{10}.

2.6. MRI Tumor Regions of Interests Analysis

Regions of interest (ROIs) were manually delineated on the metastatic lymph nodes (LNs) on b = 0 (s/mm^2) DW images and late phases of T_1w dynamic images by a team of neuroradiologists based on T_1w/T_2w images using Image J [47]. The metastatic LN volumes (V_{t-MRI}) were calculated from the T_2-weighted images as detailed elsewhere [23]. The AIF was extracted from the carotid artery in each patient [48]. Equations (2) and (6) were fitted on a voxel-wise basis with a nonlinear least-square curve fitting method [49,50]. T_{10} values were estimated on a voxel-wise basis from the multiple angles as described elsewhere [51,52]. DW and DCE post-image processing, including parametric map generation, were conducted using MRI-QAMPER (MRI Quantitative Analysis of Multi-Parameter Evaluation Routines) [42,50].

2.7. Statistical Analysis

QI metric values derived from MMI (FDG-PET/CT, FMISO-PET/CT, and DW- and DCE-MRI) were reported as mean ± standard deviation (SD). Wilcoxon signed-rank test (WSRT) was performed to compare the tumor volume obtained from MMI techniques. A nonparametric measure of the correlation, the Spearman's rank (ρ) analysis, was performed to examine the relationship among MMI-derived QI metrics. The correlation coefficient (ρ) of <0.3 was considered weak, 0.3–0.5 moderate, and 0.5–1.0 strong. The significance level was set at $p < 0.05$.

To determine how and to what extent the MMI-derived QI metrics were interconnected on the network, the CDA algorithm based on the "spin-glass" model was employed for the QI metrics whose Spearman's rank test p-value was <0.05 [39]. The spin-glass is a unique community detection algorithm based on the statistical mechanics of spin around the networks [39]. The CDA-based "spin-glass" model approach splits MMI-derived QI metrics into distinct communities [53]. Links or edges heavily or sparsely connect the groups that can also reveal strong or weak, including positive or negative correlations [53]. All statistical analyses were performed using R-4.0.3 software [54].

3. Results

Ninety-two imaging datasets (FDG-PET/CT, FMSIO-PET/CT, DW-, and DCE-MRI) were successfully analyzed from 27 metastatic LNs. The median Karnofsky Performance Status (KPS) was 90 (range 80–90).

The representative signal versus b-values curve for DW data is displayed in Figure 1. The signal time representative curves for FMISO and DCE data are displayed in Figure 2A,B, respectively. The corresponding arterial input functions are also displayed. The FMISO data was taken from the metastatic LN displayed in Figure 3. Similarly, DW- and DCE-MRI data were extracted from ROIs shown in Figure 4.

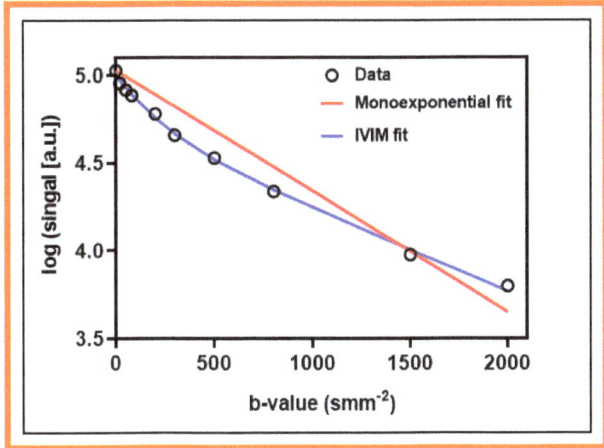

Figure 1. Representative mean semilogarithmic signal intensity decay curve as a function of the multiple b-value (black circle). The data were fitted with the monoexponential model (solid red line) and intravoxel incoherent motion (IVIM) model (solid blue line).

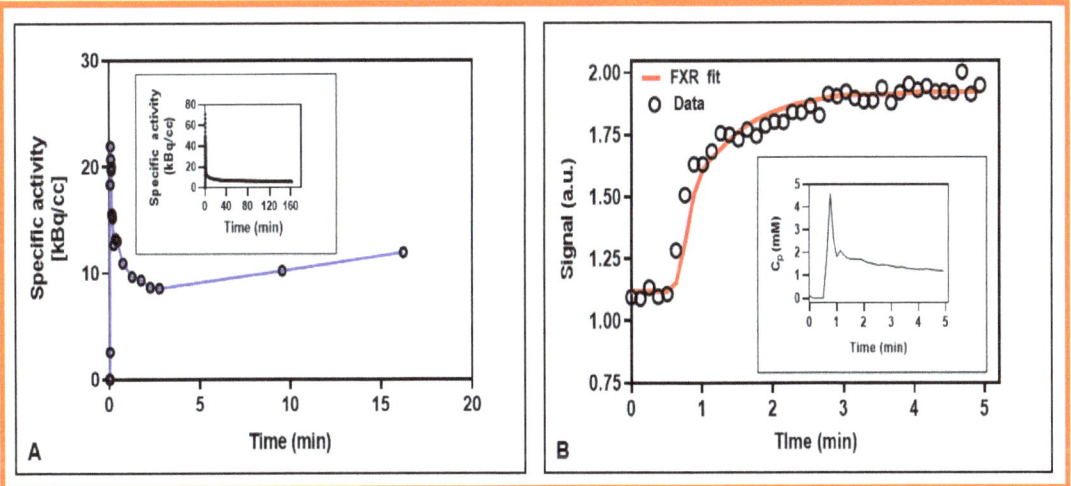

Figure 2. Representative multimodality imaging signal plots with time for data obtained from the metastatic neck lymph node in a patient with head and neck squamous cell carcinomas. (**A**) Measured mean FMISO-PET/CT time-activity curve (circles) data connected with a solid line (blue), and the corresponding input function (in the inset). (**B**) Signal intensity time curves fitted with the fast exchange regime (FXR) model. The circle (black) and solid line (red) represent the data and FXR model fit. Insert: Plasma contrast agent concentration, C_p with time.

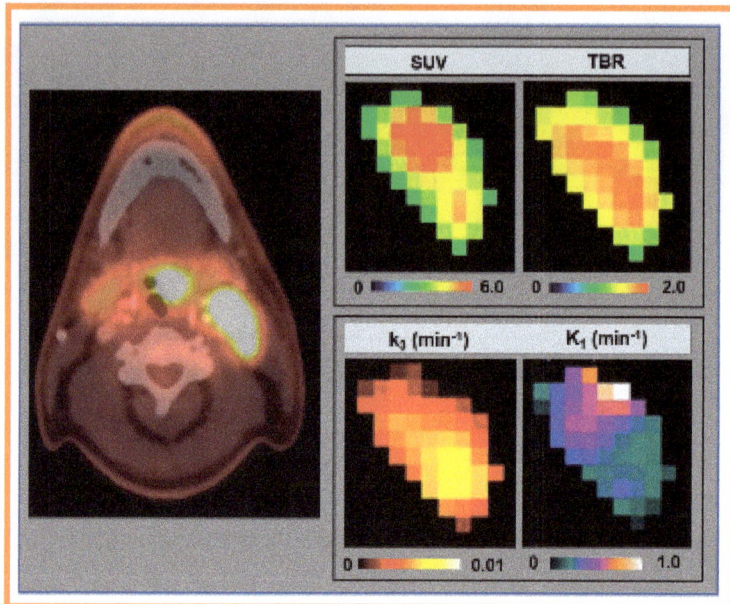

Figure 3. Left column: Representative axial images of ^{18}F-fluoromisonidazole (^{18}F-FMISO) positron emission tomography (PET/CT) from HPV-positive head and neck squamous carcinoma patient. Right column: ^{18}F-fluorodeoxyglucose-PET/CT derived standard uptake value (SUV) and FMISO-PET derived tumor to blood ratio (TBR), k_3, and K_1 maps.

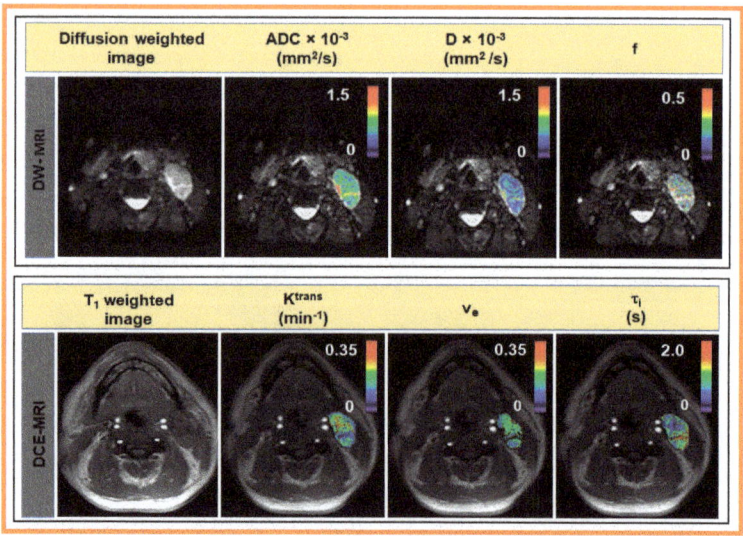

Figure 4. Top: Representative diffusion-weighted image (b = 0 s/mm^2) and monoexponential and intravoxel incoherent motion models-derived parametric maps overlaid on diffusion-weighted image (b = 0 s/mm^2). Bottom: Representative precontrast T_1 weighted (T_1w) image and fast exchange regime model-derived parametric maps overlaid on precontrast T_1w images.

Figure 3 shows the representative PET/CT image and QI metrics extracted from the FDG-PET/CT and FMISO-PET/CT.

Representative DW, T_1-weighted image, and QI metrics derived from IVIM and FXR model are displayed in Figure 4. The representative MRI images were from the same patient shown in Figure 2.

The mean tumor ROI volume and QI metrics values from MMI are given in Table 1.

Table 1. Summary of multimodality imaging derived quantitative imaging metrics values.

Method	Model Parameter	Value [1]
^{18}F-FDG-PET/CT	SUL_{max}	8.91 ± 3.94
	SUL_{mean}	5.26 ± 2.76
^{18}F-FMISO-PET/CT	K_1 (min^{-1})	0.33 ± 0.15
	$k_{3\,max}$ (min^{-1})	0.0087 ± 0.0049
	$k_{3\,mean}$ (min^{-1})	0.0034 ± 0.0021
	TBR_{max}	1.76 ± 0.53
	TBR_{mean}	1.29 ± 0.27
	DV	0.89 ± 0.14
DW	ADC $\times 10^{-3}$ (mm^2/s)	0.93 ± 0.14
	D $\times 10^{-3}$ (mm^2/s)	0.67 ± 0.13
	D* $\times 10^{-3}$ (mm^2/s)	9.02 ± 1.80
	f	0.16 ± 0.06
DCE	K^{trans} (min^{-1})	0.18 ± 0.06
	v_e	0.32 ± 0.09
	τ_i (s)	0.670 ± 0.15
FDG-PET tumor volume	$V_{t\text{-PET}}$ (cm^3)	13.59 ± 7.65
T_{2w} MRI tumor volume	$V_{t\text{-MRI}}$ (cm^3)	11.41 ± 10.09

Note: [1] Data are represented as mean $\pm$ SD.

Mean metastatic LN volumes obtained from PET ($V_{t\text{-PET}}$) and MRI ($V_{t\text{-MRI}}$) were significantly different ($V_{t\text{-PET}} = 13.59 \pm 7.65$ cm^3 vs. $V_{t\text{-MRI}} = 11.41 \pm 10.09$ cm^3, $p = 0.005$, WSRT) and were strongly positively correlated ($\rho = 0.85$, $p < 0.0001$) in HNSCC. Mean $V_{t\text{-MRI}}$ was strongly positively correlated with ^{18}F-FDG-PET/CT-derived metrics SUL_{mean} ($\rho = 0.48$, $p = 0.01$) and SUL_{max} ($\rho = 0.57$, $p = 0.0001$) (Figure 5). The metrics SUL_{max} and SUL_{mean} derived from FDG-PET/CT represent the standardized uptake value normalized to lean body mass, respectively. No significant correlations were found between $V_{t\text{-PET}}$ and metrics obtained from ^{18}F-FMISO-PET/CT, DW-, and DCE-MRI ($p > 0.05$). $V_{t\text{-MRI}}$ also did not show a significant correlation with ^{18}F-FMISO-PET/CT, DW-, and DCE-MRI derived metrics ($p > 0.05$).

Spearman correlation analysis identified several weak, moderate, and strong statistically significant, either positive or negative, correlations between QI metrics (surrogate markers of cellularity, glucose metabolism, perfusion, and hypoxia) derived from MMI data (Table 2). Herein, a summary of the Spearman correlation results is reported.

Table 2. Summary of Spearman rank correlation analysis (ρ) results between the quantitative metrics derived from multimodality imaging data.

Quantitative metric	PET volume	MR T$_2$ weighted volume	ADC	D	D*	f	K^{trans}	v$_e$	τ$_i$	k$_{ep}$	SUL$_{max}$	SUL$_{mean}$	K$_1$	k$_{3,max}$	k$_{3,mean}$	DV	TBR Max	TBR Mean
PET volume		0.84*	−0.09	−0.10	0.28	−0.06	0.19	−0.09	0.16	0.17	0.58*	0.42*	0.26	0.29	0.13	0.16	0.30	0.20
MRI T$_2$ weighted volume			−0.17	−0.18	0.07	0.01	0.14	−0.14	0.12	0.26	0.57*	0.48*	0.17	0.30	0.31	0.04	0.25	0.27
ADC				0.95*	−0.34	−0.18	−0.48*	0.46*	−0.36	0.18	−0.29	−0.42*	−0.40*	0.26	0.15	−0.31	0.07	−0.14
D					−0.26	−0.18	−0.43*	0.32	−0.41*	0.23	−0.31	−0.41*	−0.40*	0.32	0.23	−0.32	0.14	−0.08
D*						0.39*	0.39*	−0.11	0.01	0.04	0.21	0.24	0.40*	−0.25	−0.35	0.49*	0.09	0.13
f							0.31	0.18	0.14	−0.14	0.06	0.20	0.20	−0.45*	−0.30	0.40*	−0.18	0.12
K^{trans}								−0.10	0.43*	0.12	0.17	0.28	0.48*	−0.41*	−0.27	0.44*	−0.17	−0.03
v$_e$									−0.41*	−0.15	0.17	0.15	0.02	−0.20	−0.26	0.40*	0.14	0.13
τ$_i$										−0.03	0.06	0.11	0.08	−0.17	0.05	−0.04	−0.23	−0.12
k$_{ep}$											−0.11	−0.16	0.20	0.34	0.20	−0.23	−0.09	−0.20
SUL$_{max}$												0.94*	−0.01	−0.09	−0.02	0.42*	0.36	0.44*
SUL$_{mean}$													0.003	−0.15	−0.02	0.48*	0.38	0.53*
K$_1$														−0.26	−0.46*	0.59*	−0.18	−0.19
k$_{3,max}$															0.79*	−0.57*	0.57*	0.34
k$_{3,mean}$																−0.60*	0.57*	0.54*
DV																	0.13	0.23
TBR$_{max}$																		0.88*
TBR$_{mean}$																		

The p-value < 0.05 is denoted by an asterisk *. ADC: Apparent diffusion coefficient, D: true diffusion coefficient, D*: pseudo-diffusion constant, f: perfusion fraction, K^{trans}: volume transfer constant, v$_e$: volume fraction of extravascular extracellular space (EES), τ$_i$: mean lifetime of water molecules, k$_{ep}$: transport constant for contrast agent form EES to blood plasma space, SUL: standardized uptake values of ^{18}F-fluorodeoxyglucose divided by lean body mass, K$_1$: transport rate constant of tracer from the plasma to the tissue for ^{18}F-fluoromisonidazole (FMISO), k$_3$: kinetic rate constant approximating the rate of irreversible binding of FMISO, TBR: Tumor-to-Blood Ratio, and DV: total ^{18}F-FMISO distribution volume.

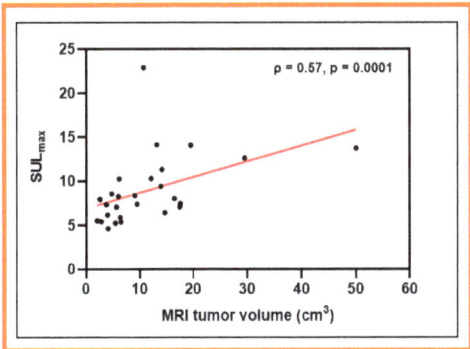

Figure 5. Scatter plot showing a correlation between ^{18}F-FDG-PET/CT-derived maximum standardized uptake value normalized to lean body mass (SULmax) and metastatic lymph node volumes from T$_2$ weighted MRI (V$_{t\text{-MRI}}$). Circles represent the data, and the solid line denotes the line of best fit.

The metrics ADC and D, markers of tumor cellularity, exhibited a significant moderate negative correlation with SUL$_{mean}$, a feature of glycolytic activity ($\rho = -0.42$, $p = 0.03$ for ADC and $\rho = -0.41$, $p = 0.03$ for D). Additionally, there was a significant moderate negative correlation between D and K^{trans}, a marker of tumor perfsuion//permeability ($\rho = -0.43$, $p = 0.03$), and D and τ_i, a maker of cell metabolic activity ($\rho = -0.41$, $p = 0.04$). ADC and v$_e$, a leakage space for CA, showed a significant positive correlation ($\rho = 0.46$, $p = 0.02$). D showed a moderate negative correlation with K$_1$, a measure of perfusion for FMISO ($\rho = -0.40$, $p = 0.04$).

The metric D*, a marker of capillary perfusion in tissue, showed a moderate positive correlation with K^{trans} and K$_1$ ($\rho = 0.39$, $p = 0.04$ for K^{trans} and $\rho = 0.40$, $p = 0.04$ for K$_1$). The perfusion fraction, f (the volume fraction occupied by capillaries), showed a moderate positive correlation with DV, a distribution volume of FMISO ($\rho = 0.40$, $p = 0.04$). In contrast, it showed a moderate negative correlation with k$_{3max}$ ($\rho = -0.40$, $p = 0.02$). The metrics K^{trans} and K$_1$ were moderately positively correlated ($\rho = 0.48$, $p = 0.01$). K^{trans} and k$_{3max}$, a marker of tumor hypoxia, were moderately negatively correlated ($\rho = -0.41$, $p = 0.03$). K^{trans} and DV exhibited a moderate positive correlation ($\rho = 0.44$, $p = 0.02$). The metric v$_e$ and DV were moderately positively correlated ($\rho = 0.40$, $p = 0.04$).

Figure 6 shows the representative scatter plots between MMI-derived QI metrics.

The network as a graph constructed from 16 MMI-derived QI metrics, including T$_2$ weighted tumor volume (V$_{t\text{-MRI}}$), using the CDA-based "spin-glass" analysis, is illustrated in Figure 7. The CDA approach resulted in four communities with 33 edges in the network. As a note, the edges were constructed between the nodes that yielded a Spearman rank correlation value $p < 0.05$ (Table 2). The nodes within the community are densely coupled to each other. In contrast, these nodes are relatively sparsely connected with other communities in the same graph. The solid blue line represents the negative correlation. In contrast, the positive correlation is represented by the orange and red colors, respectively. The thickness of the lines representing the extent of correlation ranging from weak to strong between them.

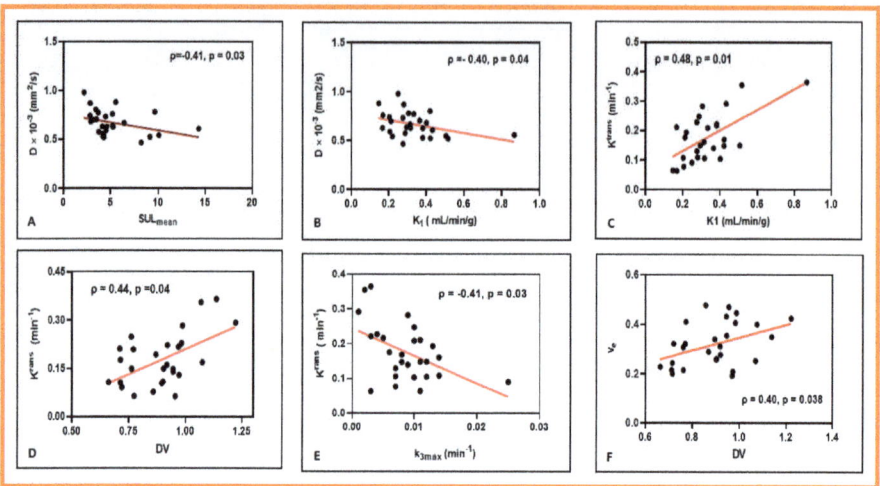

Figure 6. Representative scatter plots showing the relationships between quantitative imaging metrics derived from multimodality imaging methods. (**A**) True diffusion coefficient (D) vs. mean of the maximum standardized uptake value normalized to lean body mass (SULmean). (**B**) D vs. K_1 (Perfusion constant for FMISO). (**C**) K^{trans} (Volume transfer constant for Gd-based contrast agent) vs. K_1. (**D**) K^{trans} vs. DV (FMISO distribution volume). (**E**) K^{trans} vs. k_{3max}. (**F**) v_e (Volume fraction of the extravascular extracellular space) vs. DV.

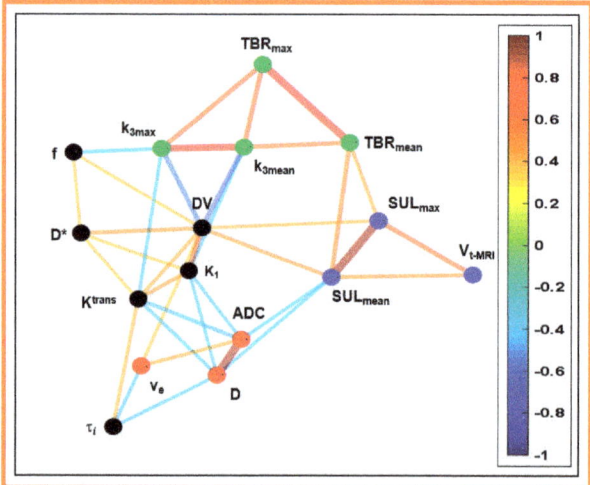

Figure 7. Sample network with 16 nodes and 33 edges constructed from a community detection algorithm (CDA) based on the spin-glass model. The nodes represent the quantitative imaging (QI) metrics derived from four multimodality imaging which are connected by lines or edges in the graph. The perfusion metric, K_1, and distribution volume (DV) derived from the ^{18}FMISO-PET/CT overlap with DW- and DCE-MRI metrics and are densely interconnected compared to other metrics in the network (blue color: 3 nodes [$V_{t\text{-MRI}}$, SULmax, mean], green color: 4 nodes [TBRmax, mean, and $k_{3max,mean}$] black color 6 nodes [K_1, DV, D* and f, K^{trans} and τ_i], and red color: 3 nodes [ADC, D, and v_e]). A solid blue line represents the negative correlation, whereas the orange and red colors represent the positive correlation among the QIs. The thickness of lines indicates the extent of a correlation (weak, moderate, and strong). The value in the color bar scale represents either negative or positive links detected by the CDA approach in networks.

$V_{t\text{-MR}}$ is a community member in the network formed by FDG-PET/CT-derived metrics ($SUL_{max,mean}$ [3 nodes, blue color]). The quantitative metrics ADC, D, and v_e formed the 2nd community network (3 nodes, red color). The metrics $k_{3max,mean}$, and $TBR_{max,mean}$ created the 3rd community (4 nodes, green color). The fourth community consisted of 6 nodes (black color), including K_1 and DV (FMISO), f and D^* (DW-MRI), and K^{trans} and τ_i (DCE-MRI). CDA approach yielded 8, 7, and 6 edges for the metrics DV, K^{trans}, and K_1, respectively.

K^{trans} is regarded as one of the most influential metrics to assess tumor microvasculature. K^{trans} (a member of the black community) exhibits distinct relationships with nearby nodes (red community [ADC and D] and green community [$k_{3.max}$]). In contrast, K^{trans} did not directly link FDG-PET/CT-derived metrics and tumor volume in the network. The extent of the K^{trans} relationship with nearby nodes (K_1, DV, $k_{3.max}$, and D^*) was further evaluated using regression analysis. The combination of three nodes (K_1, DV, and k_{3max}) yielded a significant correlation ($R^2 = 0.45$, adjusted $R^2 = 0.38$, $p = 0.002$). In contrast, linear regression analysis between K^{trans} and k_{3max} yielded a meaningful inverse relationship ($R^2 = 0.23$, adjusted $R^2 = 0.19$, $p = 0.011$), indicating the influence of vascular permeability on radiotracer diffusion in hypoxic tumors.

4. Discussion

Integration of metabolic (^{18}F-FDG-PET/CT and ^{18}FMISO- PET/CT) and functional imaging (DW-, and DCE-MRI) aggregate the complementary information of tumor physiology [10,23,41,42]. The present study investigated a correlation at pre-TX between QIs obtained from MMI characterizing tumor = physiology, including glucose metabolism, perfusion, hypoxia, pseudo-diffusion in the capillary network, cellularity, and perfusion/permeability and metabolic activity markers using a CDA-based "spin-glass model" in addition to Spearman correlation in HNSCC patients. The CDA approach identified the four communities and revealed that K^{trans}, a measure of perfusion/vascular permeability, links to seven edges in the community. Thus, detecting communities and identifying their relationship is an essential step to investigate robust imaging biomarkers for precision medicine in HNSCC. Our previous two separate studies used ^{18}F-FMISO dynamic PET (dPET) to assess the tumor hypoxia and perfusion and monitor early response to chemo-RT in HNSCC [41]. The first study with ^{18}F-FMISO dPET data provided parametric maps of tumor hypoxia, perfusion, and radiotracer distribution volume, improving the characterization of a tumor lesion [40]. The other study concluded that kinetic modeling of FMISO dPET data reveals a more detailed description of the tumor microenvironment and improved assessment of response to chemo-RT than a single static image [10]. In DW-MRI, IVIM derived QI metrics obtained at pre-TX and intra-TX weeks 1, 2, and 3 were used to characterize and monitor response to chemo-RT. Hierarchical clustering performed using the intra-TX IVIM derived QI metrics demonstrated the subtypes in HPV + patients in HNSCC [23].

Jansen et al. found a correlation between tumor volume and ^{18}F-FMISO SUV in 13 HNSCC patients [36]. The present study also found a strong correlation between pre-TX MRI tumor volume with $SUL_{max,mean}$. A moderate negative correlation between SUL_{mean} and ADC was consistent with previous studies in HNSCC [6,55]. FDG-PET/CT-derived SUV and DWI-MRI-derived ADC represent different aspects of the tumor cells. The glycolytic activity of tumor cells (reflected by FDG uptake) is related to high tumor cell density, consequently restricting water molecule diffusion and lowering ADC values. It has been reported that there was a strong negative correlation between the mean of pre-TX ADC and ^{18}F-FDG PET SUV [56]. The present study did not find a significant positive correlation between K_1 and $SUL_{max,mean}$. In contrast, Vidiri et al. reported a significant negative correlation between K^{trans} and ^{18}F-FDG-PET/CT parameters in LNs of oropharyngeal squamous cell carcinoma [13]. Surov et al. reported a moderate positive correlation between SUVmax and k_{ep} [11]. In contrast, in the present study, SUL exhibited a nonsignificant negative correlation with k_{ep} derived from the FXR model. Chen et al.

study concluded that qMRI could provide additional value in distinguishing metastatic nodes, particularly among small nodes, when used with FDG-PET [53].

Dynamic FMISO-PET/CT and DCE-MRI-derived QI metrics capture the tumor physiology through various mechanisms. The molecular weights of FMISO (189.14 Daltons) and Gd-based CA (Gd-DTPA ~ 547 Daltons) are different, and the transport mechanism across the vasculature is assessed differently. The FMISO is lipophilic, and its uptake is driven by passive diffusion out of the vasculature and through the cell membranes. The radiotracer eventually accumulates in hypoxic regions, largely independently of the perfusion. In contrast, the K^{trans} measures the influx of a CA entering the EES, altering the T_1 relaxation of the tissue water protons, but CA does not enter the cell. As τ_i is associated with cell size, $\tau_i = [(v_i/A) \times 1/P]$, where v_i/A is the ratio of volume to the cell's surface area and P is the cell membrane's permeability. Thus, a decrease in metric τ_i value associated with shrinkage of a cell would correspond to an increase in ADC/D values. Previous studies reported the inconsistent correlation between τ_i and SUV in breast cancer [57] and hepatocellular carcinoma [58]. As a note, τ_i is mainly representing a cell metabolic activity characterized by adenosine triphosphate production [30]. In the present study, K^{trans} and k_{3max} exhibited a strong negative Spearman correlation.

Identifying the precise dose (e.g., dose escalation or de-escalation) for HNSCC patients is difficult because of heterogeneous populations of various disease sites, stages, and prognoses. HPV+ oropharyngeal cancer is a distinct biologic entity that shows a favorable prognosis with standard chemo-RT [59]. In contrast, HPV-negative tumors continue to have a poor prognosis despite treatment intensification. Thus, patient selection is vital for treating less aggressive radiotherapy regimens to maintain excellent standard therapy outcomes [60]. The utilities of MMI-derived biomarkers have been considerably improving tumor delineation accuracy, subvolume determination, longitudinal tracking of treatment response, permitting dose escalation or de-escalation to target tissues, and reducing toxicity to nearby tissues and organs [16], thus highlighting the need for robust biomarkers to be included in clinical trials.

Despite the significant advances in MMI methods, findings of reliable biomarkers that can effectively assess changes in tumor physiology after RT are still challenging, especially for precision therapy in HNSCC, given that we do not yet know which one of these imaging modalities is the gold standard. The present study CDA "spin-glass"-based analysis resulted in four communities for 16 MMI-derived metrics, clustering related metrics together in a network. This indicates a preferential linking between nodes to the other groups in the network exhibiting similar characteristics [39]. K_1 and K^{trans}, measures of the tumor perfusion and permeability for FMISO and Gd-based CA, showed a strong connection in the CDA network. Similarly, DV and v_e, distribution volume for FMISO and CA, exhibited a similar relationship. In contrast, k_{3max}, a hypoxia marker, was negatively correlated with the K^{trans} and f. The metric k_3 is related to the diffusive compartment, which is hypoxic, consistent with the view that tumor hypoxia results from inadequate oxygen supply to the tumor [61]. As a note, K^{trans} represents a passive transport of CA across the capillary wall driven by diffusion, whereas k_{3max} is the FMISO uptake in hypoxic tissues caused by convective transport [62]. Therefore, ^{18}F-MISO-PET/CT and DCE-MRI can provide complementary information for characterizing the tumor microenvironments [63]. The community structure displayed by a CDA approach is visually interpretable to identify important biomarker metrics and infer their relationships. Thus, the CDA approach may improve in identifying the surrogate biomarkers for prognostication at pre-TX in HNSCC patients.

The present study is limited by the sample size for CDA analysis, which warrants validation in a larger sample. Motion artifacts in the MR images due to the voluntary and involuntary movements in the neck region, such as swallowing and breathing, can be minimized by carefully setting up the scan. Respiratory motion artifacts can be minimized with proper breath-holding and shortened scan duration. A robust co-registration method could improve the correlation between QIs. The present study was also limited to assessing the correlation between mean QI values rather than a voxel-by-voxel basis. A B_1 non-uniformity due to varying the flip angle influences the accuracy and precision of DCE-MRI-derived QIs at higher field strength. Hence, acquiring the B_1 mapping sequence can improve the accuracy of DCE-MRI-derived QI metrics. Despite these limitations, the CDA approach demonstrated its potential in assessing the correlation between the QI metrics.

5. Conclusions

Significant Spearman correlations, ranging from moderate to strong, were observed between few QI metrics. The CDA approach illustrated how and to what extent MMI-derived QI metrics were associated in the network. After validation in a larger HNSCC population, the present preliminary findings may help identify potential biomarkers in individualized patient care.

Author Contributions: Conceptualization, N.Y.L., J.L.H. and A.S.-D.; Methodology, R.P., M.G. and J.H.O.; validation, R.P., M.G. and J.H.O.; formal analysis, R.P., M.G., D.A.N. and J.H.O.; investigation, N.Y.L., J.L.H. and A.S.-D.; resources, N.Y.L. and J.L.H.; data curation, R.P., M.G. and J.H.O.; writing—original draft preparation, all authors; writing—review and editing, all authors; visualization, N.Y.L. and J.L.H.; supervision, N.Y.L., A.S.-D. and J.L.H.; funding acquisition, N.Y.L. All authors have read and agreed to the published version of the manuscript.

Funding: This research was funded by NIH, R01 CA238392-01A1 (NYL).

Institutional Review Board Statement: The study was approved by the Institutional Review Board (IRB protocol # 06-007, approved on 02/14/2006).

Informed Consent Statement: Informed consent was obtained from all subjects involved in the study.

Data Availability Statement: The data presented in this study will be provided upon reasonable request.

Acknowledgments: We are thankful to Alyssa Duck for editing the full manuscript.

Conflicts of Interest: The authors declare no conflict of interest.

References

1. Lo Nigro, C.; Denaro, N.; Merlotti, A.; Merlano, M. Head and neck cancer: Improving outcomes with a multidisciplinary approach. *Cancer Manag. Res.* **2017**, *9*, 363–371. [CrossRef] [PubMed]
2. Gillison, M. HPV and its effect on head and neck cancer prognosis. *Clin. Adv. Hematol. Oncol.* **2010**, *8*, 680–682. [PubMed]
3. Psyrri, A.; Cohen, E. Oropharyngeal cancer: Clinical implications of the HPV connection. *Ann. Oncol. Off. J. Eur. Soc. Med. Oncol. ESMO* **2011**, *22*, 997–999. [CrossRef]
4. King, A.D. Multimodality imaging of head and neck cancer. *Cancer Imaging* **2007**, *7*, S37–S46. [CrossRef]
5. Rajendran, J.G.; Krohn, K.A. F-18 Fluoromisonidazole for Imaging Tumor Hypoxia: Imaging the Microenvironment for Personalized Cancer Therapy. *Semin. Nucl. Med.* **2015**, *45*, 151–162. [CrossRef]
6. Leibfarth, S.; Simoncic, U.; Monnich, D.; Welz, S.; Schmidt, H.; Schwenzer, N.; Zips, D.; Thorwarth, D. Analysis of pairwise correlations in multi-parametric PET/MR data for biological tumor characterization and treatment individualization strategies. *Eur. J. Nucl. Med. Mol. Imaging* **2016**, *43*, 1199–1208. [CrossRef]
7. Goel, R.; Moore, W.; Sumer, B.; Khan, S.; Sher, D.; Subramaniam, R.M. Clinical Practice in PET/CT for the Management of Head and Neck Squamous Cell Cancer. *Am. J. Roentgenol.* **2017**, *209*, 289–303. [CrossRef]
8. Vidiri, A.; Gangemi, E.; Ruberto, E.; Pasqualoni, R.; Sciuto, R.; Sanguineti, G.; Farneti, A.; Benevolo, M.; Rollo, F.; Sperati, F. Correlation between histogram-based DCE-MRI parameters and 18F-FDG PET values in oropharyngeal squamous cell carcinoma: Evaluation in primary tumors and metastatic nodes. *PLoS ONE* **2020**, *15*, e0229611. [CrossRef] [PubMed]
9. Kikuchi, M.; Yamane, T.; Shinohara, S.; Fujiwara, K.; Hori, S.Y.; Tona, Y.; Yamazaki, H.; Naito, Y.; Senda, M. 18F-fluoromisonidazole positron emission tomography before treatment is a predictor of radiotherapy outcome and survival prognosis in patients with head and neck squamous cell carcinoma. *Ann. Nucl. Med.* **2011**, *25*, 625–633. [CrossRef]
10. Grkovski, M.; Lee, N.Y.; Schoder, H.; Carlin, S.D.; Beattie, B.J.; Riaz, N.; Leeman, J.E.; O'Donoghue, J.A.; Humm, J.L. Monitoring early response to chemoradiotherapy with (18)F-FMISO dynamic PET in head and neck cancer. *Eur. J. Nucl. Med. Mol. Imaging* **2017**, *44*, 1682–1691. [CrossRef] [PubMed]
11. Surov, A.; Leifels, L.; Meyer, H.J.; Winter, K.; Sabri, O.; Purz, S. Associations Between Histogram Analysis DCE MRI Parameters and Complex F-18-FDG-PET Values in Head and Neck Squamous Cell Carcinoma. *Anticancer Res.* **2018**, *38*, 1637–1642. [CrossRef]
12. Simoncic, U.; Leibfarth, S.; Welz, S.; Schwenzer, N.; Schmidt, H.; Reischl, G.; Pfannenberg, C.; la Fougere, C.; Nikolaou, K.; Zips, D.; et al. Comparison of DCE-MRI kinetic parameters and FMISO-PET uptake parameters in head and neck cancer patients. *Med. Phys.* **2017**, *44*, 2358–2368. [CrossRef]

13. Minosse, S.; Marzi, S.; Piludu, F.; Boellis, A.; Terrenato, I.; Pellini, R.; Covello, R.; Vidiri, A. Diffusion kurtosis imaging in head and neck cancer: A correlation study with dynamic contrast enhanced MRI. *Phys. Med.* **2020**, *73*, 22–28. [CrossRef] [PubMed]
14. Rajendran, J.G.; Schwartz, D.L.; O'Sullivan, J.; Peterson, L.M.; Ng, P.; Scharnhorst, J.; Grierson, J.R.; Krohn, K.A. Tumor hypoxia imaging with [F-18] fluoromisonidazole positron emission tomography in head and neck cancer. *Clin. Cancer Res.* **2006**, *12*, 5435–5441. [CrossRef] [PubMed]
15. Bandurska-Luque, A.; Lock, S.; Haase, R.; Richter, C.; Zophel, K.; Abolmaali, N.; Seidlitz, A.; Appolda, S.; Krause, M.; Steinbach, J.; et al. FMISO-PET-based lymph node hypoxia adds to the prognostic value of tumor only hypoxia in HNSCC patients. *Radiother. Oncol.* **2019**, *130*, 97–103. [CrossRef] [PubMed]
16. Riaz, N.; Sherman, E.; Pei, X.; Schoder, H.; Grkovski, M.; Paudyal, R.; Katabi, N.; Selenica, P.; Yamaguchi, T.N.; Ma, D.; et al. Precision Radiotherapy: Reduction in Radiation for Oropharyngeal Cancer in the 30 ROC Trial. *J. Natl. Cancer Inst.* **2021**. [CrossRef] [PubMed]
17. Le Bihan, D.; Breton, E.; Lallemand, D.; Grenier, P.; Cabanis, E.; Laval-Jeantet, M. MR imaging of intravoxel incoherent motions: Application to diffusion and perfusion in neurologic disorders. *Radiology* **1986**, *161*, 401–407. [CrossRef]
18. Vandecaveye, V.; Dirix, P.; De Keyzer, F.; Op de Beeck, K.; Poorten, V.V.; Delaere, P.; Verbeken, E.; Hermans, R.; Nuyts, S. Accuracy of Diffusion-Weighted Mri for Nodal Staging and Radiotherapy Planning of Head and Neck Squamous Cell Carcinoma. *Radiother. Oncol.* **2008**, *88*, S152–S153.
19. Kim, S.; Loevner, L.; Quon, H.; Sherman, E.; Weinstein, G.; Kilger, A.; Poptani, H. Diffusion-weighted magnetic resonance imaging for predicting and detecting early response to chemoradiation therapy of squamous cell carcinomas of the head and neck. *Clin. Cancer Res.* **2009**, *15*, 986–994. [CrossRef]
20. Le Bihan, D. Intravoxel incoherent motion imaging using steady-state free precession. *Magn. Reson. Med.* **1988**, *7*, 346–351. [CrossRef]
21. Hauser, T.; Essig, M.; Jensen, A.; Laun, F.B.; Munter, M.; Maier-Hein, K.H.; Stieltjes, B. Prediction of treatment response in head and neck carcinomas using IVIM-DWI: Evaluation of lymph node metastasis. *Eur. J. Radiol.* **2014**, *83*, 783–787. [CrossRef]
22. Ding, Y.; Hazle, J.D.; Mohamed, A.S.; Frank, S.J.; Hobbs, B.P.; Colen, R.R.; Gunn, G.B.; Wang, J.; Kalpathy-Cramer, J.; Garden, A.S.; et al. Intravoxel incoherent motion imaging kinetics during chemoradiotherapy for human papillomavirus-associated squamous cell carcinoma of the oropharynx: Preliminary results from a prospective pilot study. *NMR Biomed.* **2015**. [CrossRef] [PubMed]
23. Paudyal, R.; Oh, J.H.; Riaz, N.; Venigalla, P.; Li, J.; Hatzoglou, V.; Leeman, J.; Nunez, D.A.; Lu, Y.; Deasy, J.O.; et al. Intravoxel incoherent motion diffusion-weighted MRI during chemoradiation therapy to characterize and monitor treatment response in human papillomavirus head and neck squamous cell carcinoma. *J. Magn. Reson. Imaging* **2017**, *45*, 1013–1023. [CrossRef]
24. Hou, B.L.; Hu, J. MRI and MRS of human brain tumors. *Methods Mol. Biol.* **2009**, *520*, 297–314. [CrossRef]
25. King, A.D.; Chow, S.K.; Yu, K.H.; Mo, F.K.; Yeung, D.K.; Yuan, J.; Law, B.K.; Bhatia, K.S.; Vlantis, A.C.; Ahuja, A.T. DCE-MRI for Pre-Treatment Prediction and Post-Treatment Assessment of Treatment Response in Sites of Squamous Cell Carcinoma in the Head and Neck. *PLoS ONE* **2015**, *10*, e0144770. [CrossRef]
26. Chawla, S.; Kim, S.; Dougherty, L.; Wang, S.; Loevner, L.A.; Quon, H.; Poptani, H. Pretreatment diffusion-weighted and dynamic contrast-enhanced MRI for prediction of local treatment response in squamous cell carcinomas of the head and neck. *AJR Am. J. Roentgenol.* **2013**, *200*, 35–43. [CrossRef] [PubMed]
27. Shukla-Dave, A.; Lee, N.Y.; Jansen, J.F.; Thaler, H.T.; Stambuk, H.E.; Fury, M.G.; Patel, S.G.; Moreira, A.L.; Sherman, E.; Karimi, S.; et al. Dynamic contrast-enhanced magnetic resonance imaging as a predictor of outcome in head-and-neck squamous cell carcinoma patients with nodal metastases. *Int. J. Radiat. Oncol. Biol. Phys.* **2012**, *82*, 1837–1844. [CrossRef] [PubMed]
28. Kim, S.; Loevner, L.A.; Quon, H.; Kilger, A.; Sherman, E.; Weinstein, G.; Chalian, A.; Poptani, H. Prediction of response to chemoradiation therapy in squamous cell carcinomas of the head and neck using dynamic contrast-enhanced MR imaging. *AJNR Am. J. Neuroradiol.* **2010**, *31*, 262–268. [CrossRef]
29. Quon, H.; Kim, S.; Loevner, L.; Rosen, M.; Sherman, E.; Kilger, A.; Poptani, H. DCE-MRI perfusion imaging of head and neck squamous cell carcinoma nodal metastasis: Identifying radioresistance and the distant metastatic phenotype. *J. Clin. Oncol.* **2008**, *26*, 6041. [CrossRef]
30. Nath, K.; Paudyal, R.; Nelson, D.; Pickup, S.; Zhou, R.; Leeper, D.; Heitjan, D.; Poptani, H.; Glickson, J. Acute changes in cellular-interstitial water exchange rate in DB-1 melanoma xenografts after lonidamine administration as a marker of tumor energetics and ion transport. *Proc. Intl. Soc. Mag. Reson. Med.* **2014**, *22*, 2757.
31. Springer, C.S., Jr.; Li, X.; Tudorica, L.A.; Oh, K.Y.; Roy, N.; Chui, S.Y.; Naik, A.M.; Holtorf, M.L.; Afzal, A.; Rooney, W.D.; et al. Intratumor mapping of intracellular water lifetime: Metabolic images of breast cancer? *NMR Biomed.* **2014**, *27*, 760–773. [CrossRef]
32. Chawla, S.; Loevner, L.A.; Kim, S.G.; Hwang, W.T.; Wang, S.; Verma, G.; Mohan, S.; LiVolsi, V.; Quon, H.; Poptani, H. Dynamic Contrast-Enhanced MRI-Derived Intracellular Water Lifetime (tau i): A Prognostic Marker for Patients with Head and Neck Squamous Cell Carcinomas. *AJNR Am. J. Neuroradiol.* **2018**, *39*, 138–144. [CrossRef]
33. Choi, S.H.; Paeng, J.C.; Sohn, C.H.; Pagsisihan, J.R.; Kim, Y.J.; Kim, K.G.; Jang, J.Y.; Yun, T.J.; Kim, J.H.; Han, M.H.; et al. Correlation of 18F-FDG uptake with apparent diffusion coefficient ratio measured on standard and high b value diffusion MRI in head and neck cancer. *J. Nucl. Med.* **2011**, *52*, 1056–1062. [CrossRef] [PubMed]

34. Nakamatsu, S.; Matsusue, E.; Miyoshi, H.; Kakite, S.; Kaminou, T.; Ogawa, T. Correlation of apparent diffusion coefficients measured by diffusion-weighted MR imaging and standardized uptake values from FDG PET/CT in metastatic neck lymph nodes of head and neck squamous cell carcinomas. *Clin. Imaging* **2012**, *36*, 90–97. [CrossRef] [PubMed]
35. Zwirner, K.; Thorwarth, D.; Winter, R.M.; Welz, S.; Weiss, J.; Schwenzer, N.F.; Schmidt, H.; la Fougere, C.; Nikolaou, K.; Zips, D.; et al. Voxel-wise correlation of functional imaging parameters in HNSCC patients receiving PET/MRI in an irradiation setup. *Strahlenther. Onkol.* **2018**, *194*, 719–726. [CrossRef] [PubMed]
36. Jansen, J.F.; Schoder, H.; Lee, N.Y.; Wang, Y.; Pfister, D.G.; Fury, M.G.; Stambuk, H.E.; Humm, J.L.; Koutcher, J.A.; Shukla-Dave, A. Noninvasive assessment of tumor microenvironment using dynamic contrast-enhanced magnetic resonance imaging and 18F-fluoromisonidazole positron emission tomography imaging in neck nodal metastases. *Int. J. Radiat. Oncol. Biol. Phys.* **2010**, *77*, 1403–1410. [CrossRef]
37. Wiedenmann, N.; Grosu, A.L.; Buchert, M.; Rischke, H.C.; Ruf, J.; Bielak, L.; Majerus, L.; Ruhle, A.; Bamberg, F.; Baltas, D.; et al. The utility of multiparametric MRI to characterize hypoxic tumor subvolumes in comparison to FMISO PET/CT. Consequences for diagnosis and chemoradiation treatment planning in head and neck cancer. *Radiother. Oncol. J. Eur. Soc. Ther. Radiol. Oncol.* **2020**, *150*, 128–135. [CrossRef] [PubMed]
38. Girvan, M.; Newman, M.E. Community structure in social and biological networks. *Proc. Natl. Acad. Sci. USA* **2002**, *99*, 7821–7826. [CrossRef] [PubMed]
39. Reichardt, J.; Bornholdt, S. Statistical mechanics of community detection. *Phys. Rev. E* **2006**, *74*, 016110. [CrossRef]
40. Grkovski, M.; Schoder, H.; Lee, N.Y.; Carlin, S.D.; Beattie, B.J.; Riaz, N.; Leeman, J.E.; O'Donoghue, J.A.; Humm, J.L. Multiparametric Imaging of Tumor Hypoxia and Perfusion with (18)F-Fluoromisonidazole Dynamic PET in Head and Neck Cancer. *J. Nucl. Med.* **2017**, *58*, 1072–1080. [CrossRef]
41. Beichel, R.R.; Smith, B.J.; Bauer, C.; Ulrich, E.J.; Ahmadvand, P.; Budzevich, M.M.; Gillies, R.J.; Goldgof, D.; Grkovski, M.; Hamarneh, G. Multi-site quality and variability analysis of 3D FDG PET segmentations based on phantom and clinical image data. *Med. Phys.* **2017**, *44*, 479–496. [CrossRef]
42. Paudyal, R.; Konar, A.S.; Obuchowski, N.A.; Hatzoglou, V.; Chenevert, T.L.; Malyarenko, D.I.; Swanson, S.D.; LoCastro, E.; Jambawalikar, S.; Liu, M.Z.; et al. Repeatability of Quantitative Diffusion-Weighted Imaging Metrics in Phantoms, Head-and-Neck and Thyroid Cancers: Preliminary Findings. *Tomogr. A J. Imaging Res.* **2019**, *5*, 15–25. [CrossRef]
43. Yankeelov, T.E.; Rooney, W.D.; Li, X.; Springer, C.S., Jr. Variation of the relaxographic "shutter-speed" for transcytolemmal water exchange affects the CR bolus-tracking curve shape. *Magn. Reson. Med.* **2003**, *50*, 1151–1169. [CrossRef] [PubMed]
44. Paudyal, R.; Bagher-Ebadian, H.; Nagaraja, T.N.; Fenstermacher, J.D.; Ewing, J.R. Modeling of Look-Locker estimates of the magnetic resonance imaging estimate of longitudinal relaxation rate in tissue after contrast administration. *Magn. Reson. Med.* **2011**, *66*, 1432–1444. [CrossRef]
45. McConnell, H.M. Reaction Rates by Nuclear Magnetic Resonance. *J. Chem. Phys.* **1958**, *28*, 430–431. [CrossRef]
46. Paudyal, R.; Poptani, H.; Cai, K.; Zhou, R.; Glickson, J.D. Impact of transvascular and cellular–interstitial water exchange on dynamic contrast-enhanced magnetic resonance imaging estimates of blood to tissue transfer constant and blood plasma volume. *J. Magn. Reson. Imaging* **2013**, *37*, 435–444. [CrossRef] [PubMed]
47. Schneider, C.A.; Rasband, W.S.; Eliceiri, K.W. NIH Image to ImageJ: 25 years of image analysis. *Nat. Methods* **2012**, *9*, 671–675. [CrossRef]
48. Shukla-Dave, A.; Lee, N.; Stambuk, H.; Wang, Y.; Huang, W.; Thaler, H.T.; Patel, S.G.; Shah, J.P.; Koutcher, J.A. Average arterial input function for quantitative dynamic contrast enhanced magnetic resonance imaging of neck nodal metastases. *BMC Med. Phys.* **2009**, *9*, 4. [CrossRef]
49. Lu, Y.; Jansen, J.F.; Mazaheri, Y.; Stambuk, H.E.; Koutcher, J.A.; Shukla-Dave, A. Extension of the intravoxel incoherent motion model to non-gaussian diffusion in head and neck cancer. *J. Magn. Reson. Imaging* **2012**, *36*, 1088–1096. [CrossRef]
50. Paudyal, R.; Chen, L.; Oh, J.; Zakeri, K.; Hatzoglou, V.; Tsai, C.; Lee, N.; Shukla-Dave, A. Nongaussian intravoxel Incoherent motion diffusion weighted and fast exchange regime dynamic contrast-enhanced-MRI of nasopharyngeal carcinoma: Preliminary study for predicting locoregional failure. *Cancers* **2021**, *15*, 1158. [CrossRef]
51. LoCastro, E.; Paudyal, R.; Mazaheri, Y.; Hatzoglou, V.; Oh, J.H.; Lu, Y.; Konar, A.S.; Vom Eigen, K.; Ho, A.; Ewing, J.R.; et al. Computational Modeling of Interstitial Fluid Pressure and Velocity in Head and Neck Cancer Based on Dynamic Contrast-Enhanced Magnetic Resonance Imaging: Feasibility Analysis. *Tomogr. A J. Imaging Res.* **2020**, *6*, 129–138. [CrossRef]
52. Bagher-Ebadian, H.; Jain, R.; Nejad-Davarani, S.P.; Mikkelsen, T.; Lu, M.; Jiang, Q.; Scarpace, L.; Arbab, A.S.; Narang, J.; Soltanian-Zadeh, H.; et al. Model selection for DCE-T1 studies in glioblastoma. *Magn. Reson. Med.* **2012**, *68*, 241–251. [CrossRef] [PubMed]
53. Newman, M.E.J. Detecting community structure in networks. *Eur Phys. J. B* **2004**, *38*, 321–330. [CrossRef]
54. R Development Core Team. *A Language and Environment for Statistical Computing*; R Foundation for Statistical Computing: Vienna, Austria, 2020; Available online: http://www.R-project.org.
55. Nakajo, M.; Nakajo, M.; Kajiya, Y.; Tani, A.; Kamiyama, T.; Yonekura, R.; Fukukura, Y.; Matsuzaki, T.; Nishimoto, K.; Nomoto, M.; et al. FDG PET/CT and Diffusion-Weighted Imaging of Head and Neck Squamous Cell Carcinoma Comparison of Prognostic Significance Between Primary Tumor Standardized Uptake Value and Apparent Diffusion Coefficient. *Clin. Nucl. Med.* **2012**, *37*, 475–480. [CrossRef]

56. Aramburu, D.N.; Medina, A.L.; Iglesias, M.M.; Gomez, F.S.; Dave, A.; Hatzoglou, V.; Paudyal, R.; Calzado, A.; Deasy, J.O.; Shukla-Dave, A.; et al. Multimodality functional imaging using DW-MRI and F-18-FDG-PET/CT during radiation therapy for human papillomavirus negative head and neck squamous cell carcinoma: Meixoeiro Hospital of Vigo Experience. *World J. Radiol.* **2017**, *9*, 17–26. [CrossRef]
57. Inglese, M.; Cavaliere, C.; Monti, S.; Forte, E.; Incoronato, M.; Nicolai, E.; Salvatore, M.; Aiello, M. A multi-parametric PET/MRI study of breast cancer: Evaluation of DCE-MRI pharmacokinetic models and correlation with diffusion and functional parameters. *NMR Biomed.* **2019**, *32*, e4026. [CrossRef] [PubMed]
58. Hectors, S.J.; Wagner, M.; Besa, C.; Huang, W.; Taouli, B. Multiparametric FDG-PET/MRI of Hepatocellular Carcinoma: Initial Experience. *Contrast Media Mol. Imaging* **2018**, *2018*, 5638283. [CrossRef]
59. Chen, T.C.; Wu, C.T.; Ko, J.Y.; Yang, T.L.; Lou, P.J.; Wang, C.P.; Chang, Y.L. Clinical characteristics and treatment outcome of oropharyngeal squamous cell carcinoma in an endemic betel quid region. *Sci. Rep.* **2020**, *10*, 526. [CrossRef]
60. O'Sullivan, B.; Huang, S.H.; Siu, L.L.; Waldron, J.; Zhao, H.; Perez-Ordonez, B.; Weinreb, I.; Kim, J.; Ringash, J.; Bayley, A.; et al. Deintensification candidate subgroups in human papillomavirus-related oropharyngeal cancer according to minimal risk of distant metastasis. *J. Clin. Oncol.* **2013**, *31*, 543–550. [CrossRef]
61. Koch, C.J.; Jenkins, W.T.; Jenkins, K.W.; Yang, X.Y.; Shuman, A.L.; Pickup, S.; Riehl, C.R.; Paudyal, R.; Poptani, H.; Evans, S.M. Mechanisms of blood flow and hypoxia production in rat 9L-epigastric tumors. *Tumor Microenviron. Ther.* **2013**, *1*, 1–13. [CrossRef]
62. Asgari, H.; Soltani, M.; Sefidgar, M. Modeling of FMISO [F(18)] nanoparticle PET tracer in normal-cancerous tissue based on real clinical image. *Microvasc. Res.* **2018**, *118*, 20–30. [CrossRef] [PubMed]
63. Gertsenshteyn, I.; Epel, B.; Barth, E.; Leoni, L.; Markiewicz, E.; Tsai, H.M.; Fan, X.; Giurcanu, M.; Bodero, D.; Zamora, M.; et al. Improving Tumor Hypoxia Location in (18)F-Misonidazole PET with Dynamic Contrast-enhanced MRI Using Quantitative Electron Paramagnetic Resonance Partial Oxygen Pressure Images. *Radiol. Imaging Cancer* **2021**, *3*, e200104. [CrossRef] [PubMed]

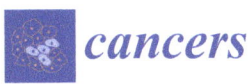

Article

HPV Infection Leaves a DNA Methylation Signature in Oropharyngeal Cancer Affecting Both Coding Genes and Transposable Elements

Diego Camuzi [1,†], Luisa Aguirre Buexm [1,†], Simone de Queiroz Chaves Lourenço [2], Davide Degli Esposti [3], Cyrille Cuenin [3], Monique de Souza Almeida Lopes [1], Francesca Manara [3], Fazlur Rahman Talukdar [3], Zdenko Herceg [3], Luis Felipe Ribeiro Pinto [1] and Sheila Coelho Soares-Lima [1,*]

[1] Molecular Carcinogenesis Program, Brazilian National Cancer Institute, Rio de Janeiro CEP 20231-050, Brazil; camuzi.diego@gmail.com (D.C.); labuexm@id.uff.br (L.A.B.); monique.lopes@inca.gov.br (M.d.S.A.L.); lfrpinto@inca.gov.br (L.F.R.P.)
[2] Department of Pathology, Dental School, Fluminense Federal University, Rua Mario Santos Braga, 30, Centro, Niterói CEP 24040-110, Brazil; silourenco@id.uff.br
[3] Epigenetics Group, International Agency for Research on Cancer, 150 Cours Albert Thomas, CEDEX 08, 69372 Lyon, France; davide.degli-esposti@inrae.fr (D.D.E.); cuenin@iarc.fr (C.C.); manaraf@students.iarc.fr (F.M.); TalukdarF@fellows.iarc.fr (F.R.T.); HercegZ@iarc.fr (Z.H.)
* Correspondence: sheila.lima@inca.gov.br or sheilacoelho@gmail.com; Tel.: +55-213-207-6520
† Co-first author, these authors contributed equally to this work.

Simple Summary: The HPV oncoproteins E6 and E7 can modulate the expression and activity of the maintenance DNA methyltransferase 1, suggesting that HPV carcinogenic mechanisms may include aberrant DNA methylation. Some studies previously proposed both gene-associated DNA methylation signatures and a global hypermethylation profile in HPV-positive head and neck cancer, but the validation of such signatures and a more detailed analysis of the methylation profile of transposable elements (TEs) in oropharyngeal squamous cell carcinoma (OPSCC) are still missing. TEs account for approximately 50% of the human genome and their hypomethylation and reactivation have been consistently reported in cancer, usually being associated with worse prognosis. Based on this, this study aimed at validating a previously established 5-CpG methylation signature in FFPE OPSCC from a middle-income population, in which the frequency of HPV infection is only 6.1%, and dissecting the methylation profile of TEs, focusing on their impact on gene expression and overall survival.

Abstract: HPV oncoproteins can modulate DNMT1 expression and activity, and previous studies have reported both gene-specific and global DNA methylation alterations according to HPV status in head and neck cancer. However, validation of these findings and a more detailed analysis of the transposable elements (TEs) are still missing. Here we performed pyrosequencing to evaluate a 5-CpG methylation signature and Line1 methylation in an oropharyngeal squamous cell carcinoma (OPSCC) cohort. We further evaluated the methylation levels of the TEs, their correlation with gene expression and their impact on overall survival (OS) using the TCGA cohort. In our dataset, the 5-CpG signature distinguished HPV-positive and HPV-negative OPSCC with 66.67% sensitivity and 84.33% specificity. Line1 methylation levels were higher in HPV-positive cases. In the TCGA cohort, Line1, Alu and long terminal repeats (LTRs) showed hypermethylation in a frequency of 60.5%, 58.9% and 92.3%, respectively. *ZNF541* and *CCNL1* higher expression was observed in HPV-positive OPSCC, correlated with lower methylation levels of promoter-associated Alu and LTR, respectively, and independently associated with better OS. Based on our findings, we may conclude that a 5-CpG methylation signature can discriminate OPSCC according to HPV status with high accuracy and TEs are differentially methylated and may regulate gene expression in HPV-positive OPSCC.

Keywords: oropharyngeal squamous cell carcinoma; HPV; DNA methylation; transposable elements; gene expression; overall survival

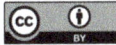

1. Introduction

Head and neck squamous cell carcinomas (HNSCC) comprise aggressive malignant neoplasms often late diagnosed with already high local invasion and metastatic dissemination [1,2]. However, given the awareness that Human Papillomavirus (HPV) infection is an important etiological factor correlating with a better therapeutic response and prognosis compared to the HPV-negative counterpart (mostly related to tobacco and alcohol), an in-depth investigation of the most relevant infection-related molecular signatures may provide new opportunities for early diagnosis and targeted therapeutic interventions [3]. HPV-positive HNSCC already represents an epidemic in high-income countries, while in low- and middle-income countries the numbers are expected to increase [4–7].

HPVs are known double-strand DNA tumor viruses, with a tropism for the basal layer of squamous epithelia, in which the completion of the viral life cycle is highly coordinated with the host keratinocyte differentiation program [8]. Among the more than 200 existing HPVs, high-risk genotype (such as HPV16 and HPV18) persistent infections progress into cancer, and in the majority of HPV-driven carcinomas, type 16 is involved [9]. Most of the HPV16-induced head and neck cancers affect the palatine tonsils, that often metastasize to nearby lymph nodes [10,11]. Crucial in the pathogenesis of HPV-driven carcinomas is the expression of early genes-encoded E6 and E7 oncoproteins which, by targeting host cell tumor suppressors p53 and pRB, provide the infected keratinocyte with a growth advantage, with enhanced proliferation rate, impaired apoptosis and progressive immune evasion [12,13]. In addition, HPV E6 and E7 can also disrupt cancer-related gene expression patterns by altering host cell transcriptional programs epigenetically, e.g., by modulating DNA methyltransferase activity [14].

DNA methylation is an epigenetic mechanism of gene expression control, and its dysregulation has been largely reported in cancer [15–17]. DNA methylation reactions are catalyzed by DNMTs, which in humans include four different enzymes [18]. DNMT3L lacks catalytic activity, while DNMT3A and 3B are classified as de novo DNMTs, by their capacity of methylating previously unmethylated CpG sites [18]. DNMT1, contrarily, is responsible for the maintenance of DNA methylation marks in the newly synthesized strand during DNA replication [18]. Both E6 and E7 oncoproteins affect the expression of DNMT1 (either through complex formation with E7 or as a consequence of E6-induced p53 suppression), but also of DNMT3A and DNMT3B [19–23]. As we recently showed, DNA methylation signatures are capable of discriminating HPV-positive and HPV-negative HNSCC, and given the different prognosis, a thorough investigation of potentially useful biomarkers allowing more effective therapeutic approaches is essential [24,25].

Although some studies reported a genome-wide hypermethylation profile based on the evaluation of transposable elements (TEs) [22,26–28], we showed that, in an analysis directed to gene regions, hypomethylation is more common in HPV-positive tumors relative to HPV-negative counterparts (58% and 65%, when considering differentially methylated positions and regions, respectively) [24]. This led to the identification of a 5-CpG methylation signature able to discriminate tumors according to HPV status, but the accuracy of this signature to identify HPV-driven carcinogenesis in specific tissues was not tested due to limited sample sizes.

Another important aspect yet to be investigated is the extension of the genome-wide hypermethylation profile reported in HPV-positive tumors. So far, degenerate assays for assessing Line and Alu elements methylation levels have been applied, highlighting the need for a more detailed evaluation of which TEs are dysregulated. This is especially relevant, since global hypomethylation was already associated with genomic instability and relapse in HNSCC [27,28], representing a promising biomarker. Furthermore, transposable elements also include the so-far neglected in HSCNC Long Terminal Repeat (LTR) elements, whose relevance for tumor development is starting to be unveiled [29].

In the present study, we were interested in evaluating gene-specific and global DNA methylation differences in OPSCC according to HPV status. We validated the previously proposed 5-CpG methylation signature of HPV infection in oropharyngeal squamous cell carcinoma (OPSCC) and confirmed the hypermethylation of Line1 TE in HPV-positive tumors. This led us to further dissect the methylation status of TEs, showing that, although hypermethylation is in general more common, hypomethylation is also observed. Finally, the methylation levels of gene-associated TEs were correlated with mRNA expression and impact patients overall survival, independently of HPV status.

2. Materials and Methods

2.1. OPSCC Cohort

In this study, a previously characterized [7] OPSCC cohort from the Brazilian National Cancer Institute (INCA, Rio de Janeiro, Brazil) was used. Briefly, 346 patients with a confirmed diagnosis of OPSCC between 1999–2010 were included and tumor samples were collected before any treatment. Patients' clinical and sociodemographic information was retrieved from medical records. The median follow-up of the patients was 10.75 months. Tumor specimens were formalin-fixed and paraffin-embedded (FFPE) and representative samples from each individual were evaluated by two independent pathologists. HPV status was considered positive when a strong p16, with diffuse nuclear and cytoplasmic staining in more than 70% of the tumor cells (determined by immunohistochemistry, IHC) was observed, and HPV16 E6 DNA was detected by quantitative-PCR (qPCR). Only samples positive for the two techniques were considered HPV-positive. All other combinations, p16 negative/E6 negative, p16 positive/E6 negative, and p16 negative/E6 positive, were considered HPV-negative. This study was approved by the local Ethics Committee (60480316.0.0000.5274).

2.2. DNA Methylation Analyses

DNA extraction was performed and quality and quantity were assessed as previously described [7]. A total of 500 ng of genomic DNA were treated with sodium bisulfite (EpiTect Bisulfite Kit, Qiagen, Hilden, Germany) according to the manufacturer's instructions. PCR reactions were performed to amplify the regions of interest using Platinum Taq DNA Polymerase (Invitrogen). PCR conditions as well as primer sequences can be found in Supplementary Materials Table S1.

After confirming amplification by amplicon visualization in 2% agarose gels, PCR products were pyrosequenced using PyroMark Gold Q96 Reagents (Qiagen) in a PyroMark Q96 ID system (Qiagen, Hilden, Germany). Sequencing primers can be found in Table S1. After the reaction, intensity peaks were converted to numerical values, and the methylation level of each CpG site was calculated. For the 5-CpG methylation signature, the mean methylation of the 5 CpGs analyzed (marked in bold red in Table S1) was calculated for each sample. For Line1 analysis, 5 CpG sites were assessed and the methylation levels of this TE for each patient are represented as the mean of all sites.

2.3. TCGA Data

Data from The Cancer Genome Atlas (TCGA) patients of the TCGA-HNSC project were retrieved. Only patients with tumors in the tonsils, base of the tongue, and oropharynx were included, totalizing 79 cases. HPV status was determined according to http://firebrowse.org/ (last accessed 10 August 2020). Patient's clinical and sociodemographic characteristics and *CCNL1* amplification status were downloaded from cBioPortal (last accessed 7 April 2021). The median follow-up of the patients was 19.78 months in this cohort.

Expression data generated by RNA-sequencing, and methylation data generated by microarray (Infinium Human Methylation 450 K BeadChip) were obtained with the TCGAbiolinks package (v2.16.1). Normalized expression data was downloaded as fragments per kilobase million (FPKM). The raw methylation data (.idats files) were processed with the ChAMP package (v2.18.2), and the following filters were applied to remove bad quality probes: low quality probes (detection p-value > 0.05), cross-reactive and polymorphic probes [30]. Then, color adjustments (Lumi [31]) and normalization (BMIQ method) were applied.

2.4. Methylation Prediction of Repetitive Elements and Methylation Difference Analysis

The prediction analysis of the methylation levels of the transposable elements was performed with the REMP package (Repetitive Element Methylation Prediction, v1.12.0) [32] using the methylation beta values. The database for annotating repetitive elements (Line1, Alu and LTRs) was created with the initREMP function, with the UCSC data source and hg19 as the reference genome. Methylation values were preprocessed using the grooMethy function, default settings. The prediction of the elements was made by Random Forest method, with a window of 1000 bp and seed of 777. After prediction, we applied a quality filter on the elements (rempTrim function) of 1.7 and elements with a missing rate in at least 20% of the samples were removed. The methylation levels of the elements were then calculated considering elements with at least two predicted CpG methylation values (rempAggregate function).

The differential methylation analysis of the TEs between HPV-positive and HPV-negative tumors was carried out for each type of element independently with the limma package (v3.44.3) using the methylation M-value of the elements. The adjustment for multiple tests was made by the Benjamini–Hochberg FDR (BH) method.

2.5. Statistical Analyses

Statistical analyses were run in an R environment or in GraphPad Prism 5 software (GraphPad Software, San Diego, CA, USA). The correlation between the methylation levels of the TEs mapped to promoter regions and the expression of the associated genes was performed by Spearman's test. Comparisons between groups were performed using the Mann–Whitney test. When necessary, p-value adjustment was performed by the BH method. All these analyses were made with base (v4.0.5) and stats (v4.0.5) R packages.

Survival analyses were performed with survival (v3.2-3) and plotted with survminer (v0.4.7) packages. For survival analyses based on gene expression, the upregulated and downregulated expression groups were determined using the median expression value for each gene in all samples. Samples with expression > median were considered upregulated and samples with expression ≤ median were downregulated. Following the same approach, for the survival analysis based on Line1 methylation, hypomethylated (≤median methylation levels in all samples) and hypermethylated (>median methylation levels in all samples) cases were defined. For the estimative of univariate survival, the Kaplan–Meier survival curve was used, and statistical significance was calculated by the log-rank test. Multivariate Cox regression was applied to adjust survival for HPV status. Statistical significance was defined when $p < 0.05$.

3. Results

3.1. HPV Infection Is Associated with a Specific DNA Methylation Signature and Global Methylation in OPSCC

In this study, we used a previously characterized cohort of OPSCC patients that showed a low frequency of HPV-positive cases (6.1%), assessed by both p16 IHC and HPV DNA detection by qPCR [7]. Our data show that the mean methylation levels of 5 CpG sites located at B3GALT6-SDF4, SYCP2-FAM217B, and HLTF-HLTF-AS1 loci [24] are lower in HPV-positive relative to HPV-negative tumors (median of 60.62% vs. 78.07%, $p < 0.001$, Figure 1A). The DNA methylation levels of each CpG site composing the signature are shown in Figure S1. After applying the previously suggested DNA methylation cut-off (<75%) [24], this 5-CpG signature was able to discriminate OPSCC according to HPV status with 80.95% sensitivity and 61.2% specificity. Since the methylation cut-off was previously determined in HNSCC in general, and the sample source differed from the present study (fresh-frozen and FFPE, respectively), we applied a receiver operating characteristic (ROC) curve analysis to test new cut-offs in our experimental settings (Figure 1B). This analysis showed that with a DNA methylation cut-off of 62.85%, the methylation signature was able to discriminate the groups with 66.67% sensitivity and 84.33% specificity ($p = 0.0001$, Figure 1B).

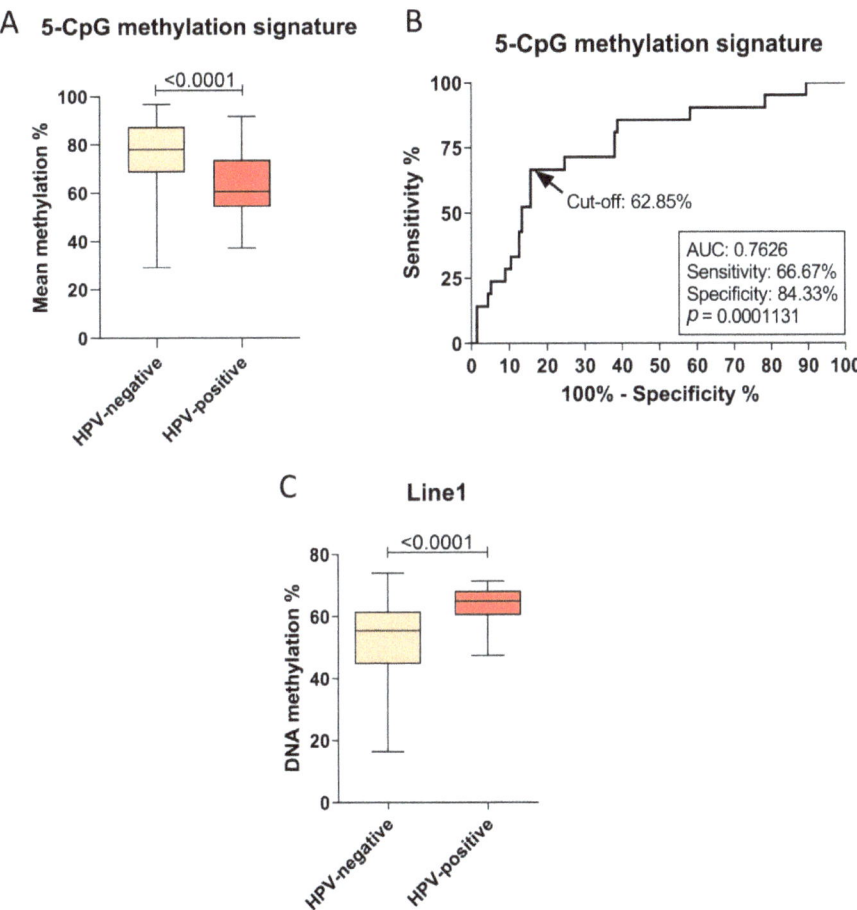

Figure 1. DNA methylation signatures of HPV-positive OPSCC. (**A**) Boxplot showing the mean methylation of 5 CpG sites in *B3GALT6-SDF4*, *SYCP2-FAM217B*, and *HLTF-HLTF-AS1* loci assessed by pyrosequencing in HPV-positive ($n = 21$) and HPV-negative ($n = 134$) OPSCC. (**B**) Receiver operating characteristic (ROC) curve showing the best DNA methylation cut-off of the 5-CpG signature to distinguish HPV-positive and HPV-negative OPSCC. (**C**) Boxplot showing the methylation levels of Line1 transposable element assessed by pyrosequencing in HPV-positive ($n = 21$) and HPV-negative ($n = 325$) OPSCC.

Apart from gene-specific signatures, HPV infection was also previously associated with global methylation dysregulation [22,26–28]. To test this hypothesis, we assessed Line1 methylation in our sample set. Figure 1C shows that Line1 methylation levels are higher in HPV-positive relative to HPV-negative OPSCC (median of 64.89% vs. 55.47%, $p < 0.0001$, Figure 1C). However, overall survival (OS) of the cases did not differ according to Line1 methylation levels (Figure S2).

Although Line1 elements have been assessed as a proxy of global methylation, other transposable elements also represent an important percentage of the human genome, including Alu and LTRs. These elements can be found both in intergenic and intragenic regions, and their methylation levels may impact prognosis. Based on this, we next evaluated the methylation levels of all these elements in OPSCC.

3.2. Transposable Elements Are Differentially Methylated According to HPV Status in OPSCC

We extracted DNA methylation information of TEs from TCGA OPSCC cohort and compared each individual element according to HPV status. Our data show that a total of 172 TEs are differentially methylated in HPV-positive relative to HPV-negative tumors (BH adjusted *p*-value ≤ 0.01), with hypermethylation being more commonly observed in HPV-positive cases. The frequency, however, varied according to TE type (Figure 2A), for Alu and Line1 a similar proportion of hypermethylated elements was observed (58.9% and 60.5%, respectively), while for LTRs this proportion was higher (92.3%).

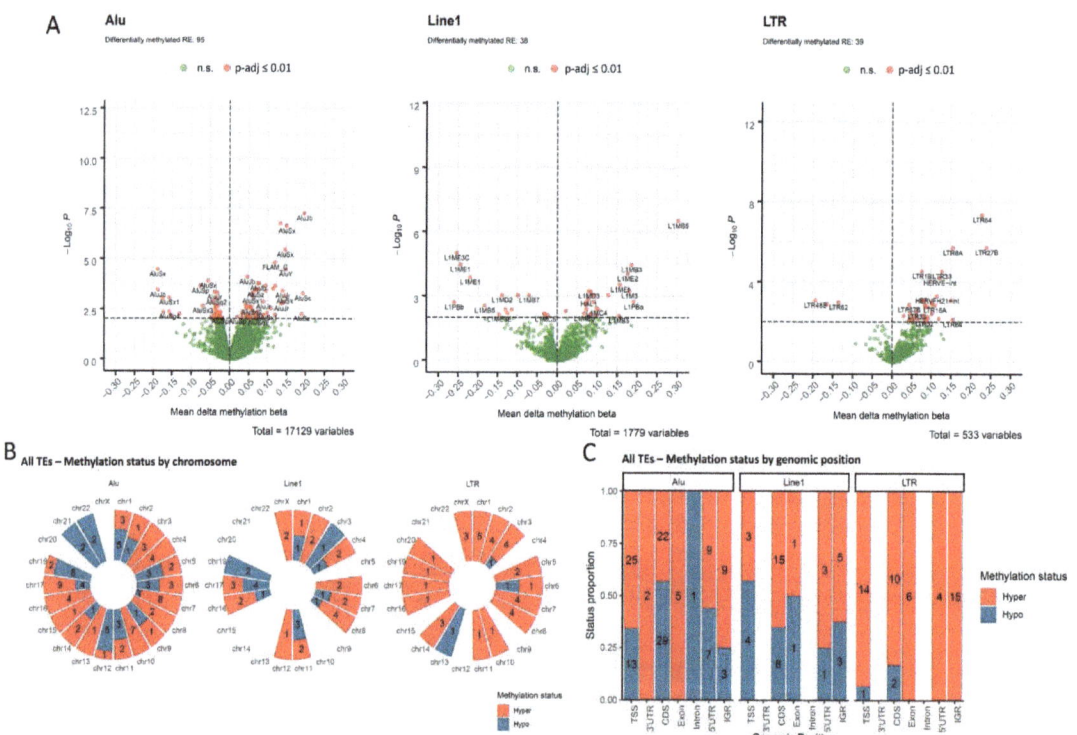

Figure 2. Transposable elements are differentially methylated in OPSCC according to HPV status. (**A**) Volcano plots showing the Line1, Alu and LTR elements differentially methylated in HPV-positive relative to HPV-negative OPSCC. The X-axis shows the mean beta value differences (mean methylation delta) between groups and the Y-axis shows the -Log Benjamini-Hochberg (BH) adjusted *p*-values. Red dots represent elements with BH adjusted *p*-value ≤ 0.01. (**B**) Chromosomal distribution and (**C**) genomic region distribution of hypermethylated (red) and hypomethylated (blue) Line1, Alu and LTR elements in HPV-positive relative to HPV-negative OPSCC. The same TE may encompass more than one genomic region.

Differentially methylated TEs were not individually enriched in any specific chromosome (Figure 2B). The stratification by genomic region reproduced the overall profile, with most of the elements showing hypermethylation in HPV-positive OPSCC in any given region (Figure 2C). The exceptions were Alu elements located in coding sequences and Line1 elements located in promoters (up to 2000 bp from transcription start sites), with 56.9% and 57.1% of the differentially methylated elements showing hypomethylation, respectively (Figure 2C). Alu, Line1 and LTR mapped to intergenic regions were mostly hypermethylated in HPV-positive relative to HPV-negative tumors (75%, 62.5% and 100%, respectively).

3.3. The Methylation Levels of Transposable Elements Mapped to Promoter Regions Are Correlated with Expression and Prognosis

Figure 3A shows the methylation profile of TEs mapped to promoter regions. Since this analysis indicated a heterogeneous profile among HPV-positive cases, we performed unsupervised clustering of these tumors (Figure S3). Although two DNA methylation clusters were identified, they were not associated with age, tobacco smoking, tumor stage or location.

We next evaluated whether DNA methylation alterations in TEs mapped to promoters were associated with gene expression. For Alu elements, the methylation levels of 13 out of 32 elements (40.6%) showed a significant correlation with the mRNA expression of the associated gene (Figure 3A). The correlation was inverse for *SNORD99*, *SLC44A2*, *ZNF541*, *NNMT*, *ZNF622* and *TSPAN10*, and positive for *ACOT7*, *TCAMP1*, *SPACA4*, *SLC45A4*, *GPLD1* and *CRACD*. From a total of six differentially methylated Line1 elements mapped to promoter regions, two (33.3%) showed a significant correlation with gene expression, being inverse for *TCEAL7* and positive for *NOTCH4* (Figure 3A). The methylation levels of LTR elements were also significantly correlated with expression in 26.7% of the genes (4 out of 15) (Figure 3A). The correlation was inverse for *CCNL1*, *MYOM3* and *MFAP2*, and positive for *TMEM67*.

Figure 3B shows the expression of those genes that showed a significant correlation with TEs methylation levels, according to HPV status in TCGA OPSCC cohort. Downregulated and hypermethylated genes in HPV-positive versus HPV-negative OPSCC included *TCEAL7*, *NNMT*, *TSPAN10*, *ZNF622*, *MYOM3* and *MFAP2*. *ACOT7* was also downregulated, but its promoter was hypomethylated in HPV-positive cases. Among the upregulated genes, *SLC44A2*, *ZNF541* and *CCNL1* were also hypomethylated, while *SPACA4*, *CRACD*, *SLC45A4*, *GPLD1*, *TCAMP1* and *TMEM67* were hypermethylated (Figure 3B). The correlation plots between DNA methylation and mRNA expression for *CCNL1* and *ZNF541* are shown in Figure S4.

Finally, the association between the expression of these genes and overall survival was assessed (Table S2). After adjustment for HPV status, patients with high *ZNF541* or *CCNL1* expression showed a median OS of 68.4 months vs. 47 months in the group with low expression (HR = 0.17, 95% CI 0.03–0.91 and HR = 0.34, 95% CI 0.13–0.93, respectively) (Figure 3C, Table S2). Since *CCNL1* amplification was previously associated with worse outcomes in head and neck cancer [33], we evaluated whether this could explain the differences we found in OPSCC. However, we did not observe a different frequency of *CCNL1* amplification according to HPV status (21% in HPV-negative and 18% in HPV-positive) nor a significant impact of *CCNL1* amplification on OS (Figure S5).

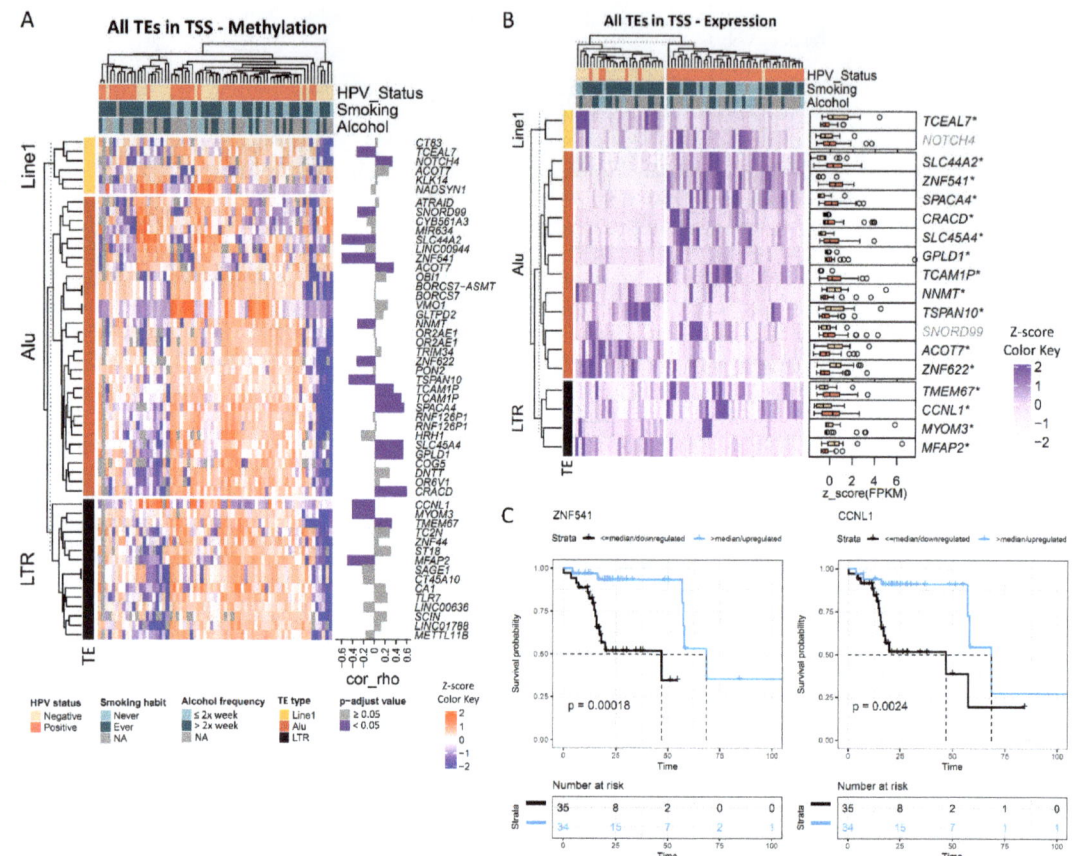

Figure 3. Differentially methylated transposable elements located at promoter regions show a correlation with gene expression and impact on prognosis. (**A**) Heatmap showing the unsupervised clustering of OPSCC TCGA samples according to the DNA methylation profile of transposable elements located up to 2000 bp of transcription start sites (promoter regions). Each line represents a transposable element and each column represents a sample. On the right, bar plots show the correlation rho (Spearman test) between the methylation levels of the element and the expression of the associated gene. Dark and light purple bars represent significant (BH adjusted $p < 0.05$) and nonsignificant correlations, respectively. (**B**) Heatmap showing the clustering of OPSCC TCGA samples according to the expression levels of genes correlated with the methylation levels of transposable elements in their promoter regions. Each line represents a transposable element and each column represents a sample. On the right, boxplots showing the expression of each gene in HPV-positive (dark pink) and HPV-negative (light pink) OPSCC. * Genes differentially expressed according to HPV status (BH adjusted $p < 0.05$). (**C**) Kaplan–Meier curves showing the overall survival of OPSCC patients from TCGA cohort according to the expression of *ZNF541* and *CCNL1*. High and low expression were defined according to the median expression of each gene in all samples.

4. Discussion

HPV oncoproteins were shown to modulate DNMT1 levels [19,20,34] and some studies have been developed to identify HPV-associated alterations of DNA methylation in cervical cancer [35–37]. This led to the design of gene panels whose methylation levels can discriminate tumors from non-tumor tissues as well as predict preneoplastic lesions more likely to progress, with high accuracy [35,38–40]. However, in head and neck cancer, the association between HPV infection and DNA methylation aberration has been less explored, both genome-wide and in target genes. Although DNA methylation signatures of infection and a global hypermethylation phenotype have been proposed in HNSCC [22,24–26,28], the validation of these signatures, and a more detailed characterization of the affected regions are still missing. Here we show that a previously proposed 5-CpG methylation signature can discriminate HPV-positive and HPV-negative OPSCC from a population with a low frequency of HPV positivity (which usually hampers biomarker sensitivity) and using a different sample source. We also show that transposable elements are mostly hypermethylated in HPV-positive relative to HPV-negative OPSCC. However, hypomethylated TEs mapped to promoter regions lead to the upregulation of associated genes, with an impact on OS, independent of HPV infection.

P16 IHC is the most widely used biomarker in the context of HPV-associated carcinogenesis. In a recent meta-analysis, its sensitivity and specificity to detect cervical intraepithelial neoplasia of grade 2 (CIN2$^+$), 3 or worse (CIN3$^+$) ranged from 82–86% and 49–71%, respectively [41]. When combined with Ki67 IHC, p16 showed a sensitivity of 75.2% to detected CIN2$^+$, compared to 61.0% achieved by cytology alone [42]. In HNSCC, p16 IHC sensitivity to detect HPV-positive cases is high (92%, 95% CI 82–97%), while its specificity seems to be moderate (72%, 95% CI 45–89%) [43]. In OPSCC, p16 was able to identify HPV-driven transformation with a sensitivity of 94% (95% CI 91–97%) and a specificity of 83% (95% CI 78–88%) [44]. Although the sensitivity of the 5-CpG methylation signature tested here was lower when compared to p16 IHC, we were able to reproduce the previous results obtained in high-income populations [24] in a middle-income population, in which the frequency of HPV-positive cases is more modest [7]. This was also the first time this signature established in all HNSCC subsites was tested in OPSCC and FFPE samples. This is relevant because an optimal biomarker should perform well independently of sample source or experimental assay. By assessing the methylation levels of a diagnostic signature in paired exfoliated cells and FFPE biopsies from women referred to colposcopy, Reuter and colleagues showed a correlation ranging from 0.379–0.550 between tests. FFPE cut-off adjustments were also necessary to improve the signature accuracy [45]. Therefore, the previously proposed HPV 5-CpG methylation signature is reproducible in OPSCC from a population with a low frequency of HPV infection and in FFPE, a more easily available source of tumor samples.

DNA methylation signatures have emerged as promising biomarkers in oncology capable of measuring risk factor exposure [35,46,47], discriminating different types of primary tumors [48,49], predicting the progression of preneoplastic lesions [50,51], predicting response to treatment and prognosis [35,52–54], and even detecting malignant tumors years before conventional diagnosis [55]. Although different DNA methylation signatures are usually assessed for different tissues and outcomes, a common feature of cancers is global hypomethylation [17,56,57], in general associated with poor OS [58–61]. Therefore, we also assessed this profile in our samples, and showed higher Line1 methylation levels in HPV-positive relative to HPV-negative OPSCC, corroborating previous data [22,26–28]. Although we did not observe an association between Line1 methylation levels and OS, it is important to mention that for the same population studied here, HPV was not associated with prognosis, likely due to the high frequency of smokers [7].

The association between global DNA hypomethylation and poor prognosis is usually linked to genomic instability [28,62–64]. Almost 50% of the human genome is composed of transposable elements, which are silenced by hypermethylation in normal cells [65,66]. During transformation, TEs lose methylation, and are therefore reactivated, leading to their mobilization [65,67]. Based on this, we evaluated whether the global hypermethylation in HPV-positive relative to HPV-negative OPSCC assessed by Line1 methylation was common to all TEs. In general, hypermethylation in HPV-positive tumors was observed for Line1, Alu and LTR. The frequency, however, differed among these classes of TEs. LTRs, which include the endogenous retrovirus (ERVs), showed the highest hypermethylation proportion. ERV activation by demethylating agents was shown to induce viral mimicry and, therefore, activate the immune response [68–70]. Since these elements were shown here to be widely hypermethylated in HPV-positive OPSCC, although speculative, this might be a mechanism by which HPV guarantees immune escape.

Although the majority of TEs are mapped to intergenic regions, their participation in regulating gene expression has been proposed [71]. Different mechanisms such as control of transcription by DNA methylation, chromatin remodeling, recruitment of transcription factors, generation of new isoforms, and even the regulation of translation put TEs as relevant regulators of cell behavior [66,71]. As an example, Line1 methylation was already associated with the regulation of the expression of genes with specialized functions, while SINEs methylation regulated the expression of genes involved in housekeeping activities in embryonic stem cells [72]. By assessing whether the methylation of these elements was correlated with gene expression, we showed a significant correlation for about one third of the genes analyzed. This was further corroborated by the differential expression of these genes in HPV-positive relative to HPV-negative OPSCC. These results suggest that the differential methylation of TEs according to HPV status may have an impact on tumor cells that goes beyond genetic instability.

Among the hypermethylated and downregulated genes, *TCEAL7* is a putative tumor suppressor gene downregulated by DNA methylation in ovarian cancer [73]. It associates with promoters containing MYC and NF-κB binding sites, such as *cyclin D1* promoter, repressing transcription. Therefore, *TCEAL7* downregulation was proposed as an alternative mechanism for the activation of MYC and NF-κB target genes [73,74]. NNMT upregulation was already reported in oral squamous cell carcinoma [75], but its downregulation was associated with increased sensitivity to 5-fluorouracil in esophageal squamous cell carcinoma cells [76]. In contrast, *MFAP2* upregulation was reported in head and neck cancer [77] and associated with poor prognosis in gastric and hepatocellular carcinomas [78,79]. Therefore, the downregulation of these genes in HPV-positive relative to HPV-negative OPSCC may contribute to the better prognosis and response to therapy observed in the first group of patients. Although an association between *ZNF622* and cancer has not been reported yet, its role as an antiviral protein upon adenovirus infection was proposed [80]. Based on these evidences, the dysregulation of gene expression via the differential methylation of TEs in HPV-positive OPSCC may contribute to successful HPV infection and carcinogenicity, but future studies are necessary to corroborate this hypothesis.

The expression of *ZNF541* and *CCNL1*, both upregulated and hypomethylated in HPV-positive cases, were associated with OS independently of HPV status. *ZNF541* encodes a zinc finger protein supposed to be a component of chromatin remodeling complexes and previously suggested to play a role in the differential expression of genes according to HPV status in cervical cancer tissues and cell lines [81]. *CCNL1* encodes Cyclin L1 and its role as an oncogene in head and neck cancer by promoting cell cycle entry was previously proposed [82]. The so far recognized mechanism behind *CCNL1* overexpression was gene amplification, which was associated with lymph node metastasis in HNSCC [33]. However, the expression differences we observed in OPSCC according to HPV status do not seem to be associated with *CCNL1* amplification, but with promoter-associated LTR methylation, suggesting a new mechanism behind its transcriptional regulation. Recently, *CCNL1* promoter differential methylation was associated with platinum resistance in ovarian cancer, but its impact on gene expression was not evaluated [83]. Therefore, our results bring a new connection between HPV infection, TEs methylation, regulation of gene expression and prognosis.

Finally, we also observed DNA methylation differences of promoter-associated TEs within HPV-positive cases, but no significant associations with age, tobacco smoking, tumor stage or location were found. However, the sample size included was limited and other biological mechanisms not evaluated here might contribute to these differences. For example, HPV integration was already associated with a specific DNA methylation signature in HNSCC [84]. Future studies are necessary to explore whether HPV integration also affects the methylation profile of transposable elements.

5. Conclusions

Here we validated a previously proposed 5-CpG methylation signature of HPV infection. This signature was originally established in head and neck cancer from high-income populations using snap frozen samples, and we were able to replicate the original findings in OPSCC from a middle-income population (which shows a frequency of HPV positivity of only 6.1%) using FFPE samples. We also showed that global methylation, estimated by Line1 assessment, is higher in HPV-positive relative to HPV-negative OPSCC. This led us to investigate the methylation profile of transposable elements in depth, showing that not only Line1, but also Alu and LTRs are hypermethylated in HPV-positive cases. However, the hypermethylation frequency varied according to TE class and genomic region. Finally, we evaluated the correlation between the methylation levels of TEs mapped to promoter regions and the expression of the associated genes, showing significant correlations for approximately one third of the genes. Among those genes differentially expressed according to HPV status, *ZNF541* and *CCNL1* (harboring Alu and LTR in their promoters, respectively) higher expression was significantly associated with a better overall survival, independent of HPV status.

Supplementary Materials: The following are available online at https://www.mdpi.com/article/10.3390/cancers13143621/s1, Figure S1: Boxplot showing the methylation levels of the individual CpG sites that compose the 5-CpG methylation signature, according to HPV status in INCA cohort. Figure S2: Kaplan–Meier plot showing the overall survival of OPSCC patients from our cohort according to Line1 methylation. Figure S3: DNA methylation profile of TEs mapped to promoters in HPV-positive OPSCC. Figure S4: Analysis of the correlation between the DNA methylation levels of the transposable elements mapped to the promoters of *CCNL1* and *ZNF541* and the mRNA expression of the associated genes in TCGA cohort. Figure S5: Kaplan–Meier plot showing the overall survival of OPSCC patients from TCGA cohort according to the presence of *CCNL1* amplification. Table S1: Primers sequences and PCR conditions used in the present study. Table S2: Multivariate Cox regression analysis of the impact of the expression of genes harboring transposable elements in their promoters on overall survival of OPSCC patients from TCGA cohort.

Author Contributions: Conceptualization, D.C., L.A.B., S.d.Q.C.L., Z.H., L.F.R.P. and S.C.S.-L.; methodology, D.C., L.A.B., D.D.E., C.C. and S.C.S.-L.; software, D.C., D.D.E. and F.R.T.; validation, D.C., L.A.B., D.D.E., C.C., M.d.S.A.L., F.M. and F.R.T.; formal analysis, D.C., L.A.B. and D.D.E.; investigation, D.C., L.A.B., M.d.S.A.L. and S.C.S.-L.; resources, S.d.Q.C.L., Z.H., L.F.R.P. and S.C.S.-L.; data curation, D.C., L.A.B., D.D.E., C.C., F.M. and F.R.T.; writing—original draft preparation, D.C., L.A.B. and S.C.S.-L.; writing—review and editing, D.C., L.A.B., S.d.Q.C.L., D.D.E., F.M., F.R.T., Z.H., L.F.R.P. and S.C.S.-L.; visualization, D.C., L.A.B. and S.C.S.-L.; supervision, S.d.Q.C.L., Z.H., L.F.R.P. and S.C.S.-L.; project administration, Z.H., L.F.R.P. and S.C.S.-L.; funding acquisition, Z.H., L.F.R.P. and S.C.S.-L. Where authors are identified as personnel of the International Agency for Research on Cancer/World Health Organization, the authors alone are responsible for the views expressed in this article and they do not necessarily represent the decisions, policy or views of the International Agency for Research on Cancer/World Health Organization. All authors have read and agreed to the published version of the manuscript.

Funding: This work was funded by the Swiss Bridge Award, Fundação Carlos Chagas Filho de Amparo à Pesquisa do Estado do Rio de Janeiro, Conselho Nacional de Desenvolvimento Científico e Tecnológico and Ministério da Saúde.

Institutional Review Board Statement: The study was conducted according to the guidelines of the Declaration of Helsinki, and approved by the Ethics Committee of Instituto Nacional de Câncer (protocol code CAAE 60480316.0.0000.5274 approved on 9 December 2016).

Informed Consent Statement: Informed consent was obtained from all subjects involved in the study.

Data Availability Statement: Publicly available RNA-seq and DNA methylation data from oropharyngeal cancer patients from the Cancer Genome Atlas (TCGA-HNSC project) were retrieved from cBioPortal.

Acknowledgments: The authors would like to thank the Pathology Division and the Head and Neck Section from the Brazilian National Cancer Institute (INCA) for all the support with patient enrollment and sample collection.

Conflicts of Interest: The authors declare no conflict of interest. The funders had no role in the design of the study; in the collection, analyses, or interpretation of data; in the writing of the manuscript, or in the decision to publish the results.

References

1. Chhabra, N.; Chhabra, S.; Sapra, N. Diagnostic modalities for squamous cell carcinoma: An extensive review of literature-considering toluidine blue as a useful adjunct. *J. Maxillofac. Oral Surg.* **2015**, *14*, 188–200. [CrossRef]
2. Ndiaye, C.; Mena, M.; Alemany, L.; Arbyn, M.; Castellsagué, X.; Laporte, L.; Bosch, F.X.; de Sanjosé, S.; Trottier, H. HPV DNA, E6/E7 mRNA, and p16INK4a detection in head and neck cancers: A systematic review and meta-analysis. *Lancet Oncol.* **2014**, *15*, 1319–1331. [CrossRef]
3. Ragin, C.C.; Taioli, E. Survival of squamous cell carcinoma of the head and neck in relation to human papillomavirus infection: Review and meta-analysis. *Int. J. Cancer* **2007**, *121*, 1813–1820. [CrossRef]
4. Anantharaman, D.; Abedi-Ardekani, B.; Beachler, D.C.; Gheit, T.; Olshan, A.F.; Wisniewski, K.; Wunsch-Filho, V.; Toporcov, T.N.; Tajara, E.H.; Levi, J.E.; et al. Geographic heterogeneity in the prevalence of human papillomavirus in head and neck cancer. *Int. J. Cancer* **2017**, *140*, 1968–1975. [CrossRef]
5. Jemal, A.; Simard, E.P.; Dorell, C.; Noone, A.M.; Markowitz, L.E.; Kohler, B.; Eheman, C.; Saraiya, M.; Bandi, P.; Saslow, D.; et al. Annual Report to the Nation on the Status of Cancer, 1975–2009, featuring the burden and trends in human papillomavirus(HPV)-associated cancers and HPV vaccination coverage levels. *J. Natl. Cancer Inst.* **2013**, *105*, 175–201. [CrossRef]
6. Bettampadi, D.; Villa, L.L.; Ponce, E.L.; Salmeron, J.; Sirak, B.A.; Abrahamsen, M.; Rathwell, J.A.; Reich, R.R.; Giuliano, A.R. Oral human papillomavirus prevalence and type distribution by country (Brazil, Mexico and the United States) and age among HPV infection in men study participants. *Int. J. Cancer* **2020**, *146*, 3026–3033. [CrossRef]
7. Buexm, L.A.; Soares-Lima, S.C.; Brennan, P.; Fernandes, P.V.; de Souza Almeida Lopes, M.; Nascimento de Carvalho, F.; Santos, I.C.; Dias, L.F.; de Queiroz Chaves Lourenço, S.; Ribeiro Pinto, L.F. Hpv impact on oropharyngeal cancer patients treated at the largest cancer center from Brazil. *Cancer Lett.* **2020**, *477*, 70–75. [CrossRef]
8. Doorbar, J. The papillomavirus life cycle. *J. Clin. Virol.* **2005**, *32* (Suppl. S1), S7–S15. [CrossRef] [PubMed]
9. Tumban, E. A Current Update on Human Papillomavirus-Associated Head and Neck Cancers. *Viruses* **2019**, *11*, 922. [CrossRef] [PubMed]
10. Nakagawa, T.; Kurokawa, T.; Mima, M.; Imamoto, S.; Mizokami, H.; Kondo, S.; Okamoto, Y.; Misawa, K.; Hanazawa, T.; Kaneda, A. DNA Methylation and HPV-Associated Head and Neck Cancer. *Microorganisms* **2021**, *9*, 801. [CrossRef] [PubMed]
11. Chow, L.Q.M. Head and Neck Cancer. *N. Engl. J. Med.* **2020**, *382*, 60–72. [CrossRef]
12. Ghittoni, R.; Accardi, R.; Hasan, U.; Gheit, T.; Sylla, B.; Tommasino, M. The biological properties of E6 and E7 oncoproteins from human papillomaviruses. *Virus Genes* **2010**, *40*, 1–13. [CrossRef]
13. Gheit, T. Mucosal and Cutaneous Human Papillomavirus Infections and Cancer Biology. *Front. Oncol.* **2019**, *9*, 355. [CrossRef]
14. Soto, D.; Song, C.; McLaughlin-Drubin, M.E. Epigenetic Alterations in Human Papillomavirus-Associated Cancers. *Viruses* **2017**, *9*, 248. [CrossRef]
15. Herceg, Z.; Ushijima, T. Introduction: Epigenetics and cancer. *Adv. Genet.* **2010**, *70*, 1–23. [CrossRef]
16. Klutstein, M.; Nejman, D.; Greenfield, R.; Cedar, H. DNA Methylation in Cancer and Aging. *Cancer Res.* **2016**, *76*, 3446–3450. [CrossRef]
17. Kulis, M.; Esteller, M. DNA methylation and cancer. *Adv. Genet.* **2010**, *70*, 27–56. [CrossRef] [PubMed]
18. Li, E.; Zhang, Y. DNA methylation in mammals. *Cold Spring Harb. Perspect Biol.* **2014**, *6*, a019133. [CrossRef]
19. Burgers, W.A.; Blanchon, L.; Pradhan, S.; de Launoit, Y.; Kouzarides, T.; Fuks, F. Viral oncoproteins target the DNA methyltransferases. *Oncogene* **2007**, *26*, 1650–1655. [CrossRef] [PubMed]
20. McCabe, M.T.; Davis, J.N.; Day, M.L. Regulation of DNA methyltransferase 1 by the pRb/E2F1 pathway. *Cancer Res.* **2005**, *65*, 3624–3632. [CrossRef] [PubMed]
21. Yeung, C.L.; Tsang, T.Y.; Yau, P.L.; Kwok, T.T. Human papillomavirus type 16 E6 suppresses microRNA-23b expression in human cervical cancer cells through DNA methylation of the host gene C9orf3. *Oncotarget* **2017**, *8*, 12158–12173. [CrossRef]
22. Sartor, M.A.; Dolinoy, D.C.; Jones, T.R.; Colacino, J.A.; Prince, M.E.; Carey, T.E.; Rozek, L.S. Genome-wide methylation and expression differences in HPV(+) and HPV(−) squamous cell carcinoma cell lines are consistent with divergent mechanisms of carcinogenesis. *Epigenetics* **2011**, *6*, 777–787. [CrossRef]
23. Leonard, S.M.; Wei, W.; Collins, S.I.; Pereira, M.; Diyaf, A.; Constandinou-Williams, C.; Young, L.S.; Roberts, S.; Woodman, C.B. Oncogenic human papillomavirus imposes an instructive pattern of DNA methylation changes which parallel the natural history of cervical HPV infection in young women. *Carcinogenesis* **2012**, *33*, 1286–1293. [CrossRef]
24. Degli Esposti, D.; Sklias, A.; Lima, S.C.; Beghelli-de la Forest Divonne, S.; Cahais, V.; Fernandez-Jimenez, N.; Cros, M.P.; Ecsedi, S.; Cuenin, C.; Bouaoun, L.; et al. Unique DNA methylation signature in HPV-positive head and neck squamous cell carcinomas. *Genome Med.* **2017**, *9*, 33. [CrossRef] [PubMed]

25. Kostareli, E.; Holzinger, D.; Bogatyrova, O.; Hielscher, T.; Wichmann, G.; Keck, M.; Lahrmann, B.; Grabe, N.; Flechtenmacher, C.; Schmidt, C.R.; et al. HPV-related methylation signature predicts survival in oropharyngeal squamous cell carcinomas. *J. Clin. Investig.* **2013**, *123*, 2488–2501. [CrossRef]
26. Furniss, C.S.; Marsit, C.J.; Houseman, E.A.; Eddy, K.; Kelsey, K.T. Line region hypomethylation is associated with lifestyle and differs by human papillomavirus status in head and neck squamous cell carcinomas. *Cancer Epidemiol. Biomark. Prev.* **2008**, *17*, 966–971. [CrossRef] [PubMed]
27. Furlan, C.; Polesel, J.; Barzan, L.; Franchin, G.; Sulfaro, S.; Romeo, S.; Colizzi, F.; Rizzo, A.; Baggio, V.; Giacomarra, V.; et al. Prognostic significance of LINE-1 hypomethylation in oropharyngeal squamous cell carcinoma. *Clin. Epigenetics* **2017**, *9*, 58. [CrossRef] [PubMed]
28. Richards, K.L.; Zhang, B.; Baggerly, K.A.; Colella, S.; Lang, J.C.; Schuller, D.E.; Krahe, R. Genome-wide hypomethylation in head and neck cancer is more pronounced in HPV-negative tumors and is associated with genomic instability. *PLoS ONE* **2009**, *4*, e4941. [CrossRef] [PubMed]
29. Bannert, N.; Hofmann, H.; Block, A.; Hohn, O. HERVs New Role in Cancer: From Accused Perpetrators to Cheerful Protectors. *Front. Microbiol.* **2018**, *9*, 178. [CrossRef]
30. Chen, Y.A.; Lemire, M.; Choufani, S.; Butcher, D.T.; Grafodatskaya, D.; Zanke, B.W.; Gallinger, S.; Hudson, T.J.; Weksberg, R. Discovery of cross-reactive probes and polymorphic CpGs in the Illumina Infinium HumanMethylation450 microarray. *Epigenetics* **2013**, *8*, 203–209. [CrossRef]
31. Du, P.; Kibbe, W.A.; Lin, S.M. lumi: A pipeline for processing Illumina microarray. *Bioinformatics* **2008**, *24*, 1547–1548. [CrossRef] [PubMed]
32. Zheng, Y.; Joyce, B.T.; Liu, L.; Zhang, Z.; Kibbe, W.A.; Zhang, W.; Hou, L. Prediction of genome-wide DNA methylation in repetitive elements. *Nucleic Acids Res.* **2017**, *45*, 8697–8711. [CrossRef] [PubMed]
33. Sticht, C.; Hofele, C.; Flechtenmacher, C.; Bosch, F.X.; Freier, K.; Lichter, P.; Joos, S. Amplification of Cyclin L1 is associated with lymph node metastases in head and neck squamous cell carcinoma (HNSCC). *Br. J. Cancer* **2005**, *92*, 770–774. [CrossRef] [PubMed]
34. Au Yeung, C.L.; Tsang, W.P.; Tsang, T.Y.; Co, N.N.; Yau, P.L.; Kwok, T.T. HPV-16 E6 upregulation of DNMT1 through repression of tumor suppressor p53. *Oncol. Rep.* **2010**, *24*, 1599–1604. [CrossRef] [PubMed]
35. Yang, S.; Wu, Y.; Wang, S.; Xu, P.; Deng, Y.; Wang, M.; Liu, K.; Tian, T.; Zhu, Y.; Li, N.; et al. HPV-related methylation-based reclassification and risk stratification of cervical cancer. *Mol. Oncol.* **2020**, *14*, 2124–2141. [CrossRef]
36. Fang, J.; Zhang, H.; Jin, S. Epigenetics and cervical cancer: From pathogenesis to therapy. *Tumour. Biol.* **2014**, *35*, 5083–5093. [CrossRef] [PubMed]
37. Verlaat, W.; Van Leeuwen, R.W.; Novianti, P.W.; Schuuring, E.; Meijer, C.J.L.M.; Van Der Zee, A.G.J.; Snijders, P.J.F.; Heideman, D.A.M.; Steenbergen, R.D.M.; Wisman, G.B.A. Host-cell DNA methylation patterns during high-risk HPV-induced carcinogenesis reveal a heterogeneous nature of cervical pre-cancer. *Epigenetics* **2018**, *13*, 769–778. [CrossRef]
38. Saavedra, K.P.; Brebi, P.M.; Roa, J.C. Epigenetic alterations in preneoplastic and neoplastic lesions of the cervix. *Clin. Epigenetics* **2012**, *4*, 13. [CrossRef]
39. Jiao, X.; Zhang, S.; Jiao, J.; Zhang, T.; Qu, W.; Muloye, G.M.; Kong, B.; Zhang, Q.; Cui, B. Promoter methylation of SEPT9 as a potential biomarker for early detection of cervical cancer and its overexpression predicts radioresistance. *Clin. Epigenetics* **2019**, *11*, 120. [CrossRef]
40. Schmitz, M.; Eichelkraut, K.; Schmidt, D.; Zeiser, I.; Hilal, Z.; Tettenborn, Z.; Hansel, A.; Ikenberg, H. Performance of a DNA methylation marker panel using liquid-based cervical scrapes to detect cervical cancer and its precancerous stages. *BMC Cancer* **2018**, *18*, 1197. [CrossRef]
41. Peeters, E.; Wentzensen, N.; Bergeron, C.; Arbyn, M. Meta-analysis of the accuracy of p16 or p16/Ki-67 immunocytochemistry versus HPV testing for the detection of CIN2+/CIN3+ in triage of women with minor abnormal cytology. *Cancer Cytopathol.* **2019**, *127*, 169–180. [CrossRef]
42. Giorgi Rossi, P.; Carozzi, F.; Ronco, G.; Allia, E.; Bisanzi, S.; Gillio-Tos, A.; Marco, L.; Rizzolo, R.; Gustinucci, D.; Del Mistro, A.; et al. p16/ki67 and E6/E7 mRNA Accuracy and Prognostic Value in Triaging HPV DNA-Positive Women. *J. Natl. Cancer Inst.* **2021**, *113*, 292–300. [CrossRef] [PubMed]
43. Gipson, B.J.; Robbins, H.A.; Fakhry, C.; D'Souza, G. Sensitivity and specificity of oral HPV detection for HPV-positive head and neck cancer. *Oral Oncol.* **2018**, *77*, 52–56. [CrossRef]
44. Prigge, E.S.; Arbyn, M.; von Knebel Doeberitz, M.; Reuschenbach, M. Diagnostic accuracy of p16. *Int. J. Cancer* **2017**, *140*, 1186–1198. [CrossRef] [PubMed]
45. Reuter, C.; Preece, M.; Banwait, R.; Boer, S.; Cuzick, J.; Lorincz, A.; Nedjai, B. Consistency of the S5 DNA methylation classifier in formalin-fixed biopsies versus corresponding exfoliated cells for the detection of pre-cancerous cervical lesions. *Cancer Med.* **2021**, *10*, 2668–2679. [CrossRef] [PubMed]
46. Ghantous, Y.; Schussel, J.L.; Brait, M. Tobacco and alcohol-induced epigenetic changes in oral carcinoma. *Curr. Opin. Oncol.* **2018**, *30*, 152–158. [CrossRef]
47. Liu, C.; Marioni, R.E.; Hedman, Å.; Pfeiffer, L.; Tsai, P.C.; Reynolds, L.M.; Just, A.C.; Duan, Q.; Boer, C.G.; Tanaka, T.; et al. A DNA methylation biomarker of alcohol consumption. *Mol. Psychiatry* **2018**, *23*, 422–433. [CrossRef]

48. Shen, S.Y.; Singhania, R.; Fehringer, G.; Chakravarthy, A.; Roehrl, M.H.A.; Chadwick, D.; Zuzarte, P.C.; Borgida, A.; Wang, T.T.; Li, T.; et al. Sensitive tumour detection and classification using plasma cell-free DNA methylomes. *Nature* **2018**, *563*, 579–583. [CrossRef]
49. Nassiri, F.; Chakravarthy, A.; Feng, S.; Shen, S.Y.; Nejad, R.; Zuccato, J.A.; Voisin, M.R.; Patil, V.; Horbinski, C.; Aldape, K.; et al. Detection and discrimination of intracranial tumors using plasma cell-free DNA methylomes. *Nat. Med.* **2020**, *26*, 1044–1047. [CrossRef]
50. Thuijs, N.B.; Berkhof, J.; Özer, M.; Duin, S.; van Splunter, A.P.; Snoek, B.C.; Heideman, D.A.M.; van Beurden, M.; Steenbergen, R.D.M.; Bleeker, M.C.G. DNA methylation markers for cancer risk prediction of vulvar intraepithelial neoplasia. *Int. J. Cancer* **2021**. [CrossRef]
51. Vink, F.J.; Dick, S.; Heideman, D.A.M.; De Strooper, L.M.A.; Steenbergen, R.D.M.; Lissenberg-Witte, B.I.; Floore, A.; Bonde, J.H.; Oštrbenk Valenčak, A.; Poljak, M.; et al. Classification of high-grade cervical intraepithelial neoplasia by p16. *Int. J. Cancer* **2021**. [CrossRef]
52. Jones, S.E.F.; Hibbitts, S.; Hurt, C.N.; Bryant, D.; Fiander, A.N.; Powell, N.; Tristram, A.J. Human Papillomavirus DNA Methylation Predicts Response to Treatment Using Cidofovir and Imiquimod in Vulval Intraepithelial Neoplasia 3. *Clin. Cancer Res.* **2017**, *23*, 5460–5468. [CrossRef] [PubMed]
53. Pan, Y.; Song, Y.; Cheng, L.; Xu, H.; Liu, J. Analysis of methylation-driven genes for predicting the prognosis of patients with head and neck squamous cell carcinoma. *J. Cell Biochem.* **2019**, *120*, 19482–19495. [CrossRef]
54. Sailer, V.; Holmes, E.E.; Gevensleben, H.; Goltz, D.; Dröge, F.; Franzen, A.; Dietrich, J.; Kristiansen, G.; Bootz, F.; Schröck, A.; et al. DNA methylation is an independent predictor of overall survival in patients with head and neck squamous cell carcinoma. *Clin. Epigenetics* **2017**, *9*, 12. [CrossRef] [PubMed]
55. Chen, X.; Gole, J.; Gore, A.; He, Q.; Lu, M.; Min, J.; Yuan, Z.; Yang, X.; Jiang, Y.; Zhang, T.; et al. Non-invasive early detection of cancer four years before conventional diagnosis using a blood test. *Nat. Commun.* **2020**, *11*, 3475. [CrossRef] [PubMed]
56. Ehrlich, M. DNA hypomethylation in cancer cells. *Epigenomics* **2009**, *1*, 239–259. [CrossRef]
57. Van Tongelen, A.; Loriot, A.; De Smet, C. Oncogenic roles of DNA hypomethylation through the activation of cancer-germline genes. *Cancer Lett.* **2017**, *396*, 130–137. [CrossRef]
58. Chen, H.C.; Yang, C.M.; Cheng, J.T.; Tsai, K.W.; Fu, T.Y.; Liou, H.H.; Tseng, H.H.; Lee, J.H.; Li, G.C.; Wang, J.S.; et al. Global DNA hypomethylation is associated with the development and poor prognosis of tongue squamous cell carcinoma. *J. Oral Pathol. Med.* **2016**, *45*, 409–417. [CrossRef]
59. Wang, T.; McCullough, L.E.; White, A.J.; Bradshaw, P.T.; Xu, X.; Cho, Y.H.; Terry, M.B.; Teitelbaum, S.L.; Neugut, A.I.; Santella, R.M.; et al. Prediagnosis aspirin use, DNA methylation, and mortality after breast cancer: A population-based study. *Cancer* **2019**, *125*, 3836–3844. [CrossRef]
60. Zelic, R.; Fiano, V.; Grasso, C.; Zugna, D.; Pettersson, A.; Gillio-Tos, A.; Merletti, F.; Richiardi, L. Global DNA hypomethylation in prostate cancer development and progression: A systematic review. *Prostate Cancer Prostatic Dis.* **2015**, *18*, 1–12. [CrossRef]
61. Li, J.; Huang, Q.; Zeng, F.; Li, W.; He, Z.; Chen, W.; Zhu, W.; Zhang, B. The prognostic value of global DNA hypomethylation in cancer: A meta-analysis. *PLoS ONE* **2014**, *9*, e106290. [CrossRef]
62. Zhang, W.; Klinkebiel, D.; Barger, C.J.; Pandey, S.; Guda, C.; Miller, A.; Akers, S.N.; Odunsi, K.; Karpf, A.R. Global DNA Hypomethylation in Epithelial Ovarian Cancer: Passive Demethylation and Association with Genomic Instability. *Cancers* **2020**, *12*, 764. [CrossRef]
63. Kawano, H.; Saeki, H.; Kitao, H.; Tsuda, Y.; Otsu, H.; Ando, K.; Ito, S.; Egashira, A.; Oki, E.; Morita, M.; et al. Chromosomal instability associated with global DNA hypomethylation is associated with the initiation and progression of esophageal squamous cell carcinoma. *Ann. Surg. Oncol.* **2014**, *21* (Suppl. S4), S696–S702. [CrossRef]
64. Ponomaryova, A.A.; Rykova, E.Y.; Gervas, P.A.; Cherdyntseva, N.V.; Mamedov, I.Z.; Azhikina, T.L. Aberrant Methylation of LINE-1 Transposable Elements: A Search for Cancer Biomarkers. *Cells* **2020**, *9*, 2017. [CrossRef] [PubMed]
65. Lee, E.; Iskow, R.; Yang, L.; Gokcumen, O.; Haseley, P.; Luquette, L.J.; Lohr, J.G.; Harris, C.C.; Ding, L.; Wilson, R.K.; et al. Landscape of somatic retrotransposition in human cancers. *Science* **2012**, *337*, 967–971. [CrossRef] [PubMed]
66. Rebollo, R.; Romanish, M.T.; Mager, D.L. Transposable elements: An abundant and natural source of regulatory sequences for host genes. *Annu. Rev. Genet.* **2012**, *46*, 21–42. [CrossRef] [PubMed]
67. Anwar, S.L.; Wulaningsih, W.; Lehmann, U. Transposable Elements in Human Cancer: Causes and Consequences of Deregulation. *Int. J. Mol. Sci.* **2017**, *18*, 974. [CrossRef]
68. Nahas, M.R.; Stroopinsky, D.; Rosenblatt, J.; Cole, L.; Pyzer, A.R.; Anastasiadou, E.; Sergeeva, A.; Ephraim, A.; Washington, A.; Orr, S.; et al. Hypomethylating agent alters the immune microenvironment in acute myeloid leukaemia (AML) and enhances the immunogenicity of a dendritic cell/AML vaccine. *Br. J. Haematol.* **2019**, *185*, 679–690. [CrossRef]
69. Attermann, A.S.; Bjerregaard, A.M.; Saini, S.K.; Grønbæk, K.; Hadrup, S.R. Human endogenous retroviruses and their implication for immunotherapeutics of cancer. *Ann. Oncol.* **2018**, *29*, 2183–2191. [CrossRef]
70. Roulois, D.; Loo Yau, H.; Singhania, R.; Wang, Y.; Danesh, A.; Shen, S.Y.; Han, H.; Liang, G.; Jones, P.A.; Pugh, T.J.; et al. DNA-Demethylating Agents Target Colorectal Cancer Cells by Inducing Viral Mimicry by Endogenous Transcripts. *Cell* **2015**, *162*, 961–973. [CrossRef]
71. Drongitis, D.; Aniello, F.; Fucci, L.; Donizetti, A. Roles of Transposable Elements in the Different Layers of Gene Expression Regulation. *Int. J. Mol. Sci.* **2019**, *20*, 5755. [CrossRef]

72. Lu, J.Y.; Shao, W.; Chang, L.; Yin, Y.; Li, T.; Zhang, H.; Hong, Y.; Percharde, M.; Guo, L.; Wu, Z.; et al. Genomic Repeats Categorize Genes with Distinct Functions for Orchestrated Regulation. *Cell Rep.* **2020**, *30*, 3296–3311.e3295. [CrossRef]
73. Chien, J.; Staub, J.; Avula, R.; Zhang, H.; Liu, W.; Hartmann, L.C.; Kaufmann, S.H.; Smith, D.I.; Shridhar, V. Epigenetic silencing of TCEAL7 (Bex4) in ovarian cancer. *Oncogene* **2005**, *24*, 5089–5100. [CrossRef]
74. Rattan, R.; Narita, K.; Chien, J.; Maguire, J.L.; Shridhar, R.; Giri, S.; Shridhar, V. TCEAL7, a putative tumor suppressor gene, negatively regulates NF-kappaB pathway. *Oncogene* **2010**, *29*, 1362–1373. [CrossRef]
75. Seta, R.; Mascitti, M.; Campagna, R.; Sartini, D.; Fumarola, S.; Santarelli, A.; Giuliani, M.; Cecati, M.; Muzio, L.L.; Emanuelli, M. Overexpression of nicotinamide N-methyltransferase in HSC-2 OSCC cell line: Effect on apoptosis and cell proliferation. *Clin. Oral Investig.* **2019**, *23*, 829–838. [CrossRef]
76. Cui, Y.; Yang, D.; Wang, W.; Zhang, L.; Liu, H.; Ma, S.; Guo, W.; Yao, M.; Zhang, K.; Li, W.; et al. Nicotinamide N-methyltransferase decreases 5-fluorouracil sensitivity in human esophageal squamous cell carcinoma through metabolic reprogramming and promoting the Warburg effect. *Mol. Carcinog.* **2020**, *59*, 940–954. [CrossRef] [PubMed]
77. Silveira, N.J.; Varuzza, L.; Machado-Lima, A.; Lauretto, M.S.; Pinheiro, D.G.; Rodrigues, R.V.; Severino, P.; Nobrega, F.G.; Silva, W.A.; de B Pereira, C.A.; et al. Searching for molecular markers in head and neck squamous cell carcinomas (HNSCC) by statistical and bioinformatic analysis of larynx-derived SAGE libraries. *BMC Med. Genom.* **2008**, *1*, 56. [CrossRef]
78. Zhu, X.; Cheng, Y.; Wu, F.; Sun, H.; Zheng, W.; Jiang, W.; Shi, J.; Ma, S.; Cao, H. MFAP2 Promotes the Proliferation of Cancer Cells and Is Associated with a Poor Prognosis in Hepatocellular Carcinoma. *Technol. Cancer Res. Treat.* **2020**, *19*, 1533033820977524. [CrossRef] [PubMed]
79. Sun, T.; Wang, D.; Ping, Y.; Sang, Y.; Dai, Y.; Wang, Y.; Liu, Z.; Duan, X.; Tao, Z.; Liu, W. Integrated profiling identifies SLC5A6 and MFAP2 as novel diagnostic and prognostic biomarkers in gastric cancer patients. *Int. J. Oncol.* **2020**, *56*, 460–469. [CrossRef] [PubMed]
80. Mun, K.; Punga, T. Cellular Zinc Finger Protein 622 Hinders Human Adenovirus Lytic Growth and Limits Binding of the Viral pVII Protein to Virus DNA. *J. Virol.* **2019**, *93*. [CrossRef] [PubMed]
81. Chen, T.; Yang, S.; Xu, J.; Lu, W.; Xie, X. Transcriptome sequencing profiles of cervical cancer tissues and SiHa cells. *Funct. Integr. Genom.* **2020**, *20*, 211–221. [CrossRef] [PubMed]
82. Redon, R.; Hussenet, T.; Bour, G.; Caulee, K.; Jost, B.; Muller, D.; Abecassis, J.; du Manoir, S. Amplicon mapping and transcriptional analysis pinpoint cyclin L as a candidate oncogene in head and neck cancer. *Cancer Res.* **2002**, *62*, 6211–6217.
83. Hua, T.; Kang, S.; Li, X.F.; Tian, Y.J.; Li, Y. DNA methylome profiling identifies novel methylated genes in epithelial ovarian cancer patients with platinum resistance. *J. Obstet. Gynaecol. Res.* **2021**, *47*, 1031–1039. [CrossRef]
84. Parfenov, M.; Pedamallu, C.S.; Gehlenborg, N.; Freeman, S.S.; Danilova, L.; Bristow, C.A.; Lee, S.; Hadjipanayis, A.G.; Ivanova, E.V.; Wilkerson, M.D.; et al. Characterization of HPV and host genome interactions in primary head and neck cancers. *Proc. Natl. Acad. Sci. USA* **2014**, *111*, 15544–15549. [CrossRef]

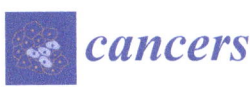

Article

Comparison of Selected Immune and Hematological Parameters and Their Impact on Survival in Patients with HPV-Related and HPV-Unrelated Oropharyngeal Cancer

Adam Brewczyński [1], Beata Jabłońska [2,*], Agnieszka Maria Mazurek [3], Jolanta Mrochem-Kwarciak [4], Sławomir Mrowiec [2], Mirosław Śnietura [5], Marek Kentnowski [1], Zofia Kołosza [6], Krzysztof Składowski [1] and Tomasz Rutkowski [1]

1. I Radiation and Clinical Oncology Department of Maria Skłodowska-Curie National Research Institute of Oncology, 44-102 Gliwice Branch, Poland; Adam.Brewczynski@io.gliwice.pl (A.B.); marek.kentnowski@io.gliwice.pl (M.K.); Krzysztof.Skladowski@io.gliwice.pl (K.S.); Tomasz.Rutkowski@io.gliwice.pl (T.R.)
2. Department of Digestive Tract Surgery, Medical University of Silesia, 40-752 Katowice, Poland; mrowasm@poczta.onet.pl
3. Centre for Translational Research and Molecular Biology of Cancer of Maria Skłodowska-Curie National Research Institute of Oncology, 44-102 Gliwice Branch, Poland; agnieszka.mazurek@io.gliwice.pl
4. The Analytics and Clinical Biochemistry Department of Maria Skłodowska-Curie National Research Institute of Oncology, 44-102 Gliwice Branch, Poland; Jolanta.Mrochem-Kwarciak@io.gliwice.pl
5. Tumor Pathology Department of Maria Skłodowska-Curie National Research Institute of Oncology, 44-102 Gliwice Branch, Poland; Miroslaw.Snietura@io.gliwice.pl
6. Department of Biostatistics and Bioinformatics of Maria Skłodowska-Curie National Research Institute of Oncology, 44-102 Gliwice Branch, Poland; zofia.kolosza@io.gliwice.pl
* Correspondence: bjablonska@poczta.onet.pl

Simple Summary: This is a research article on oropharyngeal cancer (OPC). The aim of the study was to assess and compare basic immune parameters and ratios in patients with Human Papilloma Virus (HPV)+ and HPV− OPC, before and after radiotherapy (RT) or chemoradiotherapy (CRT), and to investigate their impact on overall survival (OS) and disease-free survival (DFS). The higher neutrophil-lymphocyte ratio (NLR) and systemic immune inflammation (SII) are significant adverse prognostic factors for HPV+ OPC patients, because they are significantly associated with both inferior OS and DFS in this group, whereas the higher platelet cells (PLT) count is significant adverse prognostic factor for HPV− OPC patients, because it is significantly associated with inferior OS and DFS in this group. This study confirmed that determination of HPV etiology as well as analysis of various hematological and immune parameters should be a standard management in OPC patients in order to properly treat them for improved prognosis.

Abstract: Several immune and hematological parameters are associated with survival in patients with oropharyngeal cancer (OPC). The aim of the study was to analyze selected immune and hematological parameters of patients with HPV-related (HPV+) and HPV-unrelated (HPV−) OPC, before and after radiotherapy/chemoradiotherapy (RT/CRT) and to assess the impact of these parameters on survival. One hundred twenty seven patients with HPV+ and HPV− OPC, treated with RT alone or concurrent chemoradiotherapy (CRT), were included. Patients were divided according to HPV status. Confirmation of HPV etiology was obtained from FFPE (Formalin-Fixed, Paraffin-Embedded) tissue samples and/or extracellular circulating HPV DNA was determined. The pre-treatment and post-treatment laboratory blood parameters were compared in both groups. The neutrophil/lymphocyte ratio (NLR), platelet/lymphocyte ratio (PLR), monocyte/lymphocyte ratio (MLR), and systemic immune inflammation (SII) index were calculated. The impact of these parameters on overall (OS) and disease-free (DFS) survival was analyzed. In HPV+ patients, a high pre-treatment white blood cells (WBC) count (>8.33 /mm^3), NLR (>2.13), SII (>448.60) significantly correlated with reduced OS, whereas high NLR (>2.29), SII (>462.58) significantly correlated with reduced DFS. A higher pre-treatment NLR and SII were significant poor prognostic factors for both OS and DFS in the HPV+ group. These associations were not apparent in HPV− patients. There are

Citation: Brewczyński, A.; Jabłońska, B.; Mazurek, A.M.; Mrochem-Kwarciak, J.; Mrowiec, S.; Śnietura, M.; Kentnowski, M.; Kołosza, Z.; Składowski, K.; Rutkowski, T. Comparison of Selected Immune and Hematological Parameters and Their Impact on Survival in Patients with HPV-Related and HPV-Unrelated Oropharyngeal Cancer. *Cancers* **2021**, *13*, 3256. https://doi.org/10.3390/cancers13133256

Academic Editor: Heather Walline

Received: 26 May 2021
Accepted: 25 June 2021
Published: 29 June 2021

Publisher's Note: MDPI stays neutral with regard to jurisdictional claims in published maps and institutional affiliations.

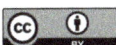

Copyright: © 2021 by the authors. Licensee MDPI, Basel, Switzerland. This article is an open access article distributed under the terms and conditions of the Creative Commons Attribution (CC BY) license (https:// creativecommons.org/licenses/by/ 4.0/).

different pre-treatment and post-treatment immune and hematological prognostic factors for OS and DFS in HPV+ and HPV− patients. The immune ratios could be considered valuable biomarkers for risk stratification and differentiation for HPV− and HPV+ OPC patients.

Keywords: oropharyngeal cancer; Human Papillomavirus (HPV); immune status; hematological parameters; radiotherapy

1. Introduction

It has been proven that significant alterations in the immunological system (IS) are observed in cancer patients. The body's specific immune response to a cancer leads to various changes in levels of basic immune parameters such as number of white blood cells (WBCs), circulating lymphocytes (CLCs), circulating neutrophils (CNCs), circulating monocytes (CMCs) and platelet cells (PLTs) [1–3]. These parameters are easy to assess in the routine peripheral blood morphology. Additionally, based on the basic abovementioned parameters, the following immune ratios can be calculated: neutrophil/lymphocyte (NLR), platelet/lymphocyte (PLR), and monocyte/lymphocyte (MLR). It is known that they strongly influence survival in cancer patients. This also applies to patients with squamous head and neck cancer, including oropharyngeal cancer (OPC) [1–3].

OPC can be associated with a typical risk factor such as smoking and alcohol abuse or with Human Papillomavirus (HPV) infection. HPV-related (HPV+) OPC is fairly responsive to radiotherapy (RT) or chemoradiotherapy (CRT) and has a better prognosis than HPV− [4,5].

Because of the different nature of HPV+ OPC, the current 8th edition of the American Joint Committee on Cancer *AJCC Staging Manual* reflected HPV infection status in determining the clinical stage of OPC [4,5]. It is interesting to note whether the difference in OPC etiology, considering HPV status, causes differences in the immune status and whether it affects the prognosis and patient survival. There are various reports regarding immune alterations in HPV+ OPC cancer in the literature [6].

The aim of the study was to assess and compare basic immune parameters and ratios in patients with HPV+ and HPV− OPC, before and after RT or CRT, and to investigate their impact on overall survival (OS) and disease-free survival (DFS).

2. Materials and Methods

2.1. Patients

The analysis included 127 adults with OPC treated at I Radiation and Clinical Oncology Department of Maria Sklodowska-Curie National Research Institute of Oncology, Gliwice Branch, Poland. There were 87 (68.5%) men and 40 (31.5%) women of the mean age of 60.62 ± 8.54 years (range: 30–80 years) in the studied group. The inclusion criteria were as follows: primary OPC (T1–T4, N0–N3, M0), age > 18 years, radical RT or CRT as sole and definitive treatment. Exclusion criteria included: cancer recurrence, initial surgery, incomplete demographic and/or clinical data.

The detailed analysis of clinicopathological parameters (age, gender, tumor grading and staging, smoking) in OPC patients is presented in Table 1.

Table 1. The patients' general clinicopathological characteristics.

Feature	All n = 127	HPV(−) n = 68	HPV(+) n = 59	p
Demographic characteristics				
Age	60.62 ± 8.54 (30–80)	60.85 ± 7.48 (37–79)	60.36 ± 9.67 (30–80)	0.745
Male	87(68.5%)	51 (75.1%)	36 (61.0%)	0.133
Female	40 (31.5%)	17 (25.0%)	23 (39.0%)	
Tumor location				
1. tonsil	91 (71.70%)	44 (64.70%)	47 (79.70%)	0.010
2. palate	10 (7.90%)	10 (14.70%)	0 (0.00%)	
3. root of the tongue	22 (17.30%)	13 (19.10%)	9 (15.30%)	
4.other oropharynx	4 (3.10%)	1 (1.50%)	3 (5.10%)	
Histopathological grading				
G1	7 (5.5%)	6 (8.8%)	1 (1.7%)	0.054
G2	55 (43.3%)	34 (50.0%)	21 (35.6%)	
G3	19 (15.0%)	7 (10.3%)	12 (20.3%)	
n.d.	46 (36.2%)	21 (30.9%)	25 (42.4%)	
Tumor depth (T)				
T1	13 (10.2%)	8 (11.8%)	5 (8.5%)	0.743
T2	42 (33.1%)	24 (35.3%)	18 (30.5%)	
T3	44 (34.6%)	22 (32.4%)	22 (37.3%)	
T4	27 (21.3%)	13 (19.1%)	14 (23.7%)	
Tx	1 (0.8%)	1 (1.5%)	0 (0.0%)	
Lymph node metastasis				
N 0–1	52 (40.9%)	36 (52.9%)	16 (27.1%)	0.005
N 2–3	74 (58.3%)	32 (47.1%)	42 (71.2%)	
Nx	1 (0.8%)		1 (1.7%)	
General treatment regimen				
Radiotherapy	31 (24.4%)	24 (35.3%)	7 (11.9%)	0.003
Radiochemotherapy	96 (75.6%)	44 (64.7%)	52 (88.1%)	

Values are presented as means ± standard deviations. n.d., not determined. Significant p values are marked in bold.

2.2. Study Design

2.2.1. The Information on Grant and Ethical Standards

This study was supported by a grant from the National Centre of Research and Development, Poland (grant TANGO2/340829/NCBR/2017). All procedures performed in studies involving human participants were in accordance with the ethical standards of the institutional research committee (the Bioethics Committee at Maria Skłodowska-Curie National Research Institute of Oncology, Gliwice Branch, KB/43018/13) and with the 1964 Helsinki Declaration and its later amendments or comparable ethical standards. Informed consent was obtained from all individual participants included in the study.

2.2.2. Laboratory Blood Investigations and Analysis

The blood was obtained under standard conditions, the patients in fasting state, between 7:00 and 9:00, by means of a vacuum Becton Dickinson (Franklin Lakes, NJ, USA) system, in sample tubes with anticoagulant ethylenediaminetetraacetic acid (EDTA). The full blood count was determined using the Sysmex XN-2000 analyzer (Sysmex, Kobe, Japan).

The pre-treatment (0) and post-treatment (1) basic laboratory blood parameters, including hemoglobin (Hb) and ret-hemoglobin (RetHb) levels, red blood cell count (RBC), reticulocyte count (Ret), white blood cell count (WBC), circulating lymphocyte count (CLC), circulating neutrophil count (CNC), and circulating monocyte count (CMC) were compared in both groups and the impact of immune and hematological parameters on survival was analyzed. The neutrophil/lymphocyte ratio (NLR), platelet/lymphocyte ratio (PLR), and monocyte/lymphocyte ratio (MLR), and systemic immune inflammation index (SII) were calculated and correlated with survival in both groups. The SII index was calculated according to the following formula: SII = platelet counts × neutrophil counts/lymphocyte counts [7]. Patients were divided into two groups depending on the HPV status: HPV-negatives (HPV−) and HPV-positives (HPV+).

Additionally, the patients were divided into two subgroups according to the cut-off value of the mean NLR, MLR, PLR, and SII. The mean values of the NLR, MLR, and PLR among the entire study population, as well as HPV− and HPV+ patients, were set as the border value to divide high and low NLR, MLR, and PLR subgroups in order to perform statistical comparisons of clinicopathological findings between these subgroups. Clinicopathological factors were compared between these low and high immune ratio subgroups.

2.2.3. Confirmation of the HPV Etiology

Confirmation of the HPV etiology was obtained from tissue material and/or extracellular circulating HPV DNA.

Tissue Material

Formalin-fixed paraffin-embedded tumor samples were examined for high-risk HPV (HR-HPV) infection using a double-check algorithm including immunohistochemical assessment of P16(INK4A) protein expression followed by detection of HR-HPV DNA in tumor tissue using real-time PCR. Only cases with both p16(INK4A) expression and HR-HPV DNA amplification were classified as truly HR-HPV-positive [7].

Analysis of cfHPV16 DNA in Plasma

Peripheral blood (12 mL) was collected into K3EDTA tubes (Becton Dickinson, Franklin Lakes, NJ, USA). Plasma was separated within an hour by double centrifugation at $300 \times g$ and $1000 \times g$, both at 4 °C for 10 min. DNA was extracted (according to the manufacturer's instructions) from 1 mL of plasma by the Genomic Mini AX Body Fluids kit (A&A Biotechnology, Gdynia, Poland). Each measurement consisted of a standard curve of three dilutions of plasmid construct containing HPV16 genome, negative control and a samples. For HPV16 detection, reaction was performed using primers and probe set for the HPV16 genome. PCR reactions were performed using the Bio-Rad CFX96 qPCR instrument (Bio-Rad Laboratories, Hemel Hempstead, UK). If HPV16 was found, its presence would be confirmed with a second independent DNA isolation.

2.2.4. Histopathological Staging and Grading Classification

The stage of OPC was classified according to the 8th edition of the American Joint Committee on Cancer (AJCC) TNM classification system [4,5].

2.2.5. Follow-Up

The median follow-up was 74.58 (0.1–165.58) months. Overall survival (OS) and disease-free survival (DFS) were analyzed in both groups.

The flowchart diagram of our study is presented in Figure 1.

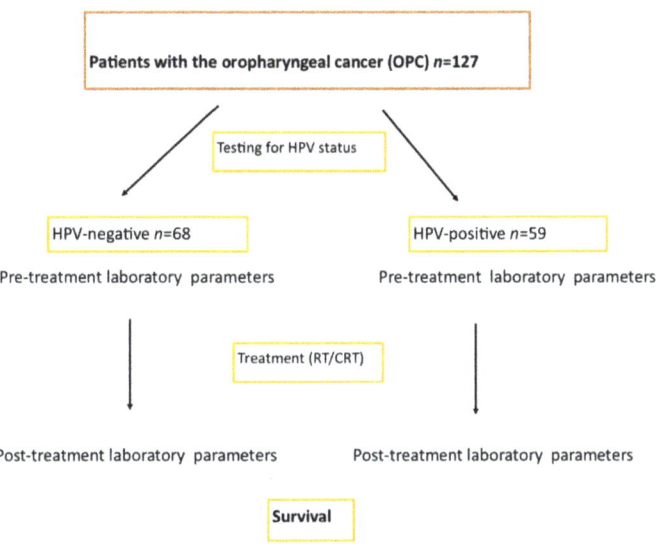

Figure 1. Flowchart diagram for the study.

2.3. Statistical Analysis

The categorical variables were presented as numbers and percentages. Continuous variables with normal distribution were expressed as the means and standard deviations. The Shapiro–Wilk test was used to determine statistical distribution in the analyzed patients. The Mann–Whitney U test was used to compare HPV+ and HPV− groups. The Wilcoxon test was used to compare pre- and post-treatment parameters in all patients and both HPV groups separately. Prevalence and frequency were expressed as number and percentage. Cox proportional-hazards models were used to estimate hazard ratios (HRs) for OS and DFS. Receiver operating characteristic (ROC) curve analysis was performed to determine the optimal cut-off values for prognostic factors related to DFS and OS. Youden's index was selected as the approximate cut-off value for each parameter. The Kaplan–Meier curves were constructed for comparison of OS and DFS between the two groups.

The log-rank test was used to assess the equality of survival distributions across different strata. The hazard ratio for death among patients with HPV− and HPV+ was determined. A p-value of equal or less than 0.05 was considered to be statistically significant. The statistical analyses were performed using the Statistica® software program, version 13.0 (StatSoft).

3. Results

3.1. General Characteristics

The general clinical characteristics of 127 patients is presented in Table 1.

Both groups were comparable regarding the age and gender structure. The mean age was 60.85 ± 7.48 (37–79) and 60.36 ± 9.67 (30–80) years in the HPV− and HPV+ groups, respectively ($p = 0.745$). The male gender was predominant in the both groups. There were 51 (75.1%) and 36 (61.0%) males in the HPV− and HPV+ groups, respectively ($p = 0.133$).

The tonsil was the most common OPC location in both groups, but the incidence of the tumor location was different depending the HPV status. The tonsil location was the most frequent (47 (79.7%)) in HPV+ patients, and this location was noted in only 44 (64.7%) HPV− patients ($p = 0.010$). The palate location was not observed in HPV+ patients, and this location was noted in 10 (14.7%) HPV− patients.

Concerning the histopathological findings, in both groups, G2 grading and T2/T3 staging were the most common. G2 grading was reported in 34 and 21 patients who were

HPV− and HPV+, respectively. G3 grading was more frequently noted in HPV+ patients compared to HPV− ones (20.3% vs. 10.3%; $p = 0.054$). The tumor depth was similar in both groups. It should be emphasized that the HPV+ patients had the more advanced nodal status compared to HPV− patients (71.2% vs. 47.1% N2–3; $p = 0.005$).

The significantly higher regional advancement of the HPV+ tumors was associated with the difference in the treatment regimen in the both groups. RCT was significantly more frequently used in the HPV+ patients compared to HPV− patients (88.1% vs. 64.7%; $p = 0.003$).

3.2. Laboratory Results before and after Treatment

The basic laboratory results in all patients and in both HPV− and HPV+ groups before and after treatment are presented and compared in Table S1.

Most pre-treatment (0) and post-treatment (1) laboratory results were comparable in both groups. Moreover, a decrease of the most parameters following RT/CRT was noted in our study. Only ret-hemoglobin (RetHb) increased after the treatment in HPV+ patients. Therefore, a significantly higher RetHb1 level was noted in HPV+ patients (35.01 ± 1.43) compared to HPV− patients (33.50 ± 3.38). A reticulocyte count (Ret) before (51.97 ± 24.96 vs. 60.56 ± 22.73, $p = 0.052$) and after treatment (51.20 ± 25.29 vs. 48.62 ± 23.88; $p = 0.574$) was comparable in HPV− and HPV+ groups, respectively, but the Ret decrease was significantly greater in HPV+ patients compared to HPV− ones (0.89 ± 29.78 vs. 12.30 ± 30.51, $p = 0.044$). A lower WBC0 was reported in HPV+ patients compared to HPV− participants (6.45 ± 1.91 vs. 7.15 ± 2.03, $p = 0.048$), while the difference in WBC1 between both groups was not statistically significant (4.35 ± 2.25 vs. 5.12 ± 2.29, $p = 0.059$). The WBC decrease was observed in both groups. CLC1 ($p = 0.004$) and CMC1 ($p = 0.012$) were significantly lower in HPV+ patients, while these pre-treatment parameters were comparable in HPV− and HPV+ groups ($p = 0.842$ for CLC0, $p = 0.057$ for CMC0). A significantly lower PLT1 count was recorded in HPV+ patients compared to HPV− ones (208.15 ± 65.18 vs. 250.31 ± 118.11, $p = 0.016$), while PLT0 was similar in HPV+ and HPV− groups (236.76 ± 57.94 vs. 256.93 ± 77.16, $p = 0.103$). It was associated with a greater PLT decrease in HPV+ patients ($p = 0.218$).

The NLR 0/1, MLR 0/1, PLR 0/1, and SII 0/1 were comparable in both groups. The results are presented in Table S2.

3.3. Comparison of Clinical and Pathological Characteristics Depending on the Values of Immune Ratios in HPV− and HPV+ Patients

The differences between low and high pre-treatment immune ratios groups (NLR 0/1, MLR 0/1, PLR 0/1 and SII 0/1) were analyzed.

In the low NLR HPV− subgroup, the significantly greater incidence of tonsil location compared to the incidence in the high NLR subgroup was reported (73.9% vs. 45.5%; $p = 0.039$). In HPV+ patients, the incidence of tonsil location was comparable in both NLR subgroups (81.1% vs. 77.3%; $p = 0.872$, respectively). There was no significant difference in terms of the other clinicopathological parameters between the two NLR groups regardless of HPV status (Table S3).

In the low MLR HPV− subgroup, the highest G3 grading was significantly more frequent compared to the high MLR subgroup (25.0% vs. 0.0%; $p = 0.026$). In a comparison of the determined grading, G2 was the commonest grading in both subgroups. In HPV+ patients, histological grading was comparable in both MLR subgroups. The other clinicopathological parameters were similar in both MLR subgroups (Table S4).

In the low PLR HPV+ subgroup, smoking was observed significantly more frequently compared to the high PLR subgroup (43.6% vs. 15.0%; $p = 0.042$). This difference was not noted in HPV− patients. The other clinicopathological parameters were comparable in both PLR subgroups (Table S5).

In HPV− patients, a higher initial BMI was noted in patients with the low SII compared to patients with the high SII (26.6 ± 4.8 vs. 24.1 ± 4.1 kg/m^2; $p = 0.028$). In HPV+ patients, G3 grading was more frequent in the low SII group compared to patients with the high SII

(47.8% vs. 9.1%; $p = 0.021$). Moreover, smoking was seen significantly more frequently in the low SII HPV+ subgroup compared to patients with the high SII (43.6% vs. 15.0%; $p = 0.042$) (Table S6). All comparisons are presented in Tables S3–S6.

3.4. Overall Survival and Disease-Free Survival Depending on HPV Status

OS and DFS in both HPV groups are presented in Tables 2–5, Tables S1–S6, and Figure 2, as well as Figures S1A–C and S2A–C. OS and DFS depending on HPV status were assessed using Cox regression univariate (UVA) and multivariate analysis (MVA). The prognostic factors determined in UVA were confirmed and presented using Kaplan–Meier curves. Generally, HPV status was a very strong prognostic factor for OS and DFS in our patients. OS and DFS were significantly better in HPV+ patients compared to HPV− ones ($p = 0.0008$ and $p = 0.0009$, respectively) (Figure 2). The treatment strategy (RT/CRT) was not a prognostic factor for both HPV− and HPV+ patients, in UVA and MVA ($p > 0.05$). Therefore, the treatment regimen did not impact survival in our patients (Tables 3 and 4).

Table 2. Overall survival (OS) depending on pre-treatment parameters in HPV−/HPV+ patients: univariate and multivariate analysis.

Variable	OS HPV−				OS HPV+			
	Univariate Analysis		Multivariate Analysis		Univariate Analysis		Multivariate Analysis	
	HR (95% CI)	p-Value	HR (95% CI)	p-Value	HR (95% CI)	p-Value	HR (95% CI)	p-Value
Hb 0 [g/dL] >11.8 vs. <11.8	0.65 (0.15–2.79)	0.563			1.65 (0.21–12.86)	0.635		
RetHb 0 [/mm³] >34.0 vs. <34.0	0.9 (0.39–2.06)	0.803			2.42 (0.65–9.08)	0.190	4.33 (0.91–20.51)	0.065
RBC 0 [/mm³] >4.6 vs. <4.6	0.46 (0.18–1.13)	0.091			0.76 (0.25–2.37)	0.641		
Ret 0 [/mm³] >37.9 vs. <37.9	0.6 (0.26–1.38)	0.229			**0.22 (0.06–0.82)**	**0.025**		
WBC 0 [/mm³] >8.33 vs. <8.33	2.33 (0.99–5.47)	0.053			**4.17 (1.25–13.93)**	**0.020**		
CLC 0 [/mm³] >1.10 vs. <1.10	0.7 (0.28–1.74)	0.442			0.42 (0.11–1.56)	0.197		
CNC 0 [/mm³] >4.96 vs. <4.96	1.82 (0.78–4.22)	0.166			2.54 (0.75–8.52)	0.132		
CMC 0 [/mm³] >0.93 vs. <0.93	**2.41 (1.01–5.74)**	**0.048**	**4.24 (1.52–11.84)**	**0.006**	3.37 (0.72–15.72)	0.122	**17.8 (1.89–167.47)**	**0.012**
PLT 0 [/mm³] >240 vs. <240	**2.53 (1.07–5.99)**	**0.035**			1.1 (0.34–3.58)	0.872	0.29 (0.07–1.18)	0.085
NLR 0 >2.13 vs. <2.13	1.44 (0.65–3.18)	0.364	0.36 (0.12–1.10)	0.074	**4.76 (1.29–17.57)**	**0.019**		
MLR 0 >0.43 vs. <0.43	**3.73 (1.71–8.15)**	**0.001**	**3.83 (1.46–10.02)**	**0.006**	0.47 (0.06–3.64)	0.470	0.07 (0.00–1.17)	0.064
PLR 0 >131.29 vs. <131.29	1.67 (0.76–3.69)	0.204	**3.6 (1.15–11.31)**	**0.028**	1.89 (0.59–6.03)	0.281		
SII 0 >448.60 vs. <448.60	1.95 (0.81–4.68)	0.135			**5.67 (1.24–25.94)**	**0.025**	**11.1 (2.02–60.97)**	**0.006**
Treatment regimen RT/CRT	0.93 (0.42–2.06)	0.858			0.60 (0.08–4.64)	0.623		

0, before treatment; Hb, hemoglobin level; RetHb, ret-hemoglobin level; RBC, red blood cells; Ret, reticulocyte count; WBC, white blood cell count; CLC, circulating lymphocyte count; CNC, circulating neutrophil count; CMC, circulating monocyte count; PLT, platelet cell count. NLR, neutrophil/lymphocyte ratio; LMR, lymphocyte/monocyte ratio; PLR, platelet/lymphocyte ratio; SII, systemic immune inflammation index; RT, radiotherapy; CRT, chemoradiotherapy. Significant p values are marked in bold.

Table 3. Disease-free survival (DFS) depending on pre-treatment parameters in HPV−/HPV+ patients: univariate and multivariate analysis.

Variable	DFS HPV−				DFS HPV+			
	Univariate Analysis		Multivariate Analysis		Univariate Analysis		Multivariate Analysis	
	HR (95% CI)	p-Value	HR (95% CI)	p-Value	HR (95% CI)	p-Value	HR (95% CI)	p-Value
Hb 0 [g/dL] >13.5 vs. <13.5	0.38 (0.17–0.87)	0.021			1.15 (0.27–4.82)	0.848	10.44 (1.31–83.38)	0.027
RetHb 0 [/mm³] >36.4 vs. <36.4	1.47 (0.57–3.78)	0.423			1.30 (0.26–6.43)	0.750		
RBC 0 [/mm³] >4.6 vs. <4.6	0.39 (0.15–0.97)	0.043	0.21 (0.07–0.66)	0.008	0.43 (0.1–1.81)	0.252	0.07 (0.01–0.60)	0.015
Ret 0 [/mm³] >54.7 vs. <54.7	0.64 (0.26–1.56)	0.323			0.23 (0.05–1.12)	0.068		
WBC 0 [/mm³] >8.33 vs. <8.33	1.57 (0.67–3.71)	0.301			2.42 (0.49–12.03)	0.280		
CLC 0 [/mm³] >1.28 vs. <1.28	0.61 (0.25–1.47)	0.271			0.19 (0.05–0.77)	0.020	0.17 (0.03–0.97)	0.046
CNC 0 [/mm3] >4.23 vs. <4.23	1.23 (0.56–2.72)	0.609			1.57 (0.38–6.6)	0.534		
CMC 0 [/mm³] >0.46 vs. <0.46	0.77 (0.32–1.85)	0.557			0.16 (0.03–0.8)	0.026	0.20 (0.04–1.07)	0.060
PLT 0 [/mm³] >319 vs. <319	2.77 (1.18–6.52)	0.020			1.59 (0.19–12.91)	0.667		
NLR 0 >2.29 vs. <2.29	1.63 (0.73–3.63)	0.232			6.02 (1.21–29.87)	0.028		
MLR 0 >0.27 vs. <0.27	0.62 (0.28–1.38)	0.242	0.20 (0.06–0.62)	0.006	0.46 (0.11–1.94)	0.291		
PLR 0 >173.20 vs. <173.20	2.88 (1.30–6.38)	0.009	2.74 (1.02–7.41)	0.046	1.77 (0.36–8.75)	0.487		
SII 0 >462.58 vs. <462.58	2.22 (0.92–5.35)	0.075	3.11 (0.90–10.77)	0.074	8.48 (1.04–68.98)	0.046		
Treatment regimen	0.71 (0.31–1.64)	0.422			0.00	0.993		

0, before treatment; Hb, hemoglobin level; RetHb, ret-hemoglobin level; RBC, red blood cells; Ret, reticulocyte count; WBC, white blood cell count; CLC, circulating lymphocyte count; CNC, circulating neutrophil count; CMC, circulating monocyte count; PLT, platelet cell count. NLR, neutrophil/lymphocyte ratio; LMR, lymphocyte/monocyte ratio; PLR, platelet/lymphocyte ratio; SII, systemic immune inflammation index; RT, radiotherapy; CRT, chemoradiotherapy. Significant p values are marked in bold.

Table 4. Overall survival (OS) depending on post-treatment parameters in HPV−/HPV+ patients: univariate and multivariate analysis.

Variable	OS HPV−				OS HPV+			
	Univariate Analysis		Multivariate Analysis		Univariate Analysis		Multivariate Analysis	
	HR (95% CI)	p-Value	HR (95% CI)	p-Value	HR (95% CI)	p-Value	HR (95% CI)	p-Value
Hb 1 [g/dL] >10.1 vs. <10.1	0.27 (0.08–0.93)	0.037			0.47 (0.06–3.77)	0.478		
RetHb 1 [/mm³] >37.8 vs. <37.8	1.37 (0.50–3.77)	0.537			0.67 (0.14–3.17)	0.613		
RBC 1 [/mm³] >3.75 vs. <3.75	0.53 (0.24–1.17)	0.118	0.32 (0.12–0.86)	0.024	0.72 (0.23–2.29)	0.580		
Ret 1 [/mm³] >27.5 vs. <27.5	4.15 (0.56–30.94)	0.166	11.24 (0.99–127.94)	0.051	0.48 (0.14–1.65)	0.245		
WBC 1 [/mm³] >3.74 vs. <3.74	0.83 (0.36–1.93)	0.664	0.16 (0.03–0.93)	0.042	2.60 (0.70–9.64)	0.152		

Table 4. Cont.

Variable	OS HPV−				OS HPV+			
	Univariate Analysis		Multivariate Analysis		Univariate Analysis		Multivariate Analysis	
	HR (95% CI)	p-Value	HR (95% CI)	p-Value	HR (95% CI)	p-Value	HR (95% CI)	p-Value
CLC 1 [/mm^3] >0.83 vs. <0.83	0.90 (0.36–2.27)	0.823			8.70 (2.26–33.54)	**0.002**	11.37 (2.61–49.64)	**0.001**
CNC 1 [/mm^3] >2.32 vs. <2.32	1.15 (0.43–3.06)	0.782	7.48 (1.00–56.06)	0.050	1.51 (0.40–5.61)	0.541		
CMC 1 [/mm^3] >0.42 vs. <0.42	1.70 (0.68–4.27)	0.260			0.94 (0.30–2.90)	0.908		
PLT 1 [/mm^3] >313 vs. <313	2.06 (0.89–4.77)	0.092	3.37 (1.18–9.62)	**0.023**	2.05 (0.26–16.14)	0.495		
NLR 1 >6.45 vs. <6.45	1.15 (0.48–2.79)	0.754			0.43 (0.12–1.60)	0.209		
MLR 1 >0.63 vs. <0.63	0.85 (0.38–1.91)	0.697	0.35 (0.12–1.03)	0.057	0.36 (0.09–1.39)	0.138		
PLR 1 >404.17 vs. <404.17	2.55 (1.13–5.77)	**0.024**			0.87 (0.28–2.72)	0.815		
SII 1 >2763 vs. <2763	3.54 (1.28–9.80)	**0.015**	4.69 (1.23–17.97)	**0.024**	2.12 (0.46–9.81)	0.338	4.17 (0.76–22.88)	0.100

0, before treatment; Hb, hemoglobin level; RetHb, ret-hemoglobin level; RBC, red blood cells; Ret, reticulocyte count; WBC, white blood cell count; CLC, circulating lymphocyte count; CNC, circulating neutrophil count; CMC, circulating monocyte count; PLT, platelet cell count. NLR, neutrophil/lymphocyte ratio; LMR, lymphocyte/monocyte ratio; PLR, platelet/lymphocyte ratio; SII, systemic immune inflammation index. Significant p values are marked in bold.

Table 5. Disease-free survival (DFS) depending on post-treatment parameters in HPV−/HPV+ patients: univariate and multivariate analysis.

Variable	DFS HPV−				DFS HPV+			
	Univariate Analysis		Multivariate Analysis		Univariate Analysis		Multivariate Analysis	
	HR (95% CI)	p-Value	HR (95% CI)	p-Value	HR (95% CI)	p-Value	HR (95% CI)	p-Value
Hb 1 [g/dL] >10.8 vs. <10.8	0.37 (0.15–0.89)	**0.027**			2.35 (0.29–19.11)	0.424		
RetHb 1 [/mm^3] >38.0 vs. <38.0	2.28 (0.76–6.82)	0.142			0.72 (0.09–5.98)	0.761		
RBC 1 [/mm^3] >3.75 vs. <3.75	0.42 (0.19–0.93)	**0.033**	0.26 (0.11–0.66)	**0.004**	1.56 (0.31–7.71)	0.589		
Ret 1 [/mm^3] >27.5 vs. <27.5	4.03 (0.54–30.11)	0.174			0.39 (0.09–1.76)	0.221		
WBC 1 [/mm^3] >3.21 vs. <3.21	0.57 (0.23–1.44)	0.233			17780630	0.994		
CLC 1 [/mm^3] >0.37 vs. <0.37	0.56 (0.22–1.42)	0.226			4.03 (0.50–32.73)	0.193		
CNC 1 [/mm^3] >2.69 vs. <2.69	0.98 (0.40–2.35)	0.956			1.66 (0.40–6.95)	0.488		
CMC 1 [/mm^3] >0.47 vs. <0.47	0.50 (0.22–1.11)	0.087			1.31 (0.33–5.22)	0.706		
PLT 1 [/mm^3] >261 vs. <261	1.07 (0.48–2.39)	0.873			4.26 (1.06–17.07)	**0.041**	7.97 (1.55–41.00)	**0.013**
NLR 1 >13.24 vs. <13.24	3.16 (1.18–8.50)	**0.022**			1.17 (0.14–9.52)	0.882		
MLR 1 >0.63 vs. <0.63	0.66 (0.29–1.51)	0.325	0.40 (0.15–1.03)	0.058	0.48 (0.10–2.38)	0.368	0.21 (0.04–1.31)	0.095
PLR 1 >380 vs. <380	2.17 (0.95–4.99)	0.068	3.96 (1.46–10.77)	**0.007**	0.80 (0.20–3.18)	0.747		
SII 1 >2730 vs. <2730	3.25 (1.27–8.28)	**0.014**			1.33 (0.16–10.81)	0.790		

0, before treatment; Hb, hemoglobin level; RetHb, ret-hemoglobin level; RBC, red blood cells; Ret, reticulocyte count; WBC, white blood cell count; CLC, circulating lymphocyte count; CNC, circulating neutrophil count; CMC, circulating monocyte count; PLT, platelet cell count. NLR, neutrophil/lymphocyte ratio; LMR, lymphocyte/monocyte ratio; PLR, platelet/lymphocyte ratio; SII, systemic immune inflammation index. Significant p values are marked in bold.

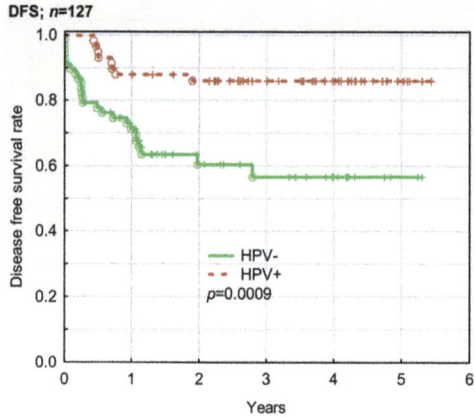
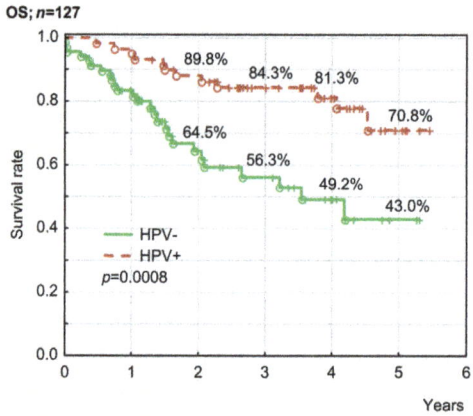

Figure 2. Comparison of overall survival (OS) and disease-free survival (DFS) between Human Papilloma Virus (HPV)− and HPV+ groups.

3.4.1. Overall Survival Depending on Pre-Treatment Parameters

HPV−

In UVA, poor prognostic factors for OS in HPV− patients were as follows: A higher CMC (HR 2.41, 95% CI 1.01–5.74, $p = 0.048$), a higher PLT (HR 2.53, 95% CI 1.07–5.99, $p = 0.035$), and a higher MLR (HR 3.73, 95% CI 1.71–8.15, $p = 0.001$). A higher WBC (HR 2.33, 95% CI 0.99–5.47, $p = 0.053$) marginally predicted inferior OS in HPV− patients.

In MVA, a higher CMC (HR 4.24, 95% CI 1.52–11.84, $p = 0.006$), a higher MLR (HR 3.83, 95% CI 1.46–10.02, $p = 0.006$), and a higher PLR (HR 3.60, 95% CI 1.15–11.31, $p = 0.028$) were poor prognostic factors for OS.

HPV+

In UVA, poor prognostic factors for OS in HPV+ patients were as follows: A higher WBC (HR 4.17, 95% CI 1.25–13.93, $p = 0.020$), a higher NLR (HR 4.76, 95% CI 1.29–17.57, $p = 0.019$), and a higher SII (HR 5.67, 95% CI 1.24–25.94, $p = 0.025$). A higher Ret was associated with higher OS (HR 0.22, 95% CI 0.06–0.82, $p = 0.025$),

In MVA, a higher CMC (HR 17.18, 95% CI 1.89–167.47, $p = 0.012$), and a higher SII (HR 11.10, 95% CI 2.02–60.97, $p = 0.006$) were poor prognostic factors for OS.

All described prognostic factors are presented in Table 2.

3.4.2. Disease-Free Survival Depending on Pre-Treatment Parameters

HPV−

In UVA, poor prognostic factors for DFS in HPV− patients were as follows: A higher PLT (HR 2.77, 95% CI 1.18–6.52, $p = 0.020$), and higher PLR (HR 2.88, 95% CI 1.30–6.38, $p = 0.009$), whereas a higher RBC (HR 0.39, 95% CI 0.15–0.97, $p = 0.043$) predicted better DFS.

In MVA, a higher PLR (HR 2.74, 95% CI 1.02–7.41, $p = 0.046$) was a poor prognostic factor for DFS, whereas a higher RBC (HR 0.21, 95% CI 0.07–0.66, $p = 0.008$), a higher MLR (HR 0.20, 95% CI 0.06–0.62, $p = 0.006$) were associated with higher DFS.

HPV+

In UVA, poor prognostic factors for DFS in HPV+ patients were as follows: A higher NLR (HR 6.02, 95% CI 1.21–29.87, $p = 0.028$), and a higher SII (HR 8.48, 95% CI 1.04–68.98, $p = 0.046$), whereas a higher CLC (HR 0.19, 95% CI 0.05–0.77, $p = 0.020$), a higher CMC (HR 0.16, 95% CI 0.03–0.8, $p = 0.026$) predicted higher DFS.

In MVA, a higher Hb (HR 10.44, 95% CI 1.31–83.38, $p = 0.027$) was a poor prognostic factor for DFS, whereas a higher CLC (HR 0.17, 95% CI 0.03–0.97, $p = 0.046$) was associated with higher DFS. A higher CMC (HR 0.20, 95% CI 0.04–1.07, $p = 0.060$) marginally predicted higher DFS in HPV+ patients.

All described prognostic factors are presented in Table 3.

3.4.3. Overall Survival Depending on Post-Treatment Parameters

HPV−

In UVA, poor prognostic factors for OS in HPV− patients were as follows: A higher PLR (HR 2.55, 95% CI 1.13–5.77, $p = 0.024$), and a higher SII (HR 3.54, 95% CI 1.28–9.80, $p = 0.015$). A higher Hb (HR 0.27, 95% CI 0.08–0.93, $p = 0.037$) predicted better OS in HPV−patients.

In MVA, higher PLT (HR 3.37, 95% CI 1.18–9.62, $p = 0.023$) and a higher SII (HR 4.69, 95% CI 1.23–17.97, $p = 0.024$) were poor prognostic factors for OS. A higher RBC (HR 0.32, 95% CI 0.12–0.86, $p = 0.024$), a higher WBC (HR 0.16, 95% CI 0.03–0.93, $p = 0.042$) were associated with better OS.

HPV+

In UVA, only a higher CLC (HR 8.70, 95% CI 2.26–33.54, $p = 0.002$) was a poor prognostic factor for OS in HPV+ patients.

In MVA, also a higher CLC (HR 11.37, 95% CI 2.61–49.64, $p = 0.001$) was a poor prognostic factor for OS in HPV+ patients.

All described prognostic factors are presented in Table 4.

3.4.4. Disease-Free Survival Depending on Post-Treatment Parameters

HPV−

In UVA, poor prognostic factors for DFS in HPV− patients were as follows: A higher NLR (HR 3.16, 95% CI 1.18–8.50, $p = 0.022$) and a higher SII (HR 3.25, 95% CI 1.27–8.28, $p = 0.014$), whereas a higher Hb (HR 0.37, 95% CI 0.15–0.89, $p = 0.027$) and a higher RBC (HR 0.42, 95% CI 0.19–0.93, $p = 0.033$) were associated with better DFS.

In MVA, a higher PLR (HR 3.96, 1.46–10.77, $p = 0.007$) was a poor prognostic factor for DFS, whereas a higher RBC (HR 0.26, 95% CI 0.11–0.66, $p = 0.004$) was associated with higher DFS.

HPV+

In UVA, only a higher PLT (HR 4.26, 95% CI 1.06–17.07, $p = 0.041$) was a poor prognostic factor for OS in HPV−+ patients.

In MVA, also a higher PLT (HR 7.97, 95% CI 1.55–41.00, $p = 0.013$) was the only poor prognostic factor for DFS.

All described prognostic factors are presented in Table 5.

3.4.5. Summary of the Analysis of OS and DFS in HPV− and HPV+ Patients

In summary, our study showed different pre-treatment and post-treatment parameters predicting OS and DFS in HPV− and HPV+ patients. HPV status was the strongest predictor for OS and DFS. Generally, there were more immune and hematological parameters predicting survival in HPV− patients compared to HPV+ participants. In HPV+ patients, a high pre-treatment WBC, NLR, and SII significantly correlated with reduced OS, whereas a high NLR and SII significantly correlated with reduced DFS. A higher pre-treatment NLR and SII were significant poor prognostic factors for both OS and DFS in the HPV+ group. These associations were not apparent in HPV− patients.

Thus, there are different pre-treatment and post-treatment immune and hematological prognostic factors for OS and DFS in HPV+ and HPV− patients.

A summary of differences regarding the impact of immune and hematological pre-treatment and post-treatment parameters on OS and DFS depending on HPV status is presented in Table 6.

Table 6. Pre-treatment and post-treatment prognostic factors for OS and DFS in HPV−/HPV+ patients.

Prognostic Factors	OS HPV−	DFS HPV−	OS HPV+	DFS HPV+
Poor prognostic factors in UVA (before treatment)	Higher CMC Higher PLT Higher MLR	Higher PLT Higher PLR Lower Hb Lower RBC	Higher WBC Higher NLR Higher SII Lower Ret	Higher NLR Higher SII Lower CLC Lower CMC
Poor prognostic factors in MVA (before treatment)	Higher CMC Higher MLR Higher PLR	Higher PLR Lower RBC Lower MLR	Higher CMC Higher SII	Higher Hb Lower RBC Lower CLC
Poor prognostic factors in UVA (after treatment)	Higher PLR Higher SII Lower Hb	Higher NLR Higher SII Lower Hb Lower RBC	Higher CLC	Higher PLT
Poor prognostic factors in MVA (after treatment)	Higher PLT Higher SII Lower RBC Lower WBC	Higher PLR Lower RBC	Higher CLC	Higher PLT

OS, overall survival; DFS, disease-free survival; UVA, univariate analysis; MVA, multivariate analysis; Hb, hemoglobin level; RetHb, ret-hemoglobin level; RBC, red blood cell count; WBC, white blood cell count; CLC, circulating lymphocyte count; CNC, circulating neutrophil count; CMC, circulating monocyte count; PLT, platelet cell count. NLR, neutrophil/lymphocyte ratio; LMR, lymphocyte/monocyte ratio; PLR, platelet/lymphocyte ratio; SII, systemic immune inflammation index.

4. Discussion

Both neutrophils and monocytes are derived from a myelocytic lineage, whereas lymphocytes are derived from a lymphoid lineage [1]. The association of high baseline myeloid-derived cells (neutrophils and monocytes) with poor clinical outcomes has been observed in various cancer types, including head and neck cancers and OPC. This concerns both the blood and tumor cell counts [1,8–10]. In Huang et al.'s study [1], both high pre-treatment CNC and CMC values independently predicted poor survival and disease control, whereas a high CLC was associated with better recurrence-free survival (RFS) and marginally better OS in HPV+ OPC patients. A similar association was not reported in HPV− OPC patients. It is proof that the host immune system significantly influences treatment outcome in HPV+ OPC individuals [1]. Also, it has been shown that pre-treatment anemia is an independent poor prognostic factor for survival in HPV+ OPC patients [11].

In recent years, various peripheral blood inflammation factors, such as counts of neutrophils, lymphocytes, monocytes, platelet cells, either as individual values or ratios, have been proposed as prognostic markers of head and neck squamous cell carcinoma

(HNSCC) [12–15]. Therefore, we decided to analyze their impact on prognosis in our OPC patients considering the status of high-risk HPV.

In our study, PLT count was a significant poor prognostic factor for both OS and DFS survival in HPV− patients. This association of the higher PLT count with inferior survival in OPC patients is in accordance with observations of other authors. Shoultz-Henley et al. [13] evaluated associations between increased PLT and anemia and oncologic outcomes in OPC patients receiving concurrent CRT. The authors noted that locoregional control (LRC), freedom from distant metastasis (FDM), and OS were significantly decreased for patients with a pre-treatment PLT value of $\geq 350 \times 10^9$ /L. Anemic patients demonstrated comparatively decreased LRC, FDM, and OS. Additionally, patients with simultaneous PLT elevation and anemia had significantly worse oncologic outcomes for LRC, FDM, and OS than those with anemia or platelet elevation alone or those with no alteration. It should be emphasized, that Shoultz-Henley's study did not stratify patients according to HPV status [13]. Gorphe et al. [11] investigated the prognostic value of pre-treatment hematological parameters in patients with HPV+ OPC. In their study, Hb < 12 g/dL was associated with impaired OS and PFS, pre-treatment NLR > 5 was associated with decreased OS. Patients with NLR > 5 had a significantly higher rate of disease recurrence. The authors explained the association between a low Hb level and poor prognosis in OPC patients as follows: low Hb concentration might exacerbate the preexisting hypoxia that is often present in tumors by decreasing oxygen-carrying capacity and so hampering the response of tumor cells to cytotoxic therapy [11]. In our study, with HPV status stratification, we showed a significant association between the pre-treatment Hb level and DFS only in HPV− patients. A similar association was not shown for HPV+ patients. In another study, Ye et al. reported that pre-treatment NLR elevation and PLT > 248×10^9 /L were promising predictors of prognosis in patients with operable HNSCC. Explanation of the association between increased PLT and poor survival in OPC patients is the theory that PLTs direct tumor cell growth, vascular invasion, hematogenous dissemination, immune system evasion, and creation of metastasis site [12]. There are scant publications regarding associations between PLT and prognosis in OPC patients, but second factor NLR is the most frequently studied immune parameter. In many publications, it has been noted that increased CNC and decreased CLC were correlated with poor prognosis in OPC patients. This is due to the proven fact that an increased CNC in an inflammatory microenvironment contributes to tumor angiogenesis. It induces the resistance to anti-vascular endothelial growth factor (anti-VEGF) therapy. Additionally, the decreased CLC plays important roles in inflammatory reaction against tumor. Therefore, increased NLR is an independent prognostic factor for survival in cancer patients [12]. Rachidi et al. [14] reported that the CNC and LCC are strong biomarkers for poor prognosis and the NLR is a strong predictor of OS in oral, pharyngeal, and laryngeal squamous cell cancers. Additionally, the authors noted that a higher CNC correlated with a lower CLC. In these authors' study, a higher CNC was associated with shorter OS, whereas a higher CLC was associated with longer OS. Also, their study demonstrated a bigger magnitude of correlation between NLR > 4.39 and survival within the HPV+ group than that seen in the HPV− group [14]. This phenomenon was also observed in many studies, including our research.

Charles et al. [15] compared patients with oropharyngeal and non-oropharyngeal HNSCC. With univariate analysis, the authors demonstrated associations between NLR and RFS and OS in both sub-populations. Multivariable analysis showed that patients with an NLR > 5 had shortened OS in both sub-populations but an NLR > 5 only predicted RFS in oropharyngeal patients [15]. Kano et al. [16] in a study conducted on patients with oropharyngeal, hypopharyngeal, and laryngeal cancers, demonstrated that a high NLR > 1.92, high PLR, and low LMR were all significantly associated with decreased OS and DFS. Valero et al. [17] reported that an increased NLR > 1.35 was independently related to inferior DFS in patients with HNSCC. Selzer et al. reported that a high NLR > 5 is associated with inferior OS in locally advanced head and neck cancer patients who were treated with curative intent by primary RT alone, or by RCT [18]. Moon et al., in HNSCC patients who underwent definitive RCT, observed that a higher NLR was associated with shortened progression-free survival (PFS) and OS [19]. In our study, an NLR above 2.13 for OS and above 2.29 for DFS was a significant poor prognostic factor in HPV+ patients. Yao et al. in a study conducted on patients with nasopharyngeal cancer, showed that an NLR > 2.50 was significantly associated with inferior OS, distant metastasis-free survival (DMFS), and PFS [20]. Lu et al. reported that an NLR $\geq$ 2.28, LMR < 2.26, and PLR $\geq$ 174 were significantly associated with a shorter OS, and an NLR $\geq$ 2.28 was significantly associated with a shorter PFS in patients with nasopharyngeal cancer [21].

The SII was the second independent prognostic factor for both OS and DFS in HPV+ patients in our study. The significant prognostic SII cut-off in the HPV+ group was >448.60 for OS and 462.58 for DFS. The SII as a prognostic factor for survival in cancer patients is less frequently described. Gao et al. described the SII, NLR, and PLR as independent prognostic factors for OS and DFS in patients with surgically resected esophageal squamous cell carcinoma (ESCC). The optimal cut-off values for the prediction of survival were 479.72 for the SII, 2.27 for NLR, 117.07 for PLR, and 0.19 for MLR [22]. Thus, the values of significant factors (NLR, SII) were similar to our findings. Among another immune ratios, our study showed only the statistical significance of MLR > 0.425 for OS in the HPV− group, and PLR > 173.2 for DFS in HPV− patients. The statistical analysis did not show significant associations for the other ratios, but observations of tendency within these parameters were comparable with the literature data. The mechanism of the SII contribution to a worse prognosis in patients with solid cancer is still unclear. There are some theories explaining the prognostic significance of the SII. According to the first hypothesis, the CNC expands both in the tumor microenvironment and systemically, and it is known that it is associated with poor prognosis in cancer patients [22,23]. The CNC may activate endothelium and parenchymal cells to enhance circulating tumor cell adhesion for distant metastasis [22,24]. The second theory is that PLTs may act as protective "cloaks" for circulating tumor cells (CTCs), protecting them from immune destruction. Additionally, PLTs and endothelial cell adhesion proteins may facilitate metastasis by augmenting tumor cell extravasation [22,25]. Thirdly, tumor-infiltrating lymphocytes (TILs) are associated with better response to cytotoxic treatment and prognosis in cancer patients [22,26,27]. The CLC can also secrete several cytokines, such as IFN-γ and TNF-α, in order to block tumor growth and improve the prognosis of cancer patients [22,28]. According to Gao et al. [22] and in our opinion, the SII should be a more objective marker, because it reflects the balance between host inflammatory and immune response status better than all the other immunological ratios, such as the NLR, PLR, and MLR. In our opinion, the SII is the best systemic inflammatory marker, superior to immune ratios (NLR, PLR, and MLR) and singular hematological parameters (CNC, CLC, CMC, and PLT). The SII involves three singular parameters (CNC, PLT, and CLC), more than the others (NLR, PLR and MLR), which include only two singular parameters. The more parameters we consider simultaneously, the better the parameter will reflect the systemic immune response.

The SII in the role of an adverse prognostic factor was described in various cancers as follows: oral squamous cell carcinoma [28], esophageal squamous cell carcinoma [22,29–31], colorectal cancer [32,33], lung cancer [34], pancreatic cancer [35], prostate cancer [36], hepatocellular cancer [37], gastric cancer [38], bladder cancer [39], renal cancer [40], cervical cancer [41], and breast cancer [42], but there is no report regarding the SII in OPC. To our knowledge, the present research is the first study on the SII in OPC patients in the worldwide literature, additionally with stratification based on HPV status. Association of the SII with OS and DFS was comparable to the NLR in our patients. Both ratios were significant poor prognostic factor for OS and DFS in HPV+ OPC patients, without such an association in the HPV− group.

Huang et al. [1] compared prognostic significance in HPV− and HPV− OPC patients. The authors noted that HPV+ OPC patients with a higher CNC, a higher CMC, and a lower CLC had inferior survival and an increased risk of disease recurrence. They did not show a similar association in HPV− patients. This observation only partially correlates with our results, because our study, conducted on 127 patients, showed a significant association between a lower CMC and CLC and inferior DFS in HPV+ patients, but did not show any correlation in the HPV− group similar to Huang's report conducted on 510 adults. This phenomenon requires further observation in a larger patient group.

Generally, our study showed significantly better OS and DFS in HPV+ patients compared to HPV− ones ($p = 0.0008$ and $p = 0.0009$, respectively). Thus, HPV status was a very strong prognostic factor for OS and DFS. Survival of HPV+ patients was better despite the higher regional disease advancement. These results are in full accordance with the literature data. Patients with HPV-related OPC have a better prognosis and longer survival compared to patients without HPV-related OPC with typical risk factors (smoking, alcohol abuse) [43,44]. A better prognosis was also observed in HPV+ patients with more advanced OPC with lymph node involvement [5,6]. Moreover, the HPV+ OPC is more responsive to radiotherapy (RT) and chemoradiotherapy (CRT) [4,5,45]. It allows for treatment de-escalation in HPV+ patients [45–47]. In our opinion, this strong impact of HPV status on survival is associated with the presence of different prognostic factors in HPV− and HPV patients. The better survival in HPV+ OPC patients is associated with a greater locoregional control, higher sensitivity to radiation, or better radio-sensitization with the use of cisplatin [48]. The association between the superior survival of HPV+ OPC patients and the administered therapy is unclear. According to numerous authors, tumor HPV status is a strong and consistent determinant of better survival, regardless of treatment strategy (surgery, radiation therapy, concurrent CRT, or induction chemotherapy plus concurrent CRT) with five year survival rates among HPV+ patients of approximately 75 to 80%, versus 45 to 50% among HPV− patients [48–52].

Our patients were treated under standard department protocols definitively with radiotherapy (stage I-II) and chemoradiotherapy (stage III-IV). The difference in treatment strategy was determined by tumor stage rather than HPV status. The fact that more patients with HPV-related tumors presented more advanced stages was associated with a different tumor biology and clinical outcome. There was a significantly higher number of more advanced N2–3 tumors in HPV+ patients compared to HPV− ones. RT was significantly more frequent in N0–1 tumors, whereas CRT was more common in N2–3 tumors in an analysis of all patients together. The greater nodal involvement is characteristic for HPV+ OPC patients, and it has been confirmed by numerous studies. Moreover, according to the literature, typically HPV OPC presents in a younger, healthier population with a different set of risk factors and good prognosis for survival. Moreover, the majority of analyses showed that patients with HPV+ tumors had significantly better responses to treatment than those with HPV− tumors. HPV− OPC patients are usually older, with numerous comorbidities [43,53,54]. Therefore, in HPV− OPC patients CRT was not possible due to a general status and comorbidities, and accelerated RT was used in this patient group. The aim of our study was a comparison of immune and hematological parameters and their impact on survival in all HPV− and HPV+ OPC patients. Exclusion of any treatment strategy would reduce the possibility of a real clinical evaluation and would distort conclusions relevant to clinical practice. After all, total effective treatment strategy in clinical practice includes both RT and CRT use depending on the tumor staging. In addition, we compared OS and DFS depending on immune and hematological parameters in HPV− and HPV+ groups separately (not between HPV− and HPV+ patients). Moreover, the treatment strategy in low and high NLR, MLR, PLR, and SII groups in both HPV− and HPV+ patients was comparable ($p > 0.05$). Thus, treatment strategy had no impact the final results. Additionally, the impact of RT and CRT on survival has been assessed in univariate (UVA) and multivariate (MVA) Cox analysis. In both UVA and MVA, for HV- and HPV+ patients, the treatment strategy was not a significant prognostic factor. There are studies with a comparative analysis of survival depending on various parameters in head and neck cancer patients despite the statistical difference of the treatment strategies between compared groups in the literature [15,31,55].

To our knowledge, there is only one study regarding a similar topic. In this study, Huang et al. [1] investigated the prognostic value of the pre-treatment circulating neutrophil count (CNC), circulating monocyte count (CMC), and circulating lymphocyte count (CLC) in HPV− and HPV+ OPC patients. Although there are numerous reports regarding the prognostic role of the NLR, MLR, PLR, SII in various cancers, including OPC, there are no reports with a detailed and comprehensive comparison of these parameters between HPV− and HPV+ patients as well as analysis of their impact on survival in both HPV− and HPV+ patients. Our study included a detailed and comprehensive comparative analysis of numerous immune and hematological parameters. Our study is a Polish/Central European voice in the discussion regarding the prognostic role of hematological and immune parameters in HPV− and HPV+ OPC patients. It can be used in a further meta-analysis on this subject. So far, there are only a few original reports in this field, and there is no meta-analysis summarizing all cohort studies. Our study presents simple and widely available blood parameters that may be used in the clinical practice. Taking into account all the above mentioned arguments, the novelty of our study is considerable.

The single center observation and retrospective analysis of a prospectively collected database are limitations of our study. A prospective randomized multi-center study is needed to understand the biology of our observation and potentially to identify new therapeutic targets based on our findings.

5. Conclusions

The higher NLR and SII are significant adverse prognostic factors for HPV+ OPC patients because they are significantly associated with both inferior OS and DFS in this group, whereas the higher PLT is a significant adverse prognostic factor for HPV− OPC patients because it is significantly associated with inferior OS and DFS in this group. Further studies are needed in order to validate our findings. The knowledge of differences in immune parameters between HPV− and HPV+ OPC patients can be useful for the identification of new targeted immunotherapy in the HPV+ OPC treatment.

Supplementary Materials: The following are available online at https://www.mdpi.com/article/10.3390/cancers13133256/s1. Table S1. Pre-treatment and post-treatment laboratory (peripheral blood morphology parameters) results. Table S2. Pre-treatment and post-treatment immune ratios. Table S3. Comparison of low and high neutrophil/lymphocyte ratio (NLR) groups according to selected clinicopathological factors in HPV(+) and HPV(−) patients. Table S4. Comparison of low and high monocyte/lymphocyte ratio (MLR) groups according to selected clinicopathological factors in HPV(+) and HPV(−) patients. Table S5. Comparison of low and high platelet/lymphocyte (PLR) groups according to selected clinicopathological factors in HPV(+) and HPV(−) patients. Table S6. Comparison of low and high systemic immune inflammation (SII) groups according to selected clinicopathological factors in HPV(+) and HPV(−) patients. Figure S1. A. Overall survival (OS) in HPV− and HPV+ depending on hemoglobin (Hb), ret-hemoglobin (RetHb), reticulocyte count (Ret), red blood cell count (RBC). B. Overall survival (OS) in HPV− and HPV+ depending on circulating lymphocyte count (CLC), circulating neutrophil count (CNC), circulating monocyte count (CMC), platelet cell count (PLT). C. Overall survival (OS) in HPV− and HPV+ patients depending on the neutrophil/lymphocyte ratio (NLR), platelet/lymphocyte ratio (PLR), and monocyte/lymphocyte ratio (MLR), and the systemic immune inflammation index (SII). Figure S2. A. Disease-free survival (DFS) in HPV− and HPV+ patients depending on hemoglobin (Hb), ret-hemoglobin (RetHb), reticulocyte count (Ret), red blood cell count (RBC). B. Disease-free survival (DFS) in HPV− and HPV+ patients depending on circulating lymphocyte count (CLC), circulating neutrophil count (CNC), circulating monocyte count (CMC), platelet cell count (PLT). C. Disease-free survival (DFS) in HPV− and HPV+ patients depending on the neutrophil/lymphocyte ratio (NLR), platelet/lymphocyte ratio (PLR), monocyte/lymphocyte ratio (MLR), and the systemic immune inflammation index (SII).

Author Contributions: Conceptualization, A.B. and B.J.; methodology, A.M.M., J.M.-K. and M.Ś.; formal analysis, A.B., B.J. and Z.K.; investigation, A.B., J.M.-K., M.Ś., M.K. and T.R.; writing—original draft preparation, A.B. and B.J.; writing—review and editing, M.Ś. and T.R.; visualization, M.K. and Z.K.; supervision, S.M., K.S. and T.R.; funding acquisition, A.M.M. All authors have read and agreed to the published version of the manuscript.

Funding: This research was funded by National Centre of Research and Development, Polan, grant number TANGO2/340829/NCBR/2017. The APC was funded by Maria Skłodowska-Curie National Research Institute of Oncology, Gliwice Branch.

Institutional Review Board Statement: The study was conducted according to the guidelines of the Declaration of Helsinki, and approved by the Bioethics Committee at Maria Skłodowska-Curie National Research Institute of Oncology, Gliwice Branch (protocol code KB/43018/13).

Informed Consent Statement: Informed consent was obtained from all subjects involved in the study.

Data Availability Statement: The data presented in this study are available in this article and supplementary materials.

Conflicts of Interest: The authors have no conflict of interest to declare.

References

1. Huang, S.H.; Waldron, J.; Milosevic, M.; Shen, X.; Ringash, J.; Su, J.; Tong, L.; Perez-Ordonez, B.; Weinreb, I.; Bayley, A.J.; et al. Prognostic value of pretreatment circulating neutrophils, monocytes, and lymphocytes in oropharyngeal cancer stratified by human papillomavirus status. *Cancer* **2014**, *121*, 545–555. [CrossRef] [PubMed]
2. Takahashi, H.; Sakakura, K.; Tada, H.; Kaira, K.; Oyama, T.; Chikamatsu, K. Prognostic significance and population dynamics of peripheral monocytes in patients with oropharyngeal squamous cell carcinoma. *Head Neck* **2019**, *41*, 1880–1888. [CrossRef] [PubMed]
3. Meshman, J.; Velez, M.A.; Wang, P.-C.; Abemayor, E.; John, M.S.; Wong, D.; Bhuta, S.; Chen, A.M. Immunologic mediators of outcome for irradiated oropharyngeal carcinoma based on human papillomavirus status. *Oral Oncol.* **2019**, *89*, 121–126. [CrossRef] [PubMed]
4. Yamashita, Y.; Ikegami, T.; Hirakawa, H.; Uehara, T.; Deng, Z.; Agena, S.; Uezato, J.; Kondo, S.; Kiyuna, A.; Maeda, H.; et al. Staging and prognosis of oropharyngeal carcinoma according to the 8th Edition of the American Joint Committee on Cancer Staging Manual in human papillomavirus infection. *Eur. Arch. Oto. Rhino. Laryngol.* **2019**, *276*, 827–836. [CrossRef]
5. Mallen-St Clair, J.; Ho, A.S. American Joint Committee on Cancer 8th edition staging-an improvement in prognostication in HPV-associated oropharyngeal cancer? *Ann. Transl. Med.* **2019**, *7* (Suppl. 1), S10.
6. Lechien, J.R.; Seminerio, I.; Descamps, G.; Mat, Q.; Mouawad, F.; Hans, S.; Julieron, M.; Dequanter, D.; Vanderhaegen, T.; Journe, F.; et al. Impact of HPV Infection on the Immune System in Oropharyngeal and Non-Oropharyngeal Squamous Cell Carcinoma: A Systematic Review. *Cells* **2019**, *8*, 1061. [CrossRef]
7. Snietura, M.; Vanderhaegen, T.; Brewczynski, A.; Kopec, A.; Rutkowski, T. Infiltrates of M2-Like Tumour-Associated Macrophages Are Adverse Prognostic Factor in Patients with Human Papillomavirus-Negative but Not in Human Papillomavirus-Positive Oropharyngeal Squamous Cell Carcinoma. *Pathobiology* **2020**, *87*, 75–86. [CrossRef]
8. Rajjoub, S.; Basha, S.R.; Einhorn, E.; Cohen, M.C.; Marvel, D.M.; Sewell, D.A. Prognostic significance of tumor-infiltrating lymphocytes in oropharyngeal cancer. *Ear Nose Throat J.* **2007**, *86*, 506–511. [CrossRef]
9. Ward, M.J.; Thirdborough, S.M.; Mellows, T.; Riley, C.; Harris, S.B.; Suchak, K.; Webb, A.A.R.; Hampton, C.L.; Patel, N.N.; Randall, C.J.; et al. Tumour-infiltrating lymphocytes predict for outcome in HPV-positive oropharyngeal cancer. *Br. J. Cancer* **2014**, *110*, 489–500. [CrossRef]
10. King, E.V.; Ottensmeier, C.H.; Thomas, G.J. The immune response in HPV+oropharyngeal cancer. *Oncoimmunology* **2014**, *3*, e27254. [CrossRef]
11. Gorphe, P.; Idrissi, Y.C.; Tao, Y.; Schernberg, A.; Ou, D.; Temam, S.; Casiraghi, O.; Blanchard, P.; Mirghani, H. Anemia and neutrophil-to-lymphocyte ratio are prognostic in p16-positive oropharyngeal carcinoma treated with concurrent chemoradiation. *Papillomavirus Res.* **2018**, *5*, 32–37. [CrossRef]
12. Ye, J.; Liao, B.; Jiang, X.; Dong, Z.; Hu, S.; Liu, Y.; Xiao, M. Prognosis Value of Platelet Counts, Albumin and Neutrophil-Lymphocyte Ratio of Locoregional Recurrence in Patients with Operable Head and Neck Squamous Cell Carcinoma. *Cancer Manag. Res.* **2020**, *12*, 731–741. [CrossRef]
13. Shoultz-Henley, S.; Garden, A.; Mohamed, A.S.; Sheu, T.; Kroll, M.H.; Rosenthal, D.; Gunn, G.B.; Hayes, A.J.; French, C.; Eichelberger, H.; et al. Prognostic value of pretherapy platelet elevation in oropharyngeal cancer patients treated with chemoradiation. *Int. J. Cancer* **2015**, *138*, 1290–1297. [CrossRef]
14. Rachidi, S.; Wallace, K.; Wrangle, J.M.; Day, T.A.; Alberg, A.J.; Li, Z. Neutrophil-to-lymphocyte ratio and overall survival in all sites of head and neck squamous cell carcinoma. *Head Neck* **2016**, *38*, E1068–E1074. [CrossRef]

15. Charles, K.A.; Harris, B.D.W.; Haddad, C.R.; Clarke, S.J.; Guminski, A.; Stevens, M.; Dodds, T.; Gill, A.J.; Back, M.; Veivers, D.; et al. Systemic inflammation is an independent predictive marker of clinical outcomes in mucosal squamous cell carcinoma of the head and neck in oropharyngeal and non-oropharyngeal patients. *BMC Cancer* **2016**, *16*, 124. [CrossRef]
16. Kano, S.; Homma, A.; Hatakeyama, H.; Mizumachi, T.; Sakashita, T.; Kakizaki, T.; Fukuda, S. Pretreatment lymphocyte-to-monocyte ratio as an independent prognostic factor for head and neck cancer. *Head Neck* **2016**, *39*, 247–253. [CrossRef]
17. Valero, C.; Pardo, L.; López, M.; García, J.; Camacho, M.; Quer, M.; León, X. Pretreatment count of peripheral neutrophils, monocytes, and lymphocytes as independent prognostic factor in patients with head and neck cancer. *Head Neck* **2017**, *39*, 219–226. [CrossRef]
18. Selzer, E.; Grah, A.; Heiduschka, G.; Kornek, G.; Thurnher, D. Primary radiotherapy or postoperative radiotherapy in patients with head and neck cancer: Comparative analysis of inflammation-based prognostic scoring systems. *Strahlenther. Onkol.* **2015**, *191*, 486–494. [CrossRef]
19. Moon, H.; Roh, J.-L.; Lee, S.-W.; Kim, S.-B.; Choi, S.-H.; Nam, S.Y.; Kim, S.Y. Prognostic value of nutritional and hematologic markers in head and neck squamous cell carcinoma treated by chemoradiotherapy. *Radiother. Oncol.* **2016**, *118*, 330–334. [CrossRef]
20. Yao, J.-J.; Zhu, F.-T.; Dong, J.; Liang, Z.-B.; Yang, L.-W.; Chen, S.-Y.; Zhang, W.-J.; Lawrence, W.R.; Zhang, F.; Wang, S.-Y.; et al. Prognostic value of neutrophil-to-lymphocyte ratio in advanced nasopharyngeal carcinoma: A large institution-based cohort study from an endemic area. *BMC Cancer* **2019**, *19*, 37. [CrossRef]
21. Lu, A.; Li, H.; Zheng, Y.; Tang, M.; Li, J.; Wu, H.; Zhong, W.; Gao, J.; Ou, N.; Cai, Y. Prognostic Significance of Neutrophil to Lymphocyte Ratio, Lymphocyte to Monocyte Ratio, and Platelet to Lymphocyte Ratio in Patients with Nasopharyngeal Carcinoma. *BioMed Res. Int.* **2017**, *2017*, 30478022. [CrossRef]
22. Gao, Y.; Guo, W.; Cai, S.; Zhang, F.; Shao, F.; Zhang, G.; Liu, T.; Tan, F.; Li, N.; Xue, Q.; et al. Systemic immune-inflammation index (SII) is useful to predict survival outcomes in patients with surgically resected esophageal squamous cell carcinoma. *J. Cancer* **2019**, *10*, 3188–3196. [CrossRef]
23. Coffelt, S.B.; Wellenstein, M.D.; De Visser, S.B.C.M.D.W.K.E. Neutrophils in cancer: Neutral no more. *Nat. Rev. Cancer* **2016**, *16*, 431–446. [CrossRef]
24. De Larco, J.E.; Wuertz, B.R.; Furcht, L.T. The potential role of neutrophils in promoting the metastatic phenotype of tumors releasing interleukin-8. *Clin. Cancer Res.* **2004**, *10*, 4895–4900. [CrossRef]
25. Stanger, B.Z.; Kahn, M.L. Platelets and Tumor Cells: A New Form of Border Control. *Cancer Cell* **2013**, *24*, 9–11. [CrossRef]
26. Gooden, M.J.; de Bock, G.H.; Leffers, N.; Daemen, T.; Nijman, H.W. The prognostic influence of tumour-infiltrating lymphocytes in cancer: A systematic review with meta-analysis. *Br. J. Cancer* **2011**, *105*, 93. [CrossRef]
27. Jia, Q.; Yang, Y.; Wan, Y. Tumor-infiltrating memory T-lymphocytes for prognostic prediction in cancer patients: A meta-analysis. *Int. J. Clin. Exp. Med.* **2015**, *8*, 1803–1813.
28. Diao, P.; Wu, Y.; Li, J.; Zhang, W.; Huang, R.; Zhou, C.; Wang, Y.; Cheng, J. Preoperative systemic immune-inflammation index predicts prognosis of patients with oral squamous cell carcinoma after curative resection. *J. Transl. Med.* **2018**, *16*, 365. [CrossRef]
29. Wang, L.; Wang, C.; Wang, J.; Huang, X.; Cheng, Y. A novel systemic immune-inflammation index predicts survival and quality of life of patients after curative resection for esophageal squamous cell carcinoma. *J. Cancer Res. Clin. Oncol.* **2017**, *143*, 2077–2086. [CrossRef]
30. Geng, Y.; Shao, Y.; Zhu, D.; Zheng, X.; Zhou, Q.; Zhou, W.; Ni, X.; Wu, C.; Jiang, J. Systemic Immune-Inflammation Index Predicts Prognosis of Patients with Esophageal Squamous Cell Carcinoma: A Propensity Score-matched Analysis. *Sci. Rep.* **2016**, *6*, 39482. [CrossRef] [PubMed]
31. Feng, J.-F.; Chen, S.; Yang, X. Systemic immune-inflammation index (SII) is a useful prognostic indicator for patients with squamous cell carcinoma of the esophagus. *Medicine* **2017**, *96*, e5886. [CrossRef] [PubMed]
32. Chen, J.-H.; Zhai, E.-T.; Yuan, Y.; Wu, K.-M.; Xu, J.-B.; Peng, J.-J.; Chen, C.-Q.; He, Y.-L.; Cai, S.-R. Systemic immune-inflammation index for predicting prognosis of colorectal cancer. *World J. Gastroenterol.* **2017**, *23*, 6261–6272. [CrossRef] [PubMed]
33. Xie, Q.-K.; Chen, P.; Hu, W.-M.; Sun, P.; He, W.-Z.; Jiang, C.; Kong, P.-F.; Liu, S.-S.; Chen, H.-T.; Yang, Y.-Z.; et al. The systemic immune-inflammation index is an independent predictor of survival for metastatic colorectal cancer and its association with the lymphocytic response to the tumor. *J. Transl. Med.* **2018**, *16*, 273. [CrossRef] [PubMed]
34. Tong, Y.-S.; Tan, J.; Zhou, X.-L.; Song, Y.-Q.; Song, Y.-J. Systemic immune-inflammation index predicting chemoradiation resistance and poor outcome in patients with stage III non-small cell lung cancer. *J. Transl. Med.* **2017**, *15*, 221. [CrossRef]
35. Zhang, K.; Hua, Y.-Q.; Wang, D.; Chen, L.-Y.; Wu, C.-J.; Chen, Z.; Liu, L.-M.; Chen, H. Systemic immune-inflammation index predicts prognosis of patients with advanced pancreatic cancer. *J. Transl. Med.* **2019**, *17*, 30. [CrossRef]
36. Man, Y.-N.; Chen, Y.-F. Systemic immune-inflammation index, serum albumin, and fibrinogen impact prognosis in castration-resistant prostate cancer patients treated with first-line docetaxel. *Int. Urol. Nephrol.* **2019**, *51*, 2189–2199. [CrossRef]
37. Hu, B.; Yang, X.-R.; Xu, Y.; Sun, Y.-F.; Sun, C.; Guo, W.; Zhang, X.; Wang, W.-M.; Qiu, S.-J.; Zhou, J.; et al. Systemic Immune-Inflammation Index Predicts Prognosis of Patients after Curative Resection for Hepatocellular Carcinoma. *Clin. Cancer Res.* **2014**, *20*, 6212–6222. [CrossRef]
38. Shi, H.; Jiang, Y.; Cao, H.; Zhu, H.; Chen, B.; Ji, W. Nomogram Based on Systemic Immune-Inflammation Index to Predict Overall Survival in Gastric Cancer Patients. *Dis. Markers* **2018**, *2018*, 1787424. [CrossRef]
39. Zhang, W.; Wang, R.; Ma, W.; Wu, Y.; Maskey, N.; Guo, Y.; Liu, J.; Mao, S.; Zhang, J.; Yao, X.; et al. Systemic immune-inflammation index predicts prognosis of bladder cancer patients after radical cystectomy. *Ann. Transl. Med.* **2019**, *7*, 431. [CrossRef]

40. De Giorgi, U.; Procopio, G.; Giannarelli, D.; Sabbatini, R.; Bearz, A.; Buti, S.; Basso, U.; Mitterer, M.; Ortega, C.; Bidoli, P.; et al. Association of Systemic Inflammation Index and Body Mass Index with Survival in Patients with Renal Cell Cancer Treated with Nivolumab. *Clin. Cancer Res.* **2019**, *25*, 3839–3846. [CrossRef]
41. Huang, H.; Liu, Q.; Zhu, L.; Zhang, Y.; Lu, X.; Wu, Y.; Liu, L. Prognostic Value of Preoperative Systemic Immune-Inflammation Index in Patients with Cervical Cancer. *Sci. Rep.* **2019**, *9*, 3284. [CrossRef]
42. Van Der Willik, K.D.; Koppelmans, V.; Hauptmann, M.; Compter, A.; Ikram, M.A.; Schagen, S.B. Inflammation markers and cognitive performance in breast cancer survivors 20 years after completion of chemotherapy: A cohort study. *Breast Cancer Res.* **2018**, *20*, 135. [CrossRef]
43. De Felice, F.; Tombolini, V.; Valentini, V.; De Vincentiis, M.; Mezi, S.; Brugnoletti, O.; Polimeni, A. Advances in the Management of HPV-Related Oropharyngeal Cancer. *J. Oncol.* **2019**, *2019*, 9173729. [CrossRef]
44. Malm, I.-J.; Fan, C.J.; Yin, L.; Li, D.X.; Koch, W.M.; Gourin, C.G.; Pitman, K.T.; Richmon, J.D.; Westra, W.H.; Kang, H.; et al. Evaluation of proposed staging systems for human papillomavirus-related oropharyngeal squamous cell carcinoma. *Cancer* **2017**, *123*, 1768–1777. [CrossRef]
45. Masterson, L.; Moualed, D.; Liu, Z.W.; Howard, J.E.; Dwivedi, R.C.; Tysome, J.R.; Benson, R.; Sterling, J.C.; Sudhoff, H.; Jani, P.; et al. De-escalation treatment protocols for human papillomavirus-associated oropharyngeal squamous cell carcinoma: A systematic review and meta-analysis of current clinical trials. *Eur. J. Cancer* **2014**, *50*, 2636–2648. [CrossRef]
46. Petar, S.; Marko, S.; Ivica, L. De-escalation in HPV-associated oropharyngeal cancer: Lessons learned from the past? A critical viewpoint and proposal for future research. *Eur. Arch. Oto. Rhino. Laryngol.* **2021**. [CrossRef]
47. Harrowfield, J.; Isenring, E.; Kiss, N.; Laing, E.; Lipson-Smith, R.; Britton, B. The Impact of Human Papillomavirus (HPV) Associated Oropharyngeal Squamous Cell Carcinoma (OPSCC) on Nutritional Outcomes. *Nutrients* **2021**, *13*, 514. [CrossRef]
48. Ang, K.K.; Harris, J.; Wheeler, R.; Weber, R.; Rosenthal, D.I.; Nguyen-Tân, P.F.; Westra, W.H.; Chung, C.H.; Jordan, R.C.; Lu, C.; et al. Human Papillomavirus and Survival of Patients with Oropharyngeal Cancer. *N. Engl. J. Med.* **2010**, *363*, 24–35. [CrossRef]
49. Licitra, L.; Perrone, F.; Bossi, P.; Suardi, S.; Mariani, L.; Artusi, R.; Oggionni, M.; Rossini, C.; Cantu', G.; Squadrelli, M.; et al. High-Risk Human Papillomavirus Affects Prognosis in Patients With Surgically Treated Oropharyngeal Squamous Cell Carcinoma. *J. Clin. Oncol.* **2006**, *24*, 5630–5636. [CrossRef]
50. Lindquist, D.; Romanitan, M.; Hammarstedt, L.; Näsman, A.; Dahlstrand, H.; Lindholm, J.; Onelöv, L.; Ramqvist, T.; Ye, W.; Munck-Wikland, E.; et al. Human papillomavirus is a favourable prognostic factor in tonsillar cancer and its oncogenic role is supported by the expression of E6 and E7. *Mol. Oncol.* **2007**, *1*, 350–355. [CrossRef]
51. Lassen, P.; Eriksen, J.G.; Hamilton-Dutoit, S.; Tramm, T.; Alsner, J.; Overgaard, J. Effect of HPV-associated p16INK4A expression on response to radiotherapy and survival in squamous cell carcinoma of the head and neck. *J. Clin. Oncol.* **2009**, *27*, 1992–1998. [CrossRef]
52. Fakhry, C.; Westra, W.H.; Li, S.; Cmelak, A.; Ridge, J.A.; Pinto, H.; Forastiere, A.; Gillison, M.L. Improved survival of patients with human papillomavirus-positive head and neck squamous cell carcinoma in a prospective clinical trial. *J. Natl. Cancer Inst.* **2008**, *100*, 261–269. [CrossRef]
53. Ihloff, A.S.; Petersen, C.; Hoffmann, M.; Knecht, R.; Tribius, S. Human papilloma virus in locally advanced stage III/IV squamous cell cancer of the oropharynx and impact on choice of therapy. *Oral Oncol.* **2010**, *46*, 705–711. [CrossRef] [PubMed]
54. You, E.L.; Henry, M.; Zeitouni, A.G. Human papillomavirus-associated oropharyngeal cancer: Review of current evidence and management. *Curr. Oncol.* **2019**, *26*, 119–123. [CrossRef] [PubMed]
55. Du, X.J.; Tang, L.L.; Mao, Y.P.; Guo, R.; Sun, Y.; Lin, A.H.; Ma, J. Value of the prognostic nutritional index and weight loss in predicting metastasis and long-term mortality in nasopharyngeal carcinoma. *J. Transl. Med.* **2015**, *13*, 364. [CrossRef] [PubMed]

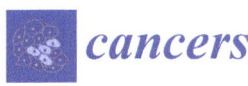

Article

Tumor-Associated Trypsin Inhibitor (TATI) as a Biomarker of Poor Prognosis in Oropharyngeal Squamous Cell Carcinoma Irrespective of HPV Status

Anni Sjöblom [1,*], Ulf-Håkan Stenman [2,†], Jaana Hagström [1,3,4,†], Lauri Jouhi [5], Caj Haglund [3,6], Stina Syrjänen [4,7], Petri Mattila [5], Antti Mäkitie [5,8,9,‡] and Timo Carpén [1,5,9,‡]

1. Department of Pathology, University of Helsinki and HUS Helsinki University Hospital, P.O. Box 21, FI-00014 Helsinki, Finland; jaana.hagstrom@hus.fi (J.H.); timo.carpen@fimnet.fi (T.C.)
2. Department of Clinical Chemistry, University of Helsinki and HUS Helsinki University Hospital, P.O. Box 63, FI-00014 Helsinki, Finland; ulf-hakan.stenman@pp.fimnet.fi
3. Research Programs Unit, Translational Cancer Biology, University of Helsinki, P.O. Box 63, FI-00014 Helsinki, Finland; caj.haglund@helsinki.fi
4. Department of Oral Pathology and Oral Radiology, University of Turku, Lemminkäisenkatu 2, FI-20520 Turku, Finland; stisyr@utu.fi
5. Department of Otorhinolaryngology—Head and Neck Surgery, University of Helsinki and HUS Helsinki University Hospital, P.O. Box 263, FI-00029 Helsinki, Finland; lauri.jouhi@helsinki.fi (L.J.); petri.mattila@hus.fi (P.M.); antti.makitie@helsinki.fi (A.M.)
6. Department of Surgery, University of Helsinki and HUS Helsinki University Hospital, P.O. Box 440, FI-00029 Helsinki, Finland
7. Department of Pathology, Turku University Hospital, Kiinamyllynkatu 10, FI-20520 Turku, Finland
8. Division of Ear, Nose and Throat Diseases, Department of Clinical Sciences, Intervention and Technology, Karolinska Institutet and Karolinska Hospital, SE-171 76 Stockholm, Sweden
9. Research Program in Systems Oncology, Faculty of Medicine, University of Helsinki, P.O. Box 63, FI-00014 Helsinki, Finland
* Correspondence: anni.sjoblom@fimnet.fi
† U.-H.S. and J.H. contributed equally to this paper.
‡ A.M. and T.C. contributed equally to this paper.

Simple Summary: Oropharyngeal squamous cell carcinoma (OPSCC) is a form of head and neck cancer in which human papillomavirus (HPV) infection has been shown to play a major role in disease development. The survival rates of HPV-positive patients are favorable compared to HPV-negative patients, but the reason for this phenomenon remains unclear. The management of OPSCC is complex, and development of novel treatment options is urgently required. Various possible factors affecting survival have been explored, including the tumor environment and cancer-related proteases. Our aim was to study a protease inhibitor known as tumor-associated trypsin inhibitor and its correlation with survival and clinical data in OPSCC patients.

Abstract: Background: We studied the role of tumor-associated trypsin inhibitor (TATI) in serum and in tumor tissues among human papillomavirus (HPV)-positive and HPV-negative OPSCC patients. Materials and methods: The study cohort included 90 OPSCC patients treated at the Helsinki University Hospital (HUS), Helsinki, Finland, in 2012–2016. TATI serum concentrations (S-TATIs) were determined by an immunofluorometric assay. Immunostaining was used to assess tissue expression. HPV status was determined with a combination of p16 immunohistochemistry and HPV DNA PCR genotyping. The survival endpoints were overall survival (OS) and disease-specific survival (DSS). Results: A significant correlation was found between S-TATI positivity and poor OS ($p < 0.001$) and DSS ($p = 0.04$) in all patients. In HPV-negative cases, S-TATI positivity was linked to poor OS ($p = 0.01$) and DSS ($p = 0.05$). In HPV-positive disease, S-TATI positivity correlated with poor DSS ($p = 0.01$). S-TATI positivity was strongly associated with HPV negativity. TATI serum was negatively linked to a lower cancer stage. TATI expression in peritumoral lymphocytes was associated with favorable OS ($p < 0.025$) and HPV positivity. TATI expression in tumor and in peritumoral lymphocytes correlated with lower cancer stages. Conclusion: Our results suggest that S-TATI positivity may be a biomarker of poor prognosis in both HPV-positive and HPV-negative OPSCC.

Citation: Sjöblom, A.; Stenman, U.-H.; Hagström, J.; Jouhi, L.; Haglund, C.; Syrjänen, S.; Mattila, P.; Mäkitie, A.; Carpén, T. Tumor-Associated Trypsin Inhibitor (TATI) as a Biomarker of Poor Prognosis in Oropharyngeal Squamous Cell Carcinoma Irrespective of HPV Status. *Cancers* **2021**, *13*, 2811. https://doi.org/10.3390/cancers13112811

Academic Editor: Heather Walline

Received: 29 April 2021
Accepted: 2 June 2021
Published: 4 June 2021

Publisher's Note: MDPI stays neutral with regard to jurisdictional claims in published maps and institutional affiliations.

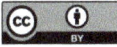

Copyright: © 2021 by the authors. Licensee MDPI, Basel, Switzerland. This article is an open access article distributed under the terms and conditions of the Creative Commons Attribution (CC BY) license (https://creativecommons.org/licenses/by/4.0/).

Keywords: OPSCC; HPV; TATI; survival

1. Introduction

The incidence of OPSCC has been increasing in recent years, particularly in Western countries [1]. Although over 100,000 new cases of oropharyngeal cancers are diagnosed yearly worldwide, the majority is diagnosed in developed countries [2,3]. Squamous cell carcinomas form over 90% of the newly diagnosed oropharyngeal cancers [2–6]. The median overall 5-year survival in Finland is 64% among men and 70% among women [7]. The most significant risk factors for OPSCC are smoking, heavy alcohol use, and HPV infection. Today, more than half of the new OPSCC cases are associated with HPV [8] and HPV-positive OPSCC and HPV-negative OPSCC are considered as separate disease entities. In HPV-positive OPSCC, the symptom profile and tumor characteristics differ from HPV-negative OPSCC, and the treatment response and the prognosis are usually substantially more favorable in HPV-related disease [9–11]. The prognosis for HPV-negative OPSCC remains relatively poor [12,13], and the explanation for poor survival rates remains unclear. To improve treatments and diagnostics, it is important to discover novel information on previously undiscovered prognostic factors and mechanisms affecting survival.

Various biomarkers have previously been associated with OPSCC, such as p16 [9,14,15]. Other potential biomarkers with possible prognostic value in OPSCC include Cyclin D1 and matrix metalloproteinases 1 and 2 [16–19]. Furthermore, recent studies have shown that HPV16 E6 and E7 serum antibody levels may predict OPSCC in advance [20,21]. However, to our knowledge there are currently no prognostic biomarkers or diagnostic serological biomarkers that are used for individualization of treatments for head and neck squamous cell cancers. Thus, further research on promising biomarkers is warranted. This study is focused on a biomarker known as tumor-associated trypsin inhibitor (TATI), which is associated with multiple malignancies, but has rarely been studied in oropharyngeal cancer [22,23].

TATI, also known as pancreatic secretory trypsin inhibitor (PSTI) or serine peptidase inhibitor Kazal 1 type (SPINK1), is a trypsin inhibitor that functions mainly in the pancreas, where it serves as a suppressor of premature trypsinogen activation [24]. The mechanisms regulating extrapancreatic TATI secretion are only partially known. The reference range of TATI concentration in serum (S-TATI) is 3.2–16 µg/L in healthy individuals [25]. S-TATI has been shown to increase in several non-malignant conditions, such as acute pancreatitis and various other severe inflammatory diseases. Elevated secretion of TATI in cancer patients was first found in the urine of patients with ovarian cancer [26,27] and it has since been detected in serum and tumor tissue in various malignancies [25].

In addition to the role if TATI as a diagnostic tumor marker, it may have value as a prognostic marker [28], and as a target for cancer treatment [29]. The purpose of this study was to evaluate the significance of TATI as a biomarker in HPV-positive and HPV-negative OPSCC based on its expression in cancer tissue and its serum concentrations and to investigate its value as a prognostic factor.

2. Materials and Methods

2.1. Study Population

This study was based on an existing database used in previous studies [30,31] and it is consisted of a cohort of 224 patients with newly diagnosed oropharyngeal squamous cell carcinoma at the HUS, Helsinki, Finland in 2012–2016.

Inclusion criteria for this study were a prospectively collected serum sample analyzed for TATI concentration, and the previously determined HPV status in tissue samples. Altogether, 90 of the 224 patients fulfilled these criteria and were included in the final analysis.

Data were collected from electronic patient records and were updated during the study for assessment of prognosis. The data included clinical characteristics such as age, gender, smoking, use of alcohol, TNM class, stage, grade of differentiation, tumor localization,

HPV status using an algorithm described by Smeets et al. [32] As a treatment modality, patients received either (chemo)radiotherapy or surgery with or without post-operative (chemo)radiotherapy. All patients were treated with curative intent. The median follow-up time was 47.5 months (range 0.0–60.0). The survival endpoints were overall survival (OS) and disease-specific survival (DSS).

The study was approved by the Research Ethics Board at the HUS and an institutional permission for the study was granted (Dnr: 51/13/03/02/2013).

2.2. Tissue Microarrays

Tissue microarray (TMA) blocks were prepared from primary tumors with the assistance from digital software by Auria Biobank (Turku, Finland). Representative areas were selected from hematoxylin and eosin-stained slides and six 1-mm thick core biopsies from each tumor were detached from paraffin blocks. The cores were then placed in another block with a semiautomatic tissue microarrayer (Beecher Instruments, Silver Spring, MD, USA).

2.3. HPV Status Determination

In our study, HPV status was determined by Smeets's algorithm using a combination of p16 immunohistochemistry (IHC) and HPV DNA detection.

All the paraffin-embedded samples were immunostained with p16-INK4a antibody. A positive control was included. HPV expression was considered as positive in samples where more than 70% of the tumor cells were positive.

For HPV DNA detection, DNA was first extracted from the tumor tissue samples followed by PCR-based genotyping using a Multiplex HPV Genotyping kit® (DiaMex GmbH, Heidelberg, Germany) as previously described [30]. Positivity of the high-risk (hr) HPV genotypes (subtypes 16, 18, 31, 33, 35, 39, 45, 51, 52, 56, 58, and 66) in the samples was considered as a positive result for hrHPV DNA in the tumor.

The methodology of these procedures has been described in detail previously [30,31,33].

2.4. Determination of TATI Serum Concentrations

All serum samples ($n = 90$) were collected prior to treatment. S-TATI was determined by a time-resolved immunofluorometric assay (IFMA) using monoclonal antibodies (MAbs) produced in-house [34]. The capture antibody was coated onto microtitration wells and the detector antibody labeled with a europium chelate. TATI purified from the urine of a patient with ovarian cancer was used as a calibrator [27]. The calibrators covered the concentration range of 0.5–150 µg/L. The sample volume was 25 µg/L and the total assay volume was 200 µL. The detection limit of the assay was 0.15 µg/L and the CV < 10% was at concentrations in the range of 1–50 µg/L [34]. The reference range for S-TATI was 3.2–16 µg/L and it was determined based on the central 95% reference interval in a group of 152 apparently healthy subjects. The lower reference limit was 3.1 µg/L and the upper reference limit was 16 µg/L [34]. The upper reference limit was lower than that for the initially used radioimmunoassay (21 µg/L) [27]. This was attributed to the higher non-specific background of the RIA. Samples, where S-TATI exceeded the selected cut-off value 17 µg/L [24,25,35,36] were considered S-TATI positive.

2.5. IHC of TATI

IHC staining of TATI was analyzed in TMA slides. Deparaffinization and rehydration of the tissue slides was performed with Sakura Tissue-Tek DRS. The HIER method (heat induced epitope retrieval) was performed with the Pretreatment Module, Agilent Dako (Dako Denmark Aps, Glostrup, Denmark) to improve antigen retrieval in the samples. Endogenous peroxidase blocking was performed with EnVision Flex peroxidase-blocking reagent (Dako). A monoclonal TATI antibody (MAb 6E8) [37] was used as the primary antibody. Dako REAL Antibody Diluent S2022 (Dako) was used for antibody dilution. EnVision Flex/HRP SM802 DM827 (Dako) was used as a secondary antibody. The chromogen was EnVision Flex DAB (Dako). Hematoxylin was used for counterstaining. Staining was performed with Autostainer 480 (Thermo Fisher Scientific, Vantaa, Finland). After the staining procedure, the specimen was dehydrated and then mounted with Pertex Histolab mounting media (Histolab Products Oy, Gothenburg, Sweden). We have not found evidence of non-specific staining while previously applying this method for TATI IHC and the specificity of the TATI antibody is described in earlier studies [34,36,37].

2.6. Sample Scoring

Scoring of TMA blocks was performed by two researchers (Anni Sjöblom and Jaana Hagström). A consensus was achieved in case of disagreements. TATI expression was assessed in the tumor tissue as well as in the peritumoral lymphocytes. The scoring of TATI in the samples was graded as described in Table S1.

2.7. Data Analysis

Data were collected and analyzed with IBM SPSS Statistics software program version 25. S-TATI and TATI expression in tumor tissues were compared with age, gender, smoking status, alcohol use, TNM class, stage, histological grade, tumor site and HPV status. Crosstab comparisons were performed with the χ^2-test and for normally distributed continuous variables, independent sample t test was used. For the survival analysis, the selected endpoints were 5-year OS and DSS. OS was defined as the time from the last day of treatment to death from any cause. DSS was defined as the time from the last day of treatment to the date of OPSCC-related death. OS and DSS were assessed with the log-rank-test and illustrated with the Kaplan–Meier-estimator using GraphPad Prism-software version 9. For the univariable and multivariable analysis, the Cox regression analysis was performed. TATI serum concentrations were logarithmically transformed to obtain normal distribution. Variables receiving p-values under 0.05 in the univariable analysis were included to the multivariable analysis.

3. Results

3.1. TATI Serum Concentrations and Clinical Characteristics

S-TATI was determined in 90 serum samples. Based on a selected cut-off value of 17 μg/L, 21 (23.3%) of the patients were considered TATI positive and 69 (76.7%) S-TATI negative. The crosstab comparisons of S-TATI according to clinical parameters are presented in Table 1.

The correlation between S-TATI and HPV status was statistically significant ($p < 0.001$). Most (90.60%) of the HPV-positive patients were S-TATI negative. Furthermore, S-TATI negativity was linked to lower cancer stage and higher histological grade (82.5% of the patients had cancer stages I-II and 83.3% of the patients were grade III). In addition, S-TATI negativity correlated with tonsil as tumor site (90.6% of the patients).

A majority (96.4%) of the non-smokers were S-TATI negative. Additionally, most (83.3%) of the former smokers were S-TATI negative. Among the smokers, 53.3% were S-TATI negative and 46.6% were S-TATI positive.

S-TATI positive patients had reduced OS during the 5-year follow-up and S-TATI positivity was linked to poor OS ($p < 0.001$) and DSS ($p = 0.04$) in the whole cohort. Furthermore, S-TATI positivity correlated with poor OS ($p = 0.01$) and DSS ($p = 0.05$) in HPV-negative patients and with poor DSS ($p = 0.01$) in HPV-positive patients. The survival curves according to S-TATI and OS are presented in Figure 1.

In the multivariate Cox regression analysis, poorer OS correlated significantly with age (adjusted Hazard ratio (HR) 1.08, 95% Confidence interval (CI) 0.03–1.13, $p = 0.004$) and S-TATI (adjusted HR 2.47, 95% CI 1.26–4.84, $p = 0.009$). In addition, poorer DSS was associated with age (adjusted HR 1.07, 95% CI 0.01–1.14, $p = 0.018$) and S-TATI (adjusted HR 2.54, 95% CI 1.07–6.02, $p = 0.034$) in the Cox regression multivariate model. The results of the multivariable analysis are presented in Table 2. In the multivariate Cox regression analysis with p16 as a separate variable, S-TATI correlated significantly with OS (adjusted

HR 2.49, 95% CI 1.28–4.83, $p = 0.007$) and DSS (adjusted HR 2.54, 95% CI 1.09–5.94, $p = 0.031$) and the results are presented in Table S2.

Table 1. Clinicopathological data according to S-TATI.

Variable	S-TATI−	%	S-TATI+	%	p-Value	Missing/% (n = 90)
Number of patients	69	76.7	21	23.3		
Age	60.8		65.1		0.054	
Gender						
Male	52	78.8	14	21.2		
Female	17	70.8	7	29.2	0.4	
Smoking						
Never	27	96.4	1	3.6		
Former	25	83.3	5	16.7		
Current	17	53.1	15	46.9	<0.001 **	
Heavy alcohol use						16/17.8
Never	36	83.7	7	16.3		
Former	6	60.0	4	40.0		
Current	13	61.9	8	38.1	0.09	
T class						
T1-T2	46	51.1	12	13.3		
T3-T4	23	25.6	9	10.0	0.4	
N class						
N0–N1	59	79.7	15	20.3		
N2–N3	10	62.5	6	37.4	0.2	
Stage						
I-II	52	82.5	11	17.5		
III-IV	17	63.0	10	37.0	0.04 *	
Grade						
I	1	33.3	2	66.7		
II	8	53.3	7	46.7		
III	60	83.3	12	16.7	0.009 *	
Localization						
Tonsil	48	90.6	5	9.4		
Base of tongue	17	77.3	5	22.7		
Soft palate	3	30.0	7	70.0		
Posterior wall of oropharynx	1	20.0	4	80.0	<0.001 **	
HPV						
HPV−	21	56.8	16	43.2		
HPV+	48	90.6	5	9.4	<0.001 **	

Abbreviations: TATI: Tumor-associated trypsin inhibitor; HPV: Human papillomavirus. $p < 0.05$ *, $p < 0.001$ **.

3.2. TATI Immunoexpression and Clinical Characteristics

Both serum and tissue data were available for 90 patients. For TATI IHC, adequate samples with HPV status determination were available for 77 (85.6%) patients. TATI was assessed in the tumor tissue in all 77 samples and in the tumor-adjacent lymphocytes in 76 samples (Figure 2a–c). Most of the samples showed moderate or strong IHC staining of TATI in both the tumor (63.3%) and in the peritumoral lymphocytes (60.5%). TATI-immunopositivity was cytoplasmic. TATI expression in IHC was associated with certain patient characteristics but not with S-TATI. Crosstab comparisons of TATI IHC and clinical characteristics are presented in Tables 3 and 4.

Table 2. Multivariate Cox regression analysis for overall-survival (OS) and disease-specific survival (DSS).

Variable	OS			DSS		
	HR	95% CI	p-Value	HR	95% CI	p-Value
Age	1.08	1.03–1.13	0.004 *	1.07	1.01–1.14	0.018 *
Smoking			0.034 *			0.205
Ex-smoker versus never	1.20	0.27–5.40	0.816	0.62	0.10–3.98	0.615
Current smoker versus never	4.14	1.22–14.06	0.023 *	2.43	0.64–9.18	0.192
Stage III–IV versus Stage I–II	1.71	0.70–4.20	0.243	2.19	0.72–6.64	0.168
HPV- versus HPV+	1.01	0.36–2.83	0.988	0.96	0.27–3.43	0.955
S-TATI	2.47	1.26–4.84	0.009 *	2.54	1.07–6.02	0.034 *

HR: Hazard ratio; CI: Confidence interval. S-TATI values are log-transformed. $p < 0.05$ *.

Moderate or strong expression of TATI in tumor tissue and in peritumoral lymphocytes (Figure 2a,b) was observed in 83% and 69.8% of patients with stage I–II disease, respectively. Expression of TATI in tumor tissue did not significantly correlate with other clinical parameters. However, elevated expression of TATI in peritumoral lymphocytes was linked to HPV positivity (66.6%) and lower T class (71.4%). In addition, patients with moderate or strong expression of TATI in peritumoral lymphocytes had a favorable OS ($p = 0.025$). However, this result was only observed in the whole patient cohort and the comparisons between HPV status and survival was not statistically significant. No correlation was seen between DSS and TATI tissue expression.

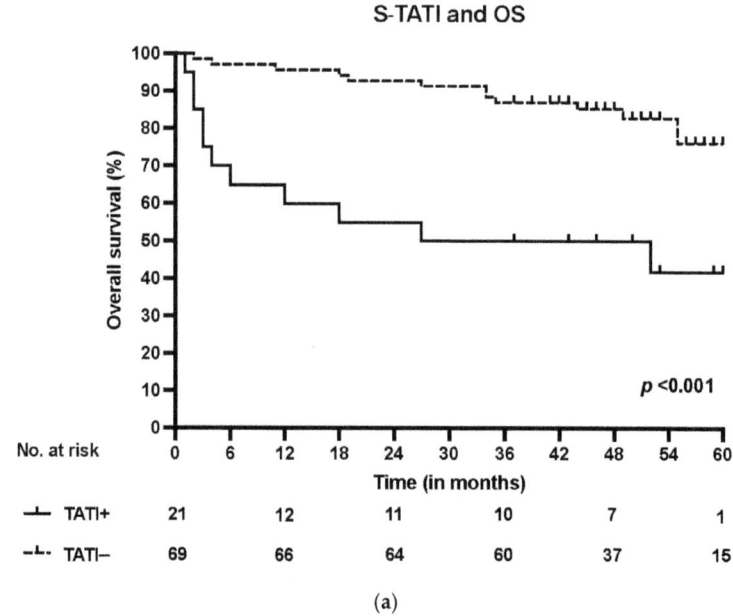

(a)

Figure 1. Cont.

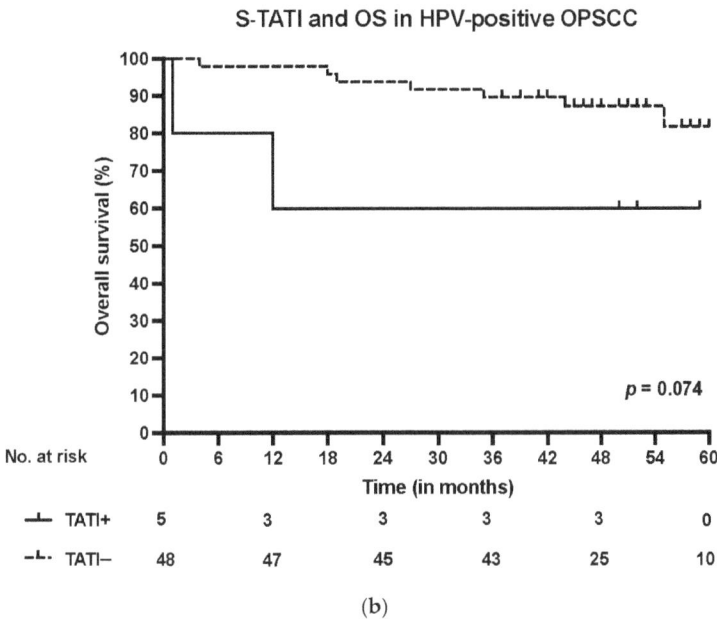

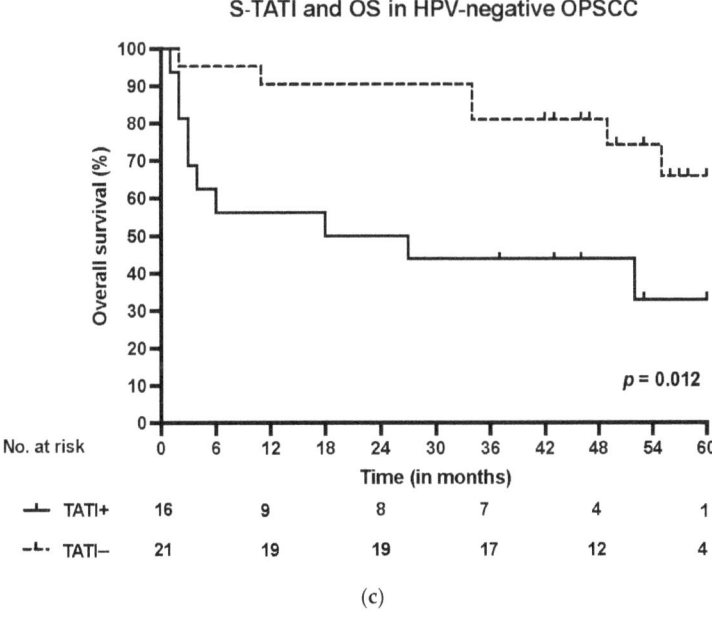

Figure 1. (a) Overall survival (OS) according to positive (>17 µg/L) and negative (<17 µg/L) S-TATI in the whole patient cohort. (b) Overall survival (OS) according to positive and negative S-TATI in HPV-positive OPSCC patients. (c) Overall survival (OS) according to positive and negative S-TATI in HPV-negative OPSCC patients.

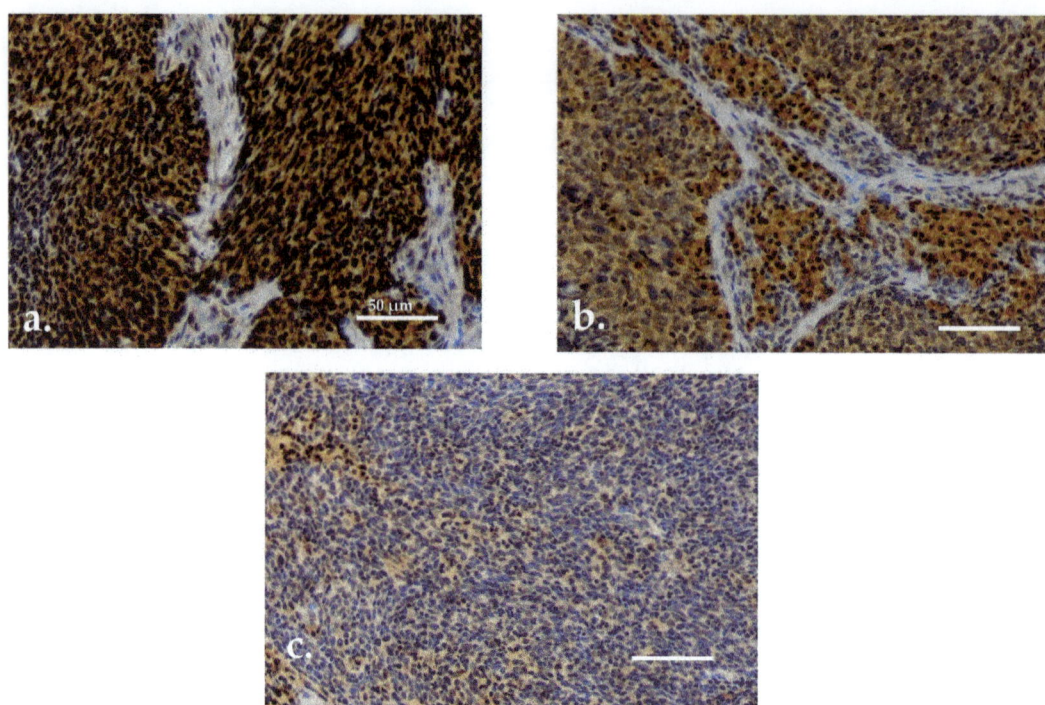

Figure 2. (**a**) Moderate/strong TATI expression in tumor tissue. (**b**) Moderate/strong TATI expression in peritumoral lymphocytes and mild expression in the tumor tissue. (**c**) Negative TATI expression in the tumor tissue. Scale bar length 50 µm. Magnification ×200.

Table 3. Clinicopathological data according to TATI expression in tumor tissue.

Variable	TATI in Tumor 0–1	%	TATI in Tumor 2–3	%	p-Value	Missing/% (n = 77)
Number of patients	20	26.0	57	63.3		
Age	64.4		61.1		0.2	
Gender						
Male	15	25.4	44	74.6		
Female	5	27.8	13	72.2	0.8	
Smoking						
Never	8	33.3	16	66.7		
Former	7	28.0	18	72.0		
Current	5	17.9	23	82.1	0.4	
Heavy alcohol use						14/18.2
Never	14	35.9	25	64.1		
Former	1	16.7	5	83.3		
Current	4	22.2	14	77.8	0.4	
T class						
T1–T2	11	22.4	38	77.6		
T3–T4	9	32.1	19	67.9	0.4	
N class						
N0–N1	12	19.0	51	81.0		
N2–N3	8	57.1	6	42.9	0.006 *	

Table 3. Cont.

Variable	TATI in Tumor 0–1	%	TATI in Tumor 2–3	%	p-Value	Missing/% (n = 77)
Stage						
I–II	9	17.0	44	83.0		
III–IV	11	45.8	13	54.1	0.007 *	
Grade						
I	0	0.0	2	100.0		
II	3	23.0	10	77.0		
III	17	27.4	45	72.6	0.7	
Localization						
Tonsil	10	21.7	36	78.3		
Base of tongue	6	35.3	11	64.7		
Soft palate	3	33.3	6	66.7		
Posterior wall of oropharynx	1	20.0	4	80.0	0.7	
HPV						
HPV−	9	29.0	22	71.0		
HPV+	11	23.9	35	76.1	0.6	

Abbreviations: TATI: tumor-associated trypsin inhibitor; HPV: Human papillomavirus, TATI immunoexpression was scored in the tumor tissue, TATI in tumor 0–1: mild positivity, TATI in tumor 2–3: moderate-strong positivity, $p < 0.05$ *.

Table 4. Clinicopathological data according to TATI expression in tumor-adjacent lymphocytes.

Variable	TATI in Lymphocytes 0–1	%	TATI in Lymphocytes 2–3	%	p-Value	Missing/% (n = 76)
Number of patients	30	39.5	46	60.5		
Age	62.6		61.3		0.6	
Gender						
Male	23	39.7	35	60.3		
Female	7	38.9	11	61.1	0.9	
Smoking						
Never	10	43.5	13	56.5		
Former	5	20.0	20	80.0		
Current	15	53.6	13	46.4	0.04 *	
Heavy alcohol use						14/18.4
Never	17	44.7	21	55.3		
Former	1	16.7	5	83.3		
Current	9	50.0	9	50.0	0.4	
T Class						
T1–T2	14	28.6	35	71.4		
T3–T4	16	59.3	11	40.7	0.009 *	
N Class						
N0–N1	23	36.5	40	63.5		
N2–N3	7	53.8	6	46.2	0.2	
Stage						
I–II	16	30.2	37	69.8		
III–IV	14	60.9	9	39.1	0.01 *	
Grade						
I	1	50.0	1	50.0		
II	6	46.2	7	53.8		
III	23	37.7	38	62.3	0.8	
Localization						
Tonsil	15	32.6	31	67.4		
Base of tongue	6	37.5	10	62.5		
Soft palate	6	66.7	3	33.3		
Posterior wall of oropharynx	3	60.0	2	40.0	0.2	
HPV						
HPV−	18	60.0	12	40.0		
HPV+	12	33.3	34	66.6	0.003 *	

Abbreviations: TATI: Tumor-associated trypsin inhibitor; HPV: Human papillomavirus, TATI immunoexpression was scored in the inflammatory cells adjacent to the tumor tissue, TATI in lymphocytes 0–1: mild positivity, TATI in lymphocytes 2–3: moderate-strong positivity, $p < 0.05$ *.

4. Discussion

Our study revealed novel information on TATI in both serum and in tumor tissue among OPSCC patients. Our findings suggest that S-TATI positivity is linked with poor prognosis of OPSCC irrespective of HPV status. In recurrent HPV-negative disease managed with primary definitive oncological treatment, the prognosis is usually considerably impaired. Therefore, determining the S-TATI could provide an advantage for the patient when establishing the treatment plan. Additionally, S-TATI determination could be valuable in monitoring purposes during posttreatment follow-up. In earlier studies TATI was shown to have prognostic value in other cancers [35,38]. Considering our results, further research with larger cohorts assessing TATI as a prognostic biomarker in OPSCC is warranted.

To the best of our knowledge, there are no studies on TATI in OPSCC. Interestingly, we found that S-TATI was associated with survival in both HPV-negative and HPV-positive disease, particularly in HPV-negative OPSCC. Given the limitations of the small sample size, we were not able to thoroughly analyze the effect of HPV status on S-TATI levels. As S-TATI positivity was associated with HPV negativity, it is likely that the association between poor prognosis and S-TATI positivity in the whole OPSCC group is strongly related to concurrent HPV negativity. Interestingly, we found a correlation between S-TATI positivity and poor DSS in HPV-positive patients. According to these findings, S-TATI positivity may have individual effects on survival unrelated to HPV negativity, although our sample size in this analysis was small. Studies on larger cohorts are needed to determine the role of HPV status and S-TATI for prognostication purposes. However, we observed that elevated S-TATI appears to function as an independent prognostic biomarker in OPSCC (Table 2). Similar results were observed in other malignancies [28,39,40].

In our study, previous and present smoking correlated strongly with S-TATI positivity ($p < 0.001$). Interestingly, similar results were observed in a previous study [41]. Furthermore, evidence of possibly smoking-related mutations in TATI has been found in chronic pancreatitis [42]. We speculate that smoking could increase mutations in TATI, possibly impairing its functions and thus leading to poor prognosis, TATI upregulation in serum, or both. Further research is required to establish the connection between smoking and TATI upregulation in OPSCC.

The mechanisms regulating TATI secretion in cancer are not known. Thus, the cause of the elevated TATI levels in serum and tissue in OPSCC and other malignancies is unclear. In general, it appears that TATI may have different effects on prognosis and pathogenesis depending on the type of malignancy [24]. There are several theories concerning the regulation of TATI in cancer and one of most frequently encountered is the connection of TATI with the protease tumor-associated trypsin (TAT) [43–45]. TAT and TATI are often produced simultaneously, and TAT has previously been linked to several malignancies and pathological conditions [46]. We speculate that TATI is acting through TAT, which is known to activate other proteinases mediating tissue destruction and invasion [43,47]. Low tissue expression of TATI could increase TAT activity due to the lack of inhibition. This phenomenon may facilitate local tumor invasion, which is associated with poor prognosis. This theory would support our findings of S-TATI positivity signaling impaired survival but does not align with our IHC results. Overexpression of TAT along with low TATI expression has previously been associated with enhanced tumor-cell invasion in oral and gastric cancer [47]. These results conflict with our findings regarding S-TATI positivity linked with poor prognosis. This contradiction might reflect the fact that their study was done in vitro with cell lines and is not directly comparable with our clinical study.

Recent studies on other malignancies have provided compelling theories on TATI and its effects on cancer aggressiveness and survival. The importance of the tumor microenvironment and the tumorigenic abilities of stromal cells is associated with prognosis [29,45]. The senescence-associated secretory phenotype (SASP), a known feature of cellular senescence, is associated with cancer and stromal cells [48]. It has been suggested that SASP in stromal cells is a mediator of paracrine S-TATI upregulation and of various cancer-promoting mechanisms (such as invasiveness), and it is associated with poor prognosis in prostate cancer [29]. Although SASP was observed after chemoradiation by Chen et al., similar events might stimulate S-TATI expression in OPSCC. Furthermore, SASP has previously been shown to trigger various cancer-promoting features with different mechanisms in oral squamous cell carcinomas [49]. Therefore, we speculate that SASP may be an important contributor to S-TATI upregulation in OPSCC and these events may also lead to poor prognosis as well. Our findings of S-TATI positivity being linked to poor prognosis support this theory. These explanations do not completely align with our IHC results.

Although we did not observe any correlation between S-TATI and TATI expression in tumor tissues, there was a moderate correlation between S-TATI negativity and tissue positivity. Interestingly, it has not been possible to establish an association between elevated S-TATI and tumor tissue in previous studies [28,50]. It has been speculated that TATI protects tissues against cancer invasion [43]. This would be consistent with our observations of TATI positivity of tumor-adjacent lymphocytes and several favorable associated factors, i.e., lower T class and stage. We speculate that while TATI expression is mainly increased in tumors and their surrounding tissues, TATI protein possibly locates in the tissues, which might reduce secretion into the blood. According to our results both negative S-TATI and high TATI expression in the peritumoral lymphocytes were linked to lower disease stage.

Several previous studies have failed to show elevated S-TATI and TATI expression in tumor tissues as associated prognostic factors [43,44,50]. Our findings indicate a significant association between poor prognosis and S-TATI positivity and these results appear to be more distinct compared to the IHC results. Further research is required to establish correlation between TATI expression in tissues and S-TATI as prognostic factors in cancer.

The present results could provide a novel path for future OPSCC research. To the best of our knowledge, there are no other serum biomarker assays for diagnostic and monitoring purposes of oral and oropharyngeal cancers.

5. Conclusions

Based on the present results, serum TATI appears to be a promising prognostic biomarker in HPV-positive and HPV-negative OPSCC. Prospective studies and further research in larger cohorts are warranted to determine the functions and physiology of TATI in OPSCC more thoroughly.

Supplementary Materials: The following are available online at https://www.mdpi.com/article/10.3390/cancers13112811/s1; Table S1: TATI immunoscoring, Table S2: Multivariate Cox regression analysis for overall-survival (OS) and disease-specific survival (DSS) with p16 as a separate variable.

Author Contributions: Conceptualization, U.-H.S., T.C. and L.J.; methodology, A.S., T.C., L.J., J.H. S.S. and U.-H.S.; software, T.C. and L.J.; validation, T.C., L.J., J.H., U.-H.S., A.M. and C.H.; formal analysis, T.C. and L.J.; investigation, A.S.; resources, data curation, A.S.; writing—original draft preparation, A.S.; writing—review and editing, A.S., T.C., L.J., J.H., U.-H.S., A.M., C.H., S.S. and P.M.; visualization, J.H. and A.S.; supervision, T.C., J.H. and A.M.; project administration T.C., J.H. and A.M., funding acquisition, A.M. All authors have read and agreed to the published version of the manuscript.

Funding: This research was funded by the Helsinki University Hospital Research Fund and the Sigrid Juselius Foundation.

Institutional Review Board Statement: The study was conducted according to the guidelines of the Declaration of Helsinki and was approved by the Ethics Committee of HUS (Dnr: 51/13/03/02/2013).

Informed Consent Statement: Informed consent was obtained from all subjects involved in the study.

Data Availability Statement: The data presented in this study are available on request from the corresponding author. The data are not publicly available due to patient data security.

Acknowledgments: Open access funding provided by University of Helsinki including Helsinki University Hospital. The authors thank Pia Saarinen (HUS) for technical assistance.

Conflicts of Interest: The authors declare no conflict of interest.

Abbreviations

HIER	Heat-induced epitope retrieval
HPV	Human papillomavirus
HUS	Helsinki University Hospital
IFMA	Immunofluorometric assay
Mab	Monoclonal antibody
OPSCC	Oropharyngeal squamous cell carcinoma
OS	Overall survival
SASP	Senescence-associated secretory phenotype
S-TATI	Serum concentration of tumor-associated trypsin inhibitor
TAT	Tumor-associated trypsin
TATI	Tumor-associated trypsin inhibitor
TMA	Tissue microarray

References

1. Bray, F.; Ferlay, J.; Soerjomataram, I.; Siegel, R.L.; Torre, L.A.; Jemal, A. Global cancer statistics 2018, GLOBOCAN estimates of incidence and mortality worldwide for 36 cancers in 185 countries. *CA Cancer J. Clin.* **2018**, *68*, 394–424. [CrossRef]
2. Warnakulasuriya, S. Global epidemiology of oral and oropharyngeal cancer. *Oral Oncol.* **2009**, *45*, 309–316. [CrossRef] [PubMed]
3. Lambert, R.; Sauvaget, C.; de Camargo Cancela, M.; Sankaranarayanan, R. Epidemiology of cancer from the oral cavity and oropharynx. *Eur. J. Gastroenterol. Hepatol.* **2011**, *23*, 633–641. [CrossRef] [PubMed]
4. Sinevici, N.; O'sullivan, J. Oral cancer: Deregulated molecular events and their use as biomarkers. *Oral Oncol.* **2016**, *61*, 12–18. [CrossRef]
5. Koneva, L.A.; Zhang, Y.; Virani, S.; Hall, P.B.; McHugh, J.B.; Chepeha, D.B.; Wolf, G.T.; Carey, T.E.; Rozek, L.S.; Sartor, M.A. HPV Integration in HNSCC Correlates with Survival Outcomes, Immune Response Signatures, and Candidate Drivers. *Mol. Cancer Res.* **2018**, *16*, 90–102. [CrossRef] [PubMed]
6. Gooi, Z.; Chan, J.Y.K.; Fakhry, C. The epidemiology of the human papillomavirus related to oropharyngeal head and neck cancer. *Laryngoscope* **2016**, *126*, 894–900. [CrossRef]
7. Pitkäniemi, J.; Malila, N.; Virtanen, A.; Degerlund, H.; Heikkinen, S.; Seppä, K. *Syöpä 2018. Tilastoraportti Suomen Syöpätilanteesta*; Publication no. 93 of the Cancer Society of Finland; Cancer Society of Finland: Helsinki, Finland, 2020. Available online: Https://www.epressi.com/media/userfiles/145405/1588150481/syopa-2018-pa-finska.pdf (accessed on 3 June 2021).
8. Chaturvedi, A.K.; Anderson, W.F.; Lortet-Tieulent, J.; Curado, M.P.; Ferlay, J.; Franceschi, S.; Rosenberg, P.S.; Bray, F.; Gillison, M.L. Worldwide trends in incidence rates for oral cavity and oropharyngeal cancers. *J. Clin. Oncol.* **2013**, *31*, 4550–4559. [CrossRef]
9. Gillison, M.L.; D'Souza, G.; Westra, W.; Sugar, E.; Xiao, W.; Begum, S.; Viscidi, L. Distinct risk factor profiles for human papillomavirus type 16-positive and human papillomavirus type 16-negative head and neck cancers. *J. Natl. Cancer Inst.* **2008**, *100*, 407–420. [CrossRef] [PubMed]
10. Ramqvist, T.; Dalianis, T. An epidemic of oropharyngeal squamous cell carcinoma (OSCC) due to human papillomavirus (HPV) infection and aspects of treatment and prevention. *Anticancer Res.* **2011**, *31*, 1515–1519. [PubMed]
11. Ang, K.K.; Harris, J.; Wheeler, R.; Weber, R.; Rosenthal, D.I.; Nguyen-Tân, P.F.; Westra, W.H.; Chung, C.H.; Jordan, R.C.; Lu, C.; et al. Human papillomavirus and survival of patients with oropharyngeal cancer. *N. Engl. J. Med.* **2010**, *363*, 24–35. [CrossRef] [PubMed]
12. Fakhry, C.; Westra, W.H.; Li, S.; Cmelak, A.; Ridge, J.A.; Pinto, H.; Forastiere, A.; Gillison, M.L. Improved survival of patients with human papillomavirus-positive head and neck squamous cell carcinoma in a prospective clinical trial. *J. Natl. Cancer Inst.* **2008**, *100*, 261–269. [CrossRef] [PubMed]
13. Elrefaey, S.; Massaro, M.A.; Chiocca, S.; Chiesa, F.; Ansarin, M. HPV in oropharyngeal cancer: The basics to know in clinical practice. *Acta Otorhinolaryngol. Ital.* **2014**, *34*, 299–309.
14. Sato, F.; Ono, T.; Kawahara, A.; Kawaguchi, T.; Tanaka, H.; Shimamatsu, K.; Kakuma, T.; Akiba, J.; Umeno, H.; Yano, H. Prognostic impact of p16 and PD-L1 expression in patients with oropharyngeal squamous cell carcinoma receiving a definitive treatment. *J. Clin. Pathol.* **2019**, *72*, 542–549. [CrossRef] [PubMed]
15. Adelstein, D.J.; Ismaila, N.; Ku, J.A.; Burtness, B.; Swiecicki, P.L.; Mell, L.; Beitler, J.J.; Gross, N.; Jones, C.U.; Kaufman, M.; et al. Role of Treatment Deintensification in the Management of p16+ Oropharyngeal Cancer: ASCO Provisional Clinical Opinion. *J. Clin. Oncol.* **2019**, *37*, 1578–1589. [CrossRef] [PubMed]
16. Grimminger, C.M.; Danenberg, P.V. Update of prognostic and predictive biomarkers in oropharyngeal squamous cell carcinoma: A review. *Eur. Arch. Otorhinolaryngol.* **2011**, *268*, 5–16. [CrossRef] [PubMed]
17. Vento, S.I.; Jouhi, L.; Mohamed, H.; Haglund, C.; Mäkitie, A.A.; Atula, T.; Hagström, J.; Mäkinen, L.K. MMP-7 expression may influence the rate of distant recurrences and disease-specific survival in HPV-positive oropharyngeal squamous cell carcinoma. *Virchows Arc.* **2018**, *472*, 975–981. [CrossRef] [PubMed]

18. Umbreit, C.; Erben, P.; Faber, A.; Hofheinz, R.-D.; Aderhold, C.; Weiss, C.; Hoermann, K.; Wenzel, A.; Schultz, J.D. MMP9, Cyclin D1 and β-Catenin Are Useful Markers of p16-positive Squamous Cell Carcinoma in Therapeutic EGFR Inhibition In Vitro. *Anticancer Res.* **2015**, *35*, 3801–3810.
19. Plath, M.; Broglie, M.A.; Förbs, D.; Stoeckli, S.J.; Jochum, W. Prognostic significance of cell cycle-associated proteins p16, pRB, cyclin D1 and p53 in resected oropharyngeal carcinoma. *J. Otolaryngol. Head Neck Surg.* **2018**, *47*, 53. [CrossRef]
20. Lang Kuhs, K.A.; Wood, C.B.; Wiggleton, J.; Aulino, J.M.; Latimer, B.; Smith, D.K.; Bender, N.; Rohde, S.; Mannion, K.; Kim, Y.; et al. Transcervical sonography and human papillomavirus 16 E6 antibodies are sensitive for the detection of oropharyngeal cancer. *Cancer* **2020**, *126*, 2658–2665. [CrossRef]
21. Ren, J.; Xu, W.; Su, J.; Ren, X.; Cheng, D.; Chen, Z.; Bender, N.; Mirshams, M.; Habbous, S.; De Almeida, J.R.; et al. Multiple imputation and clinico-serological models to predict human papillomavirus status in oropharyngeal carcinoma: An alternative when tissue is unavailable. *Int. J. Cancer* **2020**, *146*, 2166–2174. [CrossRef] [PubMed]
22. Rivera, C.; Oliveira, A.K.; Costa, R.A.P.; De Rossi, T.; Paes Leme, A.F. Prognostic biomarkers in oral squamous cell carcinoma: A systematic review. *Oral Oncol.* **2017**, *72*, 38–47. [CrossRef] [PubMed]
23. Almangush, A.; Heikkinen, I.; Mäkitie, A.A.; Coletta, R.D.; Läärä, E.; Leivo, I.; Salo, T. Prognostic biomarkers for oral tongue squamous cell carcinoma: A systematic review and meta-analysis. *Br. J. Cancer* **2017**, *117*, 856–866. [CrossRef] [PubMed]
24. Itkonen, O.; Stenman, U.-H. TATI as a biomarker. *Clin. Chim. Acta* **2014**, *431*, 260–269. [CrossRef]
25. Räsänen, K.; Itkonen, O.; Koistinen, H.; Stenman, U.-H. Emerging Roles of SPINK1 in Cancer. *Clin. Chem.* **2016**, *62*, 449–457. [CrossRef]
26. Eddeland, A.; Ohlsson, K. A radioimmunoassay for measurement of human pancreatic secretory trypsin inhibitor in different body fluids. *Hoppe Seylers Z. Physiol. Chem.* **1978**, *359*, 671–675. [CrossRef]
27. Stenman, U.H.; Huhtala, M.L.; Koistinen, R.; Seppälä, M. Immunochemical demonstration of an ovarian cancer-associated urinary peptide. *Int. J. Cancer* **1982**, *30*, 53–57. [CrossRef] [PubMed]
28. Gaber, A.; Nodin, B.; Hotakainen, K.; Nilsson, E.; Stenman, U.-H.; Bjartell, A.; Birgisson, H.; Jirström, K. Increased serum levels of tumour-associated trypsin inhibitor independently predict a poor prognosis in colorectal cancer patients. *BMC Cancer* **2010**, *10*, 498. [CrossRef] [PubMed]
29. Chen, F.; Long, Q.; Fu, D.; Zhu, D.; Ji, Y.; Han, L.; Zhang, B.; Xu, Q.; Liu, B.; Li, Y.; et al. Targeting SPINK1 in the damaged tumour microenvironment alleviates therapeutic resistance. *Nat. Commun.* **2018**, *9*, 4315. [CrossRef] [PubMed]
30. Randén-Brady, R.; Carpén, T.; Jouhi, L.; Syrjänen, S.; Haglund, C.; Tarkkanen, J.; Remes, S.; Mäkitie, A.; Mattila, P.S.; Silén, S.; et al. In situ hybridization for high-risk HPV E6/E7 mRNA is a superior method for detecting transcriptionally active HPV in oropharyngeal cancer. *Hum. Pathol.* **2019**, *90*, 97–105. [CrossRef] [PubMed]
31. Carpén, T.; Syrjänen, S.; Jouhi, L.; Randen-Brady, R.; Haglund, C.; Mäkitie, A.; Mattila, P.S.; Hagström, J. Epstein–Barr virus (EBV) and polyomaviruses are detectable in oropharyngeal cancer and EBV may have prognostic impact. *Cancer Immunol. Immunother.* **2020**, *69*, 1615–1626. [CrossRef] [PubMed]
32. Smeets, S.J.; Hesselink, A.T.; Speel, E.-J.M.; Haesevoets, A.; Snijders, P.J.F.; Pawlita, M.; Meijel, C.J.L.M.; Braakhuis, B.J.M.; Leemans, C.R.; Brakenhoff, R.H. A novel algorithm for reliable detection of human papillomavirus in paraffin embedded head and neck cancer specimen. *Int. J. Cancer* **2007**, *121*, 2465–2472. [CrossRef]
33. Carpén, T.; Sjöblom, A.; Lundberg, M.; Haglund, C.; Markkola, A.; Syrjänen, S.; Tarkkanen, J.; Mäkitie, A.; Hagström, J.; Mattila, P.S. Presenting symptoms and clinical findings in HPV-positive and HPV-negative oropharyngeal cancer patients. *Acta Oto-Laryngol.* **2018**, *138*, 513–518. [CrossRef] [PubMed]
34. Osman, S.; Turpeinen, U.; Itkonen, O.; Stenman, U.H. Optimization of a time-resolved immunofluorometric assay for tumor-associated trypsin inhibitor (TATI) using the streptavidin-biotin system. *J. Immunol. Methods* **1993**, *161*, 97–106. [CrossRef]
35. Lyytinen, I.; Lempinen, M.; Nordin, A.; Mäkisalo, H.; Stenman, U.-H.; Isoniemi, H. Prognostic significance of tumor-associated trypsin inhibitor (TATI) and human chorionic gonadotropin-β (hCGβ) in patients with hepatocellular carcinoma. *Scand. J. Gastroenterol.* **2013**, *48*, 1066–1073. [CrossRef]
36. Ravela, S.; Valmu, L.; Domanskyy, M.; Koistinen, H.; Kylanpaa, L.; Lindstrom, O.; Stenman, J.; Hämäläinen, E.; Stenman, U.-H.; Itkonen, O. An immunocapture-LC-MS-based assay for serum SPINK1 allows simultaneous quantification and detection of SPINK1 variants. *Anal. Bioanal. Chem.* **2018**, *410*, 1679–1688. [CrossRef]
37. Paju, A.; Hotakainen, K.; Cao, Y.; Laurila, T.; Gadaleanu, V.; Hemminki, A.; Stenman, U.H.; Bjartell, A. Increased expression of tumor-associated trypsin inhibitor, TATI, in prostate cancer and in androgen-independent 22Rv1 cells. *Eur. Urol.* **2007**, *52*, 1670–1679. [CrossRef]
38. Kelloniemi, E.; Rintala, E.; Finne, P.; Stenman, U.-H. Tumor-associated trypsin inhibitor as a prognostic factor during follow-up of bladder cancer. *Urology* **2003**, *62*, 249–253. [CrossRef]
39. Tornberg, S.V.; Nisen, H.; Järvinen, P.; Järvinen, R.; Kilpeläinen, T.P.; Taari, K.; Stenman, U.H.; Visapää, H. Serum tumour associated trypsin inhibitor, as a biomarker for survival in renal cell carcinoma. *Scand. J. Urol.* **2020**, *54*, 413–419. [CrossRef]
40. Kozakiewicz, B.; Chądzyńska, M.; Dmoch-Gajzlerska, E.; Stefaniak, M. Monitoring the treatment outcome in endometrial cancer patients by CEA and TATI. *Tumor Biol.* **2016**, *37*, 9367–9374. [CrossRef] [PubMed]
41. Järvisalo, J.; Hakama, M.; Knekt, P.; Stenman, U.H.; Leino, A.; Teppo, L.; Maatela, J.; Aromaa, A. Serum tumor markers CEA, CA 50, TATI, and NSE in lung cancer screening. *Cancer* **1993**, *71*, 1982–1988. [CrossRef]

42. Zou, W.-B.; Tang, X.-Y.; Zhou, D.-Z.; Qian, Y.-Y.; Hu, L.-H.; Yu, F.-F.; Yu, D.; Wu, H.; Deng, S.-J.; Lin, J.-H. SPINK1, PRSS1, CTRC, and CFTR Genotypes Influence Disease Onset and Clinical Outcomes in Chronic Pancreatitis. *Clin. Transl. Gastroenterol.* **2018**, *9*, 204. [CrossRef]
43. Gaber, A.; Johansson, M.; Stenman, U.-H.; Hotakainen, K.; Pontén, F.; Glimelius, B.; Jirström, B.K.; Birgisson, H. High expression of tumour-associated trypsin inhibitor correlates with liver metastasis and poor prognosis in colorectal cancer. *Br. J. Cancer* **2009**, *100*, 1540–1548. [CrossRef]
44. Wiksten, J.-P.; Lundin, J.; Nordling, S.; Kokkola, A.; Stenman, U.-H.; Haglund, C. High tissue expression of tumour-associated trypsin inhibitor (TATI) associates with a more favourable prognosis in gastric cancer. *Histopathology* **2005**, *46*, 380–388. [CrossRef]
45. Tiwari, R.; Manzar, N.; Bhatia, V.; Yadav, A.; Nengroo, M.A.; Datta, D.; Carskadon, S.; Gupta, N.; Sigouros, M.; Khani, F.; et al. Androgen deprivation upregulates SPINK1 expression and potentiates cellular plasticity in prostate cancer. *Nat. Commun.* **2020**, *11*, 384. [CrossRef] [PubMed]
46. Soreide, K.; Janssen, E.A.; Körner, H.; Baak, J.P.A. Trypsin in colorectal cancer: Molecular biological mechanisms of proliferation, invasion, and metastasis. *J. Pathol.* **2006**, *209*, 147–156. [CrossRef]
47. Nyberg, P.; Moilanen, M.; Paju, A.; Sarin, A.; Stenman, U.-H.; Sorsa, T.; Salo, T. MMP-9 activation by tumor trypsin-2 enhances in vivo invasion of human tongue carcinoma cells. *J. Dent. Res.* **2002**, *81*, 831–835. [CrossRef]
48. Kuilman, T.; Michaloglou, C.; Mooi, W.J.; Peeper, D.S. The essence of senescence. *Genes Dev.* **2010**, *24*, 2463–2479. [CrossRef] [PubMed]
49. Prime, S.S.; Cirillo, N.; Hassona, Y.; Lambert, D.W.; Paterson, I.C.; Mellone, M.; Thomas, G.J.; James, E.N.L.; Parkinson, E.K. Fibroblast activation and senescence in oral cancer. *J. Oral Pathol. Med.* **2017**, *46*, 82–88. [CrossRef]
50. Lukkonen, A.; Lintula, S.; von Boguslawski, K.; Carpén, O.; Ljungberg, B.; Landberg, G.; Stenman, U.H. Tumor-associated trypsin inhibitor in normal and malignant renal tissue and in serum of renal-cell carcinoma patients. *Int. J. Cancer* **1999**, *83*, 486–490. [CrossRef]

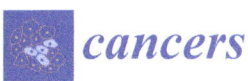

Article

Photodynamic Therapy as a Potent Radiosensitizer in Head and Neck Squamous Cell Carcinoma

Won Jin Cho [1], David Kessel [2,*], Joseph Rakowski [3,4], Brian Loughery [3,4], Abdo J. Najy [1], Tri Pham [1], Seongho Kim [3], Yong Tae Kwon [5], Ikuko Kato [3], Harold E. Kim [3,4] and Hyeong-Reh C. Kim [1,3,*]

1. Department of Pathology, Wayne State University School of Medicine, Detroit, MI 48201, USA; wcho@med.wayne.edu (W.J.C.); anajy@med.wayne.edu (A.J.N.); tpham@med.wayne.edu (T.P.)
2. Department of Pharmacology, Wayne State University School of Medicine, Detroit, MI 48201, USA
3. Department of Oncology, Karmanos Cancer Institute, Wayne State University School of Medicine, Detroit, MI 48201, USA; rakowski@karmanos.org (J.R.); lougherb@karmanos.org (B.L.); kimse@karmanos.org (S.K.); katoi@karmanos.org (I.K.); kimh@karmanos.org (H.E.K.)
4. Division of Radiation Oncology, Karmanos Cancer Institute, Wayne State University School of Medicine, Detroit, MI 48201, USA
5. Department of Biomedical Sciences, College of Medicine, Seoul National University, Seoul 03080, Korea; yok5@snu.ac.kr
* Correspondence: dhkessel@med.wayne.edu (D.K.); hrckim@med.wayne.edu (H.-R.C.K.); Tel.: +1-313-577-1766 (D.K.); +1-313-577-2407 (H.-R.C.K.)

Simple Summary: Despite the advances in multimodality treatment strategies, more than 30% of patients with advanced head and neck squamous cell carcinoma (HNSCC) experience recurrence of the disease that is usually derived from the residual tumor. The goal of our study is to understand the molecular basis underlying radiotherapy resistance in advanced HNSCC and to identify a mechanism-based radiosensitizer. We found that the autophagic cell survival pathway is upregulated in therapy-resistant HNSCC. Photodynamic therapy (PDT) directed at the endoplasmic reticulum (ER)/mitochondria induces programmed cell death such as paraptosis and apoptosis in an autophagic adaptor p62-dependent manner, promoting radiotoxicity.

Abstract: Despite recent advances in therapeutic modalities such as radiochemotherapy, the long-term prognosis for patients with advanced head and neck squamous cell carcinoma (HNSCC), especially nonviral HNSCC, remains very poor, while survival of patients with human papillomavirus (HPV)-associated HNSCC is greatly improved after radiotherapy. The goal of this study is to develop a mechanism-based treatment protocol for high-risk patients with HPV-negative HNSCC. To achieve our goal, we have investigated molecular mechanisms underlying differential radiation sensitivity between HPV-positive and -negative HNSCC cells. Here, we found that autophagy is associated with radioresistance in HPV-negative HNSCC, whereas apoptosis is associated with radiation sensitive HPV-positive HNSCC. Interestingly, we found that photodynamic therapy (PDT) directed at the endoplasmic reticulum (ER)/mitochondria initially induces paraptosis followed by apoptosis. This led to a substantial increase in radiation responsiveness in HPV-negative HNSCC, while the same PDT treatment had a minimal effect on HPV-positive cells. Here, we provide evidence that the autophagic adaptor p62 mediates signal relay for the induction of apoptosis, promoting ionizing radiation (XRT)-induced cell death in HPV-negative HNSCC. This work proposes that ER/mitochondria-targeted PDT can serve as a radiosensitizer in intrinsically radioresistant HNSCC that exhibits an increased autophagic flux.

Keywords: photodynamic therapy; ER/mitochondrial photosensitizer; paraptosis; apoptosis; autophagy

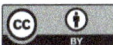

1. Introduction

Organ-sparing neoadjuvant chemoradiotherapy is an emerging treatment for patients with advanced head and neck squamous cell carcinoma (HNSCC). Despite the advances in multimodality treatment strategies, patients with advanced HNSCC often experience recurrence of the disease, usually derived from residual tumor [1]. HNSCC can be divided into two groups based on the status of human papillomavirus (HPV) infection [2–4]. Clinical characteristics of HPV-associated HNSCC are its greater sensitivity to radiotherapy [5–7] and better survival of patients compared to those with HPV-negative HNSCC [5–12]. To develop a mechanism-based radiosensitizer for intrinsically radioresistant HNSCC cells, we investigated the molecular basis underlying differential responses to ionizing radiation therapy (XRT) in radiosensitive HPV-positive and radioresistant HPV-negative HNSCC cell lines.

Radiation-induced tumor cell toxicity is attributable to cell death through mitotic catastrophe when cells attempt to divide with unrepaired DNA damage. However, increasing evidence suggest that tumor responses to radiotherapy are greatly affected by tumor cell sensitivity to programmed cell death (PCD) and their interactions with survival pathways [13,14]. Although apoptosis is a frequently observed PCD mode, recent studies have identified another PCD pathway termed paraptosis. It is characterized by a pattern of cytoplasmic vacuolization derived from the endoplasmic reticulum (ER) [15]. In addition, autophagy is sometimes associated with cell death, although it is usually a cytoprotective mechanism [16].

In this study, we show that increased autophagic flux is associated with radioresistance in HPV-negative HNSCC, while apoptosis is associated with radiosensitivity in HPV-positive HNSCC. In search for death stimuli that effectively kill radioresistant HNSCC cells, we assessed the effect of photodynamic therapy (PDT). PDT is a procedure involving the selective photosensitization of malignant cell types using agents that, upon excitation at a wavelength corresponding to an absorbance band, convert molecular oxygen to a series of reactive oxygen species (ROS). This has been used for the successful treatment of cancers and skin conditions [17–20]. In the context of PDT, ER photodamage leads to photodamaged ER proteins, which may mimic "misfolded protein"-mediated ER stress [21]. We found that ER photodamage effectively induces cytotoxicity in HPV-negative cells. In contrast, responses to ER photodamage in HPV-positive cells are minimal for reasons not yet understood. ER-targeted PDT activates the ER stress signaling pathways in HPV-negative HNSCC, leading to paraptosis followed by apoptosis. In contrast, the low degree of efficacy of lysosomal photodamage was comparable between HPV-positive and -negative HNSCC cells. We found that PDT using an ER/mitochondria photosensitizer promoted the efficacy of XRT in radioresistant HPV-negative HNSCC cells, but this effect was not observed with agents that targeted only the ER or lysosomes. Intrinsically radiosensitive and autophagy-deficient HPV-positive HNSCC cells were resistant to ER/mitochondria-targeted PDT. Lastly, we demonstrated that the autophagy adaptor p62 is critical for the induction of apoptosis and radiosensitization in intrinsically radioresistant HNSCC cells upon ER/mitochondria-targeted PDT, whereas p62 is nonfunctional and the same treatment fails to enhance radiosensitivity in HPV-positive HNSCC cells. We propose that ER/mitochondria-targeted PDT may promote therapy responses to XRT in patients with advanced HPV-negative HNSCC with increased autophagy flux.

2. Materials and Methods

2.1. Cell Culture

Human HNSCC cell lines UP-SCC-090 and UP-SCC-154 (University of Pittsburgh, Pittsburgh, PA, USA), UM-SCC-19 (University of Michigan, Ann Arbor, MI, USA) and WSU-HN-12 (Wayne State University, Detroit, MI, USA) were cultured as previously described [22].

2.2. Antibodies and Reagents

A list of antibodies and reagents and their sources used in this study is provided in Table S1.

2.3. Photodynamic Therapy

Cells (5×10^5 cells) in 35 mm tissue culture dishes were incubated at 37 °C with 0.5 µM BPD or 20 µM NPe6 for 1 h or with 1 µM hypericin for 16 h. The medium was replaced and the dishes irradiated with a 600-watt quartz-halogen source (Cat. No. 66296-600Q-R07, Newport Corp., Irvine, CA, USA). The bandwidth was confined by interference filters ($\pm$ 10 nm, Oriel, Stratford, CT, USA) to 690 (BPD), 660 (NPe6) or 600 nm (hypericin). Drug and light doses were chosen based on prior experience based on clonogenic dose-response data. Light doses were calculated using a Scientech H310 Power & Energy meter (Scientech Inc., Boulder, CO, USA).

2.4. Ionizing Radiation Treatment (XRT)

Cells were irradiated with 0, 2, 4 and 6 Gy using a gantry-mounted Best Theratronics Gammabeam 500 with a dose rate of 1 Gy/min. Irradiation was carried out at room temperature under atmospheric oxygen conditions. The delivered dose was confirmed with the use of a Farmer chamber.

2.5. Clonogenic Cell Survival Assay

Cells were grown in 6-well plates. After overnight incubation, cells were treated as indicated. After 10 days of treatments, cells were rinsed with PBS, fixed with 70% ethanol and stained with 1% Crystal violet for 2 h at room temperature. The colonies were counted using GelCount, Oxford Optronix Ltd. (Abingdon, Oxford, UK).

2.6. DEVDase Activity Assay

Cells were lysed with a 0.5% NP40 lysis buffer, and 50 µg of protein lysates were incubated with 10 mmol/L Ac-DEVD-AMC substrate (Sigma) at 37 °C for 2 h. Fluorescence was detected using a SpectraMax Gemini (Molecular Probes, Carlsbad, CA, USA): 360-nm excitation and 460 nm emission.

2.7. Detection of Splice Variants of X-Box Binding Protein-1 (XBP1) mRNA by RT-PCR Analysis

Cells treated with 0.5 µM BPD (benzoporphyrin derivative) for 1 h were exposed to the light at 22.5 mJ/cm^2, with 20 µM NPe6 for 1 h at 30 mJ/cm^2, or with 1 µM hypericin for 16 h at 15 mJ/cm^2, immediately followed by XRT at 2 Gy. One day after treatments, mRNAs were isolated using an RNeasy kit (Qiagen, Hilden, Germany) and cDNAs were synthesized with an iScriptTM cDNA Synthesis Kit (Bio-Rad, Hercules, CA, USA), followed by PCR analysis using GoTaq Flexi DNA Polymerase (Promega, Madison, WI, USA). PCR primers are listed in Table S1.

2.8. Establishment of p62-Knockdown WSU12 Cell Line

Scrambled shRNA sequence (shScram; catalog no. RHS4346) and three shRNA against p62 GIPZ (shp62; clone ID no. V3LHS-375194, -375195, -375197) were obtained from Open Biosystems (Huntsville, AL, USA). WSU12 cells were transfected with shScram or p62-targeting shRNA vectors using Lipofectamine 2000 (Invitrogen, Carlsbad, CA, USA) and selected with 0.25 µg/mL puromycin. The resulting pooled populations were referred to as shp62–94, shp62–95 and shp62–97, respectively.

2.9. Statistical Analysis

All experiments were repeated at least three times, and all data are presented as the mean $\pm$ SD. Statistical analysis was performed using Student's unpaired two-tailed t-test. The p value of <0.01(**), <0.05(*) and n.s. were considered statistically very significant, significant and not significant between studied groups, respectively. The combination index was calculated using the method of constant ratio drug combination proposed by Chou and Talalay [23]. The 95% confidence interval (CI) for the combination index was estimated using 10,000 bootstrap samples. The combination index of less than, equal to, and greater than one represented synergism, additive effect and antagonism, respectively.

Statistical analyses were performed using statistical software R version 4.0.2 (R Core Team, 2020) and RStudio version 1.4.1103 (RStudio Team, 2021).

2.10. Immunoblot Analysis

Densitometric analysis of immunoblots was performed using the NIH ImageJ program. Values were adjusted to the proper experimental control (time or treatment condition) and displayed under each panel in Supplementary Figures (Figures S1–S3) as a fold change. The uncropped whole blots with molecular weight markers are shown in the Supplemental Materials (Figure S6).

3. Results

3.1. HPV-Negative HNSCC Cell Lines Show Increased Basal Autophagy and Fail to Undergo Apoptosis after XRT, Whereas HPV-Positive HNSCC Cell Lines Are Prone to XRT-Induced Apoptosis

To investigate the molecular basis for the differential radiosensitivities between HPV-positive and-negative HNSCC cells, we utilized two HPV-positive HNSCC cell lines (UP90 and UP154) and two HPV-negative HNSCC cell lines (WSU12 and UM19). HPV status was confirmed by RT-PCR analysis of the HPV oncogenes E6 and E7 in these cell lines [22]. HPV-positive UP90 and UP154 cell lines were more responsive to XRT than the HPV-negative WSU12 and UM19 cells [22]. Apoptosis, assessed by proteolytic activation of caspase 3 and DEVDase activity assay, was detected in the HPV-positive HNSCC cell lines but not in the HPV-negative HNSCC cell lines (Figure 1A,B). Differential apoptotic sensitivity was not restricted to XRT. Tumor necrosis factor-related apoptosis-inducing ligand (TRAIL) also induced caspase activity more effectively in HPV-positive HNSCC cells than in HPV-negative HNSCC cells (Figure S4). These indicated an apoptosis-resistant phenotype in HPV-negative HNSCC cell lines. In contrast to apoptotic response, autophagy was readily detected in the radioresistant HPV-negative HNSCC cells, as indicated by conversion of LC3-I to LC3-II. No evidence of autophagic flux was detected in HPV-positive cells (Figure 1C). This observation is consistent with a literature review on cytoprotective function of autophagy [24–26].

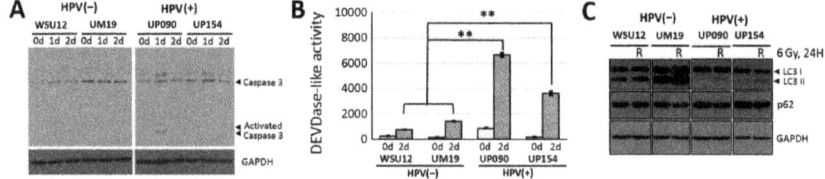

Figure 1. Radiosensitive human papillomavirus (HPV)-positive head and neck squamous cell carcinoma (HNSCC) cells were associated with apoptosis and radioresistant HPV-negative HNSCC with high autophagic flux. (**A**) Immunoblot of caspase 3 and (**B**) DEVDase activity assay at indicated day after irradiation at 6 Gy. (** $p < 0.01$) (**C**) Immunoblot of LC3 and p62 in control or one day after irradiation at 6 Gy.

3.2. PDT Directed at ER/Mitochondria Promotes Efficacy of XRT in HPV-Negative HNSCC Cells

Three different photosensitizing agents were examined: BPD targets both ER and mitochondria for photodamage, while hypericin is specific for the ER/Golgi and NPe6 is selective for lysosomes. Photodamage from either BPD or hypericin effectively reduced viability of HPV-negative WSU12 cells but had only a limited effect on HPV-positive UP154 cells, while NPe6 was ineffective against both cell lines (Figure 2A). Microscopic examination showed that photodamage from BPD or hypericin initially evoked paraptosis, with apoptosis observed at higher doses (Table 1). Figure 2B shows morphologic evidence for paraptosis and apoptosis in WSU12 cells after ER/mitochondrial photodamage. Paraptosis was characterized by highly-vacuolated cytoplasm but no nuclear fragmentation

(Figure 2B, arrowhead). Formation of apoptotic bodies was detected by phase-contrast microscopy, and the condensed and fragmented chromatin was identified by the fluorogenic probe Hö33342 (Figure 2B bottom panel, arrow). Apoptosis in WSU12 cells was confirmed by caspase activation (Figure 2D). ER photodamage-induced paraptotic vacuoles were confirmed to be derived from ER membranes, after photodamage with hypericin or BPD, using ER Tracker Green (Figure 2C). Neither paraptosis nor apoptosis was evident in HPV-positive UP154 cells (Figure 2D and additional negative data not shown). The difference in responsiveness to photodamage from BPD was not related to differences in localized accumulation of this agent in WSU12 vs. UP154 cells (Figure S5). Photodamage from BPD was found to enhance the efficacy of XRT in WSU12 cells. An LD_{20} effect by XRT alone was increased to an LD_{70} level by addition of an LD_{20} PDT dose using BPD (Figure 2E). The combination index was 0.67 (95% Ci, 0.47 to 0.97), indicating synergism.

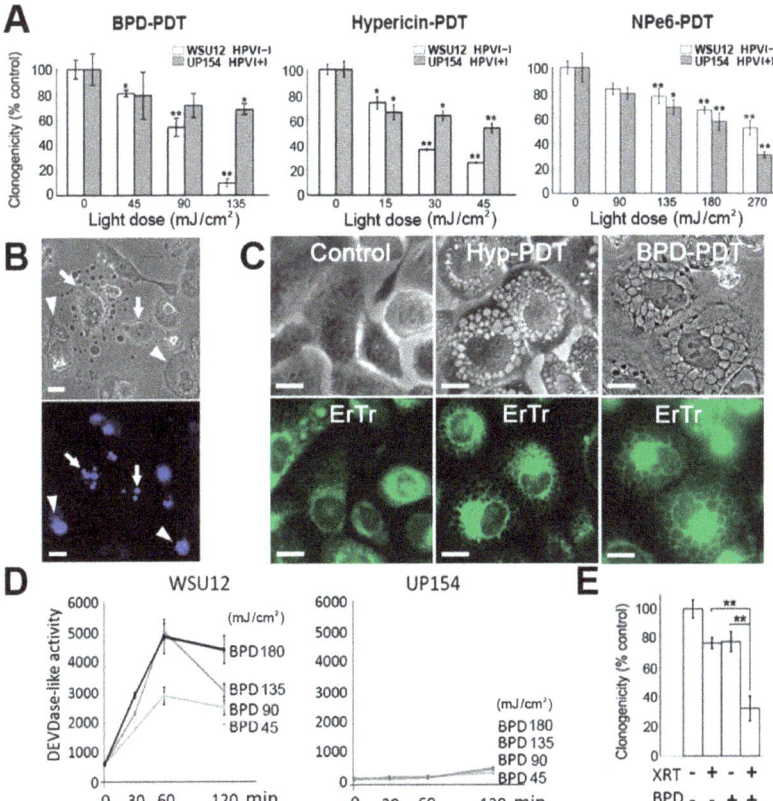

Figure 2. Endoplasmic reticulum (ER)/mitochondria-targeted PDT enhanced ionizing radiation therapy (XRT)-mediated cytotoxicity in HPV-negative WSU12 cells, but not in HPV-positive UP154 cells, via paraptosis and apoptosis. (**A**) Clonogenic cell survival assay. (* $p < 0.05$, ** $p < 0.01$). (**B**) Typical morphologies of apoptosis (arrow) and paraptosis (arrowhead) in WSU12 cells are shown one day after PDT. Top, phase-contrast; bottom, Hö33342 staining. Scale bar, 20 µm. (**C**) Formation of ER-derived paraptotic vacuoles in WSU12 cells after LD_{90} levels of photodamage with hypericin or BPD. Top panels, phase-contrast; bottom panels, ER Tracker. Scale bar, 20 µm. (**D**) DEVDase activity assay post BPD-PDT. (**E**) Clonogenic cell survival assay of WSU12 cells post BPD-PDT at 22.5 mJ/cm^2, then immediately exposed to XRT at 2 Gy. (** $p < 0.01$).

Table 1. BPD-photodynamic therapy (PDT)- and hypericin-PDT-induced cell death modes.

Photosensitizing Agent	Light Dose (mJ/cm^2)	WSU12		UP154	
		Paraptosis	Apoptosis	Paraptosis	Apoptosis
BPD	45	+	−	−	−
	90	+++	+	−	−
	135	++	+	−	−
	180	+	++	−	−
Hypericin	15	+	−	−	−
	30	+++	−	−	−
	45	++	+	−	−
	60	+	+	−	−

Percent (%) cells in each category: − (<5), + (5–10), ++ (10–30), +++ (>30).

3.3. ER/mitochondria Photodamage Induces Paraptosis via JNK Activation Followed by Apoptosis Induction

Although little is known about the molecular pathways/mechanisms underlying paraptosis, studies have suggested that ER stress signaling pathways activate the MAPK family members that play a critical role for paraptosis [27–29]. ER stress signaling is mediated by three major sensors of ER stress; inositol requiring enzyme 1α (IRE1α), protein kinase RNA-activated-like ER kinase (PERK) and activating transcription factor 6α (ATF6α), whose activation is controlled by ER-resident chaperone molecule GRP78/BiP [30]. Here, we confirmed activation of ER stress signaling by BPD-PDT or hypericin-PDT as evidenced by the presence of splice variants of X-box binding protein-1 (XBP1) mRNA (Figure 3A), known to result from activation of the IRE1α pathway [30,31], as well as by upregulation of BiP and the transcription factors C/EBP homologous protein (CHOP) (Figure 3B), a downstream mediator of the PERK pathway [30,32]. Consistently with previous reports, ER stress signaling led to activation of JNKs (c-Jun N-terminal Kinases) followed by p38 activation (Figure 3C). Next, we tested the involvement of JNKs and p38 in paraptosis and apoptosis induction. Inhibition of JNKs, but not p38, prevented paraptotic cell death (Figure 3D), while inhibition of p38 (and JNK at a later time point only) reduced caspase activation (Figure 3E).

3.4. BPD-PDT Sensitizes WSU12 Cells to XRT via Apoptosis Induction; Implication of the Involvement of ER Stress/Paraptotic Signaling Pathways

Next, we asked whether BPD-PDT enhancement of XRT-mediated cytotoxicity is associated with apoptosis and if new protein synthesis, thought to be critical for ER stress signaling and paraptosis, is involved in apoptosis induction. To this end, we measured caspase activity after BPD-catalyzed photodamage with or without XRT in the presence or absence of cycloheximide treatment. A sublethal dose of PDT was used for better detection of its synergistic effect with XRT. While XRT alone failed to induce caspase activation in HPV-negative WSU12 cells (Figure 3F,G, second bar, and Figure 1B), XRT together with BPD-PDT effectively activated caspase (fourth bar vs. second (XRT alone) or third (BPD-PDT alone) bar in Figure 3F). Interestingly, while new protein synthesis did not seem to be required for BPD-PDT-induced caspase activation (third vs. seventh bar), cycloheximide treatment significantly prevented synergistic activation of caspase induced by cotreatment of BPD-PDT and XRT (fourth vs. eighth bar). As we previously reported [33], apoptosis induced by PDT is associated with destruction of anti-bcl-2 family member Bcl-xL (Figure 3B). We surmise that while caspase activation is independent of protein synthesis and associated with the loss of antiapoptotic Bcl-xL protein, synergistic apoptosis induction by BPD-PDT and XRT requires newly synthesized protein-mediated signaling. Hypericin-PDT was ineffective in synergistically activating caspase together with XRT (Figure 3G), consistent with clonogenic cell survival assay (Figure 2E).

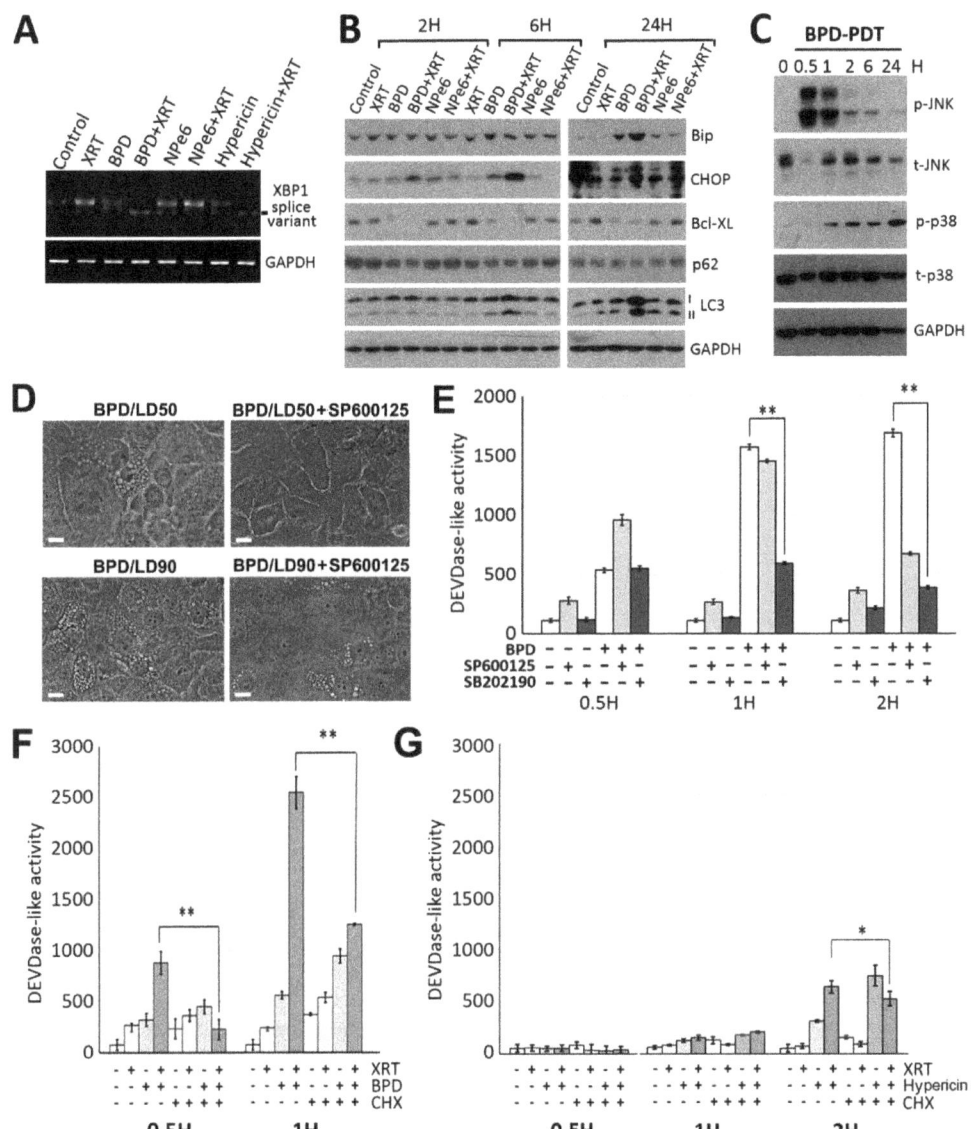

Figure 3. ER-targeted PDT induced ER stress signaling, and BPD-PDT sensitized WSU12 cells to XRT via apoptosis induction. (**A**) RT-PCR analysis of XBP1 splice variants in WSU12 cells upon indicated treatments. (**B**) Immunoblot of indicated proteins in WSU12 cells with BPD-PDT at 22.5 mJ/cm^2, NPe6-PDT at 30 mJ/cm^2 or hypericin-PDT at 15 mJ/cm^2 with/without XRT at 2 Gy. (**C**) Immunoblot of indicated phosphorylated or total proteins in WSU12 cells with BPD-PDT at 90 mJ/cm^2. (**D**) Phase contrast images of paraptotic WSU cells one day after BPD-PDT at LD$_{50}$ vs. LD$_{90}$ PDT doses with/without JNK inhibitor SP600125 (20 μM). Scale bar, 20 μm. (**E**) DEVDase activity assay in WSU12 cells after BPD-PDT at 90 mJ/cm^2 treatment with/without indicated inhibitor. (** $p < 0.01$). (**F**,**G**) DEVDase activity assay in WSU12 cells with BPD-PDT at 22.5 mJ/cm^2 (**F**) or Hypericin-PDT at 15 mJ/cm^2 (**G**) with/without XRT at 2 Gy with/without cycloheximide. (* $p < 0.05$, ** $p < 0.01$).

3.5. A Critical Role of the Autophagic Adaptor p62 in the Signal Relay for BPD-PDT-Mediated Apoptosis and Radiosensitization in Nonviral HNSCC Cells

Next, we asked whether differential interactions among cell death pathways attributable to differential regulation of ER/mitochondria photodamage-induced apoptosis and radiosensitization between HPV-positive and -negative HNSCC. Here we hypothesized that while high autophagic flux may contribute to apoptosis-resistant and radioresistant phenotypes in nonviral HNSCC cells (Figure 1), autophagy regulator(s) interact(s) with ER/mitochondria photodamage-induced stress signals, resulting in conversion of cell survival to cell death. First, we confirmed that ER photodamage further promotes the autophagic flux in HPV-negative WSU 12 cells, as detected by LC3-I conversion to LC3-II (Figure 4A), whereas HPV-positive cells were defective in inducing autophagy (Figure 1C). Since evidence supports that the autophagic adaptor p62 mediates ER stress signaling via its interaction with arginylated BiP (R-BiP) [34], we examined the involvement of the autophagic adaptor p62 in the regulation of paraptosis, apoptosis and cell fate upon ER/mitochondria photodamage. To this end, p62-knockdown WSU12 cell lines were established using three different vector-based short hairpin RNA (shRNA) constructs. Immunoblot analysis confirmed downregulation of p62 expression in cells receiving specific p62 target sequences (Figure 4B). While p62 knockdown had little effect on induction of paraptosis, this significantly impaired caspase activation (Figure 4C,D). Consistently, while p62 knockdown had little effect on low-dose BPD-PDT-induced cell toxicity (mainly paraptotic cell death), p62 knockdown significantly protected WSU12 cells from high-dose BPD PDT-induced cell apoptotic cell death (Figure 4E and Table 1). These results suggest that p62 functions as a signaling hub for the induction of apoptosis after photodamage. Further investigation of the involvement of p62 in apoptosis showed that p62 knockdown prevented synergistic caspase activation after ER/mitochondrial photodamage together with XRT (Figure 4F), providing molecular insight into p62-mediated radiosensitization upon ER/mitochondria photodamage in radioresistant HNSCC cells with high autophagy flux.

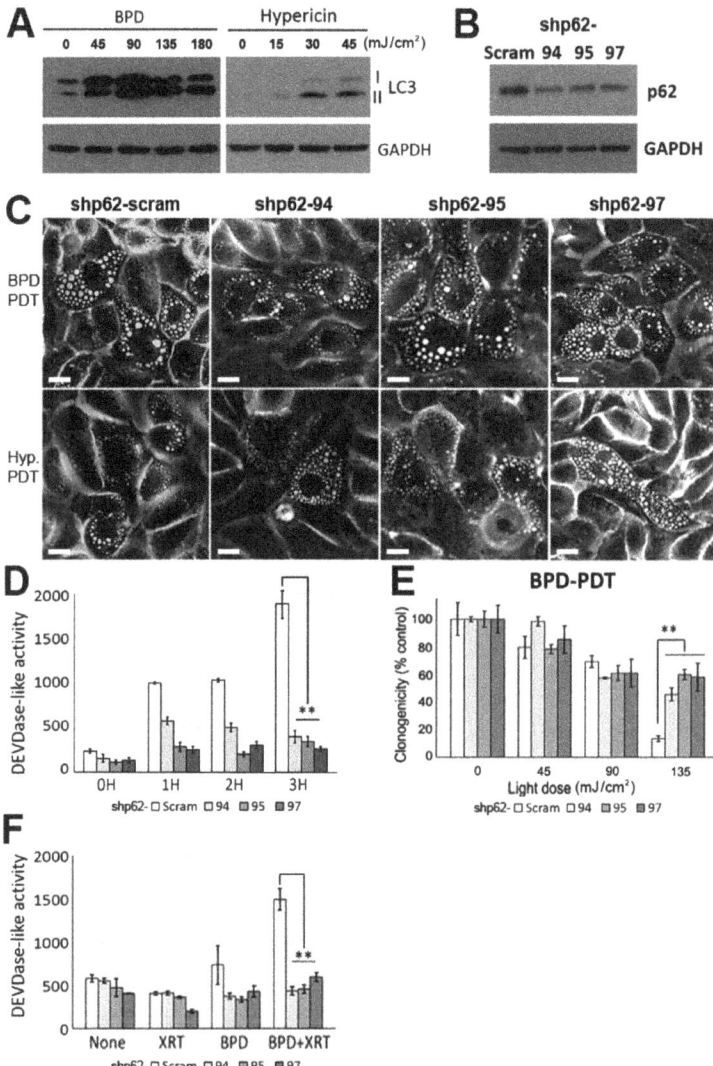

Figure 4. The autophagic adaptor p62 plays an important role in BPD-PDT-mediated apoptosis and radiosensitization. (**A**) Immunoblot analysis of LC3 in WSU12 cells at 1-day after post BPD-PDT or hypericin-PDT treatments with indicated light doses. (**B**) Immunoblot analysis of p62 in control (Scram) and p62 knockdown WSU12 cell lines (shp62–94, shp62–95 and shp62–97). (**C**) Phase contrast images of paraptotic cells in control and p62 knockdown WSU12 cells at one day after BPD-PDT at 90 mJ/cm^2 or hypericin-PDT at 45 mJ/cm^2. Scale bar, 20 µm. (**D**) DEVDase activity in control and p62 knockdown WSU12 cells upon BPD-PDT at 90 mJ/cm^2. (** $p < 0.01$). (**E**) Clonogenic cell survival of control and p62 knockdown WSU12 cells upon BPD-PDT. (** $p < 0.01$). (**F**) DEVDase activity was measured at 4 h after treatments with/without XRT at 2 Gy and/or BPD-PDT at 180 mJ/cm^2. (** $p < 0.01$).

4. Discussion

This report identifies photodamage to ER and mitochondria using BPD, an FDA-approved photosensitizer, as a means to sensitize nonviral HNSCC cells to XRT, consistent with our previous report [35]. Our results indicate that the molecular mechanism underlying BPD-PDT-induced drastic conversion of an apoptosis-resistant phenotype to an apoptotic-responsive phenotype after XRT involves the autophagy adaptor p62. As depicted in Figure 5, ER stress signaling leads to activation of JNKs and paraptosis as well as activation of p62 and autophagy. At present, it is unclear whether ER stress-induced autophagy initiated by PDT is associated with cytoprotection [36] or with cell death. After ER photodamage, ER stress signaling and autophagic regulators may interact with the mitochondrial apoptotic pathway, resulting in activation of caspase. Similarly to our study, recent findings report signal interplay between autophagy and apoptosis [37]. Dephosphorylation and cleavage of Beclin-1 disrupt R-BiP/Beclin-1/p62 complex, thereby converting autophagy to apoptosis [37]. In this study, both apoptosis and the autophagic flux are further enhanced upon photodamage and XRT (Figures 3B and 4A). These results suggest that caspase activation mediated by p62 may not occur at the expense of reducing autophagy through conversion from autophagy to apoptosis. Instead, we hypothesize that p62 functions as a signaling adaptor for apoptosis. Consistent with our hypothesis, a direct involvement of p62 in caspase activation has been suggested: the ER stress inducer tunicamycin was shown to induce apoptosis involving p62-mediated caspase-8 activation [38] and the ubiquitin-binding function of p62 promotes aggregation and activation of caspase-8 [39].

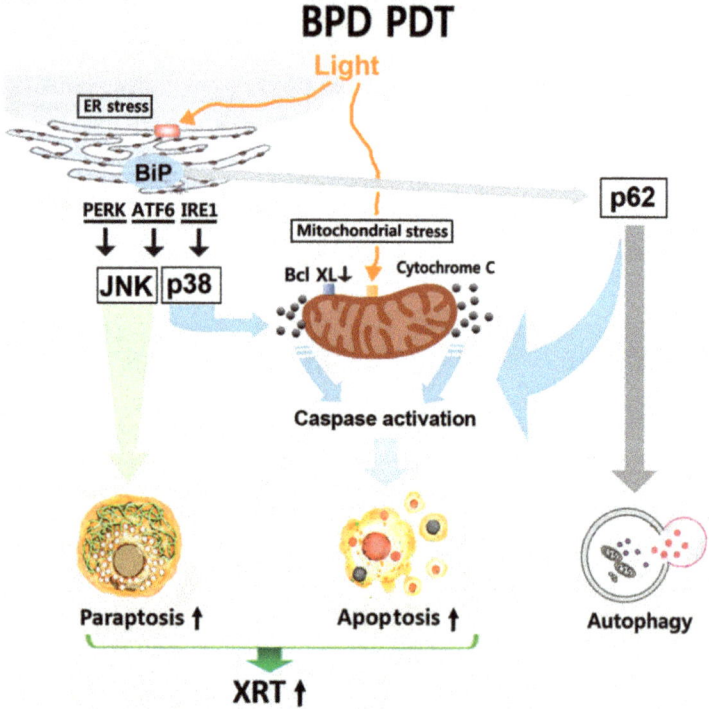

Figure 5. A working model of BPD-PDT-mediated paraptosis, apoptosis and sensitization to XRT.

We showed that ER stress-induced paraptosis preceded apoptosis in cells where apoptosis was impaired after radiotherapy. At present, it is unclear whether PDT-induced paraptosis is a prerequisite for apoptosis induction or these are two different cell death pathways independently induced by ER/mitochondria targeted PDT. Although recent studies have reported the significance of paraptosis, for instance, as an important cell death mode upon Zika virus infection [15], its presence in vivo and the functional significance in cancer therapy remain to be investigated. In light of reports demonstrating that high tumor immunogenicity is associated with nonapoptotic death of tumor cells in vivo [40], PDT-induced paraptosis warrants further investigation.

PDT is a local treatment method, known to be selective for malignant tissues and sparing normal tissues at tumor margins [16–18]. Improvement of locoregional control of HNSCC is critical for the management of patients with advanced HNSCC, and the treatment of those patients with PDT has resulted in promising outcomes [41–44]. Based on our results, we propose that ER/mitochondria-targeted PDT may serve as a part of organ-sparing multimodality treatment strategies to improve the efficacy of chemoradiotherapy for patients with advanced nonviral HNSCC with high autophagic flux.

5. Conclusions

Autophagy is associated with radioresistance in HPV-negative HNSCC, whereas apoptosis is associated with radiation sensitive HPV-positive HNSCC. The present study identified a tool to target the survival pathway in therapy-resistant HPV-negative HNSCC. Photodynamic therapy (PDT) directed at the ER/mitochondria initially induced paraptosis followed by apoptosis. This led to a substantial increase in radiation responsiveness in HPV-negative HNSCC in an autophagic adaptor p62-dependent manner. In contrast, the same PDT treatment had a minimal effect on HPV-positive cells. This work proposes that ER/mitochondria targeted PDT can serve as a radiosensitizer in intrinsically radio-resistant HNSCC that exhibits an increased autophagic flux.

Supplementary Materials: The following are available online at https://www.mdpi.com/2072-6694/13/6/1193/s1. Figure S1: Densitometric analysis of Figure 1A,C, Figure S2: Densitometric analysis of Figure 3B,C, Figure S3: Densitometric analysis of Figure 4A,B, Figure S4: Tumor necrosis factor-related apoptosis-inducing ligand (TRAIL) induces apoptosis more effectively in HPV-positive HNSCC cells compared to HPV-negative HNSCC cells, Figure S5: Uptake and localization of BPD in WSU12 and UP154 cells, Figure S6: Uncropped entire immunoblots with molecular weight markers, Table S1: List of PCR primers, Table S2: List of antibodies and reagents.

Author Contributions: W.J.C., D.K. and H.-R.C.K. designed the experiments, interpreted the results and prepared the manuscript. J.R. and B.L. performed irradiation experiments, A.J.N. and T.P. analyzed the data and prepared the manuscript, S.K. performed the statistical analysis, and H.-R.C.K., D.K., Y.T.K., I.K., and H.E.K. provided guidance, specialized reagents and expertise. All authors have read and agreed to the published version of the manuscript.

Funding: This research was funded by NIH/NCI Grants CA123362 (to H.R.C.K.) and CA 23378 (to D.K.), NIH/NIDCR DE023181 (to I.K., H.R.C.K and H.E.K.), and the Korean National Research Foundation (NRF-2016R1A2B3011389 and NRF-2020R1A5A1019023 to Y.T.K.).

Institutional Review Board Statement: Not applicable.

Informed Consent Statement: Not applicable.

Data Availability Statement: The data generated within the current study are available from the corresponding authors upon request.

Acknowledgments: The authors thank Summera Kanwal for her assistance with PDT.

Conflicts of Interest: The authors declare no conflict of interests.

References

1. Braakhuis, B.J.; Brakenhoff, R.H.; Leemans, C.R. Treatment choice for locally advanced head and neck cancers on the basis of risk factors: Biological risk factors. *Ann. Oncol.* **2012**, *23*, x173–x177. [CrossRef] [PubMed]
2. Attner, P.; Du, J.; Nasman, A.; Hammarstedt, L.; Ramqvist, T.; Lindholm, J.; Marklund, L.; Dalianis, T.; Munck-Wikland, E. The role of human papillomavirus in the increased incidence of base of tongue cancer. *Int. J. Cancer* **2010**, *126*, 2879–2884. [CrossRef] [PubMed]
3. Chaturvedi, A.K.; Engels, E.A.; Anderson, W.F.; Gillison, M.L. Incidence trends for human papillomavirus-related and -unrelated oral squamous cell carcinomas in the United States. *J. Clin. Oncol.* **2008**, *26*, 612–619. [CrossRef] [PubMed]

4. Hammarstedt, L.; Lindquist, D.; Dahlstrand, H.; Romanitan, M.; Dahlgren, L.O.; Joneberg, J.; Creson, N.; Lindholm, J.; Ye, W.; Dalianis, T.; et al. Human papillomavirus as a risk factor for the increase in incidence of tonsillar cancer. *Int. J. Cancer* **2006**, *119*, 2620–2623. [CrossRef] [PubMed]
5. Fakhry, C.; Westra, W.H.; Li, S.; Cmelak, A.; Ridge, J.A.; Pinto, H.; Forastiere, A.; Gillison, M.L. Improved survival of patients with human papillomavirus-positive head and neck squamous cell carcinoma in a prospective clinical trial. *J. Natl. Cancer Inst.* **2008**, *100*, 261–269. [CrossRef]
6. Hong, A.M.; Dobbins, T.A.; Lee, C.S.; Jones, D.; Harnett, G.B.; Armstrong, B.K.; Clark, J.R.; Milross, C.G.; Kim, J.; O'Brien, C.J.; et al. Human papillomavirus predicts outcome in oropharyngeal cancer in patients treated primarily with surgery or radiation therapy. *Br. J. Cancer* **2010**, *103*, 1510–1517. [CrossRef]
7. Sethi, S.; Ali-Fehmi, R.; Franceschi, S.; Struijk, L.; van Doorn, L.J.; Quint, W.; Albashiti, B.; Ibrahim, M.; Kato, I. Characteristics and survival of head and neck cancer by HPV status: A cancer registry-based study. *Int. J. Cancer* **2012**, *131*, 1179–1186. [CrossRef] [PubMed]
8. Ang, M.K.; Patel, M.R.; Yin, X.Y.; Sundaram, S.; Fritchie, K.; Zhao, N.; Liu, Y.; Freemerman, A.J.; Wilkerson, M.D.; Walter, V.; et al. High XRCC1 protein expression is associated with poorer survival in patients with head and neck squamous cell carcinoma. *Clin. Cancer Res.* **2011**, *17*, 6542–6552. [CrossRef]
9. Lill, C.; Kornek, G.; Bachtiary, B.; Selzer, E.; Schopper, C.; Mittlboeck, M.; Burian, M.; Wrba, F.; Thurnher, D. Survival of patients with HPV-positive oropharyngeal cancer after radiochemotherapy is significantly enhanced. *Wien. Klin. Wochenschr.* **2011**, *123*, 215–221. [CrossRef] [PubMed]
10. Mellin, H.; Friesland, S.; Lewensohn, R.; Dalianis, T.; Munck-Wikland, E. Human papillomavirus (HPV) DNA in tonsillar cancer: Clinical correlates, risk of relapse, and survival. *Int. J. Cancer* **2000**, *89*, 300–304. [CrossRef]
11. Sedaghat, A.R.; Zhang, Z.; Begum, S.; Palermo, R.; Best, S.; Ulmer, K.M.; Levine, M.; Zinreich, E.; Messing, B.P.; Gold, D.; et al. Prognostic significance of human papillomavirus in oropharyngeal squamous cell carcinomas. *Laryngoscope* **2009**, *119*, 1542–1549. [CrossRef] [PubMed]
12. Worden, F.P.; Kumar, B.; Lee, J.S.; Wolf, G.T.; Cordell, K.G.; Taylor, J.M.; Urba, S.G.; Eisbruch, A.; Teknos, T.N.; Chepeha, D.B.; et al. Chemoselection as a strategy for organ preservation in advanced oropharynx cancer: Response and survival positively associated with HPV16 copy number. *J. Clin. Oncol.* **2008**, *26*, 3138–3146. [CrossRef] [PubMed]
13. Ow, T.J.; Pitts, C.E.; Kabarriti, R.; Garg, M.K. Effective Biomarkers and Radiation Treatment in Head and Neck Cancer. *Arch. Pathol. Lab. Med.* **2015**, *139*, 1379–1388. [CrossRef]
14. Seshacharyulu, P.; Baine, M.J.; Souchek, J.J.; Menning, M.; Kaur, S.; Yan, Y.; Ouellette, M.M.; Jain, M.; Lin, C.; Batra, S.K. Biological determinants of radioresistance and their remediation in pancreatic cancer. *Biochim Biophys Acta. Rev. Cancer* **2017**, *1868*, 69–92. [CrossRef]
15. Monel, B.; Compton, A.A.; Bruel, T.; Amraoui, S.; Burlaud-Gaillard, J.; Roy, N.; Guivel-Benhassine, F.; Porrot, F.; Genin, P.; Meertens, L.; et al. Zika virus induces massive cytoplasmic vacuolization and paraptosis-like death in infected cells. *EMBO. J.* **2017**, *36*, 1653–1668. [CrossRef] [PubMed]
16. Codogno, P.; Meijer, A.J. Autophagy and signaling: Their role in cell survival and cell death. *Cell Death. Differ.* **2005**, *12*, 1509–1518. [CrossRef]
17. Agostinis, P.; Berg, K.; Cengel, K.A.; Foster, T.H.; Girotti, A.W.; Gollnick, S.O.; Hahn, S.M.; Hamblin, M.R.; Juzeniene, A.; Kessel, D.; et al. Photodynamic therapy of cancer: An update. *CA. Cancer J. Clin.* **2011**, *61*, 250–281. [CrossRef]
18. Dougherty, T.J.; Gomer, C.J.; Henderson, B.W.; Jori, G.; Kessel, D.; Korbelik, M.; Moan, J.; Peng, Q. Photodynamic therapy. *J. Natl. Cancer Inst.* **1998**, *90*, 889–905. [CrossRef]
19. Kessel, D.; Oleinick, N.L. Photodynamic therapy and cell death pathways. *Methods. Mol. Biol* **2010**, *635*, 35–46. [PubMed]
20. Del Duca, E.; Manfredini, M.; Petrini, N.; Farnetani, F.; Chester, J.; Bennardo, L.; Schipani, G.; Tamburi, F.; Sannino, M.; Cannarozzo, G.; et al. Daylight Photodynamic Therapy with 5-aminolevulinic acid 5% gel for the treatment of mild-to-moderate inflammatory acne. *G. Ital. Dermatol. Venereol.* **2019**. [CrossRef]
21. Nam, J.S.; Kang, M.G.; Kang, J.; Park, S.Y.; Lee, S.J.; Kim, H.T.; Seo, J.K.; Kwon, O.H.; Lim, M.H.; Rhee, H.W.; et al. Endoplasmic Reticulum-Localized Iridium(III) Complexes as Efficient Photodynamic Therapy Agents via Protein Modifications. *J. Am. Chem. Soc.* **2016**, *138*, 10968–10977. [CrossRef]
22. Jung, Y.S.; Najy, A.J.; Huang, W.; Sethi, S.; Snyder, M.; Sakr, W.; Dyson, G.; Huttemann, M.; Lee, I.; Ali-Fehmi, R.; et al. HPV-associated differential regulation of tumor metabolism in oropharyngeal head and neck cancer. *Oncotarget* **2017**, *8*, 51530–51541. [CrossRef] [PubMed]
23. Chou, T.C. Theoretical basis, experimental design, and computerized simulation of synergism and antagonism in drug combination studies. *Pharmacol. Rev.* **2006**, *58*, 621–681. [CrossRef]
24. Yang, Z.J.; Chee, C.E.; Huang, S.; Sinicrope, F. Autophagy modulation for cancer therapy. *Cancer Biol. Ther.* **2011**, *11*, 169–176. [CrossRef]
25. Carew, J.S.; Kelly, K.R.; Nawrocki, S.T. Autophagy as a target for cancer therapy: New developments. *Cancer Manag. Res.* **2012**, *4*, 357–365. [PubMed]
26. Sui, X.; Chen, R.; Wang, Z.; Huang, Z.; Kong, N.; Zhang, M.; Han, W.; Lou, F.; Yang, J.; Zhang, Q.; et al. Autophagy and chemotherapy resistance: A promising therapeutic target for cancer treatment. *Cell Death. Dis.* **2013**, *4*, e838. [CrossRef]

27. Sperandio, S.; Poksay, K.; de Belle, I.; Lafuente, M.J.; Liu, B.; Nasir, J.; Bredesen, D.E. Paraptosis: Mediation by MAP kinases and inhibition by AIP-1/Alix. *Cell Death. Differ.* **2004**, *11*, 1066–1075. [CrossRef] [PubMed]
28. Xue, Q.; Wang, X.; Wang, P.; Zhang, K.; Liu, Q. Role of p38MAPK in apoptosis and autophagy responses to photodynamic therapy with Chlorin e6. *Photodiagnosis. Photodyn. Ther.* **2015**, *12*, 84–91. [CrossRef] [PubMed]
29. Chen, R.; Duan, C.Y.; Chen, S.K.; Zhang, C.Y.; He, T.; Li, H.; Liu, Y.P.; Dai, R.Y. The suppressive role of p38 MAPK in cellular vacuole formation. *J. Cell Biochem.* **2013**, *114*, 1789–1799. [CrossRef]
30. Rutkowski, D.T.; Kaufman, R.J. A trip to the ER: Coping with stress. *Trends. Cell Biol.* **2004**, *14*, 20–28. [CrossRef] [PubMed]
31. Maurel, M.; Chevet, E.; Tavernier, J.; Gerlo, S. Getting RIDD of RNA: IRE1 in cell fate regulation. *Trends. Biochem. Sci.* **2014**, *39*, 245–254. [CrossRef] [PubMed]
32. Rozpedek, W.; Pytel, D.; Mucha, B.; Leszczynska, H.; Diehl, J.A.; Majsterek, I. The Role of the PERK/eIF2alpha/ATF4/CHOP Signaling Pathway in Tumor Progression During Endoplasmic Reticulum Stress. *Curr. Mol. Med.* **2016**, *16*, 533–544. [CrossRef] [PubMed]
33. Kim, H.R.; Luo, Y.; Li, G.; Kessel, D. Enhanced apoptotic response to photodynamic therapy after bcl-2 transfection. *Cancer Res.* **1999**, *59*, 3429–3432. [PubMed]
34. Cha-Molstad, H.; Sung, K.S.; Hwang, J.; Kim, K.A.; Yu, J.E.; Yoo, Y.D.; Jang, J.M.; Han, D.H.; Molstad, M.; Kim, J.G.; et al. Amino-terminal arginylation targets endoplasmic reticulum chaperone BiP for autophagy through p62 binding. *Nat. Cell Biol.* **2015**, *17*, 917–929. [CrossRef] [PubMed]
35. Kessel, D.; Cho, W.J.; Rakowski, J.; Kim, H.E.; Kim, H.C. Effects of HPV Status on Responsiveness to Ionizing Radiation vs Photodynamic Therapy in Head and Neck Cancer Cell lines. *Photochem. Photobiol.* **2020**, *96*, 652–657. [CrossRef]
36. Ogata, M.; Hino, S.; Saito, A.; Morikawa, K.; Kondo, S.; Kanemoto, S.; Murakami, T.; Taniguchi, M.; Tanii, I.; Yoshinaga, K.; et al. Autophagy is activated for cell survival after endoplasmic reticulum stress. *Mol. Cell Biol.* **2006**, *26*, 9220–9231. [CrossRef] [PubMed]
37. Song, X.; Lee, D.H.; Dilly, A.K.; Lee, Y.S.; Choudry, H.A.; Kwon, Y.T.; Bartlett, D.L.; Lee, Y.J. Crosstalk Between Apoptosis and Autophagy Is Regulated by the Arginylated BiP/Beclin-1/p62 Complex. *Mol. Cancer Res.* **2018**, *16*, 1077–1091. [CrossRef] [PubMed]
38. Ullman, E.; Pan, J.A.; Zong, W.X. Squamous cell carcinoma antigen 1 promotes caspase-8-mediated apoptosis in response to endoplasmic reticulum stress while inhibiting necrosis induced by lysosomal injury. *Mol. Cell Biol.* **2011**, *31*, 2902–2919. [CrossRef]
39. Jin, Z.; Li, Y.; Pitti, R.; Lawrence, D.; Pham, V.C.; Lill, J.R.; Ashkenazi, A. Cullin3-based polyubiquitination and p62-dependent aggregation of caspase-8 mediate extrinsic apoptosis signaling. *Cell* **2009**, *137*, 721–735. [CrossRef] [PubMed]
40. Melcher, A.; Todryk, S.; Hardwick, N.; Ford, M.; Jacobson, M.; Vile, R.G. Tumor immunogenicity is determined by the mechanism of cell death via induction of heat shock protein expression. *Nat. Med.* **1998**, *4*, 581–587. [CrossRef] [PubMed]
41. Biel, M.A. Photodynamic therapy of head and neck cancers. *Methods. Mol. Biol.* **2010**, *635*, 281–293. [PubMed]
42. Rigual, N.R.; Thankappan, K.; Cooper, M.; Sullivan, M.A.; Dougherty, T.; Popat, S.R.; Loree, T.R.; Biel, M.A.; Henderson, B. Photodynamic therapy for head and neck dysplasia and cancer. *Arch. Otolaryngol. Head Neck Surg.* **2009**, *135*, 784–788. [CrossRef] [PubMed]
43. Mimikos, C.; Shafirstein, G.; Arshad, H. Current state and future of photodynamic therapy for the treatment of head and neck squamous cell carcinoma. *World J. Otorhinolaryngol. Head Neck Surg.* **2016**, *2*, 126–129. [CrossRef] [PubMed]
44. van Doeveren, T.E.M.; Karakullukcu, M.B.; van Veen, R.L.P.; Lopez-Yurda, M.; Schreuder, W.H.; Tan, I.B. Adjuvant photodynamic therapy in head and neck cancer after tumor-positive resection margins. *Laryngoscope* **2018**, *128*, 657–663. [CrossRef]

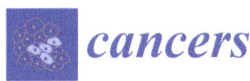

Systematic Review

Human Papillomavirus in Sinonasal Squamous Cell Carcinoma: A Systematic Review and Meta-Analysis

Kim J. W. Chang Sing Pang [1], Taha Mur [2], Louise Collins [1], Sowmya R. Rao [3,4] and Daniel L. Faden [1,5,6,*]

1. Department of Otolaryngology–Head and Neck Surgery, Massachusetts Eye and Ear, Boston, MA 02114, USA; kim.chang@hotmail.nl (K.J.W.C.S.P.); Louise_Collins@MEEI.HARVARD.EDU (L.C.)
2. Department of Otolaryngology–Head and Neck Surgery, Boston University School of Medicine, Boston, MA 02118, USA; taha.mur@bmc.org
3. Biostatistics Center, Massachusetts General Hospital, Boston, MA 02114, USA; SRRAO@mgh.harvard.edu
4. Department of Global Health, Boston University School of Public Health, Boston, MA 02118, USA
5. Massachusetts General Hospital, Boston, MA 02118, USA
6. Harvard Medical School, Boston, MA 02115, USA
* Correspondence: DFADEN@PARTNERS.ORG

Simple Summary: The causative role of human papillomavirus (HPV) in sinonasal squamous cell carcinoma (SNSCC) remains unclear and is hindered by small studies using variable HPV detection techniques. This meta-analysis aims to provide an updated overview of HPV prevalence in SNSCC stratified by detection method, anatomic subsite, and geographic region. From 60 eligible studies, an overall HPV prevalence was estimated at 26%. When stratified by detection method, HPV prevalence was lower when using multiple substrate testing compared to single substrate testing. Anatomic subsite HPV prevalence was higher in subsites with high exposure to secretion flow compared to low exposure subsites. HPV prevalence in SNSCC followed the global distribution of HPV+ oropharyngeal squamous cell carcinoma. Taken together, this meta-analysis further supports a role for HPV in a subset of SNSCCs.

Abstract: Human papillomavirus (HPV) drives tumorigenesis in a subset of oropharyngeal squamous cell carcinomas (OPSCC) and is increasing in prevalence across the world. Mounting evidence suggests HPV is also involved in a subset of sinonasal squamous cell carcinomas (SNSCC), yet small sample sizes and variability of HPV detection techniques in existing literature hinder definitive conclusions. A systematic review was performed by searching literature through March 29th 2020 using PubMed, Embase, and Web of Science Core Collection databases. Preferred Reporting Items for Systematic Reviews and Meta-Analyses (PRISMA) guidelines were followed by two authors independently. A meta-analysis was performed using the random-effects model. Sixty studies (*n* = 1449) were eligible for statistical analysis estimating an overall HPV prevalence of 25.5% (95% CI 20.7–31.0). When stratified by HPV detection method, prevalence with multiple substrate testing (20.5%, 95% CI 14.5–28.2) was lower than with single substrate testing (31.7%, 95% CI 23.6–41.1), highest in high-exposure anatomic subsites (nasal cavity and ethmoids) (37.6%, 95% CI 26.5–50.2) vs. low-exposure (15.1%, 95% CI 7.3–28.6) and highest in high HPV+ OPSCC prevalence geographic regions (North America) (30.9%, 95% CI 21.9–41.5) vs. low (Africa) (13.1%, 95% CI 6.5–24.5)). While small sample sizes and variability in data cloud firm conclusions, here, we provide a new reference point prevalence for HPV in SNSCC along with orthogonal data supporting a causative role for virally driven tumorigenesis, including that HPV is more commonly found in sinonasal subsites with increased exposure to refluxed oropharyngeal secretions and in geographic regions where HPV+ OPSCC is more prevalent.

Keywords: human papillomavirus; sinonasal squamous cell carcinoma; prevalence; detection method; anatomic subsite

Citation: Chang Sing Pang, K.J.W.; Mur, T.; Collins, L.; Rao, S.R.; Faden, D.L. Human Papillomavirus in Sinonasal Squamous Cell Carcinoma: A Systematic Review and Meta-Analysis. *Cancers* 2021, 13, 45. https://dx.doi.org/10.3390/cancers13010045

Received: 24 October 2020
Accepted: 21 December 2020
Published: 25 December 2020

Publisher's Note: MDPI stays neutral with regard to jurisdictional claims in published maps and institutional affiliations.

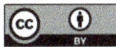

Copyright: © 2020 by the authors. Licensee MDPI, Basel, Switzerland. This article is an open access article distributed under the terms and conditions of the Creative Commons Attribution (CC BY) license (https://creativecommons.org/licenses/by/4.0/).

1. Introduction

Human papillomavirus (HPV) has been identified as an etiological factor in a subset of head and neck squamous cell carcinomas (HNSCC). HPV-driven tumors arise predominately in the oropharynx (oropharyngeal squamous cell carcinomas (OPSCC)), but also in epithelial-derived tumors of the oral cavity, larynx and nasopharynx, albeit at significantly lower prevalence [1,2]. OPSCC driven by HPV (HPV+ OPSCC) has unique biology, epidemiology, and clinical behavior compared to OPSCC driven by carcinogen exposure. Further, and perhaps most importantly, HPV+ OPSCC has improved treatment response and overall survival [3–5]. At this time, detection of HPV in OPSCC is one of the only clinically utilized biomarkers in HNSCC.

The first evidence for a potential etiological role of HPV in sinonasal squamous cell carcinoma (SNSCC) tumorigenesis arose in 1983 with the detection of HPV DNA by Syrjänen et al. [6]. Since this time, mounting histologic and epidemiologic evidence suggests a subset of SNSCCs may be HPV-driven, and that similar to HPV+ OPSCC, HPV detection in SNSCC may be a biomarker for improved survival [7–11]. However, small sample sizes and variable HPV detection techniques, each with wide ranges in sensitivity and specificity, continue to hinder definitive conclusions. Because of this, and: (1) improvements in HPV detection techniques and (2) the changing prevalence of HPV+ OPSCC in the population, we performed a meta-analysis of HPV in SNSCC, identifying 1458 cases for inclusion. In addition to establishing a new point prevalence of HPV in SNSCC, using by far the largest cohort to date, we also test orthogonal hypotheses which would support a role for HPV-driven tumorigenesis in SNSCC, including that HPV prevalence will be highest in: (1) subsites of the sinonasal cavities with the highest exposure to refluxed secretions from the oropharynx and (2) geographic regions of the world with the highest HPV+ OPSCC prevalence.

2. Materials and Methods

A systematic review was performed by a medical librarian (L.C.) following the guidelines of the Preferred Reporting Items for Systematic Reviews and Meta-Analyses (PRISMA) [12].

2.1. Literature Search

A search of published studies in Medline via Legacy PubMed (1946-), Embase.com (1947-), and Web of Science Core Collection (1900-) was performed on 6 February 2020 to identify relevant articles. Search strategies were customized for each database (Methods S1). Each search utilized a combination of controlled vocabulary and keywords focused on the concepts human papillomavirus, squamous cell carcinoma, and sinonasal. The search was constructed to exclude non-human studies. No filters for language, study design, date of publication, or country of origin were used in the search producing 1177 articles (Figure 1). All references were exported into EndNote X7.8. Duplicates were removed first by the automated process in EndNote and then manually by the librarian leaving 730 articles, which were exported into Covidence for study screening, selection, and data extraction. The search was re-run on 29 March 2020 to update for the most recent literature rendering 14 additional articles. Three subsequent articles were found through searching the references of included articles making up a total of 747 articles for screening.

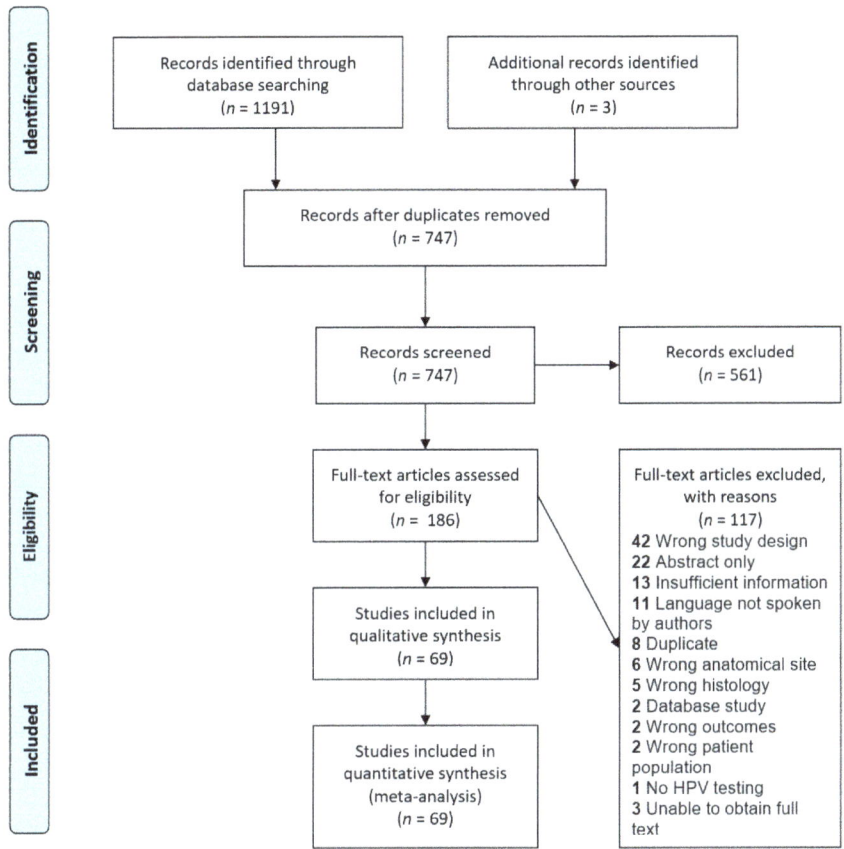

Figure 1. Preferred Reporting Items for Systematic Reviews and Meta-Analyses (PRISMA) flowchart depicting the study selection process.

2.2. Study Selection

Studies examining both SNSCC and HPV status in adult patients were considered eligible for inclusion. Included SNSCC histology subtypes were non-keratinizing, keratinizing, papillary, and basaloid squamous cell carcinoma. SCC in which the histological subtype was not further specified was also considered eligible. Other SCC subtypes such as adenosquamous and multi-phenotypic sinonasal carcinoma were excluded along with studies not listing HPV detection methods or discussing cancers originating from the nasopharynx, nasal vestibule, nasal ala or skin.

Extracted data comprised geographic region of the study, histology, anatomic subsite, HPV status, HPV genotype, and HPV detection method. During the screening, any study written in a language other than English, Dutch, Arabic, or German (languages spoken by the authors) were excluded. Titles and abstracts were screened by two authors independently (K.C.S.P. and T.M.) for full text review. The same two authors independently conducted the full text review. Any disagreements in the screening process were settled by discussion and consensus between the two authors. Disagreements that could not be settled in this manner were settled in consultation with a third author (D.F.). All eligible studies were screened for duplicate data by comparing authors, timeframe of data collection, and outcomes. After full text screening, 69 studies remained for the quantitative synthesis.

2.3. Statistical Analysis

Comprehensive Meta-Analysis (CMA) v3 (Biostat, Englewood, NJ, USA, 2013) was used to conduct the statistical analysis. To minimize distortion of the results by outliers the CMA program excludes all studies with a sample size of one patient. Using the random-effects model, HPV prevalence estimates including 95% confidence intervals (CI) were computed from sample size and event rates. In case of an event rate of 0% or 100%, the CMA program adds 0.5 to event and non-event values for computation of logit event rates and its variance. HPV prevalence was stratified by detection method, anatomic subsite, and geographic region for descriptive comparison. Subsequently, separate meta-regressions were performed to test the association of each study characteristic with HPV prevalence estimates. Interstudy variability and between-study variance were assessed by Cochran's Q statistic [13,14]. The percentage of variation explained by true heterogeneity opposed to sampling error was calculated with the I^2 statistic [13]. Potential publication bias was evaluated by generating a funnel plot and assessing its asymmetry with Egger's Test [15], Begg and Mazumdar Rank Correlation Test [16], and Duval and Tweedie's "Trim and Fill" method [17]. A sensitivity analysis was performed by removing one study at a time to assess the influence of each individual study on the combined HPV prevalence. We assume a two-sided $p < 0.05$ to be significant.

3. Results

3.1. HPV Prevalence

A total of 69 studies were included in the meta-analysis containing a total of 1458 patients with SNSCC (Table 1). There were 324/1458 HPV-positive cases comprising a crude HPV prevalence of 22.2%. After removal of all studies with a sample size of one patient, 60 studies remained for statistical analysis. Estimated HPV prevalence rates ranged from 5.0 to 94.4%. Using the random-effects model, an overall prevalence rate was estimated at 25.5% (95% CI 20.7–31.0) (Table 1).

Table 1. Overview of study characteristics. Table showing all 60 studies eligible for the statistical analysis including study characteristics, human papillomavirus (HPV) prevalence estimates using the random-effects model, and forest plot. Study characteristics of the nine excluded studies are shown in grey.

Authors	Year	Studies Included in Statistical Analysis						Event Rate	95% CI		Forest Plot of Event Rate and 95% CI	Weights (%)
		HPV+/Total	Geographic Region	Anatomic Subsite	Detection Method(s)	Substrate			Lower Limit	Upper Limit		
Syrjänen et al. [18]	1987	1/2	Europe	NC, SNNS	ISH	DNA		0.500	0.059	0.941		0.73
Klemi et al. [19]	1989	3/12	Europe	SNNS	ISH	DNA		0.250	0.083	0.552		1.77
Siivonen et al. [20]	1989	0/9	Europe	MS	ISH	DNA		0.050	0.003	0.475		0.70
Ishibashi et al. [21]	1990	1/5	Asia	NC, MS	SB	DNA		0.200	0.027	0.691		1.02
Furuta et al. [22]	1991	1/5	Asia	SNNS	PCR, ISH, DBH	DNA + RNA		0.200	0.027	0.691		1.02
Judd et al. [23]	1991	1/4	North America	MS	SB, PCR, ISH	DNA		0.250	0.034	0.762		0.98
Furuta et al. [24]	1992	5/47	Asia	SNNS	SB, PCR, SBH	DNA		0.106	0.045	0.231		2.22
Mclachlin et al. [25]	1992	1/2	North America	NC	PCR, ISH	DNA		0.500	0.059	0.941		0.73
Tyan et al. [26]	1993	1/3	Asia	SNNS	PCR	DNA		0.333	0.043	0.846		0.90
Wu et al. [27]	1993	2/4	North America	SNNS	PCR, ISH	DNA + RNA		0.500	0.123	0.877		1.18
Arndt et al. [28]	1994	3/3	Europe	SNNS	PCR	DNA		0.875	0.266	0.993		0.66
Beck et al. [29]	1995	7/10	North America	SNNS	PCR	DNA		0.700	0.376	0.900		1.72
Buchwald et al. [30]	1995	2/5	Europe	SNNS	PCR, ISH, DBH	DNA		0.400	0.100	0.800		1.31
Shen et al. [31]	1996	3/14	North America	SNNS	PCR	DNA		0.214	0.071	0.494		1.80
Bernauer et al. [32]	1997	1/2	Unknown	ES, MS	PCR	DNA		0.500	0.059	0.941		0.73
Caruana et al. [33]	1997	3/9	North America	SNNS	PCR	DNA		0.333	0.111	0.667		1.69
Mineta et al. [34]	1998	3/19	Asia	SNNS	PCR	DNA		0.158	0.052	0.392		1.85
Saegusa et al. [35]	1999	32/48	Asia	ES, MS, FS	PCR	DNA		0.667	0.523	0.785		2.60
Buchwald et al. [36]	2001	7/33	Europe	SNNS	PCR, DBH	DNA		0.212	0.105	0.383		2.33
Schwerer et al. [37]	2001	2/5	Europe	SNNS	NCL-PVp antibody detection	Protein		0.400	0.100	0.800		1.31
Fischer et al. [38]	2003	4/4	Europe	SNNS	PCR	DNA		0.900	0.326	0.994		0.68
Schwerer et al. [39]	2003	8/8	Europe	SNNS	p16	Protein		0.944	0.495	0.997		0.70
El-Mofty et al. [40]	2005	8/29	North America	SNNS	PCR, p16	DNA + Protein		0.276	0.144	0.462		2.35
Katori et al. [41]	2005	5/12	Asia	SNNS	ISH	DNA		0.417	0.185	0.692		1.95
McKay et al. [42]	2005	2/3	North America	SNNS	PCR	DNA		0.667	0.154	0.957		0.90
Hoffmann et al. [43]	2006	4/20	Europe	NC, ES, MS	SB, PCR	DNA		0.200	0.077	0.428		2.01
Kim et al. [44]	2007	0/7	Asia	SNNS	PCR	DNA		0.063	0.004	0.539		0.70
Alos et al. [11]	2009	12/60	Europe	NC, SNNS	PCR, p16	DNA + Protein		0.200	0.117	0.320		2.57
Jo et al. [45]	2009	2/4	North America	SNNS	ISH, p16	DNA + Protein		0.500	0.123	0.877		1.18
Cheung et al. [46]	2010	2/5	Asia	SNNS	PCR, ISH, p16	DNA + Protein		0.400	0.100	0.800		1.31
But-Hadzic et al. [47]	2011	3/5	Europe	NC	PCR	DNA		0.600	0.200	0.900		1.31
Jenko et al. [48]	2011	3/5	Europe	SNNS	PCR	DNA		0.600	0.200	0.900		1.31
Kim et al. [49]	2011	3/18	Asia	SNNS	p16	Protein		0.167	0.055	0.409		1.85

Table 1. Cont.

	Studies Included in Statistical Analysis								95% CI			
Authors	Year	HPV+/Total	Geographic Region	Anatomic Subsite	Detection Method(s)	Substrate	Event Rate	Lower Limit	Upper Limit	Forest Plot of Event Rate and 95% CI	Weights (%)
Bishop et al. [50]	2012	2/9	North America	SNNS	ISH, p16	DNA + RNA + Protein	0.222	0.056	0.579		1.50
Doxtader et al. [51]	2012	1/5	North America	SNNS	ISH, p16	DNA + Protein	0.200	0.027	0.691		1.02
Bishop et al. [52]	2013	23/82	North America	SNNS	ISH, p16	DNA + Protein	0.280	0.194	0.387		2.72
Deng et al. [53]	2013	3/11	Asia	SNNS	PCR, RT-PCR	DNA + RNA	0.273	0.090	0.586		1.75
Larque et al. [54]	2014	14/70	Europe	NC, SNNS	PCR, RT-PCR, ISH, p16	DNA + RNA + Protein	0.200	0.122	0.310		2.62
Takahashi et al. [55]	2014	6/70	North America	NC, ES, MS, FS	ISH, p16	DNA + Protein	0.086	0.039	0.178		2.33
Cheung et al. [46]	2015	14/26	North America	NC, SNNS	PCR	DNA + Protein	0.538	0.350	0.716		2.41
Doescher et al. [56]	2015	3/44	Europe	NC, SNNS	ISH, p16	RNA + Protein	0.068	0.022	0.191		1.92
Laco et al. [57]	2015	17/47	Europe	NC, ES, MS	PCR, RT-PCR, ISH, p16	DNA + RNA + Protein	0.362	0.238	0.507		2.61
Yamashita et al. [58]	2015	6/21	Asia	SNNS	PCR, p16	DNA + Protein	0.286	0.134	0.508		2.19
Beigh et al. [59]	2016	2/9	Asia	SNNS	PCR	DNA	0.222	0.056	0.579		1.50
Becker et al. [60]	2016	4/38	Europe	NS, NC	SB, PCR	DNA	0.105	0.040	0.249		2.08
Liu et al. [61]	2016	5/90	Asia	SNNS	ISH, p16	DNA + Protein	0.056	0.023	0.127		2.25
Oga et al. [62]	2016	0/2	Africa	NC	PCR	DNA	0.167	0.010	0.806		0.64
Chowdhury et al. [8]	2017	16/26	North America	NC, SNNS	ISH, p16	DNA + Protein	0.615	0.421	0.779		2.38
Paul et al. [63]	2017	2/6	Asia	SNNS	p16	Protein	0.333	0.084	0.732		1.39
Rooper et al. [64]	2017	2/22	North America	NC, ES, MS, SS, FS, SNNS	ISH, p16	RNA + Protein	0.091	0.023	0.300		1.62
Beigh et al. [65]	2018	2/10	Asia	SNNS	PCR	DNA	0.200	0.050	0.541		1.52
Owusu-Afriyie et al. [66]	2018	3/31	Africa	SNNS	p16	Protein	0.097	0.032	0.261		1.90
Udager et al. [67]	2018	10/36	North America	SNNS	PCR	DNA	0.278	0.156	0.444		2.45
Jiromaru et al. [10]	2019	9/101	Asia	NC, ES, MS, SS	ISH, p16	RNA + Protein	0.089	0.047	0.162		2.51
Kim et al. [68]	2019	3/6	Asia	NC	PCR, p16	DNA + Protein	0.500	0.168	0.832		1.47
Quan et al. [69]	2019	18/96	Asia	NC, MS	p16	Protein	0.188	0.121	0.278		2.69
Sahmane et al. [70]	2019	3/31	Europe	SNNS	PCR, ISH, p16	DNA + Protein	0.097	0.032	0.261		1.90
Bulane et al. [71]	2020	4/25	Africa	SNNS	PCR	DNA	0.160	0.061	0.357		2.04
Cabal et al. [72]	2020	6/74	Europe	NC, MS, ES, SS	PCR	DNA	0.081	0.037	0.169		2.33
Cohen et al. [73]	2020	5/40	North America	SNNS	ISH, p16	RNA + Protein	0.125	0.053	0.267		2.20
Random-effects model							0.255	0.207	0.310		
Studies excluded from statistical analysis											
Brandwein et al. [74]	1989	1/1	North America	SNNS	ISH	DNA					
Bradford et al. [75]	1991	0/1	North America	MS	SB	DNA					
Gaffey et al. [76]	1996	1/1	North America	SNNS	SB, PCR, ISH	DNA + RNA					
Miguel et al. [77]	1998	0/1	South America	MS	PCR, DBH	DNA					
Badaracco et al. [78]	2007	1/1	Europe	SNNS	PCR	DNA					
Mirza et al. [79]	2009	1/1	North America	SNNS	ISH	DNA					
McLemore et al. [80]	2010	1/1	North America	NC	PCR, DBH	DNA					
Singhi et al. [81]	2010	0/1	North America	SNNS	ISH, p16	DNA + Protein					
El-Salem et al. [82]	2019	1/1	North America	SNNS	PCR, p16	DNA + Protein					

Abbreviations: NC = nasal cavity, SNNS = sinonasal area not specified, MC = maxillary sinus, ES = ethmoid sinus, FS = frontal sinus, NS = nasal septum, SS = sphenoid sinus.

3.2. HPV Detection Method

There were 32 DNA-based studies, six protein-based studies, 12 DNA + protein-based studies, two DNA + RNA-based studies, four RNA + protein-based studies, and two DNA + RNA + protein-based studies. There were no studies using only RNA-based detection methods. DNA-based detection methods included DNA in situ hybridization (ISH), Southern blotting (SB), polymerase chain reaction (PCR), dot-blot-hybridization (DBH), and slot-blot-hybridization (SBH). RNA-based detection methods included RNA ISH and reverse transcriptase PCR (RT-PCR). Protein-based detection methods included p16 IHC and NCL-PVp antibody detection. Due to the small sample size in the majority of the subgroups, we categorized studies as either detecting a single HPV substrate (DNA-based or protein-based) or detecting a combination of HPV substrates (DNA + protein-, DNA + RNA-, RNA + protein-, or DNA + RNA + protein-based). Two studies, Deng et al., (2013) [53] and Larque et al., (2014) [54], first assessed HPV-positivity using DNA-based testing and only conducted additional RNA-based testing on the HPV-positive tumors. Since these studies show selection bias, both were excluded from this analysis. Additionally, when looking at the distributions of other variables in the two subgroups, only the single-agent testing group contained studies conducted in Africa. Since the three African studies reported a low HPV prevalence and thereby bias the results, they were also excluded from this analysis. The results of the 55 remaining studies are shown in Table 2.

Table 2. HPV Prevalence estimates stratified by detection method. (**A**). HPV prevalence stratified by single-agent testing and multi-agent testing. (**B**). HPV prevalence stratified by single-agent testing, multi-agent testing using RNA, and all multi-agent testing not using RNA.

Groups		Random-Effects Analysis			Heterogeneity		
Detection Method	No. of Studies	Events/Total	Point Estimate	95% CI	Q-Value	p-Value	I²
A Single testing	35	152/583	0.317	0.236–0.411	-	-	-
Multi-testing	20	142/727	0.205	0.145–0.282	-	-	-
Total between study	-	-	-	-	3.878	0.049	-
B Single testing	35	152/583	0.317	0.236–0.411	-	-	-
Multi-testing without RNA	12	101/455	0.233	0.150–0.343	-	-	-
Multi-testing with RNA	8	41/272	0.165	0.088–0.287	-	-	-
Total between study	-	-	-	-	4.595	0.101	-
Overall	55	294/1310	0.261	0.208–0.322	-	-	70.452 ^

^ Only calculated using the fixed-effects model.

As expected, HPV prevalence was lower when a combination of detection methods was used, reflecting fewer false positives, compared to when DNA- or protein-detection was used alone (Table 2A)—this difference was of border-line significance (Q = 3.88, p = 0.05, I^2 = 70.5%). Since the gold standard for determining a tumor is HPV-driven in OPSCC is RNA-based testing, we also wanted to compare RNA-based to DNA- and protein-based detection techniques. This is of particular importance as the diagnostic utility of p16 overexpression in SNSCC remains unclear. As there were no single RNA-testing studies, we split the multi-agent testing group into either RNA (RNA + DNA, RNA + protein, DNA + RNA + protein) or no RNA (DNA + protein). Again, in line with our expectations, the RNA group yielded the lowest HPV prevalence (Table 2B); however, the difference across the three groups was not statistically significant (Q = 4.60, p = 0.10, I^2 = 70.5%).

3.3. Anatomic Subsite

We next considered HPV prevalence stratified by sinonasal subsite. These data existed in 20 studies. The remaining 40 studies did not specify sinonasal subsite. We categorized anatomic subsites as either high-exposure to refluxed oropharyngeal secretion flow (nasal cavity and ethmoids), or low-exposure (maxillary, frontal, and sphenoid sinuses).

In line with our hypothesis, analysis using the random-effects model yielded the highest HPV prevalence in high-exposure subsites (37.6%, 95% CI 26.5–50.2) and lower prevalence in less exposed subsites (15.1%, 95% CI 7.3–28.6) (Figure 2A) with the prevalence of unspecified sinonasal area (likely a combination of all subsites) in the middle (25.6%, 95% CI 20.1–31.7) (Figure 2B).

A.

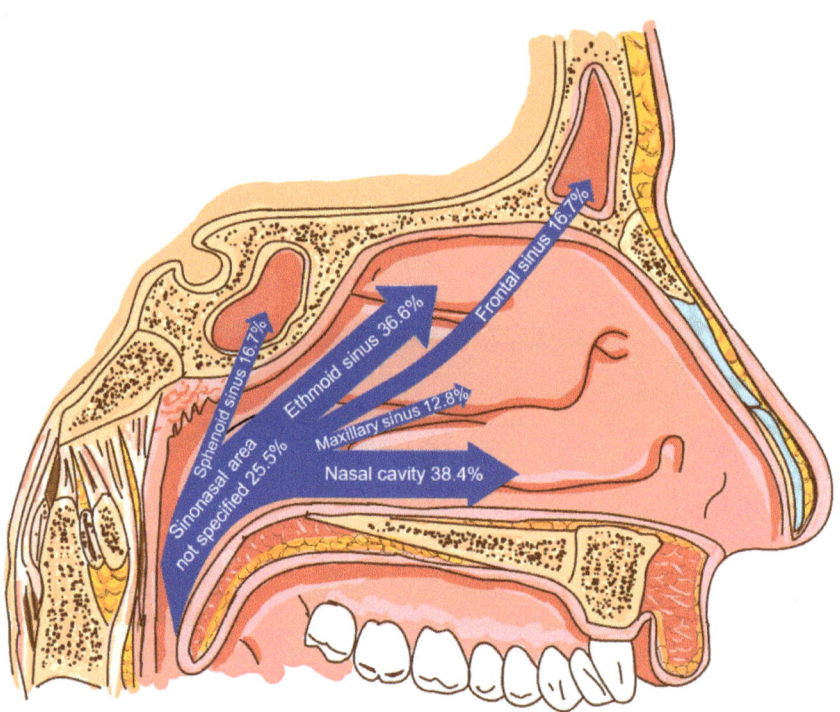

B.

Groups			Random-effects analysis				
Anatomic subsite	No. of studies	Events/Total	Point estimate	95% CI	Heterogeneity		
					Q-value	p-value	I²
High-exposure areas	15	55/175	0.376	0.265–0.502	-	-	-
Low-exposure areas	9	10/134	0.151	0.073–0.286	-	-	-
Sinonasal area not specified	47	251/1133	0.256	0.201–0.317	-	-	-
Total between subgroups	-	-	-	-	6.813	0.033	63.508^
Overall	71*	316/1442	0.271	0.224–0.323	-	-	-

Figure 2. HPV prevalence distribution by sinonasal anatomic subsite. (**A**). Sagittal section of the nasal cavity with arrows displaying the entry and distribution of HPV prevalence estimates by anatomic subsite using the random-effects model. (**B**). HPV prevalence estimates stratified by high- and low-exposure anatomic subsites. * With multiple subgroups in one study, Comprehensive Meta-Analysis (CMA) program will see each subgroup as a separate study. Hence, a total of 71 studies here. ^ Only calculated using the fixed-effects model.

3.4. Geographic Region

Data for HPV prevalence stratified by geographic region were available for 59 studies. Three studies were conducted in Africa, 18 in North America, 19 in Asia, and 19 in Europe.

No studies were available for analysis from South America or Oceania. Using the random-effects model, the highest HPV prevalence estimate was found in North America (30.9%, 95% CI 21.9–41.5), in line with existing literature using the National Cancer Database (32.0%) [9,83], and the lowest in Africa (13.1%, 95% CI 6.5–24.5). These trends mirrored HPV prevalence of OPSCC after matching for countries of origin (Figure 3). Remarkably, when examining data from North American studies only, high risk subsites showed HPV detection rates approaching those seen in OPSCC (Figure 4B).

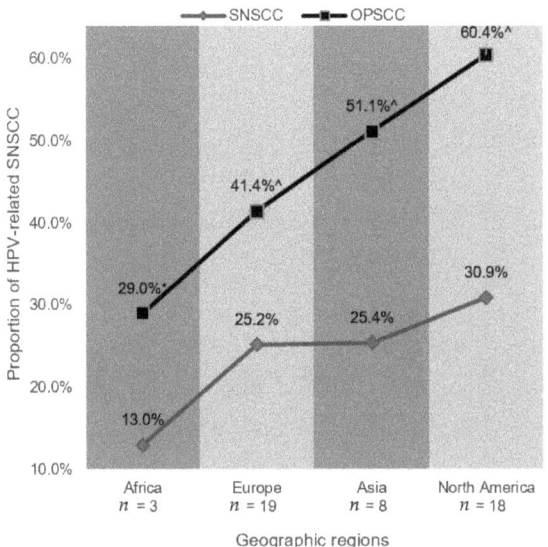

Figure 3. HPV prevalence in sinonasal squamous cell carcinoma (SNSCC) stratified by geographic region for oropharyngeal squamous cell carcinoma (OPSCC) and SNSCC demonstrating paired prevalence rates using the random-effects model. Studies from India and Japan were removed from the Asian SNSCC data as they were felt to introduce bias as these counties were not represented in the OPSCC data. * Source: Jalouli et al., (2010) [84] and Jalouli et al., (2012) [85]. ^ Source: Ndiaye et al., (2014) [86].

3.5. Analysis of Validity, Sensitivity, Data Trends and Publication Bias

The included studies show a significant amount of interstudy variability: Cochrane's $Q = 188.23$ ($p < 0.001$); $I^2 = 68.7\%$. Studies included in the subgroup analysis for detection method (single- vs. multi-agent testing) and anatomic subsite were significantly heterogeneous ($Q = 3.88$, $p = 0.05$; $I^2 = 70.5\%$ and $Q = 6.81$, $p = 0.03$, $I^2 = 63.5\%$, respectively), but not for geographic regions ($Q = 5.82$, $p = 0.12$). Meta-regression results indicated that both detection method (($Q = 3.54$, $p = 0.06$), with a border-line significance, and anatomic subsite ($Q = 6.33$, $p = 0.04$) were associated with the outcome (Table S1). However, due to limited number of studies and sample sizes we were unable to include all three covariates in one model. Our outcomes show a constant presence of interstudy variability limiting the conclusions which can be drawn. Of note, intra-study sample size increased across time, as did the use of RNA and multi-substrate testing, leading to more high yield studies (Figure S1).

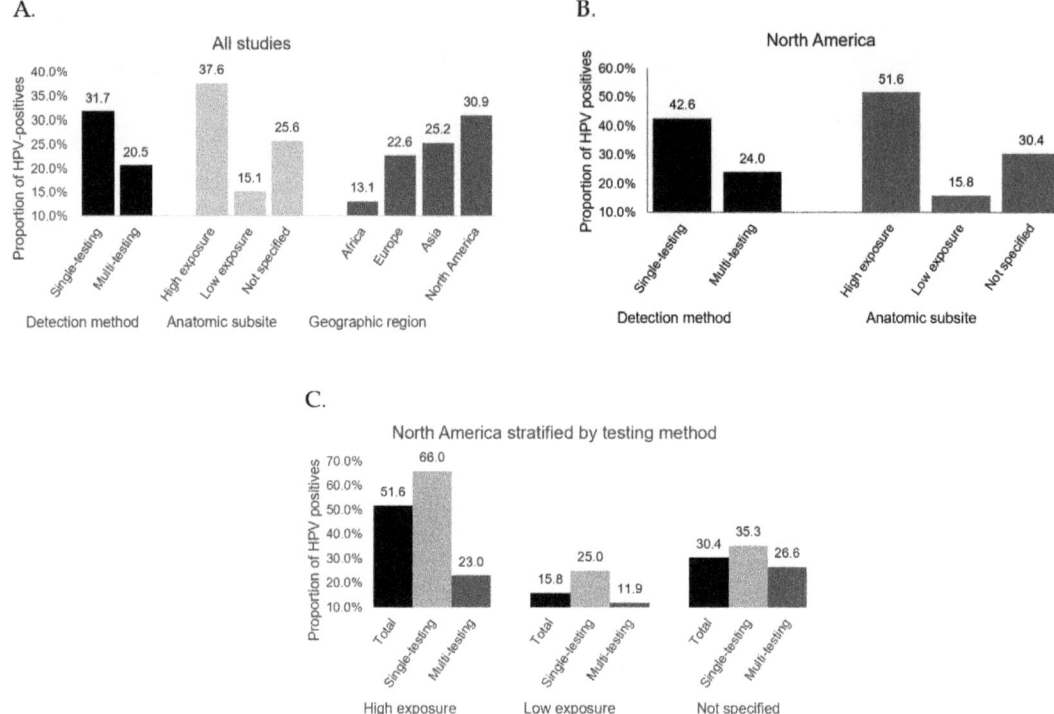

Figure 4. HPV prevalence by subgroup. (**A**). Bar chart depicting an overview of HPV prevalence per subgroup. (**B**). HPV prevalence per subgroup using only data from North America. (**C**). North American data stratified by testing method.

Sensitivity analysis conducted by removing one study at a time showed a relatively stable HPV prevalence estimate with the random-effects model with the lowest HPV prevalence of 24.3% (95% CI 19.9–29.3) when the study by Saegusa et al., (1999) [35] was removed and the highest HPV prevalence of 26.2% (95% CI 21.3–31.7) when the study of Liu et al., (2016) [61] was removed.

Begg and Mazumdar's rank correlation test yielded a Kendall's tau b with continuity correction of 0.245 with a one-tailed *p*-value of 0.003 showing significant funnel plot asymmetry (Figure S2). Duval and Tweedie's Trim and Fill method using the random-effects model imputed 14 missing studies and yielded an adjusted HPV prevalence of 19.1% (95% CI 14.8–24.3). However, Egger's test showed no statistical evidence for publication bias with an intercept (B0) of 46.3 (95% CI −0.540–1.465) with t = 0.924, df = 58, and one-tailed *p*-value of 0.180.

4. Discussion

HPV+ OPSCC is increasing in prevalence across the world and has now surpassed cervical cancer as the most common HPV-mediated malignancy. HPV status is a critical biomarker for OPSCC, signifying improved response rates to treatment and improved survival [3]. HPV+ OPSCC now necessitates its own staging criteria in the American Joint Committee on Cancer, Eighth edition, separate from the OPSCC caused by carcinogen exposure, and the rest of HNSCCs [87]. Because of the strong prognostic implications of HPV compared to carcinogen-driven tumorigenesis in HNSCC, considerable interest exists in the role of HPV in subsites outside the oropharynx. Numerous distinct cohorts of patients with HNSCC who lack carcinogen exposure have been interrogated as potential

HPV-mediated tumors, for example, oral tongue squamous cell carcinoma in young non-smoking patients. However, multiple studies have refuted this hypothesis [88–90]. Overall, less than 5% of HNSCCs outside the oropharynx appear to be HPV-driven, based on genomic interrogation of over 500 HNSCCs in The Cancer Genomes Atlas (TCGA) [91]. Of importance, the TCGA cohort excluded rare subsites, including SNSCC.

Cancer of the nasal and paranasal sinuses account for <3% of head and neck tumors, with SNSCC being the most common histologic subtype, comprising about half of cases [9,92–94]. Due to the nonspecific nature of initial symptoms, patients often present at a locally advanced stage [9,95,96]. The proximity of these malignancies to critical anatomic structures means treatment carries significant morbidity and poor overall survival [9,10,95–97]. Interest in the role of HPV in SNSCC spans back numerous decades [98]. A wide range of HPV detection rates in SNSCC have been reported, varying from 0 to 100% [8,10,20,38,44,54,67,69,99]. Major barriers to progress in defining the role of HPV in SNSCC include: (1) the relative rarity of SNSCC and thus published literature often utilizing small, single institution cohorts, (2) the use of disparate HPV detection techniques with significant variation in sensitivity and specificity for HPV, (3) few studies using "gold standard" platforms (E6/E7 mRNA detection with ISH or RT PCR) to demonstrate transcriptionally active HPV, ruling out a contamination or "bystander" infection and (4) exclusion of SNSCC from TCGA and a dearth of comprehensive genomic studies examining SNSCC at the DNA and RNA level [86,100–102].

Our systematic literature review revealed only one meta-analysis, using <500 pooled cases, from 35 studies published prior to 2012 [103]. In this study, the authors calculated an overall HPV prevalence rate of 27.0%. In addition to the small sample size, a number of critical limitations exist in applying the findings to our primary endpoints here, including: (1) a focus only on SNSCC arising from papillomas, which are a distinct subgroup of SNSCC and (2) a complete lack of RNA-based or multiple substrate testing studies, which are significantly more likely to approximate a "true" HPV-mediated cancer prevalence rate. Since 2012, significant interest in the role of HPV in SNSCC has led to a notable increase in the available pooled cohort for analysis (69 studies identified out of 747 screened, yielding 1458 cases). Additionally, the number of RNA-based and multi-substrate testing studies, and size of cohorts published have both increased across time, yielding more high quality studies.

Here, we aimed to provide an updated overall point prevalence for HPV detection in SNSCC using a larger and more contemporary cohort, and an estimate of the prevalence of SNSCCs likely to be driven by HPV, using multi-substrate testing as a benchmark, to increase specificity above DNA detection alone. Additionally, we hypothesized that if a subset of SNSCCs is indeed driven by HPV, orthogonal data should support this, including: (1) increased HPV prevalence in sinuses with more exposure to refluxed secretion flow from the oropharynx and (2) higher HPV+ SNSCC prevalence rates in regions of the world with higher HPV+ OPSCC prevalence. Using the random-effects model, we found an overall HPV point prevalence of 26%. When sub-stratified by single- vs. multi-substrate testing, we identified a prevalence of 21% for multi-substrate testing, which we posit should represent a more accurate number for estimating HPV-driven SNSCC from the cohort available here. As expected, prevalence decreased in a stepwise fashion when tests with increasing specificity were applied. Unfortunately, there were no studies using gold-standard RNA-based detection techniques alone, which met inclusion criteria for the study. This highlights the need for additional, large cohort studies using RNA-based detection methods. It should further be noted that while p16 overexpression is a widely recognized surrogate marker for high risk HPV in OPSCC, whether p16 is a sensitive and specific marker for SNSCC has not been well established. In our systematic literature review we found 18 studies using both p16 IHC and DNA- and/or RNA-based HPV testing. However, the majority of the studies were too small to make a statement on the reliability of p16 IHC. Eight studies reported correlations of 69–100% between p16 overexpression and positive HPV status [10,11,19,22,81,84,90,97]. Reported sensitivity for p16 ranged from 88 to 100%

and specificity from 67 to 100% [10,11,19,84,97]. Predictive values were calculated in three studies, all comparing p16 IHC to RNA-based HPV testing [10,84,90]. Positive predictive values ranged from 50 to 94% and negative predictive values ranged from 94 to 100%.

In line with our hypotheses, we found the highest HPV prevalence in sinonasal subsites with the greatest exposure to refluxed secretion flow from the oropharynx and the lowest prevalence in sinuses more remote from routine exposure, i.e., the more anterior, cranial and posterior sinuses, each of which also possess restrictive ostium. High-exposure subsites had HPV prevalence rates more than double low-exposure sites (38% vs. 15%). Interestingly, HPV prevalence rates by subsite mirror reported overall survival rates stratified by subsite with frontal and sphenoid sinuses having the lowest survival and nasal cavity having the highest survival [104,105]. Considering HPV+ OPSCC's improved survival compared to non-HPV OPSCC, in part due to improved responsiveness to current treatment schemas and existing studies suggesting HPV+ SNSCCs have improved survival compared to non-HPV SNSCC, additional studies will be needed to parse out the relationship between sinonasal subsite, HPV status and survival [9].

Additionally, we found considerable variation by geographic region, which aligned with HPV+ OPSCCs rates. For example, overall HPV prevalence was highest in North American studies and lowest in African studies in both OPSCC (using previously published cohorts) and SNSCC, with SNSCC HPV prevalence rates in both cohorts being approximately 50% of the OPSCC rate. Remarkably, when restricting to examination of high risk subsites in North American studies (those most likely to be HPV positive), prevalence rates approximate HPV prevalence rates in the oropharynx in some parts of the US (52%). Additional large cohort studies using RNA-based detection techniques are needed to evaluate if these findings remain true, as sample sizes available for these sub-analyses are small.

This study has a number of limitations which relate to the status of exiting literature. First, sample sizes of available studies are small, with 27 of the 60 studies included in the analysis having a sample size of under ten patients (36 of 69 studies, total). Second, there is significant heterogeneity of HPV testing methodologies, each of which have variable sensitivity and specificity. Additionally, the majority of studies (37/69) use DNA testing alone, which may not represent a tumor driven by HPV but instead contamination or a bystander infection. Small sample sizes and heterogeneity of the datasets, as highlighted by the Q and I^2 statistics make definitive conclusions challenging (Table S2). Despite this, findings of this analysis are in line with our pre-existing hypotheses, increasing confidence in our conclusions. Due to the high levels of heterogeneity between datasets and the large number of missing variables needed to accurately perform subgroup analyses, we chose not to evaluate certain factors which are likely to impact true HPV+ SNSCC prevalence rates such as association with papilloma, histologic subtypes and viral genotype [7]. Of note, recent reports have highlighted SNSCCs which arise from inverted papillomas and are associated with low risk HPV types 6/11 [106]. The role, and prevalence, of low risk HPVs in SNSCCs were not evaluated here. Future studies should focus on reporting the results of genotype-specific assays. Lastly, a recently recognized histologic variant of sinonasal cancer is HPV-related multiphenotypic sinonasal carcinoma (HMSC). HMSC is formerly known as HPV-related carcinoma with adenoid cystic-like features and is strongly associated with HPV-33 [107]. HMSC is characterized by mixed phenotypes including squamous differentiation, resembling SNSCC in some cases. While we excluded HMSC from our search, it is possible that our dataset includes HMSC mistaken for SNSCC, particularly in the studies published prior to HMSC's first description in 2012 [108].

5. Conclusions

Here, we provide a new reference point prevalence for HPV in SNSCC, stratified by detection method, along with orthogonal data supporting a causative role for virally driven tumorigenesis in SNSCC. Small sample sizes, high interstudy variability and missing data such as genotype-specific incidence highlight the need for large prospective evaluations of HPV in SNSCC and detailed genomic studies to further clarify the role of HPV in SNSCC.

Supplementary Materials: The following are available online at https://www.mdpi.com/2072-6694/13/1/45/s1, Figure S1: Sample size against year of study publication, Figure S2: Funnel plot, Table S1: Meta regression results, Table S2: Heterogeneity analyses for HPV prevalence subgroups using the fixed-effects model, Methods S1: Complete PubMed Search.

Author Contributions: Conceptualization, D.L.F.; methodology, K.J.W.C.S.P.; software, K.J.W.C.S.P., S.R.R.; validation, D.L.F., S.R.R.; formal analysis, K.J.W.C.S.P., S.R.R.; investigation, K.J.W.C.S.P., T.M.; resources, L.C.; data curation, K.J.W.C.S.P., T.M.; writing—original draft preparation, D.L.F., K.J.W.C.S.P.; writing—review and editing, D.L.F., K.J.W.C.S.P., S.R.R.; visualization, K.J.W.C.S.P.; supervision, D.L.F.; project administration, D.L.F.; funding acquisition, D.L.F. All authors have read and agreed to the published version of the manuscript.

Funding: This research received no external funding.

Institutional Review Board Statement: Not applicable.

Informed Consent Statement: Not applicable.

Data Availability Statement: All data generated or analyzed during this study are included in this published article (and its supplementary information files).

Acknowledgments: This study has been supported by the North American Skullbase Society.

Conflicts of Interest: The authors declare no potential conflict of interest. The sponsors had no role in the design, execution, interpretation, or writing of the study.

References

1. Gillison, M.L. Human papillomavirus-associated head and neck cancer is a distinct epidemiologic, clinical, and molecular entity. *Semin. Oncol.* **2004**, *31*, 744–754. [CrossRef]
2. Tumban, E. A Current Update on Human Papillomavirus-Associated Head and Neck Cancers. *Viruses* **2019**, *11*, 922. [CrossRef] [PubMed]
3. Ang, K.K.; Harris, J.; Wheeler, R.; Weber, R.; Rosenthal, D.I.; Nguyen-Tân, P.F.; Westra, W.H.; Chung, C.H.; Jordan, R.C.; Lu, C.; et al. Human Papillomavirus and Survival of Patients with Oropharyngeal Cancer. *N. Engl. J. Med.* **2010**, *363*, 24–35. [CrossRef] [PubMed]
4. Faden, D.L.; Ding, F.; Lin, Y.; Zhai, S.; Kuo, F.; Chan, T.A.; Morris, L.G.; Ferris, R.L. APOBEC mutagenesis is tightly linked to the immune landscape and immunotherapy biomarkers in head and neck squamous cell carcinoma. *Oral Oncol.* **2019**, *96*, 140–147. [CrossRef] [PubMed]
5. Faden, D.L.; Thomas, S.; Cantalupo, P.G.; Agrawal, N.; Myers, J.; DeRisi, J. Multi-modality analysis supports APOBEC as a major source of mutations in head and neck squamous cell carcinoma. *Oral Oncol.* **2017**, *74*, 8–14. [CrossRef] [PubMed]
6. Syrjänen, K.J.; Pyrhönen, S.; Syrjänen, S.M. Evidence suggesting human papillomavirus (HPV) etiology for the squamous cell papilloma of the paranasal sinus. *Arch. Geschwulstforsch.* **1983**, *53*, 77–82.
7. Elgart, K.; Faden, D.L. Sinonasal Squamous Cell Carcinoma: Etiology, Pathogenesis, and the Role of Human Papilloma Virus. *Curr. Otorhinolaryngol. Rep.* **2020**, *8*, 111–119. [CrossRef]
8. Chowdhury, N.; Alvi, S.A.; Kimura, K.; Tawfik, O.; Manna, P.; Beahm, D.; Robinson, A.; Kerley, S.; Hoover, L. Outcomes of HPV-related nasal squamous cell carcinoma. *Laryngoscope* **2017**, *127*, 1600–1603. [CrossRef]
9. Kılıç, S.S.; Ma, S.S.K.; Kim, E.S.; Baredes, S.; Mahmoud, O.; Gray, S.T.; Eloy, J.A. Significance of human papillomavirus positivity in sinonasal squamous cell carcinoma. *Int. Forum Allergy Rhinol.* **2017**, *7*, 980–989. [CrossRef]
10. Jiromaru, R.; Yamamoto, H.; Yasumatsu, R.; Hongo, T.; Nozaki, Y.; Hashimoto, K.; Taguchi, K.; Masuda, M.; Nakagawa, T.; Oda, Y. HPV-related Sinonasal Carcinoma: Clinicopathologic Features, Diagnostic Utility of p16 and Rb Immunohistochemistry, and: EGFR: Copy Number Alteration. *Am. J. Surg. Pathol.* **2019**. Publish Ahead of Print. [CrossRef]
11. Alos, L.L.; Moyano, S.; Nadal, A.; Alobid, I.; Blanch, J.L.; Ayala, E.; Lloveras, B.; Quint, W.; Cardesa, A.; Ordi, J. Human papillomaviruses are identified in a subgroup of sinonasal squamous cell carcinomas with favorable outcome. *Cancer* **2009**, *115*, 2701–2709. [CrossRef] [PubMed]
12. Moher, D.; Liberati, A.; Tetzlaff, J.; Altman, D.G. Preferred Reporting Items for Systematic Reviews and Meta-Analyses: The PRISMA Statement. *Ann. Intern. Med.* **2009**, *151*, 264–269. [CrossRef] [PubMed]
13. Deeks, J.; Higgins, J.; Altman, D. Chapter 10: Analysing data and undertaking meta-analyses. In *Cochrane Handbook for Systematic Reviews of Interventions Version 6.0 (Updated July 2019)*; Higgins, J.P.T., Chandler, J., Cumpston, M., Li, T., Page, M.J., Welch, V.A., Eds.; Cochrane: London, UK, 2019.
14. Cochran, W.G. The Combination of Estimates from Different Experiments. *Biometrics* **1954**, *10*, 101–129. [CrossRef]

15. Egger, M.; Smith, G.D.; Schneider, M.; Minder, C. Bias in meta-analysis detected by a simple, graphical test. *BMJ* **1997**, *315*, 629–634. [CrossRef] [PubMed]
16. Begg, C.B.; Mazumdar, M. Operating characteristics of a rank correlation test for publication bias. *Biometrics* **1994**, *50*, 1088–1101. [CrossRef] [PubMed]
17. Duval, S.; Tweedie, R. A Nonparametric "Trim and Fill" Method of Accounting for Publication Bias in Meta-Analysis. *J. Am. Stat. Assoc.* **2000**, *95*, 89–98.
18. Syrjänen, S.; Happonen, R.-P.; Virolainen, E.; Siivonen, L.; Syrjänen, K. Detection of human papillomavirus (HPV) structural antigens and DNA types in inverted papillomas and squamous cell carcinomas of the nasal cavities and paranasal sinuses. *Acta Oto-Laryngol.* **1987**, *104*, 334–341. [CrossRef]
19. Klemi, P.J.; Joensuu, H.; Siivonen, L.; Virolainen, E.; Syrjänen, S.; Syrjänen, K. Association of DNA Aneuploidy with Human Papillomavirus-Induced Malignant Transformation of Sinonasal Transitional Papillomas. *Otolaryngol. Neck Surg.* **1989**, *100*, 563–567. [CrossRef]
20. Siivonen, L.; Virolainen, E. Transitional Papilloma of the Nasal Cavity and Paranasal Sinuses. *ORL* **1989**, *51*, 262–267. [CrossRef]
21. Ishibashi, T.; Matsushima, S.; Tsunokawa, Y.; Asai, M.; Nomura, Y.; Sugimura, T.; Terada, M. Human Papillomavirus DNA in Squamous Cell Carcinoma of the Upper Aerodigestive Tract. *Arch. Otolaryngol. Head Neck Surg.* **1990**, *116*, 294–298. [CrossRef]
22. Furuta, Y.; Shinohara, T.; Sano, K.; Nagashima, K.; Inoue, K.; Tanaka, K.; Inuyama, Y. Molecular Pathologic Study of Human Papillomavirus Infection in Inverted Papilloma and Squamous Cell Carcinoma of the Nasal Cavities and Paranasal Sinuses. *Laryngoscope* **1991**, *101*, 79–85. [CrossRef] [PubMed]
23. Judd, R.; Zaki, S.R.; Coffield, L.M.; Evatt, B.L. Human papillomavirus type 6 detected by the polymerase chain reaction in invasive sinonasal papillary squamous cell carcinoma. *Arch. Pathol. Lab. Med.* **1991**, *115*, 1150–1153. [PubMed]
24. Furuta, Y.; Takasu, T.; Asai, T.; Shinohara, T.; Sawa, H.; Nagashima, K.; Inuyama, Y. Detection of human papillomavirus DNA in carcinomas of the nasal cavities and paranasal sinuses by polymerase chain reaction. *Cancer* **1992**, *69*, 353–357. [CrossRef]
25. McLachlin, C.M.; A Kandel, R.; Colgan, T.J.; Swanson, D.B.; Witterick, I.J.; Ngan, B.Y. Prevalence of human papillomavirus in sinonasal papillomas: A study using polymerase chain reaction and in situ hybridization. *Mod. Pathol.* **1992**, *5*, 406–409. [PubMed]
26. Tyan, Y.S.; Liu, S.T.; Ong, W.R.; Chen, M.L.; Shu, C.H.; Chang, Y.S. Detection of Epstein-Barr virus and human papillomavirus in head and neck tumors. *J. Clin. Microbiol.* **1993**, *31*, 53–56. [CrossRef] [PubMed]
27. Wu, T.C.; Trujillo, J.M.; Kashima, H.K.; Mounts, P. Association of human papillomavirus with nasal neoplasia. *Lancet* **1993**, *341*, 522–524. [CrossRef]
28. Arndt, O.; Nottelmann, K.; Brock, J.; Neumann, O.G. Inverted papilloma and its association with human papillomavirus (HPV). A study with polymerase chain reaction (PCR). *HNO* **1994**, *42*, 670–676.
29. Beck, J.C.; McCLATCHEY, K.D.; Lesperance, M.M.; Esclamado, R.M.; Carey, T.E.; Bradford, C.R. Presence of Human papillomavirus types important in progression of inverted papilloma. *Otolaryngol. Head Neck Surg.* **1995**, *113*, 558–563.
30. Buchwald, C.; Franzmann, M.-B.; Jacobsen, G.K.; Lindeberg, H. Human papillomavirus (HPV) in sinonasal papillomas: A study of 78 cases using in situ hybridization and polymerase chain reaction. *Laryngoscope* **1995**, *105*, 66–71. [CrossRef]
31. Shen, J.; E Tate, J.; Crum, C.P.; Goodman, M.L. Prevalence of human papillomaviruses (HPV) in benign and malignant tumors of the upper respiratory tract. *Mod. Pathol.* **1996**, *9*, 15–20.
32. Bernauer, H.S.; Welkoborsky, H.-J.; Tilling, A.; Amedee, R.G.; Mann, W.J. Inverted Papillomas of the Paranasal Sinuses and the Nasal Cavity: DNA Indices and HPV Infection. *Am. J. Rhinol.* **1997**, *11*, 155–160. [CrossRef] [PubMed]
33. Caruana, S.M.; Zwiebel, N.; Cocker, R.; A McCormick, S.; Eberle, R.C.; Lazarus, P. p53 alteration and human papilloma virus infection in paranasal sinus cancer. *Cancer* **1997**, *79*, 1320–1328. [CrossRef]
34. Mineta, H.; Ogino, T.; Amano, H.M.; Ohkawa, Y.; Araki, K.; Takebayashi, S.; Miura, K. Human papilloma virus (HPV) type 16 and 18 detected in head and neck squamous cell carcinoma. *Anticancer. Res.* **1999**, *18*, 4765–4768.
35. Saegusa, M.; Nitta, H.; Hashimura, M.; Okayasu, I. Down-regulation of p27Kip1 expression is correlated with increased cell proliferation but not expression of p21waf1 and p53, and human papillomavirus infection in benign and malignant tumours of sinonasal regions. *Histopathology* **1999**, *35*, 55–64. [CrossRef]
36. Buchwald, C.; Lindeberg, H.; Pedersen, B.L.; Franzmann, M.B. Human Papilloma Virus and p53 Expression in Carcinomas Associated With Sinonasal Papillomas: A Danish Epidemiological Study 1980–1998. *Laryngoscope* **2001**, *111*, 1104–1110. [CrossRef]
37. Schwerer, M.J.; Sailer, A.; Kraft, K.; Baczako, K.; Maier, H. Patterns of p21waf1/cip1 expression in non-papillomatous nasal mucosa, endophytic sinonasal papillomas, and associated carcinomas. *J. Clin. Pathol.* **2001**, *54*, 871–876. [CrossRef]
38. Fischer, M.; Von Winterfeld, F. Evaluation and application of a broad-spectrum polymerase chain reaction assay for human papillomaviruses in the screening of squamous cell tumours of the head and neck. *Acta Oto-Laryngologica* **2003**, *123*, 752–758. [CrossRef]
39. Schwerer, M.J.; Sailer, A.; Kraft, K.; Baczako, K.; Maier, H. Expression of retinoblastoma gene product in respiratory epithelium and sinonasal neoplasms: Relationship with p16 and cyclin D1 expression. *Histol. Histopathol.* **2003**, *18*, 143–151.
40. El-Mofty, S.K.; Lu, D.W. Prevalence of High-Risk Human Papillomavirus DNA in Nonkeratinizing (Cylindrical Cell) Carcinoma of the Sinonasal Tract: A Distinct Clinicopathologic and Molecular Disease Entity. *Am. J. Surg. Pathol.* **2005**, *29*, 1367–1372. [CrossRef]
41. Katori, H.; Nozawa, A.; Tsukuda, M. Markers of malignant transformation of sinonasal inverted papilloma. *Eur. J. Surg. Oncol.* **2005**, *31*, 905–911. [CrossRef]
42. McKay, S.P.; Grégoire, L.; Lonardo, F.; Reidy, P.; Mathog, R.H.; Lancaster, W.D. Human Papillomavirus (HPV) Transcripts in Malignant Inverted Papilloma are from Integrated HPV DNA. *Laryngoscope* **2005**, *115*, 1428–1431. [CrossRef] [PubMed]

43. Hoffmann, M.; Klose, N.; Gottschlich, S.; Görögh, T.; Fazel, A.; Lohrey, C.; Rittgen, W.; Ambrosch, P.; Schwarz, E.; Kahn, T. Detection of human papillomavirus DNA in benign and malignant sinonasal neoplasms. *Cancer Lett.* **2006**, *239*, 64–70. [CrossRef] [PubMed]
44. Kim, J.-Y.; Yoon, J.-K.; Citardi, M.J.; Batra, P.S.; Roh, H.-J. The Prevalence of Human Papilloma virus Infection in Sinonasal Inverted Papilloma Specimens Classified by Histological Grade. *Am. J. Rhinol.* **2007**, *21*, 664–669. [CrossRef] [PubMed]
45. Jo, V.Y.; Mills, S.E.; Stoler, M.H.; Stelow, E.B. Papillary Squamous Cell Carcinoma of the Head and Neck: Frequent Association With Human Papillomavirus Infection and Invasive Carcinoma. *Am. J. Surg. Pathol.* **2009**, *33*, 1720–1724. [CrossRef]
46. Cheung, F.M.; Lau, T.W.; Cheung, L.K.; Li, A.S.; Chow, S.K.; Lo, A.W. Schneiderian Papillomas and Carcinomas: A Retrospective Study with Special Reference to p53 and p16 tumor suppressor gene expression and association with HPV. *Ear Nose Throat J.* **2010**, *89*, E5–E12. [CrossRef]
47. But-Hadzic, J.; Jenko, K.; Poljak, M.; Kocjan, B.J.; Gale, N.; Strojan, P. Sinonasal inverted papilloma associated with squamous cell carcinoma. *Radiol. Oncol.* **2011**, *45*, 267. [CrossRef]
48. Jenko, K.; Kocjan, B.J.; Zidar, N.; Poljak, M.; Strojan, P.; Žargi, M.; Blatnik, O.; Gale, N. In Inverted Papillomas HPV more likely represents incidental colonization than an etiological factor. *Virchows Archiv* **2011**, *459*, 529. [CrossRef]
49. Kim, S.-G.; Lee, O.-Y.; Choi, J.W.; Park, Y.-H.; Kim, Y.M.; Yeo, M.-K.; Kim, J.M.; Rha, K.-S. Pattern of Expression of Cell Cycle–related Proteins in Malignant Transformation of Sinonasal Inverted Papilloma. *Am. J. Rhinol. Allergy* **2011**, *25*, 75–81. [CrossRef]
50. Bishop, J.A.; Ma, X.-J.; Wang, H.; Luo, Y.; Illei, P.B.; Begum, S.; Taube, J.M.; Koch, W.M.; Westra, W.H. Detection of Transcriptionally Active High-risk HPV in Patients With Head and Neck Squamous Cell Carcinoma as Visualized by a Novel E6/E7 mRNA In Situ Hybridization Method. *Am. J. Surg. Pathol.* **2012**, *36*, 1874–1882. [CrossRef]
51. Doxtader, E.E.; Katzenstein, A.-L.A. The relationship between p16 expression and high-risk human papillomavirus infection in squamous cell carcinomas from sites other than uterine cervix: A study of 137 cases. *Hum. Pathol.* **2012**, *43*, 327–332. [CrossRef]
52. Bishop, J.A.; Guo, T.W.; Smith, D.F.; Wang, H.; Ogawa, T.; Pai, S.I.; Westra, W.H. Human Papillomavirus-related Carcinomas of the Sinonasal Tract. *Am. J. Surg. Pathol.* **2013**, *37*, 185–192. [CrossRef] [PubMed]
53. Deng, Z.; Hasegawa, M.; Kiyuna, A.; Matayoshi, S.; Uehara, T.; Agena, S.; Yamashita, Y.; Ogawa, K.; Maeda, H.; Suzuki, M. Viral load, physical status, andE6/E7mRNA expression of human papillomavirus in head and neck squamous cell carcinoma. *Head Neck* **2012**, *35*, 800–808. [CrossRef] [PubMed]
54. Larque, A.B.; Hakim, S.; Ordi, J.; Nadal, A.; Diaz, A.; Del Pino, M.; Marimon, L.; Alobid, I.; Cardesa, A.; Alos, L. High-risk human papillomavirus is transcriptionally active in a subset of sinonasal squamous cell carcinomas. *Mod. Pathol.* **2013**, *27*, 343–351. [CrossRef] [PubMed]
55. Takahashi, Y.; Bell, D.; Agarwal, G.; Roberts, D.; Xie, T.-X.; El-Naggar, A.; Myers, J.N.; Hanna, E.Y. Comprehensive assessment of prognostic markers for sinonasal squamous cell carcinoma. *Head Neck* **2014**, *36*, 1094–1102. [CrossRef]
56. Doescher, J.; Piontek, G.; Wirth, M.; Bettstetter, M.; Schlegel, J.; Haller, B.; Brockhoff, G.; Reiter, R.; Pickhard, A.C. Epstein-Barr virus infection is strictly associated with the metastatic spread of sinonasal squamous-cell carcinomas. *Oral Oncol.* **2015**, *51*, 929–934. [CrossRef]
57. Laco, J.; Sieglová, K.; Vošmiková, H.; Dundr, P.; Němejcová, K.; Michálek, J.; Čelakovský, P.; Chrobok, V.; Mottl, R.; Mottlová, A.; et al. The presence of high-risk human papillomavirus (HPV) E6/E7 mRNA transcripts in a subset of sinonasal carcinomas is evidence of involvement of HPV in its etiopathogenesis. *Virchows Archiv* **2015**, *467*, 405–415. [CrossRef]
58. Yamashita, Y.; Hasegawa, M.; Deng, Z.; Maeda, H.; Kondo, S.; Kyuna, A.; Matayoshi, S.; Agena, S.; Uehara, T.; Kouzaki, H.; et al. Human papillomavirus infection and immunohistochemical expression of cell cycle proteins pRb, p53, and p16INK4a in sinonasal diseases. *Infect. Agents Cancer* **2015**, *10*, 23. [CrossRef]
59. Ambreen, B.; Reyaz, T.A.; Sheikh, J.; Imtiyaz, H.; Summyia, F.; Ruby, R. Histopathological study of lesions of nose and paranasal sinuses and association of Human Papilloma Virus (HPV) with sinonasal papillomas and squamous cell carcinoma. *Int. J. Med. Res. Health Sci.* **2016**, *5*, 7–16.
60. Becker, C.; Kayser, G.; Pfeiffer, J. Squamous cell cancer of the nasal cavity: New insights and implications for diagnosis and treatment. *Head Neck* **2016**, *38*, E2112–E2117. [CrossRef]
61. Liu, J.; Li, X.; Zhang, Y.; Xing, L.; Liu, H.G. Human papillomavirus-related squamous cell carcinomas of the oropharynx and sinonasal tract in 156 Chinese patients. *Int. J. Clin. Exp. Pathol.* **2016**, *9*, 1839–1848.
62. Oga, E.A.; Schumaker, L.M.; Alabi, B.S.; Obaseki, D.; Umana, A.; Bassey, I.-A.; Ebughe, G.; Oluwole, O.; Akeredolu, T.; Adebamowo, S.N.; et al. Paucity of HPV-Related Head and Neck Cancers (HNC) in Nigeria. *PLoS ONE* **2016**, *11*, e0152828. [CrossRef] [PubMed]
63. Paul, M.; Ray, S.; Sengupta, M.; Sengupta, A. Spectrum of Sinonasal Lesions with Expression of p16 and Ki-67 in Premalignant Lesions and Squamous Cell Carcinomas. *J. Clin. Diagn. Res.* **2017**, *11*, EC05–EC08. [CrossRef]
64. Rooper, L.M.; Bishop, J.A.; Westra, W.H. Transcriptionally Active High-Risk Human Papillomavirus is Not a Common Etiologic Agent in the Malignant Transformation of Inverted Schneiderian Papillomas. *Head Neck Pathol.* **2017**, *11*, 346–353. [CrossRef] [PubMed]
65. Beigh, A.; Rashi, R.; Junaid, S.; Khuroo, M.S.; Farook, S. Human Papilloma Virus (HPV) in Sinonasal Papillomas and Squamous Cell Carcinomas: A PCR-based Study of 60 cases. *Gulf J. Oncol.* **2018**, *1*, 37–42.

66. Owusu-Afriyie, O.; Owiredu, W.K.B.A.; Owusu-Danquah, K.; Larsen-Reindorf, R.; Donkor, P.; Acheampong, E.; Quayson, S.E. Expression of immunohistochemical markers in non-oropharyngeal head and neck squamous cell carcinoma in Ghana. *PLoS ONE* **2018**, *13*, e0202790.
67. Udager, A.M.; McHugh, J.; Goudsmit, C.; Weigelin, H.; Lim, M.; Elenitoba-Johnson, K.; Betz, B.; Carey, T.; Brown, N. Human papillomavirus (HPV) and somatic EGFR mutations are essential, mutually exclusive oncogenic mechanisms for inverted sinonasal papillomas and associated sinonasal squamous cell carcinomas. *Ann. Oncol.* **2018**, *29*, 466–471. [CrossRef]
68. Kim, T.; Jung, S.-H.; Kim, S.-K.; Kwon, H.J. P16 expression and its association with PD-L1 expression and FOXP3-positive tumor infiltrating lymphocytes in head and neck squamous cell carcinoma. *Mol. Cell. Toxicol.* **2019**, *15*, 137–143. [CrossRef]
69. Quan, H.; Yan, L.; Wang, S.; Wang, S.Z. Clinical relevance and significance of programmed death-ligand 1 expression, tumor-infiltrating lymphocytes, and p16 status in sinonasal squamous cell carcinoma. *Cancer Manag. Res.* **2019**, *11*, 4335–4345. [CrossRef]
70. Sahnane, N.; Ottini, G.; Turri-Zanoni, M.; Furlan, D.; Battaglia, P.; Karligkiotis, A.; Albeni, C.; Cerutti, R.; Mura, E.; Chiaravalli, A.M.; et al. Comprehensive analysis of HPV infection, EGFR exon 20 mutations and LINE1 hypomethylation as risk factors for malignant transformation of sinonasal-inverted papilloma to squamous cell carcinoma. *Int. J. Cancer* **2019**, *144*, 1313–1320. [CrossRef]
71. Bulane, A.; Goedhals, D.; Seedat, R.Y.; Goedhals, J.; Burt, F. Human papillomavirus DNA in head and neck squamous cell carcinomas in the Free State, South Africa. *J. Med Virol.* **2020**, *92*, 227–233. [CrossRef]
72. Cabal, V.; Menendez, M.; Vivanco, B.; Potes-Ares, S.; Riobello, C.; Suarez-Fernandez, L.; Garcia-Marin, R.; Blanco-Lorenzo, V.; Lopez, F.; Alvarez-Marcos, C.; et al. EGFR mutation and HPV infection in sinonasal inverted papilloma and squamous cell carcinoma. *Rhinology* **2020**, *58*, 368–376. [CrossRef] [PubMed]
73. Cohen, E.; Bs, C.C.; Menaker, S.; Martinez-Duarte, E.; Gomez, C.; Lo, K.; Kerr, D.; Franzmann, E.; Leibowitz, J.; Sargi, Z. P16 and human papillomavirus in sinonasal squamous cell carcinoma. *Head Neck* **2020**, *42*, 2021–2029. [CrossRef] [PubMed]
74. Brandwein, M.; Steinberg, B.; Thung, S.; Biller, H.; Dilorenzo, T.; Galli, R. Human papillomavirus 6/11 and 16/18 in Schneiderian inverted papillomas. In situ hybridization with human papillomavirus RNA probes. *Cancer* **1989**, *63*, 1708–1713. [CrossRef]
75. Bradford, C.R.; Zacks, S.E.; Androphy, E.J.; Gregoire, L.; Lancaster, W.D.; Carey, T.E. Human Papillomavirus DNA Sequences in Cell Lines Derived from Head and Neck Squamous Cell Carcinomas. *Otolaryngol. Neck Surg.* **1991**, *104*, 303–310. [CrossRef]
76. Gaffey, M.J.; Frierson, J.H.F.; Weiss, L.M.; Barber, M.C.M.; Baber, B.G.B.; Stoler, M.H. Human Papillomavirus and Epstein-Barr Virus in Sinonasal Schneiderian Papillomas:An In Situ Hybridization and Polymerase Chain Reaction Study. *Am. J. Clin. Pathol.* **1996**, *106*, 475–482. [CrossRef]
77. Miguel, R.E.V.; Villa, L.L.; Cordeiro, A.C.; Prado, J.C.M.; Sobrinho, J.S.P.; Kowalski, L.P. Low prevalence of human papillomavirus in a geographic region with a high incidence of head and neck cancer. *Am. J. Surg.* **1998**, *176*, 428–429. [CrossRef]
78. Badaracco, G.; Rizzo, C.; Mafera, B.; Pichi, B.; Giannarelli, D.; Rahimi, S.; Vigili, M.G.; Venuti, A. Molecular analyses and prognostic relevance of HPV in head and neck tumours. *Oncol. Rep.* **2007**, *17*, 931–939. [CrossRef]
79. Mirza, N.; Montone, K.; Sato, Y.; Kroger, H.; Kennedy, D.W. Identification of p53 and Human Papilloma Virus in Schneiderian Papillomas. *Laryngoscope* **1998**, *108*, 497–501. [CrossRef]
80. McLemore, M.S.; Haigentz, M., Jr.; Smith, R.V.; Nuovo, G.J.; Alos, L.; Cardesa, A.; Brandwein-Gensler, M. Head and Neck Squamous Cell Carcinomas in HIV-Positive Patients: A Preliminary Investigation of Viral Associations. *Head Neck Pathol.* **2010**, *4*, 97–105. [CrossRef]
81. Singhi, A.D.; Westra, W.H. Comparison of human papillomavirus in situ hybridization and p16 immunohistochemistry in the detection of human papillomavirus-associated head and neck cancer based on a prospective clinical experience. *Cancer* **2010**, *116*, 2166–2173. [CrossRef]
82. El-Salem, F.; Mansour, M.; Gitman, M.; Miles, B.; Posner, M.; Bakst, R.; Genden, E.; Westra, W. Real-time PCR HPV genotyping in fine needle aspirations of metastatic head and neck squamous cell carcinoma: Exposing the limitations of conventional p16 immunostaining. *Oral Oncol.* **2019**, *90*, 74–79. [CrossRef] [PubMed]
83. Ba, J.R.O.; Lieberman, S.M.; Tam, M.M.; Liu, C.Z.; Oliver, J.R.; Hu, K.S.; Morris, L.G.T.; Givi, B. Human papillomavirus and survival of patients with sinonasal squamous cell carcinoma. *Cancer* **2020**, *126*, 1413–1423.
84. Jalouli, J.; Ibrahim, S.O.; Sapkota, D.; Jalouli, M.M.; Vasstrand, E.N.; Hirsch, J.-M.; Larsson, P.-A. Presence of human papilloma virus, herpes simplex virus and Epstein-Barr virus DNA in oral biopsies from Sudanese patients with regard to toombak use. *J. Oral Pathol. Med.* **2010**, *39*, 599–604. [CrossRef] [PubMed]
85. Jalouli, J.; Jalouli, M.M.; Sapkota, D.; O Ibrahim, S.; Larsson, P.-A.; Sand, L. Human papilloma virus, herpes simplex virus and epstein barr virus in oral squamous cell carcinoma from eight different countries. *Anticancer. Res.* **2012**, *32*, 571–580.
86. Ndiaye, C.; Mena, M.; Alemany, L.; Arbyn, M.; Castellsagué, X.; Laporte, L.; Bosch, F.; De Sanjosé, S.; Trottier, H. HPV DNA, E6/E7 mRNA, and p16INK4a detection in head and neck cancers: A systematic review and meta-analysis. *Lancet Oncol.* **2014**, *15*, 1319–1331. [CrossRef]
87. Amin, M.B.; Edge, S.B. *American Joint Committee on C: AJCC Cancer Staging Manual*; Springer International Publishing: New York, NY, USA, 2017.
88. Faden, D.L.; Arron, S.T.; Heaton, C.M.; DeRisi, J.L.; South, A.P.; Wang, S.J. Targeted next-generation sequencing of TP53 in oral tongue carcinoma from non-smokers. *J. Otolaryngol. Head Neck Surg.* **2016**, *45*, 47. [CrossRef]
89. Li, R.; Faden, D.L.; Fakhry, C.; Langelier, C.; Jiao, Y.; Wang, Y.; Wilkerson, M.D.; Pedamallu, C.S.; Old, M.; Lang, J.; et al. Clinical, genomic, and metagenomic characterization of oral tongue squamous cell carcinoma in patients who do not smoke. *Head Neck* **2014**, *37*, 1642–1649. [CrossRef]

90. Pickering, C.R.; Zhang, J.; Neskey, D.M.; Zhao, M.; Jasser, S.A.; Wang, J.; Ward, A.; Tsai, C.J.; Alves, M.V.O.; Zhou, J.H.; et al. Squamous Cell Carcinoma of the Oral Tongue in Young Non-Smokers Is Genomically Similar to Tumors in Older Smokers. *Clin. Cancer Res.* **2014**, *20*, 3842–3848. [CrossRef]
91. TCGA. Comprehensive genomic characterization of head and neck squamous cell carcinomas. *Nature* **2015**, *517*, 576–582. [CrossRef]
92. Turner, J.H.; Reh, D.D. Incidence and survival in patients with sinonasal cancer: A historical analysis of population-based data. *Head Neck* **2012**, *34*, 877–885. [CrossRef]
93. Arnold, A.; Ziglinas, P.; Ochs, K.; Alter, N.; Geretschläger, A.; Lädrach, K.; Zbären, P.; Caversaccio, M. Therapy options and long-term results of sinonasal malignancies. *Oral Oncol.* **2012**, *48*, 1031–1037. [CrossRef] [PubMed]
94. Sanghvi, S.; Khan, M.N.; Patel, N.R.; Bs, S.Y.; Baredes, S.; Eloy, J.A. Epidemiology of sinonasal squamous cell carcinoma: A comprehensive analysis of 4994 patients. *Laryngoscope* **2014**, *124*, 76–83. [CrossRef] [PubMed]
95. Youlden, D.R.; Cramb, S.; Peters, N.; Porceddu, S.V.; Moller, H.; Fritschi, L.; Baade, P.D. International comparisons of the incidence and mortality of sinonasal cancer. *Cancer Epidemiol.* **2013**, *37*, 770–779. [CrossRef] [PubMed]
96. Jain, S.; Li, Y.; Kuan, E.C.; Tajudeen, B.A.; Batra, P.S. Prognostic Factors in Paranasal Sinus Squamous Cell Carcinoma and Adenocarcinoma: A SEER Database Analysis. *J. Neurol. Surg. Part B Skull Base* **2019**, *80*, 258–263. [CrossRef] [PubMed]
97. Hoppe, B.S.; Stegman, L.D.; Zelefsky, M.J.; Rosenzweig, K.E.; Wolden, S.L.; Patel, S.G.; Shah, J.P.; Kraus, D.H.; Lee, N. Treatment of nasal cavity and paranasal sinus cancer with modern radiotherapy techniques in the postoperative setting—the MSKCC experience. *Int. J. Radiat. Oncol.* **2007**, *67*, 691–702. [CrossRef]
98. Syrjänen, K.J.; Pyrhönen, S.; Syrjänen, S.M.; A Lamberg, M. Immunohistochemical demonstration of human papilloma virus (HPV) antigens in oral squamous cell lesions. *Br. J. Oral Surg.* **1983**, *21*, 147–153. [CrossRef]
99. Chung, C.H.; Guthrie, V.B.; Masica, D.L.; Tokheim, C.; Kang, H.; Richmon, J.; Agrawal, N.; Fakhry, C.; Quon, H.; Subramaniam, R.M.; et al. Genomic alterations in head and neck squamous cell carcinoma determined by cancer gene-targeted sequencing. *Ann. Oncol.* **2015**, *26*, 1216–1223. [CrossRef]
100. Randén-Brady, R.; Carpén, T.; Jouhi, L.; Syrjänen, S.; Haglund, C.; Tarkkanen, J.; Remes, S.; Mäkitie, A.; Mattila, P.S.; Silén, S.; et al. In situ hybridization for high-risk HPV E6/E7 mRNA is a superior method for detecting transcriptionally active HPV in oropharyngeal cancer. *Hum. Pathol.* **2019**, *90*, 97–105. [CrossRef]
101. Gao, G.; Chernock, R.D.; Gay, H.A.; Thorstad, W.L.; Zhang, T.R.; Wang, H.; Ma, X.-J.; Luo, Y.; Lewis, J.S., Jr.; Wang, X. A novel RT-PCR method for quantification of human papillomavirus transcripts in archived tissues and its application in oropharyngeal cancer prognosis. *Int. J. Cancer* **2012**, *132*, 882–890. [CrossRef]
102. Mills, A.M.; Dirks, D.C.; Poulter, M.D.; Mills, S.E.; Stoler, M.H. HR-HPV E6/E7 mRNA In Situ Hybridization: Validation Against PCR, DNA In Situ Hybridization, and p16 Immunohistochemistry in 102 Samples of Cervical, Vulvar, Anal, and Head and Neck Neoplasia. *Am. J. Surg. Pathol.* **2017**, *41*, 607–615. [CrossRef]
103. Syrjänen, K.; Syrjänen, S. Detection of human papillomavirus in sinonasal carcinoma: Systematic review and meta-analysis. *Hum. Pathol.* **2013**, *44*, 983–991. [CrossRef] [PubMed]
104. Dutta, R.; Ba, P.M.D.; Svider, P.F.; Liu, J.K.; Baredes, S.; Eloy, J.A. Sinonasal malignancies: A population-based analysis of site-specific incidence and survival. *Laryngoscope* **2015**, *125*, 2491–2497. [CrossRef] [PubMed]
105. Robin, T.P.; Jones, B.L.; Ba, O.M.G.; Phan, A.; Abbott, D.; McDermott, J.D.; Goddard, J.A.; Raben, D.; Lanning, R.M.; Karam, S.D. A comprehensive comparative analysis of treatment modalities for sinonasal malignancies. *Cancer* **2017**, *123*, 3040–3049. [CrossRef] [PubMed]
106. Mehrad, M.; Stelow, E.B.; Bishop, J.A.; Wang, X.; Haynes, W.; Oliver, D.; Chernock, R.D.; Lewis, J.S. Transcriptionally Active HPV and Targetable EGFR Mutations in Sinonasal Inverted Papilloma: An Association Between Low-risk HPV, Condylomatous Morphology, and Cancer Risk? *Am. J. Surg Pathol.* **2020**, *44*, 340–346. [CrossRef]
107. Thompson, L.D.R. HPV-Related Multiphenotypic Sinonasal Carcinoma. *Ear Nose Throat J.* **2020**, *99*, 94–95. [CrossRef]
108. Bishop, J.A.; Andreasen, S.; Hang, J.F.; Bullock, M.J.; Chen, T.Y.; Franchi, A.; Garcia, J.J.; Gnepp, D.R.; Gomez-Fernandez, C.R.; Ihrler, S.; et al. HPV-related Multiphenotypic Sinonasal Carcinoma: An Expanded Series of 49 Cases of the Tumor Formerly Known as HPV-related Carcinoma With Adenoid Cystic Carcinoma-like Features. *Am. J. Surg. Pathol.* **2017**, *41*, 1690–1701. [CrossRef]

Article

Role of Human Papillomavirus Infection in Head and Neck Cancer in Italy: The HPV-AHEAD Study

Marta Tagliabue [1,†], Marisa Mena [2,3,†], Fausto Maffini [4,†], Tarik Gheit [5,†], Beatriz Quirós Blasco [2,3], Dana Holzinger [6], Sara Tous [2,3], Daniele Scelsi [1], Debora Riva [1], Enrica Grosso [1], Francesco Chu [1], Eric Lucas [5], Ruediger Ridder [7,8], Susanne Rrehm [7], Johannes Paul Bogers [9], Daniela Lepanto [4], Belén Lloveras Rubio [10], Rekha Vijay Kumar [11], Nitin Gangane [12], Omar Clavero [2,3], Michael Pawlita [6], Devasena Anantharaman [13], Madhavan Radhakrishna Pillai [13], Paul Brennan [14], Rengaswamy Sankaranarayanan [15], Marc Arbyn [16], Francesca Lombardi [17], Miren Taberna [18], Sara Gandini [19], Fausto Chiesa [1], Mohssen Ansarin [1,‡], Laia Alemany [2,3,‡], Massimo Tommasino [5,*,‡], Susanna Chiocca [19,*,‡,§] and The HPV-AHEAD Study Group ∥

1. Division of Otolaryngology and Head and Neck Surgery, IEO, European Institute of Oncology IRCCS, 20141 Milan, Italy; marta.tagliabue@ieo.it (M.T.); daniele.scelsi@gmail.com (D.S.); deborariva88@gmail.com (D.R.); enrica.grosso@ieo.it (E.G.); francesco.chu@ieo.it (F.C.); faustochiesa@gmail.com (F.C.); mohssen.ansarin@ieo.it (M.A.)
2. Cancer Epidemiology Research Program, Catalan Institute of Oncology-Bellvitge Biomedical Research Institute (ICO-IDIBELL), L'Hospitalet de Llobregat, 08908 Barcenola, Spain; mmena.iconcologia@gmail.com (M.M.); bquiros@iconcologia.net (B.Q.B.); stous@iconcologia.net (S.T.); oclavero@iconcologia.net (O.C.); lalemany@iconcologia.net (L.A.)
3. Centro de Investigación Biomédica en Red: Epidemiología y Salud Pública (CIBERESP), Instituto de Salud Carlos III, 28029 Madrid, Spain
4. Division of Pathology, IEO, European Institute of Oncology IRCCS, 20141 Milan, Italy; fausto.maffini@ieo.it (F.M.); daniela.lepanto@ieo.it (D.L.)
5. Infections and Cancer Biology Group, International Agency for Research on Cancer (IARC), 69372 Lyon, France; ghett@iarc.fr (T.G.); LucasE@iarc.fr (E.L.)
6. Deutsches Krebsforschungszentrum (DKFZ), 69120 Heidelberg, Germany; dana.holzinger@gmx.de (D.H.); m.pawlita@dkfz.de (M.P.)
7. Roche mtm laboratories, 69117 Mannheim, Germany; ruediger.ridder@roche.com (R.R.); susanne.rehm@roche.com (S.R.)
8. Ventana Medical Systems Inc./Roche Tissue Diagnostics, Tucson, AZ 85755, USA
9. Laboratory for Cell Biology and Histology, University of Antwerp, 2610 Antwerp, Belgium; john-paul.bogers@uantwerpen.be
10. Hospital del Mar, 08003 Barcelona, Spain; BLloveras@parcdesalutmar.cat
11. Kidwai Memorial Institute of Oncology, Bangalore, Karnataka 560029, India; rekha_v_kumar@yahoo.co.in
12. Mahatma Gandhi Institute of Medical Sciences, Sevagram, Wardha, Maharashtra State 442102, India; nitingangane@gmail.com
13. Rajiv Gandhi Centre for Biotechnology, Poojappura, Thiruvananthapuram, Kerala 695012, India; devasenaa@gmail.com (D.A.); mrpillai@rgcb.res.in (M.R.P.)
14. Section of Genetics, International Agency for Research on Cancer (IARC), 69372 Lyon, France; BrennanP@iarc.fr
15. Research Triangle Institute (RTI) International India, New Delhi 110001, India; sankardr@hotmail.com
16. Unit of Cancer Epidemiology/Belgian Cancer Centre, Sciensano, 1050 Brussels, Belgium; marc.arbyn@sciensano.be
17. Data Management, IEO, European Institute of Oncology IRCCS, 20141 Milan, Italy; francesca.lombardi@ieo.it
18. Medical Oncology Department, Catalan Institute of Oncology (ICO), ONCOBELL, IDIBELL, L'Hospitalet de Llobregat, 08035 Barcelona, Spain; mtaberna@iconcologia.net
19. Department of Experimental Oncology, IEO, European Institute of Oncology IRCCS, 20141 Milan, Italy; sara.gandini@ieo.it
* Correspondence: tommasinom@iarc.fr (M.T.); susanna.chiocca@ieo.it (S.C.)
† Contributed equally as first authors.

‡ Contributed equally as senior authors.
§ Lead author: susanna.chiocca@ieo.it (S.C.).
∥ HPV-AHEAD Study Group: Cindy Simoens, Ivana Gorbaslieva (University of Antwerp, Antwerp, Belgium); Christel Herold-Mende (Departmentof Neurosurgery and Department of Otorhinolaryngology, Head and Neck Surgery, University of Heidelberg, Germany); Gerhard Dyckhoff (Department of Otorhinolaryngology, Head and Neck Surgery, University of Heidelberg, Germany); George Mosialos (Aristotle University of Thessaloniki, Greece); Heiner Boeing (German Institute of Human Nutrition, Berlin, Germany); Xavier Castellsagué (Castellsagué passed away on June 12th, 2016), Silvia de Sanjosé, Francesc Xavier Bosch (Catalan Institute of Oncology—IDIBELL, L'Hospitalet de Llobregat, Spain); Pulikottil Okkuru Esmy (Christian Fellowship Community Health Centre, Ambillikai, India); Rudrapatna S. Jayshree, Kortikere S. Sabitha, Ashok M. Shenoy (Kidwai Memorial Institute of Oncology, Bangalore, India); Manavalan Vijayakumar (YEN ONCO Centre, Yenepoya University, Deralakatte, Mangalore 575018, Karnataka, India); Aruna S. Chiwate, Ranjit V. Thorat, Girish G. Hublikar, Shashikant S. Lakshetti, Bhagwan M. Nene (Nargis Dutt Memorial Cancer Hospital, Barshi 413401, India); Amal Ch Kataki, Ashok Kumar Das (B. Borooah Cancer Institute, Guwahati, Assam, India); Subha Sankaran, Anju Krishnan, Jinu Austin (Rajiv Gandhi Centre for Biotechnology, Thiruvananthapuram, India); Kunnambath Ramadas (Regional Cancer Centre, Thiruvananthapuram, India); Christine Carreira, Sandrine McKay-Chopin (International Agency for Research on Cancer (IARC), Lyon, France), Priya Ramesh Prabhu, Madhavan Radhakrishna Pillai (Rajiv Gandhi Centre for Biotechnology, Poojappura, Thiruvananthapuram 695014, Kerala, India), Thara Somanathan (Regional Cancer Centre, Thiruvananthapuram 695011, India).

Received: 28 October 2020; Accepted: 24 November 2020; Published: 29 November 2020

Simple Summary: This is the largest and most comprehensive assessment of the role of human papillomavirus (HPV) in head and neck cancer (HNC) in Italy, which is a region currently considered bearing a low burden of HPV-driven HNC. $p16^{INK4a}$, HPV-DNA, and HPV RNA biomarkers were used to assess the HPV status in head and neck cancer in a retrospective cohort of approximately 700 patients. In our study, HPV prevalence in oropharyngeal cancers was much higher than in oral and laryngeal cancers, and HPV positivity conferred better prognosis only in oropharyngeal cancers. Importantly, we have observed an increase of the prevalence of HPV positivity in oropharyngeal cancers in the most recent calendar periods, suggesting that this disease is increasing in Italy, as has happened before in other developed regions.

Abstract: Literature on the role of human papillomavirus (HPV) in head and neck cancer (HNC) in Italy is limited, especially for non-oropharyngeal tumours. Within the context of the HPV-AHEAD study, we aimed to assess the prognostic value of different tests or test algorithms judging HPV carcinogenicity in HNC and factors related to HPV positivity at the European Institute of Oncology. We conducted a retrospective cohort study (2000–2010) on a total of 696 primary HNC patients. Formalin-fixed, paraffin-embedded cancer tissues were studied. All HPV-DNA-positive and a random sample of HPV-DNA-negative cases were subjected to HPV-E6*I mRNA detection and $p16^{INK4a}$ staining. Multivariate models were used to assess for factors associated with HPV positivity and proportional hazards for survival and recurrence. The percentage of HPV-driven cases (considering HPV-E6*I mRNA positivity) was 1.8, 2.2, and 40.4% for oral cavity (OC), laryngeal (LC), and oropharyngeal (OPC) cases, respectively. The estimates were similar for HPV-DNA/$p16^{INK4a}$ double positivity. Being a non-smoker or former smoker or diagnosed at more recent calendar periods were associated with HPV-E6*I mRNA positivity only in OPC. Being younger was associated with HPV-E6*I mRNA positivity in LC. HPV-driven OPC, but not HPV-driven OC and LC, showed better 5 year overall and disease-free survival. Our data show that HPV prevalence in OPC was much higher than in OC and LC and observed to increase in most recent years. Moreover, HPV positivity conferred better prognosis only in OPC. Novel insights on the role of HPV in HNC in Italy are provided, with possible implications in the clinical management of these patients.

Keywords: head and neck cancer; human papillomavirus; oropharyngeal cancer; virus-related cancers; human papillomavirus diagnosis

---

1. Introduction

Head and neck carcinoma (HNC) is a heterogeneous group of tumours located at the nasopharynx, oropharynx, hypopharynx, larynx, and oral cavity. Over 90% of HNC are squamous cell carcinomas (HNSCC) and are caused mainly by environmental factors such as smoking, alcohol consumption, human papillomavirus (HPV), and Epstein Barr (EBV) infections. According to the Surveillance, Epidemiology, and End Results (SEER), approximately 4% of all worldwide cancers are in the head and neck region, with more than 430,000 cases per year [1].

Globocan future estimations of HNC in Italy are projected to increase: specifically, a boost of more than 10% of new cases is estimated in all head and neck (HN) areas for both sexes, at all ages, per 100,000 people [2], within the next decade. Compared to 2018, in 2030 the incidence is predicted to increase by 10% for oropharyngeal cancers (OPC) and by 12, 14, and 16% for oral cavity (OC), larynx (LC), and hypopharynx (HPC) cancers, respectively, regardless of HPV status [2]. In addition, a cancer registry-based study assessing the incidence and survival patterns of HNC diagnosed in Italy between 1988 and 2012 found increasing incidence rates of OPC, presumably attributed to HPV infection [3]. Likewise, increasing trends of HPV-driven OPC have been observed for the last two decades in other parts of the world [4].

The HPV distribution in HNSCC largely differs by anatomical site: while the prevalence of HPV-driven OPC ranges between 30–40%, much lower are the estimated rates for the other areas, specifically 2.1–4.4% for OC and 2.7–3.5% for LC and HPC [5–9].

Italian data on HPV status in HNSCC were reported from three other studies with HPV-DNA/HPV-E6*I mRNA double positivity with variable ranges such as 37.9% in OPC (1992–2015) [6], 6% in OC, 20% in OPC, and 1% in LC (2003–2012) [10], and 32.3% in more recent years (2000–2018) for OPC [11]. Indeed, in Italy, HPV infection plays a role in HNSCC similarly to the rest of the Western world, not only for its well documented positive prognostic value but also for its mediation in carcinogenesis [12,13]. However, currently, it is crucial to fully understand how the presence of HPV interacts with other risk factors such as smoking and alcohol in HNSCC in this region [14,15]. From the etiological point of view and in terms of tumour progression and prognosis, the role of these known risk factors is still debated, and those are considered as either "HPV competitors" or as positively interacting with HPV [16–18].

The distinction between HPV-driven and non-HPV-driven OPC is underscored also in the 8th edition of the TNM, where the HPV status (as defined by $p16^{INK4a}$ staining) has been considered for the stage classification of the tumour [19]. It is thus critical to select and use robustly sensitive and specific HPV diagnostic assays in order to determine whether the tumour is truly an HPV-driven OPC. The mere detection of HPV-DNA could reflect a transient or non-related infection rather than a genuine HPV-driven oncogenic process [20–22]. Several markers have been described and are used for HPV detection in HNC, such as E6/E7 HPV mRNA RT-PCR, HPV-DNA/RNA in situ hybridisation, and $p16^{INK4a}$ immunohistochemistry (IHC) [23]. The identification of viral E6/E7 mRNA [22] is widely accepted as the present gold-standard test to elucidate the oncogenic role of HPV but is difficult to employ in everyday clinical practice. Cellular $p16^{INK4a}$ high expression detected by IHC is the most widely implemented technique in clinical settings for HPV-driven OPC diagnosis [24]. However, a significant fraction of $p16^{INK4a}$-positive OPCs are HPV-DNA-negative with no prognostic advantage with respect to HPV-DNA/$p16^{INK4a}$ double-negative tumours, as they might not be related to HPV [25]. The combination of HPV-DNA detection and $p16^{INK4a}$ IHC is starting to be recommended to diagnose HPV-related OPCs [26]. Outside the oropharynx, $p16^{INK4a}$ IHC is not recommended for the diagnosis of HPV association; however, there is limited information about the accuracy and prognostic value of dual HPV-DNA and p16^{INK4a} testing in non-oropharyngeal HNSCC.

Moreover, country-specific estimates of HPV-attributable fractions in OPC and non-oropharyngeal HNC are warranted in order to evaluate the possible protective effect of HPV vaccination.

In this study, we assessed the prognostic value of HPV positivity (as defined by HPV-E6*I mRNA positivity) in a sample of OPC and non-OPC Italian patients and compared the results with those from HPV-DNA positivity and HPV-DNA/p16^{INK4a} double positivity.

We also studied factors related to HPV positivity (as defined by different HPV-relatedness definitions) and the overall proportion and type distribution of HPV-positive at different anatomical sites, as well as the trend of the proportion of HPV-positive HNSCC in more recent years, in Italy. Finally, we highlight the differences between HPV-positive versus negative cancers at three different anatomical regions in terms of prognosis and survival in an Italian setting.

2. Results

2.1. HPV Type Distribution in HPV-Driven HN Sites According to Different Combination of Biomarkers

Supplementary Figure S1 shows the workflow of the HNSCC cases, samples collected, processed, tested, and finally included in the study.

A total of 1594 cases consecutively diagnosed with a primary HNSCC at European Institute of Oncology, IRCCS (IEO) in 2000–2010 were identified, of which 835 (52%) had unavailable formalin-fixed, paraffin-embedded (FFPE) tissue blocks at diagnosis. Some differences were observed between cases with and without available FFPE tissue blocks: specimens from younger patients, cases diagnosed with stage IV a-b (7th TNM edition) or located at sites distal to the oropharynx were over-represented among OC cases with available FFPE tissue blocks. Cases diagnosed with stage III (7th TNM edition) were over-represented among OPC cases with available FFPE tissue blocks, whereas OPC cases located at the base of the tongue were under-represented. Smokers and drinkers, as well as cases diagnosed at earlier periods and located at anatomical subsites proximal to the oropharynx, were over-represented among LC cases with available FFPE tissue blocks. A total of 696 primary cases had a valid HPV result and 675 were finally included in the analyses: 165 OC, 109 OPC, and 401 LC cases (21 pharyngeal-hypopharyngeal cancers were excluded from the analyses due to the low number of cases). The percentage of HPV-driven cases (considering HPV-E6*I mRNA positivity) was 1.8, 2.2, and 40.4% for OC, LC, and OPC cases, respectively (Table 1). The percentage of HPV-DNA/p16^{INK4a} double positivity was 2.4, 1.8, and 43.9% for OC, LC, and OPC cases, respectively. All OPC HPV-DNA-negative cases tested for p16^{INK4a} were also p16^{INK4a}-negative, but three (15.0%) OC and one (3.8%) LC HPV-DNA-negative cases were p16^{INK4a}-positive.

HPV16 was the most common type among HPV-DNA-positive cases for all HN sites, although with lower proportions in LC (59.3%) than in OC (90.0%) and OPC (96.4%) (Figure 1). The next most common HPV type was HPV18 for OC (10%) and LC (14.8%) and HPV33 (1.8%) for OPC. When only considering cases that are double-positive for HPV-DNA/p16^{INK4a}, the prevalence of HPV16 increased in LC and OPC but not in OC. When only considering HPV-E6*I mRNA-positive cases, the prevalence of HPV16 increased in OC and OPC, but not in LC. Differences in HPV type distribution by HPV relatedness definitions were statistically significant. Supplementary Tables S1–S3 show the demographic and clinical characteristics of the HNSCC cases included in the analysis, as well as the HPV prevalence and ORs for each biomarker for HPV positivity. Patients were mostly male (60.0% of OC, 78.0% of OPC, and 88.5% of LC), current or previous smokers (57.0% of OC, 67.9% of OPC, and 97.0% of LC), and current or previous drinkers (52.7% of OC, 60.6% of OPC, and 70.0% of LC). OPC patients most commonly had a locally advanced non-keratinizing SCC, whereas OC and LC had most commonly a locally advanced keratinizing grade 1 SCC and an early stage (I or II) keratinizing grade 2 SCC, respectively. Being a non-smoker or former smoker or diagnosed at more recent calendar periods were associated with HPV positivity in OPC for all three HPV-relatedness definitions. Younger ages (17–54 y) were associated with HPV-DNA positivity in OPC, but this association was not observed for HPV-DNA/p16^{INK4a} double positivity and HPV-E6*I mRNA positivity after adjusting for significant covariates such as tobacco use. Being younger was associated with HPV-DNA/p16^{INK4a} double positivity and HPV-E6*I mRNA positivity in LC. Being a non-smoker was associated with HPV-E6*I mRNA positivity in LC. None of these associations neither others were observed for OC after adjusting for significant covariates, with the exception of an anatomical location proximal to the oropharynx for HPV-DNA positivity. This association was not observed for HPV-DNA/p16^{INK4a} double positivity and HPV- E6*I mRNA positivity.

Table 1. Human papillomavirus (HPV)-attributable fractions by different combinations of biomarkers: HPV-DNA, p16^{INK4a} and E6*I mRNA detection.

Total HNC (n = 675)	Oral Cavity (OC) n = 165 (23.7%) [a]		Oropharynx (OPC) n = 109 (15.7%) [a]		Larynx (LC) n = 401 (57.6%) [a]	
	n	% [b]	n	% [b]	n	% [b]
HPV markers positivity						
HPV-DNA+	10/165	6.1%	55/109	50.5%	29/401	7.2%
p16^{INK4a}+ in HPV-DNA+ cases	4/9	44.4%	47/53	88.7%	7/28	25.0%
p16^{INK4a}+ in HPV-DNA- cases	3/20	15.0%	0/8	0.0%	1/26	3.8%
E6*I mRNA+ in HPV-DNA+ cases	3/10	30.0%	44/55	80.0%	9/29	31.0%
E6*I mRNA+ in HPV-DNA- cases	0/21	0.0%	0/8	0.0%	0/33	0.0%
HPV-DNA+ AND p16^{INK4a}+	4/164	2.4%	47/107	43.9%	7/400	1.8%
HPV-DNA+ AND E6*I mRNA+	3/165	1.8%	44/109	40.4%	9/401	2.2%
HPV-DNA+ AND [E6*I mRNA+ OR p16^{INK4a}+]	4/164	2.4%	47/107	43.9%	9/400	2.3%
HPV-DNA+ AND E6*I mRNA+ AND p16^{INK4a}+	3/164	1.8%	42/107	39.3%	6/400	1.5%

"HNC": head and neck cancer; "OC": oral cavity cancer; "OPC": oropharyngeal cancer; "LC": laryngeal cancer; HPV-DNA detection using a type-specific PCR bead-based multiplex genotyping (E7-MPG) assay that combines multiplex polymerase chain reaction (PCR) and bead-based Luminex technology (Luminex Corp., Austin, TX, USA); p16^{INK4a} considered as positive when a continuous, diffuse staining cells for p16^{INK4a} within the cancer area of the tissue sections was observed. Performed in HPV-DNA-positive cases and in a 11% of random HPV-DNA-negative cases; E6*I mRNA performed in case of HPV-DNA-positive cases for any of the 20 high-risk genotypes detectable by the technique. [a]: % of invasive cancer cases included for each anatomic head and neck (HN) sublocation among all HNC included in the study. [b]: % of positive cases for each combination of HPV-biomarker results among total cases analysed for each HPV-biomarker.

2.2. Overall and Progression-Free Survival of HPV-Driven OPC, OC, LC

HPV-driven OPC, but not HPV-driven OC or LC, showed better 5 year overall survival (OS) ($p < 0.001$), as compared to HPV-non-driven OPC (Figure 2). HPV-driven OPC also showed better 5 year progression-free survival (PFS) ($p = 0.004$), as compared to HPV-non-driven OPC (Figure 3). Both results were equivalent for HPV-DNA-positive and HPV-DNA/p16^{INK4a}-double-positive cases. Other co-variates found to have a prognostic value for OS and PFS in univariate Cox proportional hazards models are shown in Tables 2 and 3. Age was a prognostic factor for death for OPC and LC cases and for recurrence for all HNSCC. LC cases located distal to the oropharynx showed statistically significant improved OS and PFS. Clinical variables such as more advanced stages (7th TNM edition), node status > 1, multimodal treatment including surgery and positive margins for patients treated with surgery were also prognostic factors for death and recurrence for OC and LC, but not for OPC. Statistically significant improved OS among patients diagnosed in 2004–2007 was observed in OPC.

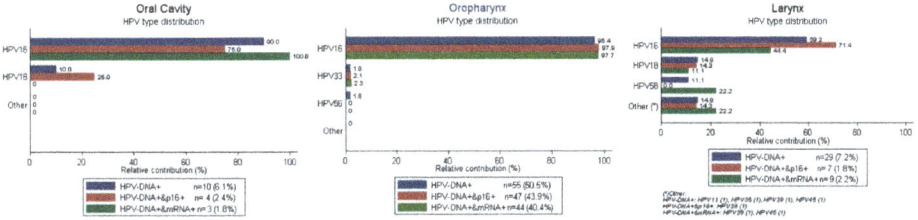

Figure 1. HPV type distribution in HPV-driven HN sites according to different combination of biomarkers: HPV-DNA, HPV-DNA/p16^{INK4a}, and HPV-DNA/E6*I mRNA detection.

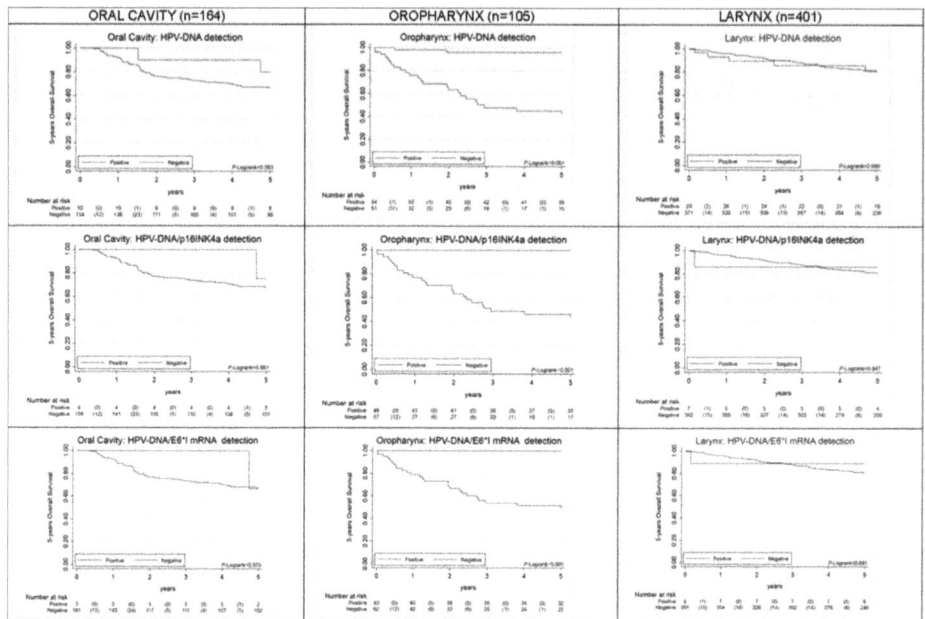

Figure 2. Five-year overall survival of OPC, OC, LC patients (stage IVc patients are excluded) by HPV positivity according to three different HPV-relatedness definitions: HPV-DNA, HPV-DNA/p16^{INK4a}, and HPV-DNA/E6*I mRNA detection.

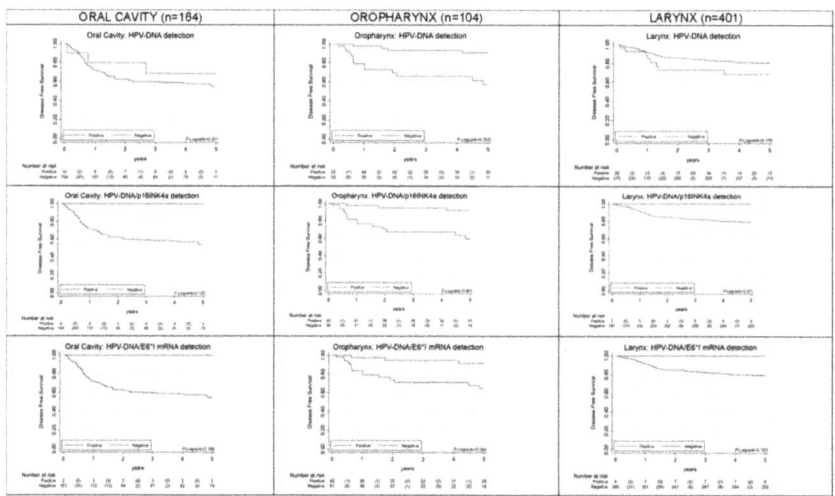

Figure 3. Five-year progression-free survival of OPC, OC, LC patients (stage IVc patients are excluded) by HPV positivity according to three different HPV-relatedness definitions: HPV-DNA, HPV-DNA/p16^{INK4a}, and HPV-DNA/E6*I mRNA detection.

Table 2. Hazard ratios and 95% CI for death for OPC, OC, LC patients (stage IVc patients are excluded) for 5 year follow-up.

Covariate	OPC Cases/Deaths	HR	Crude HR 95% CI Lower	Crude HR 95% CI Upper	p-Value	OC Cases/Deaths	HR	Crude HR 95% CI Lower	Crude HR 95% CI Upper	p-Value	LC Cases/Deaths	HR	Crude HR 95% CI Lower	Crude HR 95% CI Upper	p-Value
HPV-DNA	105/26				0.000	164/51				0.322	401/69				0.990
Other	51/24	Ref.				154/49	Ref.				372/64	Ref.			
HPV-DNA+	54/2	0.05	0.01	0.22		10/2	0.52	0.13	2.16		29/5	1.01	0.40	2.50	
HPV-E6*I mRNA	105/26				-	164/51				0.872	401/69				0.666
Other HPV-E6*I mRNA+	62/26					161/50	Ref.				392/68	Ref.			
	43/0	-	-	-		3/1	0.85	0.12	6.18		9/1	0.67	0.09	4.80	
HPV-DNA and p16	103/26				-	163/50				0.640	400/69				0.946
Other HPV-DNA+ and p16+	57/26	Ref.				159/49	Ref.				393/68	Ref.			
	46/0	-	-	-		4/1	0.64	0.09	4.67		7/1	0.93	0.13	6.73	
Age at diagnosis	105/26	1.05	1.01	1.10	0.023	164/51	1.01	0.99	1.03	0.190	401/69	1.04	1.01	1.07	0.002
17-54 y	24/3	Ref.			0.076	71/17	Ref.			0.142	70/9	Ref.			0.205
55-62 y	38/8	1.79	0.46	6.76		28/12	2.30	1.10	4.82		115/20	1.42	0.65	3.12	
63-70 y	22/7	2.64	0.68	10.20		27/11	1.85	0.87	3.95		108/16	1.28	0.57	2.90	
71-94 y	21/8	4.84	1.28	18.31		38/11	1.38	0.65	2.94		108/24	2.10	0.98	4.52	
Gender	105/26				0.778	164/51				0.898	401/69				0.906
Male	82/21	Ref.				99/31	Ref.				355/61	Ref.			
Female	23/5	0.87	0.33	2.31		65/20	1.04	0.59	1.82		46/8	1.05	0.50	2.18	
Period of diagnosis	105/26	0.87	0.76	0.99	0.028	164/51	0.98	0.90	1.07	0.725	401/69	1.00	0.92	1.08	0.914
2000-2003	38/16	Ref.			0.028	49/15	Ref.			0.447	147/24	Ref.			0.612
2004-2007	46/7	0.32	0.13	0.79		68/24	1.28	0.67	2.44		170/33	1.23	0.73	2.08	
2008-2010	21/3	0.36	0.10	1.22		47/12	0.83	0.39	1.78		84/12	0.92	0.46	1.85	
Tobacco use	105/26				0.091	164/51				0.775	401/69				0.783
Non-smoker	21/3	Ref.				61/17	Ref.				11/2	Ref.			
Former smoker	21/3	1.04	0.21	5.14		31/11	1.22	0.57	2.61		28/6	1.28	0.26	6.34	
Smoker	51/18	2.84	0.84	9.65		63/21	1.21	0.64	2.29		361/61	0.89	0.22	3.66	

Table 2. Cont.

Covariate	OPC Cases/Deaths	HR	Crude HR 95% CI Lower	Crude HR 95% CI Upper	p-Value	OC Cases/Deaths	HR	Crude HR 95% CI Lower	Crude HR 95% CI Upper	p-Value	LC Cases/Deaths	HR	Crude HR 95% CI Lower	Crude HR 95% CI Upper	p-Value
Unknown	12/2	0.99	0.17	5.95		9/2	0.65	0.15	2.83		1/0	-			
Alcohol use	105/26				0.276	164/51				0.089	401/69				0.166
Non-drinker	25/4	Ref.				66/15	Ref.				115/18	Ref.			
Former drinker	3/2	4.90	0.89	26.86		3/0	-				3/1	3.28	0.44	24.6	
Drinker	62/17	1.97	0.66	5.87		84/33	1.80	0.98	3.32		274/50	1.19	0.69	2.04	
Unknown	15/3	1.13	0.25	5.06		11/3	1.05	0.30	3.61		9/0	-			
Subsite	105/26				0.110										
Tonsil	47/9	Ref.				-					-				
BOT	29/6	1.16	0.41	3.26		-					-				
Other oropharynx	29/11	2.50	1.03	6.03		-					-				
Proximal to oropharynx	-	-			-	49/13	Ref.			0.437	97/23	Ref.			0.024
Distal to oropharynx	-	-				115/38	1.28	0.68	2.39		304/46	0.55	0.33	0.91	
Stage (7th edition TNM)	105/26				0.852	164/51				0.040	401/69				0.000
I + II	24/6	Ref.				74/17	Ref.				256/30	Ref.			
III	22/5	0.80	0.24	2.61		28/9	1.58	0.70	3.55		77/13	1.53	0.80	2.94	
IVa + IVb	59/15	1.06	0.41	2.73		62/25	2.19	1.18	4.07		68/26	4.05	2.39	6.85	
cN	105/26				0.209	164/51				0.007	401/69				0.000
0	37/12	Ref.				94/24	Ref.				339/46	Ref.			
1	22/4	0.52	0.17	1.61		37/11	1.24	0.61	2.54		16/4	2.17	0.78	6.04	
2	39/7	0.52	0.20	1.32		33/16	2.89	1.53	5.45		41/15	3.53	1.97	6.33	
3	7/3	1.93	0.54	6.89		0					5/4	7.64	2.74	21.28	
Treatment	105/26				0.204	164/51				0.000	401/69				0.025
Only surgery	22/8	Ref.				85/17	Ref.				267/37	Ref.			
Surgery + others	41/11	0.53	0.21	1.33		71/29	2.54	1.39	4.62		107/27	2.03	1.24	3.34	
Conservative	37/6	0.36	0.13	1.05		3/1	1.87	0.25	14.04		19/3	1.71	0.53	5.56	
Unknown	5/1	1.96	0.23	16.51		5/4	25.57	8.17	80.10		8/2	3.93	0.95	16.32	

Table 2. Cont.

Covariate	OPC					OC					LC				
	Cases/Deaths	HR	Crude HR 95% CI Lower	Upper	p-Value	Cases/Deaths	HR	Crude HR 95% CI Lower	Upper	p-Value	Cases/Deaths	HR	Crude HR 95% CI Lower	Upper	p-Value
Positive margins	77/18				0.299	159/49				0.041	353/68				0.039
No	60/16	Ref.				144/42	Ref.				294/43	Ref.			
Yes	17/2	0.49	0.11	2.14		15/7	2.54	1.14	5.68		59/15	1.92	1.07	3.46	
Time of follow-up															
Median (years) (Min–Max)	5.08 (0.02–18.71)					9.05 (0.02–19.05)					6.83 (0.00–18.51)				
Time since dead															
Median (years) (Min–Max)	1.97 (0.02–16.21)					1.97 (0.02–16.21)					3.43 (0.01–16.40)				

95% CI: confidence interval; OPC: oropharyngeal cancer; OC: oral cavity cancer; LC: laryngeal cancer; HR: hazard ratio; cN: clinical node status; Tonsil: C02.4 and C09.0 and C09.1 and C09.9; BOT: base of the tongue (C01); other oropharynx: C10 and C10.0 and C10.2 and C10.3 and C10.8 and C10.9; *OC Distal to oropharynx:C02 and C02.0 and C02.1 0 and C02.2 and C02.3 and C03.1 and C04.1 and C04.9 and C06.0; OC Proximal to oropharynx: C02.8 and C02.9 and C05.8 and C06.2; LC Proximal to oropharynx: C32.1 and C32.8; LC Distal to oropharynx: C32.0; Std: standard deviation; Min: minimum; Max: maximum. Stage IVc patients are excluded. Bold represents statistically significant categories.

Table 3. Hazard ratios and 95% CI for recurrence for OPC, OC, LC patients (stage IVc patients are excluded) for 5 year follow-up.

Covariate	OPC					OC					LC				
	Cases/Rec.	HR	95% CI Lower	95% CI Upper	p-Value	Cases/Rec.	HR	95% CI Lower	95% CI Upper	p-Value	Cases/Rec.	HR	95% CI Lower	95% CI Upper	p-Value
HPV-DNA	**105/20**				0.000	**164/70**				0.402	**401/75**				0.152
Other	51/15	Ref.				154/67	Ref.				372/67	Ref.			
HPV-DNA+	54/5	0.16	0.05	0.50		10/3	0.63	0.20	2.01		29/8	1.78	0.85	3.71	
HPV-E6*I mRNA	**105/20**				0.003	**164/70**				-	**401/75**				-
Other	62/16	Ref.				161/70					392/75				
HPV-E6*I mRNA+	43/4	0.19	0.06	0.67		3/0	-				9/0	-			
HPV-DNA and p16	**103/20**				0.001	**163/70**				-	**400/75**				-
Other	57/16	Ref.				159/70					393/75				
HPV-DNA+ and p16+	46/4	0.15	0.04	0.52		4/0	-				7/0	-			
Age at diagnosis	**105/20**	1.04	0.99	1.10	0.107	**164/70**	1.02	1.00	1.03	0.013	**401/75**	1.03	1.01	1.05	0.017
17–54 y	24/2	Ref.			0.097	71/25	Ref.			0.079	70/10	Ref.			0.202
55–62 y	38/7	2.21	0.45	10.94		28/16	2.08	1.11	3.90		115/18	1.16	0.54	2.52	
63–70 y	22/8	5.45	1.16	25.70		27/10	1.10	0.53	2.29		108/25	1.85	0.88	3.86	
71–94 y	21/3	2.04	0.29	14.51		38/19	1.78	0.98	3.23		108/22	1.77	0.84	3.73	
Gender	**105/20**				0.364	**164/70**				0.404	**401/75**				0.867
Male	82/13	Ref.				99/40	Ref.				355/67	Ref.			
Female	23/7	1.65	0.59	4.62		65/30	1.22	0.76	1.97		46/8	0.94	0.45	1.96	
Period of diagnosis	**105/20**	0.92	0.79	1.07	0.270	**164/70**	1.01	0.94	1.09	0.698	**401/75**	1.02	0.94	1.10	0.636
2000–2003	38/9	Ref.			0.312	49/21	Ref.			0.986	147/26	Ref.			0.799
2004–2007	46/6	0.45	0.16	1.27		68/28	1.05	0.59	1.84		170/31	1.06	0.63	1.79	
2008–2010	21/5	0.65	0.18	2.40		47/21	1.04	0.57	1.90		84/18	1.23	0.67	2.27	

Table 3. Cont.

Covariate	OPC					OC					LC				
	Cases/Rec.	HR	Crude HR 95% CI Lower	Upper	p-Value	Cases/Rec.	HR	Crude HR 95% CI Lower	Upper	p-Value	Cases/Rec.	HR	Crude HR 95% CI Lower	Upper	p-Value
Tobacco use	105/20				0.168	164/70				0.845	401/75				0.395
Non-smoker	21/5	Ref.				61/27	Ref.				11/2	Ref.			
Former smoker	21/1	0.29	0.03	2.80		31/11	0.76	0.38	1.54		28/7	1.62	0.34	7.81	
Smoker	51/12	1.69	0.48	6.00		63/27	0.93	0.55	1.59		361/66	0.98	0.24	4.01	
Unknown	12/2	0.82	0.14	4.92		9/5	1.16	0.45	3.02		1/0	-			
Alcohol use	105/20				0.388	164/70				0.829	401/75				0.062
Non-drinker	25/5	Ref.				66/26	Ref.				115/20	Ref.			
Former drinker	3/1	2.12	0.25	18.30		3/2	1.84	0.44	7.76		3/0	-			
Drinker	62/13	0.99	0.34	2.86		84/37	1.18	0.71	1.95		274/55	1.16	0.69	1.93	
Unknown	15/1	0.27	0.03	2.28		11/5	1.04	0.40	2.71		9/0	-			
Subsite	105/20				0.549										
Tonsil	47/10	Ref.													
BOT	29/4	0.81	0.24	2.68											
Other oropharynx	29/6	1.59	0.55	4.59											
Subsite						164/70				0.258	401/75				0.012
Proximal to Opx						49/17	Ref.				97/26	Ref.			
Distal to Opx						115/53	1.36	0.79	2.35		304/49	0.54	0.33	0.87	
Stage (7th edition TNM)	105/20				0.497	164/70				0.473	401/75				0.001
I + II	24/7	Ref.				74/33	Ref.				256/36	Ref.			
III	22/4	0.60	0.17	2.14		28/9	0.67	0.32	1.41		77/16	1.47	0.81	2.69	
IVa + IVb	59/9	0.52	0.18	1.51		62/28	1.04	0.63	1.71		68/23	2.94	1.74	4.97	
cN	105/20				0.111	164/70				0.033	401/75				0.001
0	37/8	Ref.				94/40	Ref.				339/50	Ref.			
1	22/4	0.90	0.26	3.08		37/11	0.64	0.33	1.25		16/7	3.18	1.36	7.042	
2	39/5	0.48	0.14	1.65		33/19	1.68	0.97	2.91		41/16	3.44	1.96	6.05	
3	7/3	3.83	0.97	14.98		0					5/2	3.95	0.96	16.26	
Treatment	105/20				0.090	164/70				0.699	401/75				0.052
Only surgery	22/6	Ref.				85/35	Ref.				267/45	Ref.			
Surgery + others	41/5	0.23	0.06	0.80		71/32	1.09	0.67	1.76		107/24	1.47	0.89	2.42	
Conservative treatment	37/9	0.65	0.22	1.86		3/1	0.72	0.10	5.26		19/6	3.00	1.27	7.05	
Unknown	5/0	-				5/2	2.50	0.59	10.51		8/0	-			
Positive margins	77/13				0.189	159/69				0.014	353/65				0.039
No	60/12	Ref.				144/59	Ref.				294/49	Ref.			
Yes	17/1	0.31	0.04	2.41		15/10	2.58	1.31	5.06		59/16	1.87	1.07	3.31	

Rec.: recurrences; 95% CI: confidence interval; OPC: oropharyngeal cancer; OC: oral cavity cancer; LC: laryngeal cancer; HR: hazard ratio; cN: clinical node status; Tonsil: C02.4 and C09.0 and C09.1 and C09.9; BOT: base of the tongue (C01); other oropharynx: C10 and C10.0 and C10.2 and C10.3 and C10.8 and C10.9; *OC Distal to oropharynx:C02 and C02.0 and C02.1 0 and C02.2 and C02.3 and C03.1 and C04.1 and C04.9 and C06.0; OC Proximal to oropharynx: C02.8 and C02.9 and C05.8 and C06.2; LC Proximal to oropharynx: C32.1 and C32.8; LC Distal to oropharynx: C32.0; Std: standard deviation; Min: minimum; Max: maximum. Stage IVc patients are excluded. Bold represents statistically significant categories.

3. Discussion

To our knowledge, this study is the largest and most comprehensive assessment of the role of HPV in HNSCC in Italy. HPV-induced carcinogenesis is mediated by the oncoviral proteins E6 and E7, which, respectively, promote the degradation of the cellular proteins p53 and Rb, leading to cell proliferation, evasion from apoptosis, immortalization, and an increase of genomic instability [27]. The importance of determining whether an HN tumour is truly HPV-driven is underscored by the notion that these cancers are currently classified into two subtypes that must be considered as distinct entities: HPV-negative and HPV-positive. HPV-positive tumours, compared to the HPV-negative ones, are characterized by multiple molecular and clinicopathological differences, including age, socioeconomic status, prognosis, genetic landscape, and tissue differentiation [28,29]. Nevertheless, patients are treated with the same therapeutic protocols consisting mainly of surgery, radiation, and platinum-based chemotherapy [30].

Herein, we assess the prognostic value of different HPV-relatedness definitions, as well as factors related to HPV positivity in a retrospective cohort of approximately 700 HNSCC patients. We estimated that 1.8% of OC, 2.2% of LC, and 40.4% of OPC were HPV-driven based on HPV-RNA detection. The results were similar for HPV-DNA/ p16^{INK4a} double positivity.

A previous study of 248 HNC cases diagnosed in 2003–2012 in Northern Italy found HPV prevalence of 1.6% in OC, 20% in OPC, and 1% in LC, when considering HPV-DNA/HPV-E6*I RNA double positivity [10]. Our estimates were equivalent for OC and LC but considerably higher for OPC. Another study of 195 OPC cases diagnosed between 1992 and 2015 in Pavia, Italy, found a HPV prevalence of 37.9% when considering HPV-DNA/p16^{INK4a} double positivity [6], similar to our estimate of HPV-DNA/p16^{INK4a} double positivity in OPC, 43.9%. The study observed a marginally non-significant increase of HPV prevalence among OPC cases diagnosed after 2010 (45 vs. 28.3%, $p = 0.06$) [6]. A more recent Italian study also evaluated the role of HPV in patients with newly diagnosed OPC during the period 2000–2018, reporting a prevalence of HPV-driven OPC of 32.3% and a higher prevalence in the most recent years [11]. We also observed that OPC cases diagnosed at more recent periods (2008–2010) were independently associated with HPV positivity for all three HPV-relatedness definitions herein considered.

A cancer registry-based Italian study assessing the incidence and survival patterns of HNC diagnosed in Italy between 1988 and 2012 [3] found increasing incidence rates of OPC. These results, together with ours and those from others [6,11], suggest that HPV-related OPCs are increasing in Italy, as has previously happened in areas where nowadays most OPC cases are HPV-related. Regarding non-OPC sites, we did not observe any association between HPV positivity and calendar period.

Our study was conducted in the context of the international HPV-AHEAD study [31–33], which aimed to perform a comprehensive analysis of approximately 8000 HNC cases from Europe and India. A standardized protocol for optimizing the use of FFPE tissue blocks was developed, and each assay was performed in a single laboratory [33]. The first results on 355 Indian cases showed results equivalent to ours for HPV-E6*I mRNA positivity in LC (1.7%) and OC (1.6%), but considerably lower for OPC (9.4%) [32]. In a comprehensive study of 3680 HNC patients from 29 different countries, geographic heterogeneity of HPV-attributable fractions (HPV-AFs) was particularly evident for OPC [7].

HPV16 was the most common type among HPV-positive cases across all HN sites and HPV-relatedness definitions. However, its predominance was far higher in OC and OPC than in LC. Moreover, when considering only cases were HPV was the truly triggering carcinogenic agent (i.e., cases HPV-E6*I mRNA-positive) the percentage of HPV16-positive cases increased for OC and OPC but decreased for LC. These results, if confirmed in other larger studies, may have implications on the estimation of HPV vaccination effects.

Being a non-smoker or former smoker was associated with HPV positivity in OPC, consistently with what is reported in the literature regardless of geographical region [25,34,35]. However, as already observed in other studies [25], we did not find any association between gender and HPV positivity in OPC. HPV-driven OPC has been consistently associated with males in US studies [35], whereas in other regions, it has been associated with females [7]. These results highlight the geographical variability of the disease and the need of country-specific population-based studies to assess possible gender differences in HPV-driven OPC carcinogenesis.

Regarding non-oropharyngeal HNSCC cases, being younger and a non-smoker were associated with HPV positivity in LC. As compared to OPC, fewer studies have analysed the factors associated with HPV positivity in non-oropharyngeal cancer sites. The ICO international study also observed that HPV-positive LC patients, as well as OC ones, showed younger ages at diagnosis than HPV-negative ones [7]. However, we did not observe this association for OC after adjusting for co-variates.

As expected, HPV-positive OPC patients showed better OS and PFS than HPV-negative OPC cases regardless of the HPV-relatedness definition herein considered. However, as it has been already observed [23,36] the prognostic advantage of HPV-positive cases was higher when considering as positive only OPC cases truly driven by HPV infection (i.e., positive for HPV-E6*I mRNA or double-positive for HPV-DNA/p16^{INK4a}). HPV-positive LC and OC cases did not show better OS and PFS than HPV-negative cases. Noteworthy, HPV-DNA/p16^{INK4a}-positive and HPV-E6*I mRNA double-positive OC cases showed a marginally non-significant better PFS than the rest of cases. The prognostic value of HPV in non-oropharyngeal HNC is still unclear. While some studies have observed a better outcome for HPV-positive HNC, others have not [24]. The most updated guidelines for HPV testing in HNC have been published by the College of American Pathologists [24]. In this context, a panel of experts conducted a systematic review of studies that investigated the clinical outcomes of HPV-positive HNSCC. The panel concluded that there is no proven prognostic difference based on the presence or absence of HPV in non-oropharyngeal cancer. Thus, there is a need for more meta-analytical work to establish survival differences by HPV-relatedness of non-oropharyngeal cancer separated by anatomic site. The HPV AHEAD studies will contribute a considerable contribution to such pooled analyses.

We acknowledge that our study has several limitations. The retrospective nature of the cohort may have limited the accuracy of data related to some risk factors such as tobacco/alcohol use. Only 11% of HPV-DNA-negative cases were further tested for HPV-E6*I mRNA and p16^{INK4a}, in accordance with the protocol established within the HPV-AHEAD consortium. For an important number of primary HNC cases consecutively diagnosed at IEO during the study period and targeted to be included in the study, no FFPE tissue blocks were available. Moreover, some differences were observed between cases with and without tissue sample, as it has been noted in other studies [25]. We had a small number of HPV-positive cases, and multivariate Cox's proportional hazards models could not be performed due to the small number of deaths and recurrences. The small number of cases also hampered the performance of Kaplan–Meier analyses on locally advanced cases only. However, stage (according to 7th edition TNM) was not found to be associated with HPV positivity. For non-OPC cases, the small number of HPV-positive cases has made it difficult to extrapolate meaning from the survival analyses and results must be taken with caution. HPV-AHEAD definition of p16^{INK4a} positivity was established before the publication of the guidelines for HPV testing in HNC by the College of American Pathologists [24], where a 70% nuclear and cytoplasmic staining cut-off was recommended and is currently widely accepted in clinical practice. However, the impact of misclassification can be considered low due to the low number of p16^{INK4a}-positive cases, which are less than 70%. A total of 15 out of 68 cases classified as p16^{INK4a}-positive did not reach the 70% nuclear and cytoplasmic staining threshold.

4. Materials and Methods

4.1. Study Design and Samples

A retrospective cohort of patients consecutively diagnosed with a primary HNC at the IEO in Milan from 2000 to 2010 was conducted within the HPV-AHEAD project [31–33]. HNC cases were identified from medical records/pathology reports of the hospital. Selected cases had a histopathological diagnosis of primary squamous cell carcinoma of the oropharynx (International Classification of Diseases for

Oncology (ICD-O) C01.9, C02.4, C05.1, C05.2, C09, C10), oral cavity (ICD-O: C02.0–C06.9, excluding C02.4, C05.1, C05.2), the hypopharynx, and larynx (ICD-O: C13, C32).

Information on demographics, smoking and alcohol consumption, and clinical and follow-up data up to 2019 was extracted from electronic medical records. The definition of a drinker was consumption of three or more drinks per week. We only considered FFPE tumour samples from the diagnosis previous to treatment.

Ethical clearance was obtained from IEO Ethical Committee (code IEO N101), Milan, Italy as well as IARC, Lyon, France. The study did not involve any contact with the patients. All clinical and pathological data were collected using well-designed case report forms (CRF) according to good clinical practice guidelines.

Adequate measures to ensure data protection, confidentiality, patients' privacy, and anonymization were taken into account. FFPE tissue blocks were used to perform several laboratory assays, as described below. Each assay was performed in a single laboratory: (i) HPV-DNA assay at IARC, (ii) HPV RNA assay at DKFZ, and (iii) p16^{INK4a} staining at Roche mtm laboratories.

Cancer samples having tested negative for both HPV-DNA and beta-globin DNA were excluded from the analyses.

4.2. Preparation of the Tissue Sections

FFPE tissues were in part processed at the International Agency for Research on Cancer, Lyon, France and at IEO, Milan, Italy, following the HPV-AHEAD sectioning protocol [33].

4.3. Histological Analysis

All sections were evaluated by the HPV-AHEAD histopathology review panel six pathologists (J.P.B., B.L.R., F.M., O.C., R.V.K., N.G.). An online pathology form was used. Each pathologist evaluated tissues from approximately 80 patients. All sections were re-evaluated by a second panel of pathologists. Only FFPE tissue blocks for which the first and last haematoxylin/eosin stained sections reflected tumour tissue were included in the study.

4.4. HPV-DNA Genotyping

DNA was purified from three consecutive FFPE sections (S6–8), as previously described [31]. HPV-DNA was detected by E7 type-specific multiplex genotyping (E7-MPG), which combines multiplex polymerase chain reaction (PCR) and hybridization to type-specific oligonucleotide probes on fluorescent beads (Luminex Corporation, Austin, TX) [37,38]. TS-MPG uses HPV type-specific primers targeting the E7 region of 19 high-risk (HR) or possible/probable HR (pHR) HPV types (HPV16, 18, 26, 31, 33, 35, 39, 45, 51, 52, 53, 56, 58, 59, 66, 68a and b, 70, 73, and 82) and two low-risk (LR) HPV types (HPV6 and 11). Detection limits range from 10 to 1000 copies of the viral genome per reaction. Two primers for amplification of the beta-globin gene were also included to control for the quality of the template DNA. A slightly modified E7-MPG with higher analytical sensitivity was performed with amplicon size of approximately 100 bp for 10 HPV types (HPV16, 18, 31, 33, 35, 52, 56, 66, 6, and 11), and 117 bp for beta-globin [20,39]. After PCR amplification, 10 µl of each reaction mixture were analysed by multiplex HPV genotyping (MPG) using Luminex technology (Luminex Corporation) as described previously [40].

All HPV-DNA-positive FFPE specimens and a random subgroup of approximately 11% of HPV-DNA-negative cases were subjected to HPV-E6*I mRNA detection and p16^{INK4a} staining.

4.5. HPV E6*I RNA Analysis

An ultra-short amplicon, E6*I mRNA RT-PCR assay was chosen for HPV-mRNA detection for its applicability to FFPE material and absolute RNA specificity by using a splice-site as identification target [20]. Total RNA was purified from three pooled consecutive sections of the same tissue block using the PureLink FFPE Total RNA Isolation Kit (Invitrogen, Carlsbad, CA) [20]. The HPV type-specific

E6*I mRNA assays are available for 20 HR- or pHR-HPV types for which presence of splice sites was demonstrated. Briefly, extracted RNA was subjected to a one-step reverse transcription PCR protocol with the QuantiTect Virus Kit (Qiagen, Hilden, Germany) using HPV type specific primers to amplify 65–75 bp cDNA sequences across the E6*I splice sites and human ubiquitin C (ubC) primers that generate a 85 bp cDNA amplicon as a control for tissue and RNA quality. The products were then hybridized to HPV and ubC specific oligonucleotide probes coupled to fluorescence-labelled Luminex beads (Luminex Corp.) as described previously [20]. Specimens that were HPV-E6*I and/or ubC mRNA-positive were considered RNA valid.

4.6. $p16^{INK4a}$ IHC

Expression of p16 was evaluated manually by IHC in FFPE sections using the CINtec p16 Histology Kit (Roche mtm laboratories AG, Mannheim, Germany) according to the manufacturer's instructions and as previously described [32]. A continuous, diffuse staining for $p16^{INK4a}$ within the cancer area of the tissue sections was considered as positive, while a focal staining or no staining was considered negative. IHC slides were analysed without knowledge of any other clinical information (including HPV-DNA and RNA status) by R.R. and F.M. Discordant cases were analysed by O.C. and consensus was reached.

4.7. Statistical Analyses

Differences in the covariate distribution (age, gender, sub-site, tobacco and alcohol use, TNM 7th Edition) between cases with and without available FFPE block were assessed by Pearson's chi2 test. We used HPV-E6*I mRNA positivity as the reference test for viral carcinogenic activity. We assumed that HPV-DNA-negative cases not tested for HPV-E6*I mRNA were HPV-E6*I mRNA-negative and HPV-DNA/HPV-E6*I mRNA double-positive cases were considered as HPV-E6*I mRNA-positive cases. HPV-prevalence and HPV-type distribution were assessed. Unconditional logistic regression analyses were performed to identify independent factors (i.e., age, sex, tobacco-alcohol use, clinical data) associated with HPV etiological involvement in each HNSCC site according to the three different HPV-relatedness definitions using backward selection of significant covariates. The likelihood ratio test (LR $p < 0.05$) and the Akaike information criterion were applied to exclude non-significant factors. Histological variables were not considered in multivariate analyses as they were considered to be intermediate variables in the carcinogenic process, as previously described [41]. Crude and adjusted ORs and their 95% confidence intervals (CI) were estimated. Survival time was defined as the period between the date of histological diagnosis and the date of death for any cause (OS) or the date of cancer recurrence (PFS). The cumulative probability of survival was estimated by Kaplan–Meier analyses. Survival curves were compared with the log-rank test for each HPV-relatedness definition and each head and neck site up to 5 years. Univariate Cox proportional hazards models were also conducted up to 5 years to assess the prognostic role of HPV status and other co-variates. Multivariate Cox proportional hazards models could not be performed due to the small number of deaths and recurrences. Metastatic patients (stage IVc, 7th edition TNM) were excluded from survival analyses. Statistical significance for all analyses was set at the 2-sided 0.05 level. Data analyses were performed with STATA software v.16 (Stata Corp., College Station, TX, USA).

5. Conclusions

Our findings from a large cohort of unselected HNSCC patients provide a comprehensive picture on the role of HPV in OPC and non-oropharyngeal cancer in a setting of Southern Europe, which is a region currently considered to bear a low burden of HPV-driven HNC. We have observed an increase of the prevalence of HPV positivity in OPC with most recent calendar periods. These results, together from previous findings of increasing incidence of OPC in Italy [3], suggest that HPV-driven OPC is increasing in Italy, as has happened before in other developed regions. However, we observed some differences with respect to published data from North America. Our results also suggest that current estimations of HPV prevalence in Southern Europe are outdated and warrant updated population-based studies. Moreover, our study provides novel insights on the type-specific contribution of HPV, not only on OPC but also on LC and OC, that may have implications when estimating the possible protective effect of HPV vaccination against HNC.

Supplementary Materials: The following are available online at http://www.mdpi.com/2072-6694/12/12/3567/s1, Figure S1: Flowchart of cases, Table S1: Association of demographics and clinical characteristics of OC cancers and HPV positivity according to three different HPV-relatedness definitions: HPV-DNA, HPV-E6*I mRNA detection, and HPV-DNA/p16^{INK4a}, Table S2: Association of demographics and clinical characteristics of OPC cancers and HPV positivity according to three different HPV-relatedness definitions: HPV-DNA, HPV-E6*I mRNA detection, and HPV-DNA/p16^{INK4a}, Table S3: Association of demographics and clinical characteristic of LC cancers and HPV positivity according to three different HPV-relatedness definitions: HPV-DNA, HPV-E6*I mRNA detection, and HPV-DNA/p16^{INK4a}.

Author Contributions: M.T. (Marta Tagliabue), M.M., F.M., T.G., J.P.B., B.L.R., O.C., R.V.K., N.G.: methodology, data curation; M.T. (Marta Tagliabue), M.M., S.C., M.T. (Massimo Tommasino), L.A., R.R.: writing—original draft preparation; D.S., D.R., E.G., F.C. (Francesco Chu), D.L., E.L., M.T. (Miren Taberna), S.G., M.A. (Marc Arbyn), D.A., M.R.P., P.B.: data curation; M.M., B.Q.B., D.H., F.L., M.P., R.S., S.T., S.R., R.R.: visualization, investigation, statistical analysis; S.C., L.A., M.A. (Mohssen Ansarin), F.C. (Fausto Chiesa) M.T. (Massimo Tommasino): study supervision; all authors: reviewing and editing. All authors have read and agreed to the published version of the manuscript.

Funding: This study was funded by European Commission HPV-AHEAD. Grant Number: FP7-HEALTH-2011–282562. This work was partially supported by the Italian Ministry of Health with Ricerca Corrente and 5 × 1000 funds. M. Ar. was supported by the Horizon 2020 Framework Programme for Research and Innovation of the European Commission, through the RISCC Network, Grant Number 847845. Research on HPV and Head and Neck Cancer in Susanna Chiocca laboratory was also supported by Associazione Italiana Ricerca sul Cancro (A.I.R.C. IG 2015 Id.16721).

Acknowledgments: We thank European Institute of Oncology Biobank and Luigi Santoro (biostatistician currently at Chiesi Group Parma). The authors alone are responsible for the views expressed in this article, and they do not necessarily represent the views, decisions, or policies of the institutions with which they are affiliated.

Conflicts of Interest: R.R. and S.R. are employees of Roche. Cancer Epidemiology Research Program (L.A., M.M., S.T., B.Q.B., O.C.) has received sponsorship for grants from Merck and Co., Roche, Reig-jofre, Integrated DNA Technologies, Seegene, Hologic, and GlaxoSmithKline. M.P. has received research support through cooperate contracts between DKFZ and Roche, Qiagen, Bosch in the field of HPV diagnostics. The remaining authors have declared no conflicts of interest.

Disclaimer: Where authors are identified as personnel of the International Agency for Research on Cancer/World Health Organization, the authors alone are responsible for the views expressed in this article, and they do not necessarily represent the decisions, policy, or views of the International Agency for Research on Cancer/World Health Organization.

References

1. Head and Neck Squamous Cell Carcinoma. Available online: https://www.sciencedirect.com/topics/medicine-and-dentistry/head-and-neck-squamous-cell-carcinoma (accessed on 26 November 2020).
2. Cancer Tomorrow. Available online: https://gco.iarc.fr/tomorrow/graphicisotype?type=0&population=900&mode=population&sex=0&cancer=39&age_group=value&apc_male=0&apc_female=0#collapse-group-0-4 (accessed on 26 November 2020).
3. Boscolo-Rizzo, P.; Zorzi, M.; Del Mistro, A.; Da Mosto, M.C.; Tirelli, G.; Buzzoni, C.; Rugge, M.; Polesel, J.; Guzzinati, S.; AIRTUM Working Group. The evolution of the epidemiological landscape of head and neck cancer in Italy: Is there evidence for an increase in the incidence of potentially HPV-related carcinomas? *PLoS ONE* **2018**, *13*, e0192621. [CrossRef]
4. Chaturvedi, A.K.; Anderson, W.F.; Lortet-Tieulent, J.; Curado, M.P.; Ferlay, J.; Franceschi, S.; Rosenberg, P.S.; Bray, F.; Gillison, M.L. Worldwide trends in incidence rates for oral cavity and oropharyngeal cancers. *J. Clin. Oncol.* **2013**, *31*, 4550–4559. [CrossRef] [PubMed]
5. Li, H.; Torabi, S.J.; Yarbrough, W.G.; Mehra, S.; Osborn, H.A.; Judson, B. Association of Human Papillomavirus Status at Head and Neck Carcinoma Subsites With Overall Survival. *JAMA Otolaryngol. Head Neck Surg.* **2018**, *144*, 519–525. [CrossRef] [PubMed]

6. Morbini, P.; Alberizzi, P.; Ferrario, G.; Capello, G.; De Silvestri, A.; Pedrazzoli, P.; Tinelli, C.; Benazzo, M. The evolving landscape of human papillomavirus-related oropharyngeal squamous cell carcinoma at a single institution in Northern Italy. *Acta Otorhinolaryngol.* **2019**, *39*, 9–17. [CrossRef]
7. Castellsagué, X.; Alemany, L.; Quer, M.; Halec, G.; Quirós, B.; Tous, S.; Clavero, O.; Alòs, L.; Biegner, T.; Szafarowski, T.; et al. HPV Involvement in Head and Neck Cancers: Comprehensive Assessment of Biomarkers in 3680 Patients. *J. Natl. Cancer Inst.* **2016**, *108*, djv403. [CrossRef] [PubMed]
8. Arbyn, M.; de Sanjosé, S.; Saraiya, M.; Sideri, M.; Palefsky, J.; Lacey, C.; Gillison, M.; Bruni, L.; Ronco, G.; Wentzensen, N.; et al. EUROGIN 2011 roadmap on prevention and treatment of HPV-related disease. *Int. J. Cancer* **2012**, *131*, 1969–1982. [CrossRef] [PubMed]
9. De Martel, C.; Georges, D.; Bray, F.; Ferlay, J.; Clifford, G.M. Global burden of cancer attributable to infections in 2018: A worldwide incidence analysis. *Lancet Glob. Health* **2020**, *8*, e180–e190. [CrossRef]
10. Baboci, L.; Holzinger, D.; Boscolo-Rizzo, P.; Tirelli, G.; Spinato, R.; Lupato, V.; Fuson, R.; Schmitt, M.; Michel, A.; Halec, G.; et al. Low prevalence of HPV-driven head and neck squamous cell carcinoma in North-East Italy. *Papillomavirus Res.* **2016**, *2*, 133–140. [CrossRef] [PubMed]
11. Del Mistro, A.; Frayle, H.; Menegaldo, A.; Favaretto, N.; Gori, S.; Nicolai, P.; Spinato, G.; Romeo, S.; Tirelli, G.; da Mosto, M.C.; et al. Age-independent increasing prevalence of Human Papillomavirus-driven oropharyngeal carcinomas in North-East Italy. *Sci. Rep.* **2020**, *10*, 9320. [CrossRef]
12. Husain, Z.A.; Chen, T.; Corso, C.D.; Wang, Z.; Park, H.; Judson, B.; Yarbrough, W.; Deshpande, H.; Mehra, S.; Kuo, P.; et al. A Comparison of Prognostic Ability of Staging Systems for Human Papillomavirus-Related Oropharyngeal Squamous Cell Carcinoma. *JAMA Oncol.* **2017**, *3*, 358–365. [CrossRef]
13. Zhan, K.Y.; Puram, S.V.; Li, M.M.; Silverman, D.A.; Agrawal, A.A.; Ozer, E.; Old, M.O.; Carrau, R.L.; Rocco, J.W.; Higgins, K.M.; et al. National treatment trends in human papillomavirus-positive oropharyngeal squamous cell carcinoma. *Cancer* **2020**, *126*, 1295–1305. [CrossRef] [PubMed]
14. Jethwa, A.R.; Khariwala, S.S. Tobacco-related carcinogenesis in head and neck cancer. *Cancer Metastasis Rev.* **2017**, *36*, 411–423. [CrossRef] [PubMed]
15. Marziliano, A.; Teckie, S.; Diefenbach, M.A. Alcohol-related head and neck cancer: Summary of the literature. *Head Neck* **2020**, *42*, 732–738. [CrossRef] [PubMed]
16. Xiao, R.; Pham, Y.; Ward, M.C.; Houston, N.; Reddy, C.A.; Joshi, N.P.; Greskovich, J.F., Jr.; Woody, N.M.; Chute, D.J.; Lamarre, E.D.; et al. Impact of active smoking on outcomes in HPV+ oropharyngeal cancer. *Head Neck* **2020**, *42*, 269–280. [CrossRef] [PubMed]
17. Fakhry, C.; Westra, W.H.; Li, S.; Cmelak, A.; Ridge, J.A.; Pinto, H.; Forastiere, A.; Gillison, M.L. Improved survival of patients with human papillomavirus-positive head and neck squamous cell carcinoma in a prospective clinical trial. *J. Natl. Cancer Inst.* **2008**, *100*, 261–269. [CrossRef] [PubMed]
18. Gillison, M.L.; Alemany, L.; Snijders, P.J.; Chaturvedi, A.; Steinberg, B.M.; Schwartz, S.; Castellsagué, X. Human papillomavirus and diseases of the upper airway: Head and neck cancer and respiratory papillomatosis. *Vaccine* **2012**, *30*, F34–F54. [CrossRef]
19. Huang, S.H.; O'Sullivan, B. Overview of the 8th Edition TNM Classification for Head and Neck Cancer. *Curr. Treat. Options Oncol.* **2017**, *18*, 40. [CrossRef]
20. Halec, G.; Schmitt, M.; Dondog, B.; Sharkhuu, E.; Wentzensen, N.; Gheit, T.; Tommasino, M.; Kommoss, F.; Bosch, F.X.; Franceschi, S.; et al. Biological activity of probable/possible high-risk human papillomavirus types in cervical cancer. *Int. J. Cancer* **2013**, *132*, 63–71. [CrossRef]
21. Jung, A.C.; Briolat, J.; Millon, R.; de Reyniès, A.; Rickman, D.; Thomas, E.; Abecassis, J.; Clavel, C.; Wasylyk, B. Biological and clinical relevance of transcriptionally active human papillomavirus (HPV) infection in oropharynx squamous cell carcinoma. *Int. J. Cancer* **2010**, *126*, 1882–1894. [CrossRef]
22. Holzinger, D.; Schmitt, M.; Dyckhoff, G.; Benner, A.; Pawlita, M.; Bosch, F.X. Viral RNA patterns and high viral load reliably define oropharynx carcinomas with active HPV16 involvement. *Cancer Res.* **2012**, *72*, 4993–5003. [CrossRef]
23. Bussu, F.; Ragin, C.; Boscolo-Rizzo, P.; Rizzo, D.; Gallus, R.; Delogu, G.; Morbini, P.; Tommasino, M. HPV as a marker for molecular characterization in head and neck oncology: Looking for a standardization of clinical use and of detection method(s) in clinical practice. *Head Neck* **2019**, *41*, 1104–1111. [CrossRef] [PubMed]

24. Lewis, J.S., Jr.; Beadle, B.; Bishop, J.A.; Chernock, R.D.; Colasacco, C.; Lacchetti, C.; Moncur, J.T.; Rocco, J.W.; Schwartz, M.R.; Seethala, R.R.; et al. Human Papillomavirus Testing in Head and Neck Carcinomas: Guideline From the College of American Pathologists. *Arch. Pathol. Lab. Med.* **2018**, *142*, 559–597. [CrossRef] [PubMed]
25. Mena, M.; Taberna, M.; Tous, S.; Marquez, S.; Clavero, O.; Quiros, B.; Lloveras, B.; Alejo, M.; Leon, X.; Quer, M.; et al. Double positivity for HPV-DNA/p16 is the biomarker with strongest diagnostic accuracy and prognostic value for human papillomavirus related oropharyngeal cancer patients. *Oral. Oncol.* **2018**, *78*, 137–144. [CrossRef] [PubMed]
26. Prigge, E.S.; Arbyn, M.; von Knebel Doeberitz, M.; Reuschenbach, M. Diagnostic accuracy of p16 immunohistochemistry in oropharyngeal squamous cell carcinomas: A systematic review and meta-analysis. *Int. J. Cancer* **2017**, *140*, 1186–1198. [CrossRef]
27. Leemans, C.R.; Snijders, P.J.F.; Brakenhoff, R.H. The molecular landscape of head and neck cancer. *Nat. Rev. Cancer* **2018**, *18*, 269–282. [CrossRef]
28. Dok, R.; Nuyts, S. HPV Positive Head and Neck Cancers: Molecular Pathogenesis and Evolving Treatment Strategies. *Cancers* **2016**, *8*, 41. [CrossRef]
29. Sabatini, M.E.; Chiocca, S. Human papillomavirus as a driver of head and neck cancers. *Br. J. Cancer* **2020**, *122*, 306–314. [CrossRef]
30. Chow, L.Q.M. Head and Neck Cancer. *N. Engl. J. Med.* **2020**, *382*, 60–72. [CrossRef]
31. Role of Human Papillomavirus Infection and Other Co-Factors in the Aetiology of Head and Neck Cancer in Europe and INDIA (HPV-AHEAD). Available online: http://hpv-ahead.iarc.fr/ (accessed on 26 November 2020).
32. Gheit, T.; Anantharaman, D.; Holzinger, D.; Alemany, L.; Tous, S.; Lucas, E.; Prabhu, P.R.; Pawlita, M.; Ridder, R.; Rehm, S.; et al. Role of mucosal high-risk human papillomavirus types in head and neck cancers in central India. *Int. J. Cancer* **2017**, *141*, 143–151. [CrossRef]
33. Mena, M.; Lloveras, B.; Tous, S.; Bogers, J.; Maffini, F.; Gangane, N.; Kumar, R.V.; Somanathan, T.; Lucas, E.; Anantharaman, D.; et al. Development and validation of a protocol for optimizing the use of paraffin blocks in molecular epidemiological studies: The example from the HPV-AHEAD study. *PLoS ONE* **2017**, *12*, e0184520. [CrossRef]
34. Taberna, M.; Mena, M.; Pavón, M.A.; Alemany, L.; Gillison, M.L.; Mesía, R. Human papillomavirus-related oropharyngeal cancer. *Ann. Oncol.* **2017**, *28*, 2386–2398. [CrossRef] [PubMed]
35. Gillison, M.L.; Chaturvedi, A.K.; Anderson, W.F.; Fakhry, C. Epidemiology of Human Papillomavirus-Positive Head and Neck Squamous Cell Carcinoma. *J. Clin. Oncol.* **2015**, *33*, 3235–3242. [CrossRef] [PubMed]
36. Coordes, A.; Lenz, K.; Qian, X.; Lenarz, M.; Kaufmann, A.M.; Albers, A.E. Meta-analysis of survival in patients with HNSCC discriminates risk depending on combined HPV and p16 status. *Eur. Arch. Otorhinolaryngol.* **2016**, *273*, 2157–2169. [CrossRef] [PubMed]
37. Gheit, T.; Vaccarella, S.; Schmitt, M.; Pawlita, M.; Franceschi, S.; Sankaranarayanan, R.; Sylla, B.S.; Tommasino, M.; Gangane, N. Prevalence of human papillomavirus types in cervical and oral cancers in central India. *Vaccine* **2009**, *27*, 636–639. [CrossRef]
38. Gheit, T.; Landi, S.; Gemignani, F.; Snijders, P.J.; Vaccarella, S.; Franceschi, S.; Canzian, F.; Tommasino, M. Development of a sensitive and specific assay combining multiplex PCR and DNA microarray primer extension to detect high-risk mucosal human papillomavirus types. *J. Clin. Microbiol.* **2006**, *44*, 2025–2031. [CrossRef]
39. Halec, G.; Schmitt, M.; Egger, S.; Abnet, C.C.; Babb, C.; Dawsey, S.M.; Flechtenmacher, C.; Gheit, T.; Hale, M.; Holzinger, D.; et al. Mucosal alpha-papillomaviruses are not associated with esophageal squamous cell carcinomas: Lack of mechanistic evidence from South Africa, China and Iran and from a world-wide meta-analysis. *Int. J. Cancer* **2016**, *139*, 85–98. [CrossRef]
40. Schmitt, M.; Dondog, B.; Waterboer, T.; Pawlita, M.; Tommasino, M.; Gheit, T. Abundance of multiple high-risk human papillomavirus (HPV) infections found in cervical cells analyzed by use of an ultrasensitive HPV genotyping assay. *J. Clin. Microbiol.* **2010**, *48*, 143–149. [CrossRef]

41. Alemany, L.; Saunier, M.; Alvarado-Cabrero, I.; Quirós, B.; Salmeron, J.; Shin, H.R.; Pirog, E.C.; Guimerà, N.; Hernandez-Suarez, G.; Felix, A.; et al. Human papillomavirus DNA prevalence and type distribution in anal carcinomas worldwide. *Int. J. Cancer* **2015**, *136*, 98–107. [CrossRef]

Publisher's Note: MDPI stays neutral with regard to jurisdictional claims in published maps and institutional affiliations.

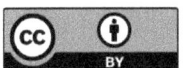

© 2020 by the authors. Licensee MDPI, Basel, Switzerland. This article is an open access article distributed under the terms and conditions of the Creative Commons Attribution (CC BY) license (http://creativecommons.org/licenses/by/4.0/).

MDPI
St. Alban-Anlage 66
4052 Basel
Switzerland
Tel. +41 61 683 77 34
Fax +41 61 302 89 18
www.mdpi.com

Cancers Editorial Office
E-mail: cancers@mdpi.com
www.mdpi.com/journal/cancers

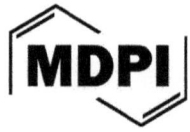